Introduction to Community-Based Nursing

5th EDITION

Roberta Hunt, RN, MSPH, PhD

Associate Professor
St. Catherine University
St. Paul, Minnesota

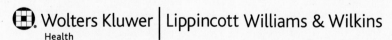

Wolters Kluwer | Lippincott Williams & Wilkins
Health

Philadelphia · Baltimore · New York · London
Buenos Aires · Hong Kong · Sydney · Tokyo

Acquisitions Editor: Hilarie Surrena
Product Manager: Annette Ferran
Editorial Assistant: Zachary Shapiro
Design Coordinator: Holly McLaughlin
Illustration Coordinator: Brett MacNaughton
Manufacturing Coordinator: Karin Duffield
Prepress Vendor: SPi Global

5th edition

Library of Congress Cataloging-in-Publication Data
Hunt, Roberta.
   Introduction to community-based nursing / Roberta Hunt. — 5th ed.
      p. ; cm.
   Includes bibliographical references and index.
   ISBN 978-1-60913-686-4
   1. Community health nursing. I. Title.
   [DNLM: 1. Community Health Nursing. 2. Health Promotion. WY 106]
   RT98.H86   2013
   610.73'43—dc23

                                                                    2011027295

Care has been taken to confirm the accuracy of the information presented and to describe generally accepted practices. However, the author, editors, and publisher are not responsible for errors or omissions or for any consequences from application of the information in this book and make no warranty, expressed or implied, with respect to the currency, completeness, or accuracy of the contents of the publication. Application of this information in a particular situation remains the professional responsibility of the practitioner; the clinical treatments described and recommended may not be considered absolute and universal recommendations.

The author, editors, and publisher have exerted every effort to ensure that drug selection and dosage set forth in this text are in accordance with the current recommendations and practice at the time of publication. However, in view of ongoing research, changes in government regulations, and the constant flow of information relating to drug therapy and drug reactions, the reader is urged to check the package insert for each drug for any change in indications and dosage and for added warnings and precautions. This is particularly important when the recommended agent is a new or infrequently employed drug.

Some drugs and medical devices presented in this publication have Food and Drug Administration (FDA) clearance for limited use in restricted research settings. It is the responsibility of the health care provider to ascertain the FDA status of each drug or device planned for use in his or her clinical practice.

LWW.com

Introduction to Community-Based Nursing

5th EDITION

To my beautiful grandchildren, Josie, Gus, Levi, Mack, Brooksley, Ashton, and Nolen, with love.

RJH

Contributors

Joan Brandt, PhD, MPH, RN
Family Health Section Manager
St. Paul Ramsey County Public Health
St. Paul, Minnesota

Barbara Champlin, PhD, RN
Associate Professor of Nursing
St. Catherine University
St. Paul, Minnesota

Marcia Derby, MSN, RN
Assistant Professor of Nursing
Nova Southeastern University
Fort Lauderdale, Florida

Paula Swiggum, MS, RN
Professor Emeritus
Gustavus Adolphus College
Saint Peter, Minnesota

Reviewers

Louise A. Aurilio, RNC, CAN, PhD
Associate Professor
Youngstown State University
Youngstown, Ohio

Joanne Bonesteel, MS, RN
Faculty
Excelsior College
Albany, New York

Wendy Bowles, MSN, RN, CPNP
Associate Professor
Kettering College of Medical Arts
Kettering, Ohio

Karen Clark, RN, EdD
Dean of Nursing and Assistant Professor
Indiana University School of Nursing at Indiana University East
Richmond, Indiana

Nancy Cooley, MSN, CAGS, FNP-BC
Associate Professor of Nursing
University of Maine at Augusta
Augusta, Maine

Sarah Covington, RN, MSN
Director of Nursing
Renton Technical College
Renton, Washington

Katherine Dewan, RN, MN, PNP
Associate Professor
Ohlone College
Fremont, California

Elizabeth A. Downes, MPH, MSN, APRN-BC, FNP
Clinical Assistant Professor
Nell Hodgson Woodruff School of Nursing, Emory University
Atlanta, Georgia

Marie O. Etienne, MSN, ARNP, PNP, FNP, GNP
Associate Professor, Senior
Miami Dade College, Medical Center Campus, School of Nursing
Miami, Florida

Sheila Grossman, PhD. APRN, FNP-BC
Professor and Coordinator, Family Nurse Practitioner Program
Fairfield University
Fairfield, Connecticut

Pamela Gwin, RNC, BSN
Director, Vocational Nursing Program
Brazosport College
Lake Jackson, Texas

Rosemary F. Hall, RN, BSN, MSN, PhD
Associate Professor of Clinical Nursing
University of Miami School of Nursing and Health Studies
Coral Gables, Florida

Vicki L. Imerman, RN, MSN
Nursing Faculty
Des Moines Area Community College
Boone, Iowa

Karen Kelley, RN, MSN
Assistant Professor of Nursing
Harding University
Searcy, Arkansas

Nancy W. Mosca, RN, PhD
Professor and Coordinator, School Nurse Program
Coordinator, MPH Program
Youngstown State University
Youngstown, Ohio

Carel Mountain, RN, MSN
Faculty
Shasta College
Redding, California

Dr. Pammla Petrucka, BScN, MN, PhD
Assistant Professor
University of Saskatchewan
Regina, Saskatchewan

Cheryl Slack, RN, MS
Adjunct Clinical Instructor
Valparaiso University
Valparaiso, Indiana

Debra Solomon
Instructor
Bethel University
St. Paul, Minnesota

Valerie South, RNC, MS, WHNP-BC, CCE
Nursing Instructor
Bon Secours Memorial School of Nursing
Richmond, Virginia

Linda Spencer, RN, MPH, PhD
Director of Public Health Nursing
    Leadership Graduate Program
Nell Hodgson Woodruff School of Nursing,
    Emory University
Atlanta, Georgia

Mary Ann Thompson, RN, DrPH
Associate Professor of Nursing
McKendree College, Louisville Campus
Louisville, Kentucky

Sandra Kay Thompson, MEd, MSN, APRN, BC
Assistant Professor of Nursing
Bluefield State College
Bluefield, West Virginia

Peggy Trewn, BS, MSN, PhD
Associate Professor/Interim Director
Eastern Michigan University
Ypsilanti, Michigan

Jeanne Ann VanFossan
Professor of Nursing
West Virginia Northern Community College
Weirton, West Virginia

Preface

As the health care delivery system changes, new challenges arise for nurses. Schools of nursing are struggling to find the best ways to restructure curriculum to meet current needs and to give students experiences in a variety of clinical situations and settings that will prepare them for their careers in the increasingly diversified field of nursing. This textbook, *Introduction to Community-Based Nursing*, fifth edition, is designed to fill that need. The fundamental concepts in this text spring from my experience of more than 30 years of teaching community health nursing and working in community settings. This revised edition was influenced by the recommendations found in Patricia Benner's book *Educating Nurses: A Call for Radical Transformation* and Institute of Medicine's report *The Future of Nursing: Leading Change, Advancing Health*.

Purpose of The Text

As the fifth edition of *Introduction to Community-Based Nursing* was developed, four major goals were considered:

1. *To give an informative and experiential introduction to nursing care in the community to develop skills in clinical reasoning.*
   In the past, most schools of nursing focused on preparing students to provide care in the hospital. Increasingly, nursing care has moved out of acute care settings into a variety of settings and specialties throughout the community. Fundamental aspects of community-based care are presented to allow the nurse to develop a knowledge base applicable in any community setting.

2. *To illustrate the variety of settings and situations in which the community-based nurse gives care to prepare the student nurse to practice to the full extend of their education and training.*
   Because of the range of settings in which a nurse may practice and the limitation of time in the curriculum of schools of nursing, it is often difficult to schedule sufficient diversified clinical experiences. A wide assortment of settings are discussed in this textbook: from home care nursing and specialized home care roles to school nursing; from emergency preparedness to chronic care; from parish nursing to advocacy in global health. One of the purposes of this text is to provide an array of opportunities for clinical applications of the concepts presented in the course to a range of settings with a diversity of populations. This is accomplished in several ways. First, examples of different settings and situations are scattered throughout the body of the text. Second, one of the special features of the text, *Client Situations in Practice*, integrates and synthesizes chapter concepts, showing the student step-by-step how the theory discussed in the chapter relates to the reality of clinical practice. Third, *Case Studies* appear in many of the *Learning Activities* at the end of each chapter and as part of the extensive instructors' resources available online at thePoint (http://thePoint.lww.com), Lippincott Williams & Wilkins' popular web-based course and content management system. These case studies give students an opportunity to practice skills while applying chapter concepts. Last, questions for reflection for use with a clinical journal or individual assignments are found in the *Learning Activities* at the end of each chapter and at thePoint. All of these activities are designed to enhance clinical reasoning skills.

3. *To clarify cultural diversity and health disparity found within the community in which nurses provide quality care.*
   Another important emphasis of this edition of *Introduction to Community-Based Nursing* is cross-cultural care. Our society is diverse, with many racial, ethnic, and

minority groups. The community-based nurse will care for clients from many different cultures and must be prepared to give quality and culturally competent care to all clients and families. Chapter 3, "Cultural Care," is written by Joan Brandt, who has extensive experience in cross-cultural nursing, in both recruiting and providing academic support for students from diverse cultural backgrounds, as well as in curriculum development. Consideration of cross-cultural issues is woven throughout the text.

4. *To integrate throughout the text the importance of the individual to the family and the family to the individual.*
Most clients are part of a family. In this text, family is defined as those whom the client has identified as family or a significant other. The client's health and the client's care during illness are influenced by the family. In some cases, the client's health is influenced by lack of family and social support. The client's health status and outlook will influence the continuous growth and development of the family. Understanding this symbiotic relationship and incorporating this knowledge into care is an important focus of the text. Special attention is also given to nursing support of the lay caregiver.

Organization of The Text

Introduction to Community-Based Nursing is divided into five units: basic concepts, nursing skills, application, settings, and implications for future practice.

- *Unit I, Basic Concepts in Community-Based Nursing,* includes the essential elements of community-based nursing. An introductory chapter discusses definitions of a community and a healthy community, components of community-based nursing, and nursing skills and competencies needed to give quality care in the community. The unit also outlines the goals of *Health People 2020* and introduces the concepts of health promotion and disease prevention, cultural care, and family care.

- *Unit II, Skills for Community-Based Nursing Practice,* reviews the basics of assessment, health teaching, case management, and continuity of care and addresses those skills specific to community-based settings.

- *Unit III, Community-Based Nursing Across the Life Span,* provides assessment guides, teaching materials, and strategies for addressing health promotion and disease and injury prevention across the life span.

- *Unit IV, Settings for Practice,* offers a wide sampling of practice settings and practice specialties. One chapter discusses home health care in depth and another focuses on specific roles in specialized home care nursing. Mental health nursing in community-based settings is also included in this unit. One chapter addressing global health and community-based care discusses health issues that extend to the larger community, including environmental health, emergency preparedness, immigrants and refugees, and nursing advocacy in global health.

- *Unit V, Implications for Future Practice,* discusses trends in health care and implications for community-based nursing.

The text was designed using a consistent approach throughout the chapters. Many chapters include a short section giving a historical perspective on the subject. Most chapters address nursing skills and competencies, with information on the nursing process or on such topics as communication, health teaching, and case management. Any repetition of information among chapters is intended to reinforce knowledge or skills in light of each chapter's subject. Documentation is covered in many chapters because of its importance to community-based nursing. All chapters conclude with *Learning Activities.*

Key Features of The Text

The following features of the book were developed as pedagogical aids for the student. They help clarify text information, give the student guidelines for actions, or require the student to use critical thinking.

- Learning Activities: several activities at the end of every chapter that form a compact study and application guide. These comprise the following exercises:
  - Journaling: to be used for a clinical journal or as individual assignments to assist the student in applying theoretical content to clinical situations and becoming a reflective practitioner.
  - Client Situations in Practice: at least one in most chapters. A client situation is described, followed by critical thinking exercises.
  - Practical Applications: appear in many chapters. Not related to a specific client, these activities prepare the student for clinical application.
  - Clinical Reasoning Exercises: in most chapter. A problem is presented in a sentence or two, with directions for developing clinical reasoning.
- Community-Based Nursing Care Guidelines: boxed information that includes specific interventions for the community-based nurse.
- Community-Based Teaching: boxed lists of information to give clients and their families.
- Research in Community-Based Nursing Care: boxed information that includes short descriptions of recent.
- Assessment Tools: many chapters provide sample assessment forms to be used in community-based nursing care.
- Healthy People 2020: health promotion and disease prevention materials in Chapters 8, 9, and 10, with addresses of Web sites from which numerous additional materials can be downloaded.
- What's on the Web: found in most chapters, this feature contains addresses and descriptions of Web sites related to the chapter material that provide additional resources. Chapter 16 includes a list of general Web sites helpful in community-based nursing.
- Other pedagogical aids: Objectives, Key Terms, Chapter Topics, References, and Bibliography.
- Glossary: helps the student review terminology or understand unfamiliar terminology used in the book.

We have tried to avoid sexist terms for the nurse and clients. Throughout the text, we have used the term "family" for consistency. However, the term refers to anyone who is concerned about and supportive of the client and can signify a relative or a significant other.

Instructor's Resources

This book is accompanied by a set of Instructor's Resources that can be accessed on thePoint. These Instructor's Resources were prepared with an ongoing emphasis on practical application of the student's knowledge base. More than 200 assignments and discussion topics, more than 700 test questions, and additional client care studies are provided, all designed to help the associate-degree nurse develop the skills and knowledge essential for the unique role of community-based nursing. Many of the assignments have been used and improved over the years that I have taught community health nursing. In addition, quizzes are provided to test students' reading comprehension and review questions to test their learning. Answers are given for all of the tests, quizzes, assignments, discussion topics, and case studies. Point-by-point lecture outlines accompanied by PowerPoint presentations, all designed to support the instructor, are provided for each chapter.

Roberta Hunt, RN, MSPH, PhD
hunthean@comcast.net

Acknowledgments

I am grateful to many individuals, especially family, friends, and colleagues, for their encouragement and assistance in the development of this textbook. It is impossible to acknowledge everyone, given the limitations of memory and space.

To all my colleagues who have given encouragement and validation and who have made the teaching of nursing an exciting and stimulating profession—you have contributed to this project. To the more than 2,500 students whom I have had the pleasure of working with in the classroom and in clinical settings in the community, who have provided feedback and suggestions about my teaching and assignments—you have each made an invaluable contribution to this book.

Thanks to Joan Brandt for sharing her expertise in Chapters 3 and 15. Chapter 3, titled "Cultural Care," is an expertly crafted and beautifully written chapter that emphasizes the importance of respectful care, which is the central premise of *Introduction to Community-Based Nursing*. The importance of developing skills in culture care through a global view of nursing is the focus of Chapter 15. To my colleague and friend, Barb Champlin, a heart-filled thanks for writing Chapter 14. In this chapter, Barb shares her knowledge and her sensitive approach to care, gained through more than 30 years of providing nursing care for adults and children experiencing difficulties with mental health issues. This chapter makes an important contribution in emphasizing that both mental and physical health are essential to comprehensive community-based care.

Finally, I am grateful to my family and friends, who provide day-to-day support and encouragement. To my colleagues at the St. Catherine University—the most professional and supportive faculty group an educator could ever hope to work with—thanks for the opportunity to work with all of you. To Rebecca von Gillern, my developmental editor, thank you for your guidance, organization, and editorial expertise. Thanks to my family, especially Becky Hunt Carmody and Steve Hunt, for your continuing encouragement. To my wonderful daughters—Jackie, for your cheerful attitude plus valuable editorial assistance, and Megan, for your thoughtful advice and balanced view of the world—a heartfelt thank you. I am grateful to my husband, Tim Heaney, who provided ongoing editorial support during the long process of completing this edition.

Roberta Hunt

Contents

UNIT I

Basic Concepts in Community-Based Nursing

Before you practice nursing in a community-based setting, you must understand the basic concepts behind community-based health care. These concepts are introduced in Unit I for further exploration as you begin to apply what you have learned. An overview of community-based nursing, beginning with a brief historical perspective of nursing, is provided in Chapter 1. Also discussed are health care reform and health care funding, which created the movement of the provision of health care out of the hospital and into the community. Finally, components of community-based care and nursing skills as well as competencies are presented to round out the chapter.

Health promotion and disease prevention, as outlined by the federal government's *Healthy People 2020* (Department of Health and Human Services, 2010), are the focus of Chapter 2.

Chapter 3 discusses the ever-changing makeup of our society and asks you to look at your own cultural background and attitudes about diversity. The chapter promotes the development of culturally competent care.

Chapter 4 discusses family involvement, an important consideration in community-based care.

The remainder of the book uses these concepts to build your knowledge base and relates it to practical experiences.

Chapter 1

Overview of Community-Based Nursing

ROBERTA HUNT

Learning Objectives

1. Explain the major issues leading to the development of community-based nursing.
2. Discuss the history of reimbursement systems for health care services and its impact on nursing.
3. Identify the factors that define community.
4. Indicate the relationship between health and community.
5. Compare acute care nursing, community-based nursing, and community health nursing.
6. Describe components of community-based care.
7. Outline the skills necessary for community-based nursing practice.

Key Terms

acute care
advance directives
community
community-based nursing
continuity of care
demographics
diagnosis-related groups (DRGs)
durable power of attorney
extended family

health impact assessment (HIA)
health maintenance organizations (HMOs)
living will
nuclear family
preferred provider organizations (PPOs)
prospective payment
self-care
vital statistics

Chapter Topics

Historical Perspectives

Health Care Reform

Health Care Funding

The Community

Community Nursing Versus Community-Based Nursing

Focus of Nursing

Components of Community-Based Care

Nursing Skills and Competencies

Nursing Interventions

Conclusions

The Nursing Student Speaks

In general, having clinical in the community has broadened my horizons of what I am able to do as a nurse. Before this community experience, my mind-set was that you had to work in a hospital or a nursing home when you graduated. Acute care was the only setting that I could think about working in, and now I realize that these people in the community need me too. Public health, I have noticed, is short staffed too, just like hospitals. They only have one nurse at the shelter to see all of the families. It seems to be overwhelming. This experience has broadened my horizons to see the different roles that I can play as a nurse, most of which I have never seen myself in.

Before this experience, I could not believe that we had to do a community rotation. Once I was out there, I was shocked at how my views of community health were distorted. After the rotation was over, I was glad that we were able to experience the community setting. Working in the homeless shelter helped me to look at people in a more holistic way, which I now believe is the only way to look at people. Before this experience, it [my focus] was always the physical aspects of a person, such as blood pressure and pain. Now I can see the whole person—the physical, the mental, and the spiritual aspects. These are all of the parts that need to be healed. I appreciate what I have learned from the community experience. It is all coming together.

Kristin Ocker, RN, Student Completing a BSN
St. Catherine University

Over the last three decades, nursing practice in the **community** has been transformed. Many of these changes arise from public pressure regarding the need for reform of our health care system. These concerns relate to quality of, access to, and cost of health care, as well as fragmentation of health care. As health care evolves, nurses have an opportunity to participate in this process (National League for Nursing [NLN], 1993, 1997). In the first decades of the 21st century, the NLN has predicted 10 trends in health care that will affect nursing education and practice (Box 1-1).

These trends and the implications for nursing educational preparation and quality nursing practice are the focus of this book. This chapter provides a historical background and overview of nursing care in the community, introduces the reader to the concept of community and **community-based nursing**, and describes components of community-based nursing practice, skills, and competencies.

Historical Perspectives

Although during most of the 20th century nursing care was associated primarily with hospital settings, historically, the setting for nursing care has been the home and community. The first written reference to care of the ill in the home is found in the New Testament, in which mention is made of visiting the sick at home to aid in their health needs.

Florence Nightingale, credited as the mother of modern nursing, developed a classic model for educating nurses in hospital-based programs. Nightingale's curriculum also included the first training programs to educate district nurses, with 1 year of training devoted to promoting **self-care** and the health of communities (Monteiro, 1991).

William Rathbone, a resident of Liverpool, England, in the 1850s, established the modern concept of the visiting nurse (Kalish & Kalish, 1995). Lillian Wald and Mary Brewster began a program for visiting nurses in the United States in the early 1900s (Fee & Bu, 2010). Wald, the founder of public health nursing, drew on contemporary ideas of the times that linked nursing, motherhood, social welfare, and the public. Her work was

---

BOX 1-1   **The Future of Nursing Education: Trends to Watch**

1. Changing demographics and increasing diversity
2. The technology explosion
3. Globalization of the world's economy and society
4. Educated consumers, alternative therapies and genomics, and palliative care
5. Shift to population-based care and increasing complexity of client care
6. Costs of health care and challenges of managed care
7. Impact of health policy and regulation
8. The growing need for interdisciplinary education for collaborative practice
9. The current nursing shortages, opportunities for lifelong learning, and workforce development
10. Significant advances in nursing science and research

Source: Heller, B., Oros, M., & Durney-Crowley, J. (2007). *The future of nursing education: Ten trends to watch*. New York: National League for Nursing. Retrieved from http://www.nln.org/nlnjournal/infotrends.htm

---

designed to respond to the needs of those populations at greatest risk by nursing the sick in their homes and communities while providing preventive instructions to reduce illness. First and foremost, Wald contended that the nurse working in the community must treat social and economic problems and not just take care of sick people. Wald understood that nurses could reach and educate their clients in the broadest sense, by drawing on diversity of cultural beliefs and societal demands of the populace.

SHIFT FROM COMMUNITY TO HOSPITAL

In 1910, approximately 90% of all nursing care was provided in the home. After World War I, care of the sick started to shift to the hospital. In the early 1950s, the growing complexity in health care technology resulted in an increased need for hospital care. During the 1960s and 1970s, a person typically stayed in the hospital for 7 to 10 days for uncomplicated conditions or for surgery (Craven & Hirnle, 2009).

This trend continued until the early 1980s, when escalating health care costs prompted changes in the health care delivery system and its financing. From 1980, this movement intensified as the number of nurses working in public and community health, ambulatory care, and other institutional settings increased (Health Resources and Services Administration [HRSA], 2010). In brief, nursing care provided in the home in the 1800s migrated to the **acute care** hospital in the middle of the 20th century and then back to the home in the 1980s.

AN ERA OF COST CONTAINMENT

Until the early 1980s, hospitals were reimbursed by Medicare on a cost basis, which meant the more the hospital spent, the more its revenue increased. In fact, improved efficiency meant less revenue for the hospital (Goldfield, 2010). President Reagan signed the Tax Equity and Fiscal Responsibility Act in 1982 and the Social Security Amendments in 1983. This legislation changed the way Medicare and Medicaid services were reimbursed, initiating a service called the **prospective payment** system. The prospective payment system calculates reimbursement to hospitals based on the client's diagnosis according to federally mandated **diagnosis-related groups (DRGs)**. The client's diagnosis is categorized according to the federal DRG coding system, and payment is bundled into one fee, which is then paid to the hospital. Payment by client diagnosis, therefore, was an attempt to contain Medicare and Medicaid costs.

Gradually, many insurance companies, **health maintenance organizations (HMOs)**, and other third-party payers adopted the DRG method of payment in the United States.

As the reimbursement system for health care evolved over three decades, the average length of stay for a hospitalized client decreased substantially. The fact that it is financially advantageous for the hospital if individuals had shorter stays resulted in a situation where clients are discharged "quicker and sicker." Over time, more and more services have been provided outside the hospital because it is more cost-effective. These trends have not been without challenges. One major issue has been an increase in hospital readmission as clients are sometimes discharged prematurely from day surgery or hospital care. These along with other problems that accompany the reduction in hospital care continue to this day.

SHIFT FROM HOSPITAL TO COMMUNITY

Acute Care Setting

Acute care is typically a term used for health care provided in the hospital, whether it is inpatient or for emergency care. But hospital care is not always synonymous with acute care. In some cases, community-based care of acute conditions is provided in the hospital where an ambulatory clinic or day surgery unit may be found. In general, individuals in acute care settings are very sick. Many are postsurgical clients or are individuals experiencing an acute exacerbation of an existing health condition requiring highly technical care. Others may have life-threatening conditions and require close monitoring and constant care. The care given to these clients is specialized and requires considerable expertise. Acute care nursing differs from community-based nursing care, as seen in the differences between hospital and home environments outlined in Table 1-1.

Community Setting

Clients and families have been profoundly impacted by the shift from hospital to community care. Care that once was considered safe only within the hospital has become routine in outpatient settings, such as ambulatory care centers, surgical centers, dialysis centers, rehabilitation centers, walk-in clinics, physicians' offices, and the home. As length of stay in the hospital has continued to decrease, family members bear of the burden of caring for loved ones who are discharged much quicker and sicker from the hospital.

As health care delivery has been transformed, so has nursing care. In the past decade, the number of nurses working in every employment setting has increased. However, the rate of increase in hospitals is less than that in previous years. The greatest growth occurred in community-based settings (Fig. 1-1). This trend of more nurses working in the community, particularly in home care, continues with home health nurses accounting for 3.8% of the workforce in 2004 and 6.4% in 2008 (HRSA, 2010).

Table 1-1 Differences Between Hospital and Home		
Factors	**Hospital**	**Home**
Resources	Predetermined	Variable
Environment	Predictable	Highly variable
Locating client	Certain with captive audience	Requires planning
Access to client	Guaranteed	Not guaranteed, but determined by client and family
Focus	Individual client	Client in family system
Family support	Helpful in accomplishing client outcomes	Critical in accomplishing client outcomes
Client role	Relatively dependent	Highly autonomous
Safety	Under the auspices of agency oversight	Multiple unpredictable threats

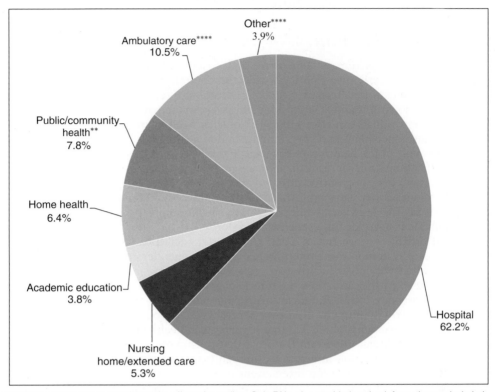

Employment settings of registered nurses*

*Percents my not add to 100 due to the effect of rounding. Only RNs who provided setting information are included in the calculations used for this figure.

**Public/community health include school and occupational health.

***Ambulatory care includes medical/ physician practices, health center and clinics, and other types of nonhospital clinical settings.

****Other includes insurance, benefits, and utilization review.

Source: 2008 National Sample Survey of Registered Nurses

Figure 1-1 Registered nurse population by employment setting, 2008. Source: Health Resources and Services Administration. (2010). *Preliminary findings: 2008 National Sample Survey of Registered Nurses.* (p. 75). Retrieved from http://bhpr.hrsa.gov/healthworkforce/rnsurveys/rnsurveyfinal.pdf

Health Care Reform

The United States is in the midst of major health care reform that few people deny is necessary. One federal initiative that has served as a road map for the health of all citizens in the United States for the last 40 years is *Healthy People*. This document, published every decade, outlines government goals and objectives for the upcoming decade. It has stirred the imagination of professionals about how to meet the health needs of all Americans. Particular populations are targeted for care. *Healthy People 2020* is discussed in more detail in Chapter 2.

Numerous discussions have been provoked by this initiative. The perception of health care as a privilege versus a right, along with the question over who bears the cost of keeping society healthy, will be at the center of the debate for some time. These issues present challenges and opportunities for the nurse in the second decade of the new century. Nurses have an important role to play in health care reform beginning by being prepared for practice in community settings where highly developed skills in assessment, communication, interdisciplinary collaboration, and working with culturally diverse populations are imperative.

Health Care Funding

Health care is extremely expensive, and costs continue to rise impacting individuals, families, and nearly every entity within the community. These pressures require that all parties must explore alternative funds, in addition to fee-for-service charges, in the form of voluntary donations and state and federal programs to pay for care.

Few individuals can afford to pay all of their health care costs out of their own pockets. Group insurance plans and government-funded health care such as Medicare and Medicaid provide most of the health care coverage in the United States. Almost all plans have numerous restrictions to care, resulting in many individuals being "underinsured" through policies that do not cover preventive care, psychiatric treatment, outpatient support services, and medications. Other plans limit the amount of service paid for a particular type of care, such as home health care visits, while some have a maximum cap for how much they will pay for an individual's care or for a specific condition.

Affordability Care Act of 2010 (ACA) is expected to have a profound impact on the health care system in the United States. This law includes comprehensive health insurance reforms that will lower health care costs while requiring insurance companies to be more accountable. At the same time the reform guarantees health care choices and improves quality of health care for all Americans. Although portions of the law took effect immediately, much of it will be implemented over several years, through 2014 and beyond. One of the greatest achievements of ACA is that it guaranteed health coverage for 32 million uninsured Americans. Another important feature is that consumers are assisted to better monitor medications and medication interactions through better access to pharmacists for consultation. Medications and medication interactions cause illness and death of thousands every year. Better access to pharmacists translates to increased opportunities for individuals to sit down with their pharmacist to determine if there should be changes or reductions in their medication regimen. Another emphasis of health care reform adds incentives for programs, processes, and procedures that enhance **continuity of care** to avoid rehospitalizations. Specific examples include models of care delivery such as medical homes and accountable care.

Registered nurses, as the largest single group of health care professionals, play an important role in this new system of care. A major benefit for nurses is that they will be able to provide care without regard for ability to pay (Robert Wood Johnson Foundation, 2010). Further, nurses are educated and practice within an inclusive, holistic framework that views individuals, families, and communities as an interconnected system that promotes wellness and healing. Registered nurses working in the community are fundamental facilitators for the critical shift needed in health services delivery, with the goal of transforming the current "sick care" system to a true "health care" system (American Nurses Association [ANA], 2010).

This legislation represents movement toward much needed, comprehensive, and meaningful reform for our nation's health care system. To learn more about ACA, consult the Web site listed on What's on the Web at the end of the chapter.

FEDERALLY FUNDED HEALTH CARE

Up to the time of health care reform in 2010, most government funding for health care was provided through Medicare and Medicaid. Under Medicare, home health care is an important service for the elderly, and concern about it will continue to grow as the elderly population increases in the United States. In the past, Medicare covered nursing; physical, speech, and occupational therapies; home care aides; medical social services; and some medical supplies. These programs will change with the ACA.

GROUP PLANS

Group plans include HMOs, **preferred provider organizations (PPOs)**, and private insurance. HMOs are prepaid, structured, managed systems in which providers deliver a comprehensive range of health care services to enrollees. Preferred provider organizations allow a network of providers to provide services at a lower fee in return for prompt payment at prenegotiated rates. Private insurance may be obtained through large, nonprofit, tax-exempt organizations or through small, private, for-profit insurance companies. This type of insurance is called third-party payment. Long-term care insurance may also be obtained through private insurance companies.

IMPACT OF THE NURSING SHORTAGE ON CARE IN THE COMMUNITY

The Bureau of Labor Statistics estimates that job opportunities for registered nurses in all specialties are expected to be excellent with employment of registered nurses predicted to grow much faster than average for all occupations through 2018. The U.S. Bureau of Labor Statistics anticipates that the need for nurses will increase by 22% by 2018, while at the same time, the number of U.S. educated nursing school graduates decreased by 10% from 1995 to 2004 (Bureau of Labor Statistics, 2010).

Not only is the need for nurses increasing faster than the supply of nurses, the educational level of nurses is not keeping up with the amplified demand for skill and knowledge as health care becomes ever more complex. Currently, nurses are not choosing to advance their education from associate degree to the baccalaureate in adequate numbers, which leaves a deficit in the number of baccalaureate-prepared nurses necessary for the more complex health needs of those seeking health care. This shortage comes at the same time as the demand for nurses in the community increased. Further, there will be fewer nurses prepared to move to the graduate level to meet the urgent need for advanced practice registered nurses and nurse educators (Tri-Council for Nursing, 2010). It is anticipated that the ensuing need for advanced practice nurses stemming from health care reform will exceed supply. At the same time, qualified applicants to nursing schools are being turned away because of a shortage of nursing faculty. The need for nursing faculty will only increase as many instructors near retirement.

The current nursing shortage has significantly impacted the supply of nurses who work in the community including public health nurses. Public health nurses are the largest component of the public health workforce in the community. Thus, aging and retirement trends of registered nurses will have a drastic effect on the health of the public. The average age of public health nurses is 47 years of age and retirements are estimated to be as high as 45% in the next 5 years (Quad Council of Public Health Nursing Organizations, 2006).

In summary, nursing is facing a growing shortage of an estimated 1 million nurses by 2020, nearly one third of the entire professional workforce (HRSA, 2009). Unlike shortages in the past, this one will be driven by a permanent shift in the labor market that is unlikely to reverse in the next few years as the average age of the population along with the average age of the registered nurse increases. At this tipping point, action is needed to put in place strategies to meet the market demand for a stronger nursing workforce.

These changes make it imperative for nursing educators to prepare graduates for practice both in and outside the walls of the acute care setting and for a variety of roles in the community. The NLN recommends that all levels of nursing education continue to prepare nurses to function in a community-based, community-focused health care system and be competent to practice in a variety of settings across the continuum of care.

The Community

Nurses who practice community-based nursing profit from understanding the community within which they practice. Knowledge of the community helps ensure nurses maintain holistic, quality care.

DEFINING COMMUNITY

Community is defined in numerous ways, depending on the application, but this text defines community as "a people, location, and social system" (Josten, 1989).

People: Families, Culture, and Community

The variety of individuals, families, and cultural groups represented in a community contributes to the overall character of that community. The simplest way to understand a community is through **vital statistics** and **demographics**. These data may be thought of as the community's vital statistics, similar to an individual's vital signs. A community consisting primarily of senior citizens has totally different vital statistics from a community of young, unmarried adults.

For example, in a community with a higher percentage of the population being over 60 years of age, there would most likely be a higher death rate than in a community with a higher population between 20 and 40 years of age. The community with the higher age wouldn't necessarily have more diseases or epidemics; rather an older person is more likely to die than a younger person. Similarly, the younger community would have a higher birth rate, not because there were bigger families but because the younger average age of the community would contribute to a higher birth rate.

The characteristics of the families living in a community contribute to the overall complexion of that community and, in turn, define the community health care needs. Older families require different services compared to families with young children. Single-headed family needs may vary from those where two parents are living in the same household. In communities where families are strong and nurturing, there is an opportunity for a more vibrant and caring strong or prosperous community. When families fail to provide an adequate basis for healthy individual growth, development, and self actualization, problems with physical abuse, neglect, substance abuse, and violence may arise. A strong family unit is the basic building block for strong communities.

Culture contributes to the overall character of a community and, in turn, influences its health needs. In most of the world, sometimes a scarcity of resources necessitates **extended family** residing together in one home. At other times, cultural norms dictate that all generations live under one roof. Included in the extended family may be grandparents, aunts, uncles, and other relatives. When living together in one household, many members may be involved with child care and care of the sick or injured. In these communities, there are different needs related to child and health care than in communities in the United States, Canada, and Western Europe, where the **nuclear family** has been the norm. It merits mentioning that in the last decade, there has been an increase in extended family living together in the United States but the nuclear family remains the dominant configuration. In the 6% of the world where nuclear family structures prevail, isolation and self-reliance affect the needs and function of the family, which, in turn, influence the design and delivery of community health services. A client, then, who has a nuclear family and no extended family often has different needs for support through community services compared to the client with numerous extended family members living in the same household or nearby.

The role of individuals within the family and community is often dictated by culture. In some cultures, older people retire from leadership and governing responsibilities, whereas in other cultures, these members are considered essential to the governing structure of the community. In this situation, the more prestigious positions of authority and responsibility are assigned to the older members of the community. In other cultures, household tasks and child care may be assigned to the older members of the family.

Health is affected by culture. For some time it has been common knowledge that that "health and illness states are strongly influenced and often primarily determined by the cultural background of an individual" (Leininger, 1970). The norms and values of the culture of the individual and his or her family determine the community's definition of health and the service needs of that community.

Location: Community Boundaries

A community is usually defined by boundaries. Boundaries may be geographic, such as those defined as a city, county, state, or nation or may be political; precincts and wards may determine them. A community may have diffuse boundaries such as those that emerge as the result of a group of people identifying or solving a problem. Consequently, a community may establish a boundary within which a problem can be defined and solved. Figure 1-2 depicts this variety of community boundaries.

Community boundaries are important because they often determine what services are available to individuals living within a particular geographic area. Eligibility for services may be limited, or denied, depending on whether one resides within a certain geographic area. It is important for the nurse to realize that community boundaries limit availability of, and eligibility for, services. For example, suppose you are a nurse working at Ramsey County Hospital. If your patient lives in Hennepin County, you will refer him or her to services in Hennepin County. The client, however, may also be eligible for services with a home health care agency that serves multiple counties but is not located in Hennepin County. Familiarity with community boundaries is important as it may have bearing on eligibility requirements of services in your community.

A working knowledge of service restrictions for agencies in a geographic area is also critical for the nurse working the community. In some counties, the first assessment visit by the county nurse is free; in other areas, this may not be the case. Not only should the nurse be familiar with boundaries and basic eligibility criteria and restrictions, but the nurse must also know about the available resources within the specific area. For most nurses, it becomes a lifelong process to remain informed about new and existing resources for the populations and health issues found in their community.

A community defined by its problems and solutions has a fluid boundary. The problems and those who are affected by those problems determine this boundary. This allows all those who may be affected by the problems to participate in the solutions and the resulting outcome. Thus, a more fluid boundary may allow for greater eligibility or opportunity for service.

The problem of air pollution in one community provides an example of a community issue with a fluid boundary. In the suburbs of Rosemount and Apple Valley (Fig. 1-2), two school nurses in different elementary schools notice that the percentage of children within their respective schools with symptoms of asthma is increasing. The school nurses consult one another and note that most of the children with asthma in both school districts live west of a large oil refinery. The school nurses consult the Department of Health as a result of this discovery and a public meeting is arranged. The parents of the children from both schools are invited to attend this public meeting to discuss the increase in the number of

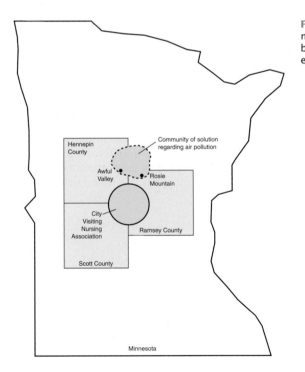

Figure 1-2 A community's boundaries may be many things: geographic, political, problem based. These boundaries are used in the example in this chapter.

children with asthma in the two schools and the potential relationship air pollution in the community may have on this change. After several meetings, through community organizing, a group of parents from both schools forms a constituency to build a coalition devoted to the identification of the problem and potential solutions. The theoretical boundaries of this community are shown in Figure 1-2. Established school boundaries or geographic boundaries become fluid in this scenario when a problem arises.

Social Systems

Social systems include a community's economic, educational, religious, political, recreational systems, as well as its legal, health care, safety and transportation, and communication systems. Social systems have an impact on a community and, consequently, the health of that community. Depending on the infrastructure, these systems may have a beneficial, neutral, or detrimental impact on the health of individuals living in a given community. A common example is that of infant mortality rate, which is lower in communities where prenatal care is available and readily accessible to all pregnant women. Here is a social system at work within a community; it has a profound impact on the quality of health of its individual members.

But health is more than access to health care. There is ample research that demonstrates the positive relationship between availability of green space and health. Where recreational facilities provide opportunities for health promotion activities, for instance, the health of the citizens will be enhanced.

Availability of certain services impacts the nutritional status and thus the health of a community. Whether a neighborhood has a grocery store including a large array of fresh fruits and vegetables or only a convenience store with no produce determines what access those living in that area have to healthy food choices. About 9% of households in the United States do not own a car, thus depend heavily on neighborhood access for food products. Further, there is a relationship between the availability of grocery stores that sell fresh produce and recreational opportunities and the rate of childhood obesity within a given community. In communities where children have diets rich in nutrition, low-calorie snacks, and safe places to participate in recreational activities, they are more likely to be of normal weight.

Social Determinants of Health

As discussed in the previous section, social systems within a community impact health. Where people live, learn, work, and play affect how long they will live and how healthy they will be. Thus, the people, place, and social systems of a community all contribute to health of those living in that community. Over the last two decades, as the concept of health has broadened so has interest in the concept of the social determinants of health. Social determinants are defined as "the circumstances, in which people are born, grow up, live, work and age, and the systems put in place to deal with illness. These circumstances are in turn shaped by a wider set of forces: economics, social policies, and politics" (World Health Organization, 2010, p. 1). There is a wide variation in the "health" of cities, counties, and states across the United States, which in turn predicts the health of the people living in that city, county, or state. This concept is discussed in more detail in Chapter 5.

A HEALTHY COMMUNITY

There is a large gap between how healthy Americans are and how healthy they could be. Although there have been major breakthroughs in medical science and a 1 trillion dollar increase in annual health care spending over the past decade, health outcomes in the. United States do not compare favorably to other developed nations. Infant mortality and life expectancy rates in the United States lag behind Japan, Canada, Australia, and most of Europe for the last two decades. Health is more than health care. Only 10% to 15% of preventable mortality has been attributed to medical care (Robert Wood Johnson Foundation,

2009). Just as there are characteristics of healthy individuals, so are there characteristics of healthy communities (Fig. 1-3).

Community, whether it is a city, county, or neighborhood, affects individual health. In this dynamic relationship between health and community, health is considered in the context of the community's people, its location, and its social system (Fig. 1-4).

Healthy citizens can contribute to the overall health, vitality, and economy of the community. Similarly, if a large portion of individuals in a community is not healthy, not

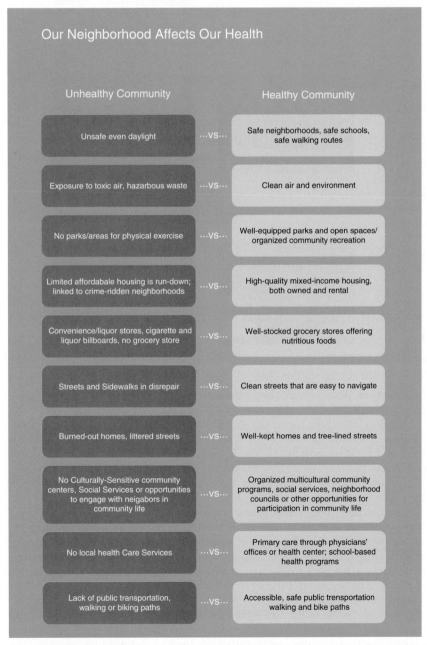

Figure 1-3 Our neighborhood affects our health. Source: Robert Wood Johnson Foundation. (2009). *Beyond health care: New directions to a healthier America*. Retrieved from www.commissiononhealth.org. © 2009 Robert Wood Johnson Foundation Commission to Build a Healthier America. (Used with permission)

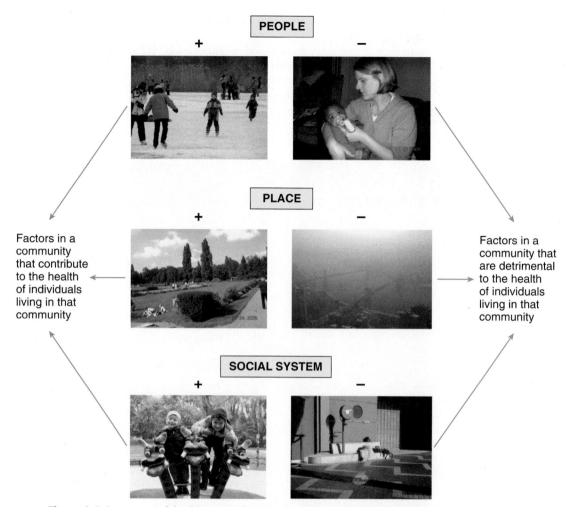

Factors in a community that contribute to the health of individuals living in that community

Factors in a community that are detrimental to the health of individuals living in that community

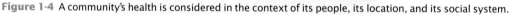

Figure 1-4 A community's health is considered in the context of its people, its location, and its social system.

productive, or poorly nourished, the community can suffer from a lack of vitality and productivity (Fig. 1-5).

Location also influences the health of a community. If a toxic landfill or refinery emissions contaminate the earth, water, or air, the health of the people in the area will obviously be detrimentally affected. Figure 1-6 illustrates the relationship between the location and the level of health in a given community.

Likewise, a relationship exists between social systems and public policy and health (Fig. 1-7).

For example, there will be fewer smokers in communities where smoking is not allowed in any public space and the sale of cigarettes to minors is restricted and strictly enforced. In a community where all pregnant women have access to prenatal care, both the rate of low birth weight infants and the infant mortality rate will be lower. In a community where immunizations are well marketed, available, and accessible to all children, the immunization rate will be higher and the corresponding communicable disease rates lower compared to communities without such services.

Lowering crime rates, strengthening families and their lifestyles, improving environmental quality, and providing behavioral or mental health care are the most critical elements to creating healthy communities. A healthy community requires adequate funding for equal access for all community members to quality education, jobs, a healthy environment, safe housing, and transportation as well as the more obvious need for health services.

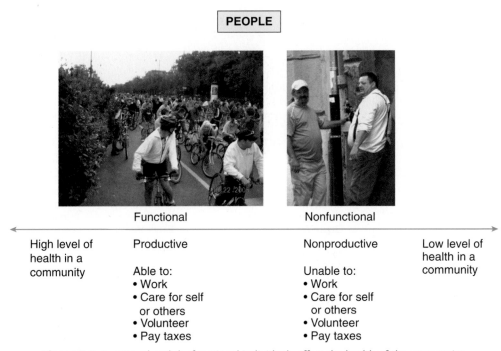

Figure 1-5 Functional and dysfunctional individuals affect the health of the community.

There is a body of evidence to support the idea that to build a healthy community individual health status and quality of life should be considered in every local government decision related to policy and resource allocation. There is a new movement to apply this concept similarly to how an environmental impact assessment is used to provide information for decision making related to the environmental consequences of proposed actions. A **health impact assessment (HIA)** evaluates the potential effects of a policy, program, or project on the health of a population (Centers for Disease Control and Prevention, 2010). This concept is discussed in more detail in Chapter 5.

Community Nursing Versus Community-Based Nursing

More employment opportunities are created for nurses in the community as the setting for nursing care continues to develop outside the acute care setting. Many of these settings, positions, and opportunities are discussed in Chapter 11. The prominent nursing role in the community in the past was that of public health or community health nurse. For over four decades, there has been a debate regarding the difference between community health and public health nursing. In this text, the term community health nursing will be used synonymously with public health nursing. Although a monumental need for provision of nursing care in the community resulted from the federal legislation that mandated changes in the health care delivery system, this need has not been for more community health nurses but rather for additional nurses prepared to give community-based care. At the same time, there are many similarities between the roles of the community based and community health nurse and currently both are in short supply.

While community health nursing practice includes nursing directed to individuals, families, and groups, the predominant responsibility is to the population as a whole (ANA, 1999). Thus, community, or public, health nursing is defined by its role in promoting the public's health. Community health nursing is a subset of community-based nursing.

Community-based nursing has a defined philosophy of practice that requires specific knowledge and skill. It is not defined by the setting or by the level of academic preparation

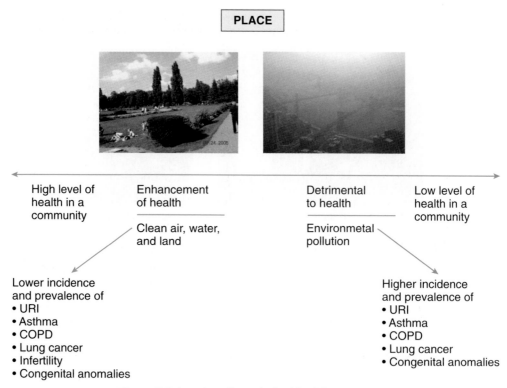

Figure 1-6 Location affects the health of the community.

but by a philosophy of practice (Hunt, 1998). It is about how the nurse practices, not where the nurse practices. Community-based nursing provides care to individuals and families across a continuum focusing on health promotion and rehabilitative primary health care through interdisciplinary collaboration for diverse populations (American Association of Colleges of Nursing, 2002; Quad Council of Public Health Nursing Organizations, 2008). Community-based nursing care can be defined as nursing care directed toward specific individuals and families within a community and designed to meet needs of people as they move between and among health care settings. The emphasis is on a "flowing" kind of care that does not necessarily occur in one setting.

Focus of Nursing

As it is broadly defined, nursing care involves four essential components: the client, the environment, health, and nursing (Fawcett, 1984). Each area is approached differently depending on whether the care is provided in the acute care setting or in the community-based setting (Table 1-1).

In the acute care setting, the client is typically identified by the medical diagnosis and is separated from the family. The environment is controlled by the facility with restriction of the family's access to the client and a limitation on the client's freedom. Health and illness are seen as separate and apart from one another. When the client is discharged, the goals of acute care are considered accomplished. Nursing functions are largely delegated medical functions that center on treatment of illness.

In community-based nursing, the client is in his or her natural environment, in the context of the family and community. Illness is seen as merely an aspect of life, and the goals of care are focused around maximizing the client's quality of life and optimizing health. Nursing in the community is an autonomous role, for the most part, with nursing interventions determined by the client, family, and health care team and based on the values of the client or family and the community. The goal is to encourage self-care in the context of the family and community with a focus on illness prevention and continuity of care.

Components of Community-Based Care

Components of community-based care include self-care, preventive health care, care within the context of the community, continuity of care, and collaborative care (NLN, 1993, 1997,2000). These are described here and expanded on throughout the text.

SELF-CARE: CLIENT AND FAMILY RESPONSIBILITY

Within the past several decades, the consumer movement has enhanced awareness of the importance of self-care. The value of taking care of oneself to remain healthy, rather than neglecting health, with the consequence of illness or injury, has become a more accepted notion. Programs, Web sites, written material, and research on stress management, nutrition, exercise and fitness, as well as smoking cessation and substance abuse prevention and treatment are examples of how health-seeking behaviors have taken a more prominent role. Self-care is also seen in disease management. Disease management programs are beginning to encompass providers across the continuum of care. This is also seen in political and government factions promoting consumer protection, pollution control, and handgun control.

Self-care charges the individual client and the family with primary responsibility for decisions and actions that impact health. Because health care is increasingly provided outside the hospital setting, by design the client, family, or other caregiver, such as a friend or neighbor, often provide care rather than a health care professional. The burden of responsibility has shifted as the insurance companies and other third-party payers claim it is too expensive to do otherwise.

Empowering individuals to make informed health care decisions is an essential component of self-care. There are numerous examples of the important role that nurses play in facilitating self-care for client with chronic illness such as congestive health failure (Cameron, Worrall-Carter, Page, & Stewart, 2009; Enç, Yigit, & Altiok, 2010; Schnell-Hoehn, Naimark, & Tate, 2009) and chronic renal disease (Ba & Mollaoglu, 2010).

One common example of empowering individuals to make informed health care decisions is **advance directives** that allow clients to participate in decisions about their care, including the right to refuse treatment. Completing this document facilitates discussions among family members about the kind of medical care would one might want if too ill or hurt to express one's own wishes. Advance directives are legal documents that allow individuals to convey decisions about end-of-life care ahead of time. They provide a way for to communicate desires to family, friends, and health care professionals and to avoid confusion later on. A **durable power of attorney** for health care is a document that names a health care proxy. A *proxy* is someone delegated to make health decisions if one is unable to do so (American Bar Association, 2010).

One type of advance directive is the **living will**, which is the client's statement regarding the medical treatment he or she chooses to omit or refuses in the event the client is unable to make those decisions for himself or herself. There are many issues to address, including but not restricted to the use of dialysis and breathing machines, resuscitation if breathing or heartbeat stops, tube feeding, and organ or tissue donation. Despite the fact that the legislation for advance directives is over a decade old, there continues to be limited use of this important strategy. The nurse plays an essential role in ensuring that the client and family are informed about this vital issue. In some cases, the nurse may facilitate securing and completing the necessary documents.

Although community-based nursing affords the opportunity for direct physical care intervention on the part of the nurse, it also requires other types of interventions such as health teaching to enhance self-care for the client and caregiver. The nurse's role in facilitating self-care requires use of the nursing process through assessment, planning, implementation, and evaluation that revolves around the question: How much care can the client and other caregivers safely provide on their own at home?

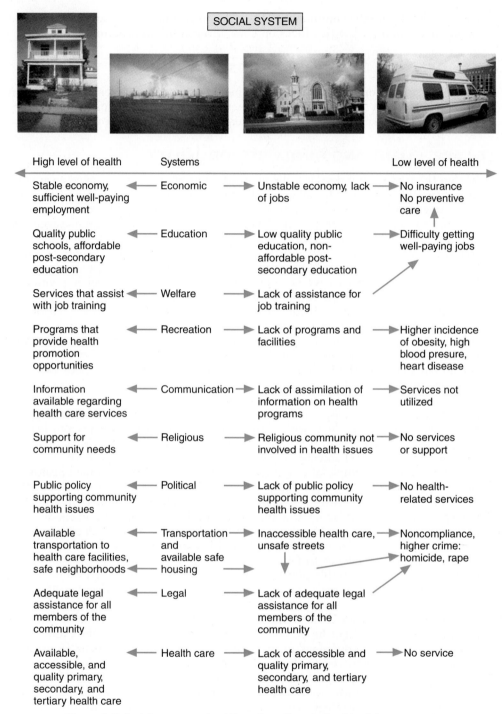

Figure 1-7 Social system and public policy affect the health of the community.

PREVENTIVE HEALTH CARE

Treatment efficacy rather than technologic imperative promotes nursing care that emphasizes prevention. America's biggest killers, heart disease, cancer, and lung disease can be addressed with prevention strategies. There is ample evidence of the need for more emphasis on prevention: only 45% of people with high blood pressure have it under control, only 29% of those with high cholesterol monitor the condition, only 2% get medication, and only 20% of smokers get help to quit (Sells, 2010).

Community-based nursing intervenes at all three levels of prevention. These concepts are discussed in greater depth in Chapter 2. Unlike community health nursing that tends to focus on primary and secondary prevention, many roles in community-based nursing call for a focus on tertiary prevention. An emphasis on prevention is evident in all settings and roles in community-based nursing.

For example, a nurse in the emergency room caring for a child who has ingested a poisonous substance considers not only the impact of the child's poisoning but also which preventive nursing interventions will maximize recovery and avoid a repeat of the incident. Diligent care of a wound in concert with vigilant teaching about wound care to avoid infection is an important preventive intervention for the client who is having a laceration sutured. Likewise, referral of a client for substance abuse assessment is an appropriate preventive nursing intervention for an intoxicated person who presents at the urgent care center after a fall.

CARE WITHIN THE CONTEXT OF THE COMMUNITY

Health and social issues are interactive. Nursing care is provided while considering the culture, values, and resources of the client, the family, and the community. If the client requests a particular religious or social ceremony before tube feeding, then the nurse attempts, within the constraints of safety, to comply with the client's request. In situations where family members want to participate in the client's care but their psychomotor skills restrict their ability to do so, the nurse will accommodate the desire within the constraints of time and safe care. If the client enjoys attending religious services every week, the visiting nurse honors that value by scheduling visits around the religious functions and if possible assisting the client to find transportation to the church, temple, or mosque. Similarly, the nurse tailors health teaching related to nutrition by considering the food preference of the culture of the family while integrating the basic principles of sound nutrition.

Care in the context of the client, family, and community is affected by the location and social systems of each community. Location often defines access and sometimes eligibility for health care services. It follows that location influences the health of a community. For instance, access to care is impeded by location when an adolescent who does not drive lives in the suburbs where there is no public transportation and seeks information about family planning services offered only in the nearby metropolitan area. In such a case, the social systems of the community affect access to care. Certainly, individual choices are important, but factors in the social environment are what determine access to health services and limit lifestyle choices in the first place.

CONTINUITY OF CARE

Fragmentation of care has long been a concern of health care professionals. For instance, a client with a variety of problems may be seen by several physicians: a family physician, cardiologist, endocrinologist, and surgeon. Other health care providers such as physical therapy, occupational therapy, social work, and respiratory therapy may also be involved in the client's care. Conflicting directions for treatments and therapies may result in overmedication or under medication. Treatment, protocols, or preparations incorrectly completed may lead to harm to the client. Continuity of care is a bridge to quality care.

Community-based care is particularly important in situations where clients are seen by several health care practitioners and move from one health care setting to another. Continuity allows quality of care to be preserved in a changing health care delivery system. If all providers follow the basic principles of continuity of care, then the possibility of a detrimental impact from a decreased length of stay in the acute care setting, to a community setting, where care is provided through a variety of individuals, can be minimized. Continuity is the adhesive that holds community-based nursing care together and is one of the fundamental concepts of this book. The evidence that nurses make a significant contribution to producing high-quality care is strong. Further, nurses are uniquely positioned to contribute to care teams, expand access to primary care, and enhance continuity (Bovbjerg, Ormond, & Pindus, 2009). Continuity of care is discussed in Chapter 7.

COLLABORATIVE CARE

Closely related to continuity of care is collaborative care. Collaborative care among health care professionals is an essential part of community-based care in that the primary goal of each practitioner is to promote wellness and restore health. These processes involve numerous interfaces and patient handoffs among multiple health care practitioners with varying levels of educational and occupational training. In the course of a 4-day hospital stay and discharge to home, transitional facility or home care, a client and family may interact with 50 different individuals, including physicians, nurses, technicians, and others. In numerous instances, critical information must be accurately communicated, making team collaboration essential (Mennenga & Smyer, 2010). When health care professionals are not communicating effectively, patient safety is at risk. Lack of critical information, misinterpretation of information, unclear orders over the telephone, and overlooked changes in status may lead to medical errors or poorly coordinated or executed discharge planning. In the last decade, the most costly consequence, unnecessary rehospitalization, has been on the rise (O'Daniel & Rosenstein, 2009).

Each team member has a role in the collaborative process. The physician or nurse practitioner is responsible primarily for diagnosing an illness and initiating required medical or surgical treatment. Nurse practitioners and physicians have the authority to admit clients into a specific health care setting and to discharge them from that setting into another setting. Further, they determine the plan of care for the medical needs of the client with input from other professional caregivers. Various therapists (physical, occupational, respiratory, and speech) may be involved in the client's care, providing therapy in the acute care setting, a rehabilitation setting, a residential care setting, or the home. The client may visit the facility, or the therapist may visit the home.

A dietitian may adapt a specialized diet to a specific individual and family or counsel and educate clients and their families. The social worker helps clients and families make decisions related to the use of community resources, life-sustaining treatments, and long-term care. A chaplain or the client's spiritual advisor will also counsel the client and family and give spiritual support. The pharmacist will dispense medications as directed by the physician and provide health education about the drug. Although each professional is responsible for a specialized concern, each is also responsible for sharing information with others or for evaluating how care is proceeding.

Currently there is a call for a new way of thinking about community care, where interprofessional collaboration is the norm (Satcher, 2010). A commitment to collaborative care recognizes that if one person in the chain fails to communicate, the bridge of continuity is weakened. Usually one person is designated as coordinator of care. In many cases this is the nurse. This role is discussed in Chapter 7.

Nursing Skills and Competencies

As mentioned, there are differences in the role of the nurse in the hospital compared to the community. For several decades, the different practice patterns among home health, community health, and hospital nurses have been understood (Hughes & Marcantonio, 1992). In acute care, nurses spend the majority of their time in direct patient care mostly with delegated medical functions and have little time for administrative, supervisory, or consultant roles. The home care and community-based nurse spends almost three times as many hours a week as the acute care nurse in consultation, health education, and counseling roles. The community-based and home care nurses also spend five times as many hours in the administrator and case manager role as the acute care nurse. In the hospital, nurses spend 84% of their time doing direct client care; in community-based and home care nursing, only about 60% of the time is spent on direct care.

Home care nursing differs in several ways from other nursing roles. First, home care nurses spend more time in supervisory and case management roles incorporating critical aspects of both the hospital and the community health nurse roles. Second, nurses in home care express more job satisfaction than those working in acute care or community health. Further, they are less likely to work weekends or nights. Cole, Ouzts, and Stepans (2010) reported that most staff nurses and managers working in the community were satisfied with their jobs.

Competencies for the nurses working in community settings require knowledge and skills in assessment, program planning, communication, and cultural competency, dimensions of communities, public health science, management, and leadership. These competencies are designed to serve as a starting point for understanding the role of the nurse in the community (Quad Council of Public Health Nursing Organizations, 2003).

COMMUNICATION

Communication skills in community care are, as in all settings, an essential element of nursing practice. However, nurses in the community rely almost completely on the concept of relationship-based care. Developing a trusting, therapeutic relationship requires that first the nurse has well-developed self-awareness. This means they understand about themselves and who they are, what they do, and how they do what they do. The heart of relationship-based care occurs when one human connects to another as compassion and care are communicated through touch, a kind act, competent clinical interventions, or through listening and seeking to understand another human being's experience. Healing is attributable to relationship-based care whether it is with individuals, families, or communities.

In practice in all settings, the nurse identifies and interprets verbal and nonverbal communications as a part of the assessment phase of the nursing process. Well-developed interpersonal skills are essential to comprehensive assessment of individuals, families, and communities. Listening to others in an unbiased manner and respecting various points of views as well as promoting the expression of diverse opinions and perspectives is the desired outcome of competent communication in the community. A working knowledge of the principles of teaching and learning is also imperative to collect and interpret information to determine the learner's need to learn and readiness to learn.

Documentation is a vital communication competency. Complete, accurate documentation is an essential element of nursing care in any setting, but it is of particular importance in community-based settings. Creating a clear account of what the nurse saw and did not only provides a record of care but also creates a log of client progress. As in the acute care setting where several caregivers may be documenting care simultaneously, the nurse is not the only person documenting care. This makes documentation an essential element for collaboration across the continuum of care.

Comprehensive charting is significant for several other reasons. Charting is used to determine eligibility for reimbursement for care provided. If services rendered by the nurse fall within the requirements of Medicaid, Medicare, or other third-party payers, then the agency will be paid for the care rendered. Because charting is a legal document, in cases in which an agency and nurse are sued, charting of the incident in question will be used as the record of care provided and client response to that care. Litigation is often avoided or readily resolved if care is accurately and completely documented.

ASSESSMENT

Analytical assessment skills applied to the nursing process are an important aspect to quality care in all settings. But because the role of the nurse in the community is often more autonomous compared to that of the nurse in the acute care setting, sound analytical assessment skills are even more essential. The nurse, client, and family all work in tandem to assemble information about the health status of the client to guide care. After systematically collecting and interpreting data related to the client's condition, the nurse collaborates with the client and family to determine the strengths and priority needs of the client as well as what care to initiate, continue, alter, or terminate. Likewise, the environmental variables in the home and community that may affect nursing care are identified and considered. With this information, the client, caregiver, and, in some cases, other family members along with the nurse determine expected outcomes and outcome criteria and develop a plan of care. After implemented, the effectiveness of the nursing care, expected outcomes, and outcome criteria is evaluated and modifications are made accordingly. The ability of other caregivers to provide adequate physical care and psychosocial support for the client is also evaluated. This same process is used to assess family and community. Throughout this book, there are opportunities to develop skills and knowledge related to assessment in Chapter 5.

PROGRAM PLANNING SKILLS

Program planning skills are more often a role function of the nurse with a graduate degree but associate and baccalaureate-prepared nurses benefit from basic program planning skills. This competency requires using the nursing process to plan educational programming. For example, in a clinic where many clients have hypertension, nurses working there may decide that rather than do individual teaching for management of hypertension, a series of three group classes should be offered. The nurses, in collaboration with a dietitian, would determine who would attend these classes, how the participants would be invited, where and when the classes would be offered, and the content covered in each class. They would develop a simple evaluation to determine how to improve the classes. This topic is covered in more detail in Chapter 6.

CULTURAL COMPETENCE

Cultural competence requires a commitment to a lifelong process of self-reflection and learning. The U.S. population is made up of a diverse mix of ethnicity and race including new Americans who are refugees and immigrants and Americans from families who have lived in the country for decades or sometimes centuries. Each ethnic and racial background has distinctive values, methods of communication, diet, and religious practices that directly affect the caregivers approach. To add further to this complex mix of needs, values, and strengths, members of different racial, ethnic, and cultural groups have varied genetic and environmental threats and risks. When working as a nurse in any setting, recognition of how culture impacts health behaviors, health beliefs, and health practices is imperative to developing cultural competence. Further, it is important for all nurses to embrace the importance of a diverse health care workforce. To practice holistically, nurses should learn about other cultures and use the information when providing care. This topic is covered in more detail in Chapter 3.

KNOWLEDGE OF COMMUNITIES

All nurses have a role in community assessment, ranging from identifying appropriate resources for referral to determining the need for a new clinic or hospital. Nurses informally establish linkages with community members and key stakeholders in the course of living and working in a community. Formally and informally, they may collaborate with community partners in projects to promote the health of large groups. Because community assessment varies in levels of complexity, the role of the nurse sometimes depends on the nurse's educational preparation and expertise. The person with an associate or baccalaureate degree in nursing uses community assessment primarily as it relates to the care of the individual client in the context of the community. For example, a nurse working in the acute care setting may want to find placement for a client with mental illness, but the agencies generally used by the referring facility are not appropriate. Thus, the nurse may conduct a simple community assessment to determine available, accessible, and appropriate community resources for referral. This topic is covered in more detail in Chapter 5.

BASIC PUBLIC HEALTH SCIENCE SKILLS

It is vital that nurses are able to define, assess, and understand the health status of populations, determinants of health and illness. Nurses also must understand factors contributing to health promotion and disease prevention, and factors contributing to the use of health services. Skills to identify and retrieve current relevant scientific evidence are also central to the provision of nursing care in the community. Because of the complexities involved in working in the community, nurses benefit from developing a lifelong commitment to learning.

MANAGEMENT SKILLS

The management competency requires the nurse use his or her leadership ability to carry out the management functions of planning, organizing, coordinating, delegating, and evaluating care for one client or a group of clients. This involves collecting and interpreting relevant data to meet the priority needs of the client. The nurse assesses individual and family resources, capabilities of other providers, and the client or family's ability to provide ongoing care as well as the resources in the community. This assessment leads to the care plan goals that tend to be more short-term and provide the foundation to develop a management plan with more long-term goals geared toward the client's recovery.

When management skills are used to oversee the care of a group of clients, the nurse delegates nursing activities to coworkers but assume responsibility for care given under his or her direction. This is commonly seen in the role of home care nurse overseeing the home health care aid. The role of nurse as manager requires that every aspect of care is evaluated. Evaluation of the client's ability to assess his or her own situation and condition and to plan and implement care is an essential component of the recovery process. The manager role extends not only to clients but also to other nursing personnel who are providing care under the direction and leadership of the registered nurse.

Care management refers to care coordination, case management, and safe transitions of care, all of which are important cost containment measures. Increasingly, case management is being recognized as a valuable service to enhance quality of care. Policy makers are beginning to understand how care coordination benefits the bottom line. Health care reform in recent years has had a heavy emphasis on the concepts of care coordination and care management. These are discussed in more depth in Chapter 7.

Ethical dilemmas in community-based care may require different leadership skills than those essential in the acute-care setting. When practicing in the community, nurses must take a leadership role in creating a culture of following ethical standards. For example, there may be lack of formal institutional support, such as an ethics committee or ethics rounds in community-based care. In the acute setting, the nurse has 24-hour contact with the client and family, whereas care is intermittent and brief in the community setting. Problem identification and problem solving are troublesome when communication is fragmented over several weeks or months. In theory, collaborating with the client and family may sound like common sense, but in reality, it can be exceedingly exasperating. Once again, the importance of clear, concise, and comprehensive charting is imperative. In all of these considerations, the nurse has a responsibility to take a leadership role.

When care is provided in the home or other community settings, respecting the client and family's desire for self-determination is foremost. This may limit the nurse's influence in the decision-making process, which may be stressful for the nurse. However, the prevailing principle is to assist the client and family to identify key values and shared vision to guide planning care. When the values of the family and nurse collide, frustrating dilemmas may result. Interdisciplinary communication is difficult in community-based care; this fact may intensify difficulties with ethical issues. One simple way that nurses take a leadership role with ethical issues is to facilitate the discussion of ethical concerns as they arise, using an ethical framework and encouraging open dialogue between the client, family, friends, and interdisciplinary team members. It is important to know one's own values. If conflicts arise when the nurse and family do not agree, the nurse may have to recommend that the family identify another party to facilitate discussions.

APPLICATION OF THE NURSING PROCESS

As in any setting for practice, the nursing process guides the nurse in thinking through assessment, planning, implementation, and evaluation and guides the nurse to replan accordingly. The nurse uses clinical decision-making skills and clinical reasoning to identify what to assess with each client, family, and community as well as determining the meaning of assessment data. This information allows the nurse to determine the strengths and needs of the client, family, and caregiver so that together they develop a problem or need statement sometimes referred to as a nursing diagnosis. All parties then identify goals, expected outcomes and outcome criteria as appropriate. Interventions are identified that are reasonable and acceptable to all parties involved in the planning process. The person who will carry out those interventions is designated. In some cases, the nurse may teach a procedure to the client or family caregiver. The client may be able to do the procedure, but a caregiver may need to buy the supplies or help set up the equipment for the procedure each time it is used.

Sometimes community-based nurses follow a standard plan of care from the physician, nurse practitioner, or agency. These set plans must be individualized by the nurse for the particular needs of each client and family. This may mean adding nursing care that may not be delineated on the standard plan or in other cases modifying the plan. In contrast to care typically provided in the hospital, in community settings, nursing process is a mutual endeavor used to plan care but also to develop therapeutic relationships with client family members and caregivers. In the chapters that follow, there are numerous opportunities to use the nursing process in client situations in community-based settings.

Nursing Interventions

Nursing interventions in the community-based setting are both similar and different from those typical in the acute care setting. Nursing interventions in the community have been defined through the work of the Public Health Nursing Section of the Minnesota Department of Health. These interventions are organized to focus on three levels of practice: community-focused practice, system-focused practice, and individual-focused practice (Keller, Schaffer, Lia-Hoagberg, & Strohschein, 2002). Although all levels of practice are covered in this book, individual care is highlighted. Nursing interventions are explained in more detail in the next chapter and integrated throughout the remainder of the text.

Conclusions

Community-based nursing is not defined by a setting but by a philosophy of practice. Increasingly, health care is provided in community settings and not in acute care facilities. As a result, clients and families require enhanced skills in self-care. The increasing cost of health care has led to more focus on prevention and health promotion. Community-based nursing averts the initial occurrence of disease or injury and provides early identification and treatment or a comprehensive rehabilitation of a disease or injury to maximize health. Continuity and collaborative care allow for quality care to be preserved in a changing health care delivery system. Community-based nurses use special skills and competencies to provide care within the context of the client's culture, family, and community.

What's on the Web?

Healthcare.gov: Taking Care into Your Own Hands
INTERNET ADDRESS: http://www.healthcare.gov/law/introduction/index.html
Health Care Reform (Affordability Care Act of 2010;ACA) is expected to have a profound impact on the health care system in the United States. ACA will not be implemented all at once. Portions of the law have already taken effect. Other changes will be implemented through 2014 and

beyond. This Web site is an important resource for all nurses and nursing students. Nurses can use this site as an educational tool to help clients understand prevention, determine how to get health care coverage, explore insurance options, determine quality of those options, and how the new law may change what their options are.

A good place to start is to watch a video tour of the Web site at http://www.healthcare.gov/news/videos/tour.html

Cultural Competence Project
INTERNET ADDRESS: **http://www.cultural-competence-project.org/en/index.html**
Through online and face-to-face educational offerings for nurses to enhance their cognitive, affective, and psychomotor cultural competencies this site offers to assist nurses to develop skills in addressing individuals, groups, and communities that are diverse, with special emphasis on those at risk for health disparities. A series of educational offerings focused on developing cultural competencies using a train-the-trainer model are available.

References

2010 may bring new career opportunities. (2010). *Case Management, Advisor, 21*(1). Retrieved from http://behavioralhealthcentral.com/index.php/20091231166183/Care/Case-Manager/cma-2010-may-bring-new-career-opportunities-for-case-managers.html

American Association of Colleges of Nursing. (2002). *Moving forward with community-based nursing education.* Washington: Author.

American Bar Association. (2010). *Living wills, health care proxies, and advance health care directives.* Retrieved from http://www.abanet.org/rppt/public/living-wills.html

American Nurses Association. (1999). *American Nurses Association standards of public health nursing practice.*

American Nurses Association. (2010). *Key provisions related to nursing: Health care reform.* Retrieved from http://www.nursingworld.org/MainMenuCategories/HealthcareandPolicyIssues/HealthSystemReform/Key-Provisions-Related-to-Nurses.aspx; http://www.nursingworld.org/MainMenuCategories/HealthcareandPolicyIssues/HealthSystemReform.aspx

Ba, E., & Mollaoglu, M. (2010). The evaluation of self-care and self-efficacy in patients undergoing hemodialysis. *Journal of Evaluation in Clinical Practice, 16*(3), 605–610.

Bovbjerg, R., Ormond, B., & Pindus, N. (2009). *The nursing workforce challenge: Public policy for a dynamic and complex market.* Report Number o8277-000-000. Urban Institute Health Care Center. Retrieved from http://www.urban.org/publications/411933.html

Bureau of Labor Statistics, U.S. Department of Labor. (2010). *Occupational outlook handbook, 2010–2011 edition: Registered nurses.* Retrieved from http://www.bls.gov/oco/ocos083.htm#projections_data

Cameron, J., Worrall-Carter, L., Page, K., & Stewart, S. (2010). Self-care behaviours and heart failure: Does experience with symptoms really make a difference? *European Journal of Cardiovascular Nursing, 9*(2), 92–100.

Centers for Disease Control and Prevention. (2010). *Health impact assessment: Fact sheet.* Retrieved from http://www.cdc.gov/healthyplaces/publications/Health_Impact_Assessment2.pdf

Cole, S., Ouzts, K., & Stepans, M. (2010). Job satisfaction in rural public health nurses. *Journal of Public Health Management and Practice, 16*(4), E1–E6. Retrieved from CINAHL Plus with Full Text database.

Craven, R. C., & Hirnle, C. J. (Eds.) (2009). *Fundamentals of nursing: Human health and function* (6th ed.). Philadelphia: Lippincott Williams & Wilkins.

Department of Health and Human Services. (2010). *Health, United States, 2010.* Washington: Author. Retrieved from http://healthypeople.gov/Default.htm

Enç, N., Yigit, Z., & Altiok, M. (2010). Effects of education on self-care behaviour and quality of life in patients with chronic heart failure. *CONNECT: The World of Critical Care Nursing, 7*(2), 115–121. Retrieved from CINAHL Plus with Full Text database.

Fawcett, J. (1984). *Analysis and evaluation of conceptual models of nursing.* Philadelphia, PA: F.A. Davis.

Fee, E., & Bu, L. (2010). The origins of public health nursing: The Henry Street Visiting Nurse Service. *American Journal of Public Health, 100*(7), 1206–1207. Retrieved from CINAHL Plus with Full Text database.

Goldfield, N. (2010). The evolution of diagnosis-related groups (DRGs): From its beginnings in case-mix and resource use theory, to its implementation for payment and now for its current utilization for quality within and outside the hospital. *Quality Management in Health Care, 19*(1), 3–16. Retrieved from CINAHL Plus with Full Text database.

Health Resources and Service Administration. (2009). *What is behind HRSA's projected supply, demand, and shortage of registered nurses?* Retrieved from http://bhpr.hrsa.gov/healthworkforce/reports/behindrnprojections/2.htm

Health Resources and Services Administration. (2010). *Preliminary findings: 2008 National sample survey of registered nurses.* Retrieved from http://bhpr.hrsa.gov/healthworkforce/rnsurvey/initialfindings2008.pdf

Heller, B., Oros, M., & Durney-Crowley, J. (2007). *The future of nursing education: Ten trends to watch.* New York: National League for Nursing. Retrieved from http://www.nln.org/nlnjournal/infotrends.htm

Hughes, K., & Marcantonio, R. (1992). Practice patterns among home health, public health, and hospital nurses. *Nursing and Health Care, 13*(10), 532–536.

Hunt, R. (1998). Community based nursing: Philosophy or setting. *American Journal of Nursing, 98*(10), 44–47.

Josten, L. (1989). Wanted: Leaders for public health. *Nursing Outlook, 37,* 230–232.

Kalish, P., & Kalish, B. (1995). *The advance of American nursing* (3rd ed.). Philadelphia, PA: Lippincott.

Keller, L., Schaffer, M., Lia-Hoagberg, B., & Strohschein, S. (2002). Assessment, program planning, and evaluation in population-based public health practice. *Journal of Public Health Management Practice, 8*(5), 30–43.

Leininger, M. (1970). *Nursing and anthropology: Two worlds to blend.* New York, NY: Wiley.

Mennenga, H., & Smyer, T. (2010). A model for easily incorporating team-based learning into nursing education. *International Journal of Nursing Education Scholarship, 7*(1), 1–16. Retrieved from CINAHL Plus with Full Text database.

Monteiro, L. (1991). Florence Nightingale on public health nursing. In B. Spradley (Ed.), *Readings in community health nursing.* Philadelphia, PA: Lippincott.

National League for Nursing. (1993). *A vision for nursing education.* New York: Author.

National League for Nursing. (1997). *Final report: Commission on a workforce for a restructured health care system.* New York: Author.

National League for Nursing, Council of Associate Degree Nursing Competencies Task Force. (2000). *Educational competencies for graduates of associate degree nursing programs.* Boston, MA: Jones & Bartlett Publisher.

O'Daniel, M., & Rosenstein, A. (2009). Professional communication and team collaboration In Hughes, R. G. (Ed.), *Patient safety and quality: An evidence-based handbook for nurses.* (Prepared with support from the Robert Wood Johnson Foundation). AHRQ Publication No. 08-0043. Rockville, MD: Agency for Healthcare Research and Quality. Retrieved on March 2008 from http://www.ahrq.gov/qual/nurseshdbk/nurseshdbk.pdf

Quad Council of Public Health Nursing Organizations. (2003). *Quad Council PHN competencies.* Retrieved from http://www.astdn.org/publication_quad_council_phn_competencies.htm

Quad Council of Public Health Nursing Organizations. (2006). *A public health nursing shortage: A threat to the public's health.* Retrieved from http://www.astdn.org

Quad Council of Public Health Nursing Organizations (2008). As cited in: Prevention, protection, and promotion: Nursing' role in public health. (2008) *Charting nursing's future.* Retrieved from http://www.rwjf.org/pr/product.jsp?id=35348

Robert Wood Johnson Foundation. (2009). *Beyond health care: New directions to a healthier America.* Retrieved from www.commissionon health.org

Robert Wood Johnson Foundation. (2010). *Health care overhaul means more opportunities, and demand for nurses.* Retrieved from http://www.rwjf.org

Satcher, D. (2010). Include a social determinants of health approach to reduce health inequities. *Public Health Reports, 125*(Suppl. 4). Retrieved from http://www.publichealthreports.org/archives/issueopen.cfm?articleID=2476

Schnell-Hoehn, K., Naimark, B., & Tate, R. (2009). Determinants of self-care behaviors in community-dwelling patients with heart failure. *Journal of Cardiovascular Nursing, 24*(1), 40–47. Retrieved from CINAHL Plus with Full Text database.

Sells, T. (2010). CDC director says prevention is the most cost effective health strategy. *The Commercial Appeal.* Retrieved from http://www.commercialappeal.com/news/2010/jul/16/ailing-health-care/?cid=xrs_rss-nd

Tri-Council for Nursing. (2010). *Educational advancement of registered nurses.* Retrieved from http://www.nln.org/governmentaffairs/pdf/workforce_supply_statement_final.pdf

World Health Organization. (2010). *Social determinants of health: Key concepts.* Retrieved from http://www.who.int/social_determinants/en/

LEARNING ACTIVITIES

JOURNALING ACTIVITY 1-1

In your clinical journal, discuss a community with which you are familiar and describe what defines that community.

1. Identify some of the health needs and strengths of the community.
2. Where do members of this community receive health care?
3. Are there people in the community who have difficulty getting access to health care? Who are they? What services are they not able to access? What services are provided for those without insurance?
4. Discuss service in the community that would help individuals and families improve self-care.
5. Describe health promotion and disease prevention services available in the community.
6. Identify services for the most common cultural groups in the community.

CLIENT CARE ACTIVITY 1-2

How can the nurse encourage self-care in the following client situations?

1. Jane is the 31-year-old mother of Jackie, a 4-month-old baby who has frequent apnea spells. Jane states, "I am afraid she will stop breathing at home. I can't figure out the monitor."
2. Stephan is a 60-year-old widower whose wife died 3 years ago. There is an increasing possibility that he will have to have his leg amputated below the knee as a result of a very large leg ulcer. Stephan has been hospitalized three times in the past 6 months because of uncontrolled diabetes. The last time, there were maggots in his leg ulcer.
3. Tim's wife of 40 years passed away 1 month ago. He comes to the clinic and does not make eye contact with you as he says, "I have no appetite and am so lonely for my wife I can't go on. I never leave the house."

How can the nurse encourage disease prevention and health promotion in the following client situations?

1. Barb and Steve have a 10-month-old baby, Andy, who requires intermittent nursing care because of oxygen therapy and tracheotomy care. They have three other children, ages 2, 4, and 6. Andy has had three bouts of respiratory flu and two colds in the last 4 months resulting in a hospitalization each time. You are the home care nurse caring for Andy. You noticed on your last visit that Andy's brothers and sister kiss him, touch his trach tube, and cough on him. One of the children went in to use the bathroom and left the door open, and you noticed that he did not wash his hands afterward. Two of the children have runny noses. Casual inspection of the children's hands reveals visual dirt on the fingers and under the finger nails.

What is your priority nursing intervention with Barb, Steve, and their family? What does the nursing literature say about the intervention that you identified? How will you proceed with your teaching using a prevention focus?

2. Meg and Bob have a 3-year-old child, Mark, who has cerebral palsy. Meg provides 24-hour care for Mark, with no assistance from anyone in her family or friends. You notice on your last home visit that Meg has lost weight, is not sleeping, and complains that she has no energy. You suspect that she may be suffering from depression. You recommend several counselors and respite care for Mark so that Meg can get out occasionally. Meg states, "I come from a very large family. We never use a babysitter in our family." What do you do and say?

PRACTICAL APPLICATION ACTIVITY 1-4

Describe an incident from your clinical experience in which you believe continuity was interrupted.

- Indicate some things that could have been done to ensure continuity in these situations. What other action may have improved continuity?
- Describe a time or circumstance that you observed or participated in where continuity of care was provided. What happened, and who and what made it happen?

PRACTICAL APPLICATION ACTIVITY 1-5

1. Contact your local or state department of health. You can either call them or visit their Web site. What are the current issues facing department of health in your city or county? How are these issues related to nursing?
2. Find an article in the paper that is related to one of the topics covered in this chapter. What new things did you learn about the issue or topic? How is the topic related to what is discussed in this chapter.

Chapter 2

Health Promotion and Disease Prevention

ROBERTA HUNT

Learning Objectives

1. Describe the health–illness continuum.
2. Relate the vision of Healthy People 2020 to community-based nursing.
3. Discuss an action a nurse could make to address one of the overarching goals of Healthy People 2020.
4. Recognize the difference between health promotion and disease prevention.
5. Identify nursing roles for each level of prevention.
6. Identify four nursing interventions important for the role of the nurse in community-based settings.

Key Terms

disease and injury prevention services
function
health
health disparity
health promotion
health protection
health–illness continuum

nursing interventions in community based settings
primary prevention
secondary prevention
social determinants of health
tertiary prevention

Chapter Topics

Health and Illness

Healthy People 2020

Health Promotion Versus Disease and Injury Prevention

The Prevention Focus

Nursing Interventions in Community-Based Care

Nursing Interventions in Community-Based Care and Levels of Prevention

Conclusions

The Nurse Speaks

When people ask me what I do, I am reluctant to disclose being a community mental health nurse. For the most part, there is a total lack of understanding for community mental health nursing. When I applied for the job that I have now, I too had a vague idea of mental health nursing and little real understanding of what I would actually be doing. Mental health had always intrigued me. I just didn't think that I would be so lucky to find my niche easily as a new nurse. I have always wanted to work with patients on many levels, as they function in real life, in the community. Additionally, I wanted to build a therapeutic relationship with people that would persist over time, through life changes, and hopefully result in positive outcomes in the management of long-term mental health.

On a whim, I applied for the job and was hired despite having no mental health experience. I can honestly say I love my job. My boss said the first 3 months would be a "trial by fire." He was not exaggerating. With a few vague guidelines, I created the position of psychiatric nurse clinician on my own. What I didn't realize until writing this is how much the public health intervention wheel really guided the development of my position. Aside from hours of reading about diagnoses, treatment, medications, and side effects and learning to integrate care for a team of four psychiatrists, I live and breathe the "wheel."

At the county-based and funded outpatient mental health clinic, everyone warned me about how sick our clients would be. In addition to a mental health diagnosis, many have a background of abuse, neglect, poor socioeconomic status, substance abuse/dependence, criminal behavior, and a host of other complications. When I first encounter new clients, I use health teaching to inform them about their illness, medications, side effects, and long-term outcomes. In my role, I spend more time with the clients than the psychiatrists do. I advocate for clients when they don't know what to say to their psychiatrist or when they just want me there. I help them access free medication programs, do prior authorizations so insurance will pay for their medications, prepare mediplanners, and assist clients in managing complex medication regimens. I collaborate a great deal with other providers and often refer clients to therapy, medical providers, and inpatient and drug recovery programs. It is my job and ultimate goal to make transitions run smoothly no matter what that may mean for the client. I try to approach each client with respect, and if a client is requesting help I do everything possible professionally to meet his or her needs. This could be anything from offering support to a client regarding a family member to presenting supportive evidence to a social service agent that a client has been compliant with medication. This position presents much variety. No day is ever the same!

Jodi Kroening RN, BSN
Psychiatric Nurse Clinician

Over the last decades, the U.S. health care system remains the most expensive in the world, using 15.3% of the U.S. gross national product (GNP), at a cost of nearly $7,290 per person. The next most expensive health care system is in Canada, where 10% of the GNP is used for health care, at a per capita cost of $3,672. A recent study found Canadians healthier than citizens in the United States despite spending almost half of what is spent on health care per person in the United States (Lasser, Himmelstein, & Woolhandler, 2006). Most industrialized nations spend 8% to 10% of their GNP on health care (World Health Organization [WHO], 2010).

Despite having the most expensive health care in the world, the United States lags behind other nations in key health indicators. The United States ranks 30th among nations in its infant mortality rate, behind most European countries The main cause of the high infant mortality rate is the very high percentage of preterm births in the United States (MacDorman & Mathews, 2009). In the United States, there is an emphasis on rescuing babies who are born premature, but not on preventing prematurity by providing universal access to health care for women of childbearing age or pregnant women of any age. Nor is attention paid to **social determinants of health** such as social and behavioral factors that influence preterm birth like smoking and alcohol and drug use.

Life expectancy at 50 in the United States ranks 29th behind Japan, Australia, Canada, France, Italy, Iceland, Spain, Switzerland, Sweden, and other countries. Twenty-three percent of the nation's 1½- to 3-year-old children are inadequately immunized against diphtheria, tetanus, pertussis, polio, measles, mumps, and rubella. Disadvantaged populations rank significantly worse than average in these and other health indicators (Federal Interagency Forum on Child and Family Statistics, 2009; WHO, 2010). Mortality trends over the last decade are not encouraging. In the United States, where 60% of adults are overweight or obese, overall rankings fell, reflecting an increase in premature death, from 34th in the world in female mortality and 41st in male mortality in 1990 to 49th for women and 45th for men in 2010, behind Chile, Tunisia, and Albania (Rajaratnam et al., 2010). In summary, Americans spend twice as much as residents of other developed countries on health care, with outcome indicators showing lower quality, less efficiency, and a less equitable system.

Health care costs are a barrier to care for both the insured and the uninsured. According to a landmark study by the Harvard School of Public Health, nearly one-quarter of Americans had problems paying medical bills in 2005, and more than 61% of those reporting problems paying medical bills were covered by health insurance (Kaiser Family Foundation & Harvard School of Public Health, 2006). Moderate- and low-income, working adults report significantly more problems paying for medical care compared with their higher-income peers. Uninsured adults (18% of the public) report more problems accessing health care because of cost. Two-thirds (66%) of the insured adults say their health insurance premiums have gone up over the past 5 years, including 38% who say that their premiums have gone up "a lot." Every large industrialized nation except the United States has a national health plan in place that covers all citizens free of charge.

The profession of nursing reflects the needs of society. Although a great deal of money is spent on health care in the United States, the level of health of U.S. citizens is disappointing. The consumer movement toward increased participation in wellness, weight loss, smoking cessation, and exercising has resulted in the preventive care movement. Settings for practice have evolved naturally as nurses focus on health rather than illness. Nursing has taken on a new look as it assumes the role of health promotion and illness and injury prevention. Community-based nursing calls for interventions distinct and different from many of those common in the acute care setting. Community-based nursing is a philosophy of care that incorporates the concepts of self-care and collaborative care that considers the context in which health occurs.

A discussion of health and its place on the health–illness continuum begins this chapter. The vision, mission, and overarching goals in the federal government's program Healthy People 2020 framework are presented. The remainder of the chapter is devoted to illustrating the difference between health promotion and disease prevention and the major strategies nurses use to meet the goals of Healthy People 2020. The emphasis is on levels of prevention related to nursing roles and common interventions appropriate in community-based nursing.

Health and Illness

Unlike most of nursing practice that focuses on "sick care" or curing illness and injury, community-based care concentrates on true "health care" activities to promote health and prevent illness and injury. This is accomplished through a collaborative model that encourages self-care within the context in which health occurs. The classic definition of **health** from the WHO (1986) is a "state of physical, mental and social well-being and not merely absence of disease or infirmity." In 2008, this definition was updated to include a person's

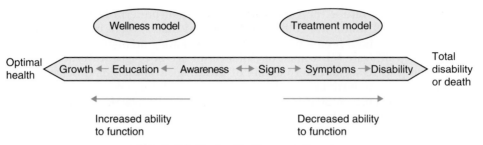

Figure 2-1 The health–illness continuum.

characteristics, behaviors, and physical, social, and economic environment (WHO). This holistic philosophy differs greatly from that of the current health care delivery system in the United States, which focuses on sick care.

Considering health—rather than illness—as the essence of care requires a shift in thinking. The **health–illness continuum** illustrates this model of care (Fig. 2-1). Health is conceptualized as a resource for everyday living. It is a positive idea that emphasizes social and personal resources and physical capabilities. Wellness is a lifestyle aimed at achieving physical, emotional, intellectual, spiritual, and environmental well-being. The use of wellness measures can increase stamina, energy, and self-esteem. These then enhance quality of life.

Improvement of health is not seen as an outcome of the amount and type of medical services or the size of the hospital. Treatment efficacy, rather than technology, drives care in this model. Here health is viewed as a function of collaborative efforts at the community level.

Care provided in acute care settings is usually directed at resolving immediate health problems. In community-based care, the focus is on maximizing individual potential for self-care. The client assumes responsibility for health care decisions and care provision. Where health is the essence of care, the client's ability to function becomes the primary concern. The intent of care is not to "fix" with treatment but to enhance the quality of life and support actions that make the client's life as comfortable and productive as possible.

Function is defined by subjective and objective measurements. Both the client's abilities to perform activities of daily living (ADL) and the client's perception of how well he or she is functioning are considered. Clients may state that they are satisfied with their ability to care for themselves; however, objective data from laboratory reports, diagnostic tests, and caregivers' observations may show that this is not the case. On the other hand, clients may report that they are concerned about their ability to perform ADLs, yet other information may indicate that they are functioning quite well. The following Client Situation in Practice reflects this dichotomy.

CLIENT SITUATIONS IN PRACTICE

Perceptions of Health and Illness

Mary had a myocardial infarction 3 days ago. After two episodes of chest pain and dizziness, she reluctantly went to the emergency room. Laboratory values showed moderate heart damage. As a 46-year-old single parent, Mary is the sole provider for three adolescents. She is a physical therapist and works at an ambulatory clinic during the week and a nursing home on weekends. She tells the nurse caring for her that she feels fine and asks to go home so she can go back to work tomorrow.

Mary's mother, Shirley, is extremely distraught about her daughter's condition and believes Mary is dying. Figure 2-2 illustrates the objective data versus Mary's subjective point of view. The dissonance between subjective perceptions and objective data can interrupt and delay recovery.

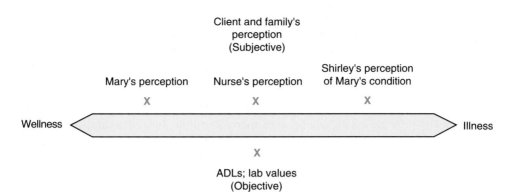

Figure 2-2 Subjective perceptions of health and function may differ from each other and from objective data.

A person's lifestyle is a dynamic process that involves needs, beliefs, assumptions, and values. Choices in life evident in self-care therefore can be seen as opportunities for moving toward optimal health or wellness.

Wellness involves more than simply good physical self-care. It also requires using one's mind constructively, expressing one's emotions effectively, interacting constructively with others, and being concerned about one's physical and psychological environment. Regardless of the setting for health care, wherever nurses practice, their concern should be for the whole person, and the care they provide holistic (Fig. 2-3).

Healthy People 2020

Every 10 years, the U.S. Department of Health and Human Services (HHS) leverages scientific insights and lessons learned from the past decade, along with new knowledge of current data, trends, and innovations through the Healthy People initiative. This road map to improve the nation's health provides science-based, 10-year national objectives for promoting health and preventing disease. Healthy People 2020 incorporates assessments of major risks to health and wellness to change public health priorities and improve our nation's health preparedness and prevention. Healthy People 2020 offers a vision of a "society in which all people live long, healthy lives" (U.S. Department of Health and Human Services [DHHS], 2010). This vision is the result of a collaborative effort of a national consortium of health care professionals, citizens, and private and public agencies from across the United States.

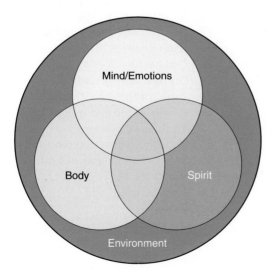

Figure 2-3 Schematic representation of holism. The system is greater than and different from the sum of the parts. Wherever the setting, the nurse's concern is for the whole person.

Healthy People 2020's missions, goals, and objectives spring from analysis of those targets set a decade ago in Healthy People 2010. Two overarching goals were articulated in 2010: increasing the quality of life and eliminating health disparities. Preliminary analyses show that life expectancy has increased by 1.2% when measured at birth and by 5.1% when measured at age 65. However, the goal of eliminating disparities remains unmet (Sondik, Huang, Klein, & Satcher, 2010).

Healthy People 2020 articulates five missions. The first is to identify nationwide health improvement priorities. The second is to increase public awareness and understanding of the determinants of health, disease, and disability and the opportunities for progress. The third mission strives to provide measurable objectives and goals applicable at the national, state, and local levels. The fourth intent is to engage multiple sectors to take actions to strengthen policies and improve practices that are driven by the best available evidence and knowledge. The fifth initiative attempts to identify critical research, evaluation, and data collection needs.

Healthy People 2020 states that its overarching goals are to

1. Attain higher quality, longer lives free of preventable disease, disability, injury, and premature death

2. Achieve health equity, eliminate disparities, and improve the health of all groups

3. Create social and physical environments that promote good health for all

4. Promote quality of life, healthy development, and healthy behaviors across all life stages

Measurable targets or objectives to be achieved are organized into 37 priority areas (see Healthy People 2020 2-1).

Healthy People 2020 ❄ *2-1*

FOCUS AREAS

1. Access to health services	19. HIV
2. Adolescent health	20. Immunization and infectious diseases
3. Arthritis, osteoporosis, and chronic back conditions	21. Injury and violence prevention
4. Blood disorders and blood safety	22. Maternal, infant and child health
5. Cancer	23. Medical product safety
6. Chronic kidney disease	24. Mental health and mental disorders
7. Diabetes	25. Nutrition and weight status
8. Disability and secondary conditions	26. Occupational safety and health
9. Early and middle childhood	27. Older adults
10. Education and community-based programs	28. Oral health
11. Environmental health	29. Physical activity and fitness
12. Family planning	30. Public health infrastructure
13. Food safety	31. Quality of life and well-being
14. Genomics	32. Respiratory diseases
15. Global health	33. Sexually transmitted diseases
16. Health communications and health literacy	34. Social determinants of health
17. Healthcare-associated infections	35. Substance abuse
18. Heart disease and stroke	36. Tobacco use
	37. Vision

ATTAIN LONGER LIVES FREE OF PREVENTABLE DEATH AND DISEASE

The first goal of Healthy People 2020 is to attain high-quality, longer lives free from preventable disease, disability, injury, and premature death. A combination of four unhealthy behaviors that include smoking, lack of exercise, poor diet, and substantial alcohol consumption greatly increase the risk of premature death when combined. (Kvaavik, Batty, Ursin, Huxley, & Gale, 2010). Modest but achievable changes to lifestyle behaviors have a considerable impact on the health of both individuals and communities. Healthy People 2020 proposes different ways to promote healthy diets and lifestyles to prevent premature death.

ACHIEVE HEALTH EQUITY, ELIMINATE DISPARITIES, AND IMPROVE THE HEALTH OF ALL GROUPS

In order to improve the health of all, individual differences in health and access to health care services by gender, age, race or ethnicity, education or income, disability, geographic location, or sexual orientation must be considered. For example, men have a life expectancy that is 5 years less than women. Likewise, information about the biologic and genetic characteristics of African Americans, Hispanics, Native Americans, Alaska Natives, Asians, Native Hawaiians, and Pacific Islanders does not explain the health disparities experienced by these groups compared with the White, non-Hispanic population in the United States. See Box 2-1 for a summary of **health disparity** in the United States.

Disparity in health in the United States is well documented with numerous federal initiatives undertaken in an attempt to reduce these disparities. One of the goals in Healthy People 2000 and Healthy People 2010 was to reduce health disparities. Analysis of disparities between non-Hispanic Black and non-Hispanic White populations nationwide widened for 6 of the 15 health status indicators from 1990 and 2005. "With more than 15 years of time and effort spent at the national and local level to reduce disparities, the impact remains negligible." (Orsi, Margelios-Anast, & Whitman, 2010)

It is believed that these disparities are a result of the complex interaction among genetic variations, environmental factors, and specific health behaviors. Inequalities in

---

BOX 2-1   Racial and Ethnic Disparities in Health Care

The overall health of Americans has improved in the last few decades, but all Americans have not shared equally in these improvements. The prevalence of diabetes among American Indians and Alaskan Natives is more than twice that for all adults in the U.S. Overall mortality was 25% higher for black Americans than for white Americans in 2009, compared with 37% higher in 1990. In 2006, age-adjusted death rates for the black population exceeded those for the white population by 48% for stroke (cerebovascular disease), 31% for heart disease, 21% for cancer (malignant neoplasm), 113% for diabetes, and 786% for HIV disease. (U.S. Department of Health and Human Services,2009) National Center for Health Statistics. 2009. Health, United States, 2009. Washington, DC: U.S. Department of Health and Human services. http://www.cdc.gov/nchs/data/hus/hus09.pdf#executivesummary

One may ask: Among people who receive health care, how much do differences in race and ethnicity contribute to disparities in that health care?

Preventive health care services improve health by protecting against disease, lessening its impact, or detecting disease at an early stage when it is easier to treat. Although Americans use many types of clinical preventive services, utilization remains suboptimal for some services. Blacks, Asians, American Indians, Alaskan Natives, and Hispanics all experience disparities in the percentage of adults age 50 and over who receive a colonoscopy, sigmoidoscopy, proctoscopy, or fecal occult blood test and in recommended hospital care for pneumonia. Some recent trends show that Blacks and Hispanics both had worsening disparities in colorectal cancer mortality in the last decade and American Indians, Alaskan Natives and Hispanics had worsening disparities in the recommended hospital care for heart failure and that Asians and Hispanics both had worsening disparities in pneumococcal vaccination for adults age 65 and over in the last decade.

income and education underlie many health disparities, with income and education often serving as a proxy measure for each other. In general, population groups that suffer the worst health status are also those that have the highest poverty rates and the least education. Disparities in health care can be eliminated through continued commitment to understanding why disparities exist. Effective strategies to eliminate and overcome disparities need to be identified. Nurses have a role in working more closely with communities to ensure that relevant research findings are implemented quickly. There is a need to evaluate transcultural competence (discussed in Chapter 3) as it relates to health care disparities. Finally, capacity for health services research among minority institutions and minority investigators is lacking.

Nurses have a role in seeing that these deficiencies are addressed. First and foremost, nursing focuses on caring—caring for individuals, families, and communities. This caring often is manifested in advocacy. When nurses care about individuals and families as they face difficulties and crisis, they enable them to heal within the context of their own abilities, opportunities, and social circumstances. This watchful state allows for openness to recognize strengths, needs, and resources of individuals and families within their respective communities but also the strengths, needs, and resources available within the community. Through this process, nurses have the opportunity to identify vulnerable populations within a community and assist within these groups the capacity to act on their own behalf. Nurses must educate themselves regarding issues related to lack of health equity and disparity within vulnerable populations. Further, evidence-based decision making must be used to analyze identified disparity and to empower individuals and families to recognize and seek high-quality care. With this knowledge, nurses work with communities to address disparity stemming from inadequate institutional policies. The end goal of this type of caring through advocacy is to not only influence individuals and families but also transform communities, institutions, and state and federal policy.

CREATE SOCIAL AND PHYSICAL ENVIRONMENTS THAT PROMOTE GOOD HEALTH FOR ALL

The fact that individual health is closely linked to community health was discussed in Chapter 1. Certainly, individual choices are important, but factors in the social environment are what determine access to health services and influence lifestyle choices in the first place. Likewise, community health is affected by the collective behaviors, attitudes, and beliefs of everyone who lives in the community. The WHO Commission on Social Determinants of Health concluded in 2008 that the social conditions in which people are born, live, and work are the single most important determinant of one's health status. The underlying premise of Healthy People 2020 is that the health of the individual is almost inseparable from the health of the larger community and that the health of every community in every state and geographic region determines the overall health status of the nation. Nurses must consider the context in which health occurs. Nurses have numerous roles in community assessment, ranging from identifying appropriate resources for referral to assessing the health and health care needs of a community. More is discussed on this topic in Chapter 5.

PROMOTE QUALITY OF LIFE, HEALTHY DEVELOPMENT, AND HEALTHY BEHAVIORS ACROSS ALL LIFE STAGES

Poor diet and physical inactivity contributed to 400,000 deaths in 2000 (16.6% of all deaths that year) (Mokdad, Marks, Stroup, & Gerberding, 2004). Promoting healthy development and healthy behaviors across the life span is one way to increase the quality and years of healthy life for communities. Nurses accomplish this by working with individuals in all care settings, whether hospital, home, clinic, school, or workplace. Another way to promote healthy development and healthy behaviors is to follow the recommendations of Healthy People 2020. This road map for improving health is based on the concepts of health promotion, disease prevention, and health protection.

HEALTH INDICATORS

The achievement of the Healthy People 2020 goals is determined through measuring and comparing health indicators. Each of the leading health indicators has one or more objectives from Healthy People 2020 associated with it. The health indicators reflect the major health concerns in the United States at the beginning of the 21st century. The health indicators were selected on the basis of their ability to motivate action, the availability of data to measure progress, and their importance as public health issues. Refer to Healthy People 2020 2-2 for a list of health indicators.

Health Promotion Versus Disease and Injury Prevention

Sometimes people confuse health promotion and disease prevention. It is easy to do, because some approaches and interventions are the same or they overlap. **Health promotion** is the science and art of helping individuals change their lifestyle to move toward a state of optimal health. Optimal health is the balance of physical, emotional, social, spiritual, and intellectual health. Strategies to facilitate lifestyle change include a combination of efforts to enhance awareness, change behavior, and create environments that support good health practices. Of these, a supportive environment is believed to have the greatest impact in producing lasting change (O'Donnell, 1989). Individual lifestyle has a powerful influence over one's long-term health. Educational and community-based programs, such as smoking cessation programs, are designed to address lifestyle through increasing awareness and changing behavior. Supportive environments to discourage smoking are those that do not allow smoking in public space and make it difficult for people to smoke. Public policies that do not allow smoking in public space create supportive environments to stop smoking. It follows that in states where there are such policies in place, a smaller percentage of the population smokes. **Disease and injury prevention strategies** attempt to avoid disease or injury or minimize the consequences. Services to prevent disease or injury include counseling, screening, immunization, and chemoprophylactic interventions. Health promotion activities are used to promote and maximize health, and disease prevention activities are intended to prevent future illness.

Health protection strategies relate to environmental or regulatory measures that confer protection on large population groups. Rather than the individual focus of health promotion, health protection involves a communitywide focus. Policy development at the state level creating laws requiring that infants and children be in infant seats or car seats is an example of a health protection strategy. One goal of the Center for Disease Control related to health protection for all people in the United States, and especially those at greater risk of health

Healthy People 2020 ✸ *2-2*

HEALTH INDICATORS
1. Physical activity
2. Overweight and obesity
3. Tobacco use
4. Substance abuse
5. Responsible sexual behavior
6. Mental health
7. Injury and violence
8. Environmental quality
9. Immunization
10. Access to health care

disparities, is that all citizens will achieve their optimal life span with the best possible quality of health in every stage of life.

The Prevention Focus

The prevention of disease and injury is a key concept of community-based nursing. Preventive services are a crucial investment that contribute to good health. Prevention is conceptualized on three levels: primary prevention, secondary prevention, and tertiary prevention. An overview of these levels of prevention appears in Table 2-1.

Different strategies are found at each level of prevention. These fall into a continuum of activities that prevents disease or injury, prolongs life, and promotes health. The following are common preventive intervention strategies: health teaching, counseling, screening, outreach, and delegated functions for clients in clinical settings.

Health protection and health promotion activities conducted by nurses in community-based settings usually occur at the primary prevention level, although they may occur at secondary and tertiary levels also.

Some of the preventive activities listed in Table 2-1 are further developed in Table 2-2, which shows the goals of these selected activities.

There are numerous reasons for adopting a preventive focus to health care; cost benefit is one. Primary prevention strategies are particularly cost-effective. For every $1 spent on water fluoridation, $38 is saved in dental restorative treatment. Children with incomplete well-child care in the first 6 months of life are significantly more likely than children with complete care to visit an emergency department for an upper respiratory tract infection, gastroenteritis, or asthma. In fact, children with incomplete care are 60% more likely to visit an emergency department for any cause compared to children who are up-to-date on their well-child care (Hakim & Ronsaville, 2002).

Table 2-1	Levels of Disease Prevention and Examples of Activities	
Level	**Description**	**Activities**[a]
Primary	Prevention of the initial occurrence of disease or injury	Immunization, family planning, retirement planning, well-child care, hygiene teaching, fluoride supplements, fitness classes, alcohol, smoking, and drug prevention, seat belts and child seat car restraints, environmental protection, school funding to support recess and physical education classes for public schools, school lunch programs with nutritious, healthy food options.
Secondary	Early identification of disease or disability with prompt intervention to prevent or limit disability	Physical assessments of height, weight, and growth,, hypertension screening, developmental screening for all toddlers, preschool, and early school age children, breast and testicular self-examinations,, mammography, pregnancy testing, school health screening programs for vision, hearing, obesity, scoliosis for preschool and school age children, mental health screening across the life span,
Tertiary	Assistance (after disease or disability has occurred) to halt further disease progress and to meet one's potential and maximize quality of life despite illness or injury	Teaching and counseling regarding lifestyle changes such as diet and exercise, stress management and home management after diagnosis of chronic illness, support groups for chronic conditions, support for caretaker, Meals On Wheels for homebound, physical therapy after stroke or accident, mental health counseling for any victim of physical or emotional abuse or those who have experienced trauma such as rape victims

[a]Some prevention activities listed above overlap into health promotion or health protection.

Table 2-2 Activities at Each Level of Prevention

Level	Activities	Goal of the Activity
Primary	Immunization clinics	Prevention of communicable diseases such as polio, pertussis, rubella
	Tobacco chewing prevention	Prevention of cancer of the mouth, tongue, and throat
	Sex education with emphasis on condom use	Prevention of acquired immunodeficiency syndrome (AIDS) and other sexually transmitted diseases (STDs)
Secondary	Programs to teach and motivate men to do self-exam for testicular masses	Early identification and treatment of testicular cancer
	Blood pressure screening hypertension to prevent strokes and	Early identification and treatment of heart disease
	Programs to teach and motivate women to do breast self-exams	Early identification and treatment of breast cancer
	Programs to motivate individuals to have recommended screenings such as colonoscopy and mammography	
Tertiary	Counseling, low-sodium diet, exercise for management of hypertension	Minimize the effects of hypertension
	Smoking cessation	Prevention of lung and heart disease, cancer

For some time, research has shown that engaging in regular physical activity is associated with taking less medication and having fewer hospitalizations and physician visits (Centers for Disease Control and Prevention [CDC], 2006). In summary, direct and indirect costs of physical inactivity are estimated as being approximately $251.11 billion and those of excess weight as $256.57 billion per year (Chenoweth & Leutzinger, 2006).

Chronic diseases are the leading causes of death and disability in the United States, accounting for 70% of all deaths in the United States. But death rates alone cannot describe the burden of chronic disease. For example, for heart disease and stroke the cost, including health care expenditures and lost productivity from deaths and disability, is estimated to be more than $503 billion in 2010. As the U.S. population ages, the economic impact of cardiovascular diseases on our nation's health care system will become even greater (CDC, 2010). Chronic diseases are the most common and costly of all health problems, but they are also the most preventable. Four common, health-damaging, but modifiable behaviors—tobacco use, insufficient physical activity, poor eating habits, and excessive alcohol use—are responsible for much of the illness, disability, and premature death related to chronic diseases. For instance, more than 43 million (about 1 in 5) U.S. adults smoke and 1 in 5 U.S. high school students are current smokers. More than one-third of all U.S. adults fail to meet minimum recommendations for aerobic physical activity based on the *2008 Physical Activity Guidelines for Americans*, and only 1 in 3 U.S. high school students participates in daily physical education classes. As for poor eating habits, more than 60% of U.S. children and adolescents eat more than the recommended daily amounts of saturated fat, and only 24% of U.S. adults and 20% of U.S. high school students eat five or more servings of fruits and vegetables per day. Patterns of alcohol consumption suggest that about 1 in 6 Americans aged 18 years and older engage in binge drinking (5 or more drinks for men and 4 or more drinks for women during a single occasion) in a 30-day period, and nearly 45% of U.S. high school students report having had at least one drink of alcohol in the past 30 days (CDC, 2010a).

As more technology and treatment choices are developed, the cost of health care and potential cost savings increase. The most cost-effective preventive health services are shown in Box 2-2. In addition to being cost-effective, appropriate prevention interventions result in enhanced client satisfaction and faster recovery. Historically, the major portions of primary, secondary, and tertiary prevention services are provided by nurses in community-based settings. This is still true today. Nursing interventions in primary,

---

BOX 2-2 Cost-Effective Preventive Health Services

1. Aspirin therapy
2. Childhood immunizations
3. Tobacco use screening, intervention
4. Colorectal cancer screening
5. Measurement of blood pressure in adults
6. Influenza immunizations
7. Pneumococcal immunization
8. Alcohol screening and counseling
9. Vision screening for adults
10. Cervical cancer screening
11. Cholesterol screening
12. Breast cancer screening
13. Chlamydia screening
14. Calcium supplement counseling
15. Vision screening in children
16. Folic acid
17. Obesity screening
18. Depression screening
19. Hearing screening
20. Injury prevention counseling
21. Osteoporosis screening
22. Cholesterol screening for high-risk patients
23. Diabetes screening
24. Diet counseling
25. Tetanus–diphtheria boosters

Coffield, A. (2006). Preventive services a good investment for health. *The Nation's Health, 36*(6),2.

---

secondary, and tertiary prevention play an important role in preventing the initial occurrence, early identification of existing conditions, and minimizing the impact of chronic conditions already present in individuals, families, communities, and nations.

PRIMARY PREVENTION

Primary prevention is commonly defined as prevention of the initial occurrence of disease or injury. Examples of primary prevention activities include health teaching and counseling about immunizations, family planning services, or classes to prepare people for retirement. Surveillance to make sure that those who need access to primary care have the information and opportunities to do so would be another example of primary prevention. Tables 2-1 and 2-2 list examples of specific primary prevention activities.

Also included in primary prevention are health promotion and health protection activities. Health promotion focuses on activities related to lifestyle choices in a social context for individuals who are already essentially healthy. Examples of health promotion include health teaching and counseling on topics related to exercise and nutrition and prevention programs for alcohol and other drug abuse. Prevention is also accomplished through health protection. Health protection focuses on activities related to environmental or regulatory measures that provide protection for large population groups. This category includes activities directed at preventing unintentional injuries through motor vehicle accidents, occupational safety and health, environmental health, and food and drug safety. An important example of health protection is infant and child safety seat restraint laws. Implementation of child car seat restraint laws has prevented a significant number of deaths and disabilities among children in the United States over the past 30 years. It has been one of the most effective health protection activities worldwide. Nurses are often involved in activities to make sure that all families in a community have access to infant and child safety seats. Policies restricting where smoking is permitted are another example of health protection. Environmental protection and pollution control are other primary prevention strategies.

SECONDARY PREVENTION

The intent of **secondary prevention** is the early identification and treatment of disease or injury to limit disability. Identification of health needs, health problems, and clients at risk is the inherent component of secondary prevention. As discussed, secondary prevention activities include screening programs for blood pressure, breast cancer, scoliosis, hearing, and vision. Obviously these interventions do not prevent hypertension, breast cancer, scoliosis, or hearing or vision deficits but provide early identification and subsequent treatment of a condition that may already exist. Typically, screening efforts should address conditions that cause significant morbidity and mortality in the target age group. To be cost-effective, secondary prevention often is directed to high-risk populations. Tables 2-1 and 2-2 list other examples of specific secondary prevention activities.

TERTIARY PREVENTION

Tertiary prevention maximizes recovery after an injury or illness to allow the individual to more quickly return to an optimal state of health. Most care provided in acute care facilities, in clinics, by home care nurses, and in skilled nursing facilities focuses on tertiary care. Rehabilitation is the major focus in this level of prevention. Rehabilitation activities assist clients to reach their maximum potential despite the presence of chronic conditions. Teaching a client who has had a hip replacement how to create a safe home environment that prevents falls is an example of tertiary prevention. Shelters for battered women and

Table 2-3 Three Levels of Public Health Practice

Levels	Definition
Population-based	Public health interventions are population-based if they consider all levels of practice. This concept is represented by the three inner rings of the Intervention Wheel. The inner rings of the model are labeled community-focused, systems-focused, and individual/family-focused. A population-based approach considers intervening at all possible levels of practice. Interventions may be directed at the entire population within a community, the systems that affect the health of those populations, and/or the individuals and families within those populations known to be at risk.
Community-focused practice	Changes community norms, community attitudes, community awareness, community practices, and community behaviors. They are directed toward entire populations within the community or occasionally toward target groups within those populations. Community-focused practice is measured in terms of what proportion of the population actually changes.
Systems-focused practice	Changes organizations, policies, laws, and power structures. The focus is not directly on individuals and communities but on the systems that impact health. Changing systems is often a more effective and long-lasting way to impact population health than requiring change from every single individual in a community.
Individual-focused practice	Changes knowledge, attitudes, beliefs, practices, and behaviors of individuals. This practice level is directed at individuals, alone or as part of a family, class, or group. Individuals receive services because they are identified as belonging to a population at risk.

From Minnesota Department of Health. Division of Community Health Services: Public Health Nursing Section. (2001). *Public health nursing interventions: Application to public health nursing practice.* Minneapolis, MN: Author. Used with permission.

counseling and therapy for abused children are further examples of tertiary prevention. Other examples are listed in Tables 2-1 and 2-2.

Nursing Interventions in Community-Based Care

Over the decades as the emphasis in health care has shifted and the setting for nursing practice has moved to more community-based care, numerous opportunities for nurses to participate in health promotion and disease prevention activities at all levels of prevention have resulted. The Public Health Nursing Interventions Model, developed by public health nurses at the Minnesota Department of Health, describes the scope of nursing practice in the community (Keller, Strohschein, Lia-Hoagberg, & Schaffer, 1998; Rippke, Briske, Keller, & Strohschein, 2000). The model provides concrete interventions appropriate for nurses working in community settings or in roles that call for collaboration between acute care and community settings. Public health interventions are population based at all levels of practice. Table 2-3 describes the three levels of population-based practice.

The interface between the levels of practice and the levels of prevention are shown in Table 2-4.

The Intervention Wheel is a practice model that encompasses three levels of practice and 17 community nursing interventions for use in community settings (Fig. 2-4).

Nursing interventions are defined as what the nurse can do at the individual, family, and community level. All 17 interventions and definitions are found in Table 2-5.

Sixteen of these interventions can be performed at three different levels of practice: individual and family-focused interventions, community-focused interventions, or systems interventions. The 17th intervention, case finding, does not apply to community or systems interventions but is appropriate for use only at the individual and family levels. The Public Health Nursing Interventions Wheel defines various roles of health professionals

Table 2-4 Community-Based Nursing at Three Levels of Prevention for Individuals, Families, Groups, and Communities			
	Levels of Prevention		
Client Served	**Primary**	**Secondary**	**Tertiary**
Individual client	Sexuality; teaching about using condoms Family planning Dietary teaching and exercise programs to assist clients with obesity	Counseling and HIV testing Early prenatal care Screening for early identification of diabetes	Nutrition teaching to the client with AIDS to maximize health Support groups for parents of low-birth-weight infants Teaching a newly diagnosed diabetic about diet and how to administer insulin
Family	Education about infection control in the home of a family member on a ventilator there	Tuberculosis screening for a family at risk	Teaching a family caregiver about how to follow sterile procedure for a dressing change
Systems	Prenatal classes for pregnant adolescents Sexuality teaching about AIDS and other STDs	Vision screening for first graders Hearing screening at a senior center	Support groups for children with asthma Swim therapy for physically disabled
Communities	Fluoride water supplementation Environmental cleanup of paint and other substances containing lead	Organized screening programs such as health fairs Lead screening of children in a community	Shelter or relocation provision for victims of natural disasters Development of programs to assist children with developmental delays caused by lead exposure

on individual, community, and systems levels and speaks to the need for multidisciplinary teams that encompass the array of skills and knowledge for all aspects of working in the community. (Keller, Strohschein, Lia-Hoagberg, & Schaffer, 1998). These are discussed in greater depth in Units II and III.

Table 2-5 Public Health Interventions With Definitions

Public Health Intervention	Definition
Surveillance	Describes and monitors health events through ongoing and systematic collection, analysis, and interpretation of health data for the purpose of planning, implementing, and evaluating public health interventions. (Adapted from Guidelines for evaluating Surveillance Systems. (1998). MMWR, 37(S-5), 1A.)
Disease and other health event investigation	Systematically gathers and analyzes data regarding threats to the health of populations, ascertains the source of the threat, identifies cases and others at risk, and determines control measures.
Outreach	Locates populations-of-interest or populations-at-risk and provides information about the nature of the concern, what can be done about it, and how services can be obtained.
Screening	Identifies individuals with unrecognized health risk factors or asymptomatic disease conditions in populations.
Case-finding	Locates individuals and families with identified risk factors and connects them with resources.
Referral and follow-up	Assists individuals, families, groups, organizations, and/or communities to identify and access necessary resources in to prevent or resolve problems or concerns.
Case management	Optimizes self-care capabilities of individuals and families and the capacity of systems and communities to coordinate and provide services.
Delegated functions	Direct care tasks a registered professional nurse carries out under the authority of a health care practitioner as allowed by law. Delegated functions also include any direct care tasks a registered professional nurse entrusts to other appropriate personnel to perform.
Health teaching	Communicates facts, ideas and skills that change knowledge, attitudes, values, beliefs, behaviors, and practices of individuals, families, systems, and/or communities.
Counseling	Establishes an interpersonal relationship with a community, a system, family or individual intended to increase or enhance their capacity for self-care and coping. Counseling engages the community, a system, family or individual at an emotional level.
Consultation	Seeks information and generates optional solutions to perceived problems or issues through interactive problem solving with a community, system, family or individual. The community, system, family or individual selects and acts on the option best meeting the circumstances.
Collaboration	Commits two or more persons or organizations to achieve a common goal through enhancing the capacity of one or more of the members to promote and protect health. [Adapted from Henneman, L., & Cohen (1995). Collaboration: A concept analysis. *Journal of Advanced Nursing, 21*, 103–109.]
Coalition building	Promotes and develops alliances among organizations or constituencies for a common purpose. It builds linkages, solves problems, and/or enhances local leadership to address health concerns.
Community organizing	Helps community groups to identify common problems or goals, mobilize resources, and develop and implement strategies for reaching the goals they collectively have set. [Adapted from Minkler, M. (Ed.) (1997). *Community organizing and community building for health.* New Brunswick, NJ: Rutgers University Press.]

Continued on following page

Table 2-5 Public Health Interventions With Definitions *(Continued)*

Public Health Intervention	Definition
Advocacy	Pleads someone's cause or act on someone's behalf, with a focus on developing the community, system, individual or family's capacity to plead their own cause or act on their own behalf.
Social marketing	Utilizes commercial marketing principles and technologies for programs designed to influence the knowledge, attitudes, values, beliefs, behaviors, and practices of the population-of-interest.
Policy development	Places health issues on decision-makers' agendas, acquires a plan of resolution, and determines needed resources. Policy development results in laws, rules and regulation, ordinances, and policies.
Policy enforcement	Compels others to comply with the laws, rules, regulations, ordinances and policies created in conjunction with policy development.

Minnesota Department of Health, Public Health Nursing Section (2001). *Public health nursing interventions: Application for public health nursing practice.* Minneapolis, MN: Author. Used with permission.

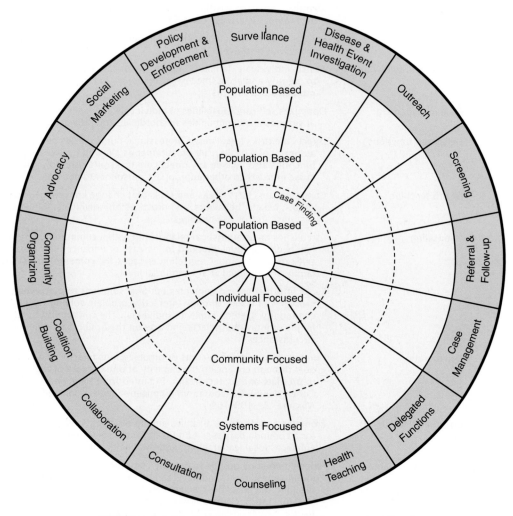

FIGURE 2-4 Public Health Intervention Model (Intervention Wheel).

Nursing Interventions in Community-Based Care and Levels of Prevention

This section describes specific examples of common nursing interventions used at each level of prevention in two types of community-based care: the ambulatory and home care settings.

PRIMARY PREVENTION

Ambulatory Health Care

Nurses have an important role in primary prevention in ambulatory settings. For example, a nurse may provide health teaching on the importance of infant seats, child restraints, and helmets to all the mothers who do not speak English at a well-child clinic. The nurse may develop teaching materials in the languages common to the community served. Considering the literacy level of the families in the school where he or she is working, a school nurse may communicate with families through written flyers sent home with the children about subjects ranging from the communicability and the methods of transmission of diseases such as chickenpox, influenza, and head lice to notification of certain disease outbreaks. Through outreach, parents of preschool children can obtain vital information and clarification from school nurses about when, where, and why their children can receive periodic checkups and immunizations.

Health teaching and counseling in clinics, schools, and occupational settings directed to individuals or groups may cover a wide range of topics including such things as immunizations, family planning, and prenatal care. At adult clinics, nurses provide current information about diet, exercise, stress management, and weight reduction. Couples of childbearing age may attend classes on family planning and prenatal topics. Occupational health nurses provide health teaching, counseling, and surveillance about injury prevention, repetitive motion injuries, and sensory losses secondary to specific job tasks. They act as consultants to disseminate information about shift work, offer strategies to avoid sleep disturbances, and provide information about the importance of health promotion activities such as exercise and stress reduction. Through organizational policies, many companies reduce fees for joining health clubs or recreational programs or offer exercise activities at work. Some provide reduced rates on health insurance if workers join a health club, regularly exercise, lose weight, or stop smoking.

Home Health Care

Clients in the home frequently require episodic care for acute health care conditions and assistance for management of chronic conditions. Opportunities for primary prevention are limited. Through health teaching, consultation, counseling, referral and follow-up, and outreach, home care nurses share information with the client and family regarding primary prevention strategies. In community-based care, the nurse assesses the client needs and strengths in the context of the family. Sometimes, the nurse influences the family's health behaviors in areas that may not directly relate to the client's condition. For example, if the client's spouse asks about immunizations for their children, the nurse has the opportunity to teach about the immunization schedule and where to get affordable care. Or if the client's adult child mentions that he or she would like to stop smoking, the nurse may provide information about resources for smoking cessation. Many caregivers need support, including referrals and follow-up, consultation, and counseling, in primary prevention of caregiver burnout.

SECONDARY PREVENTION

Ambulatory Health Care

Secondary prevention may involve alerting clients, caregivers, or family members about the time frames for health screening (e.g., mammography, Pap smears, glaucoma screening, breast examinations, and lipid levels) and encouraging them to be screened at recommended intervals. Counseling, consultation, health teaching, and referral and follow-up are additional interventions that may be used in conjunction with screening. The clinic nurse may see clients who are at risk for certain conditions, alert them to their risk, and provide information about community services that may be able to assist them.

Preschool screening, vision and hearing testing, and scoliosis screening are secondary prevention strategies provided in the school. In addition, school nurses teach secondary prevention by educating parents about the screening programs available for their children. The workplace may be the site where screening is done for hypertension, hearing loss, exposure to hazardous substances, and breast cancer. The nurse disseminates information about the services and provides educational programs.

Home Health Care

Care in the home usually involves short visits. Thus, opportunities for communicating secondary prevention information are limited. However, home health care nurses do inform the client and family about services in the community that may help them with the client's care, early identification and treatment of conditions related to the client's diagnosis, and general health promotion and disease prevention. Clients receiving home care service for a particular chronic condition that is commonly associated with other diseases may require additional screening. For example, certain medications sometimes put individuals at risk for developing another chronic condition as seen with individuals with rheumatoid arthritis who may be more likely to develop osteoporosis. This is especially true because some medications used to treat RA can contribute to osteoporosis. Thus, they may need to be screened for osteoporosis more frequently and earlier compared to the general population.

Client need determines where information may be presented. For example, with case management in the clinic, the nurse may not have the opportunity to assess the family caregiver's abilities in assisting a client with insulin injections. However, through counseling, consultation, and collaboration, the nurse in the home may be better able to assess how well the family can assist and support the client with management of therapeutic regime. Case management in the home may require the nurse to collaborate with the family caregiver to identify additional teaching to administer insulin if the caregiver could not accurately draw up the insulin during an early morning nursing visit.

TERTIARY PREVENTION

Ambulatory Health Care

Through referral and follow-up and health teaching, clinic nurses often give their clients information about community resources appropriate for the management of chronic conditions. Parents of children with celiac disease, for instance, may receive a list of organizations that provide emotional support, respite care, and information and referral. Clients with chronic conditions benefit from teaching that is directed at successful rehabilitation and prevention of related complications.

Through the schools, parents can learn about community services available for children with special health needs. In some states, children with disabilities are mainstreamed into the public schools. Often these children and their families need tertiary prevention services in the form of outreach, case finding, consultation, collaboration, health education, referral and follow-up, and case management.

Nurses working in schools may provide a significant amount of care in the form of delegated functions through school-based clinics and other school nurse services. These may include physical examinations, routine screenings, venipuncture, or other simple collection of lab samples for laboratory studies. Nurses may also provide direct nursing care to some children on an ongoing basis (e.g., children who use a mechanical ventilator or children with conditions that result in frequent urinary catheterization). The school nurse also dispenses prescription medications and provides first aid in emergencies.

In the occupational setting, most of the public health interventions are utilized in tertiary prevention. The nurse uses counseling with employees with chronic conditions or recent acute conditions about the opportunities and advantages of returning to work. Through return-to-work programs, nurses assist personnel with management of chronic injuries or illnesses and illustrate the tertiary prevention approach of maximizing individual potential for health through counseling, collaboration, consultation, health teaching, referral, and case management.

Home Health Care

Because home health care clients typically have a chronic condition for which episodic care is needed, a primary role of the home health care nurse is to teach and counsel to clients and family members about tertiary prevention. Teaching may focus on rehabilitation or restoration for those with a recent stroke, head injury, fractured hip, management of a chronic condition, or postsurgical care at home.

Delegated functions provided in the home are usually at the tertiary level of prevention. To qualify for payment for services, home health care nursing includes skilled nursing care such as a dressing change. This combined with the interventions of health teaching, collaboration, and consultation regarding infection control techniques with the client and the family illustrates multiple interventions used in tertiary preventions. Although in home care the client is the main focus of care, a holistic nursing style means that nurses also provide care for family and other support persons. Chapter 12 covers this topic in more detail.

Conclusions

Settings for nursing practice have evolved as a reflection of society's need to focus on health rather than illness. State and local health departments are using Healthy People 2020 as a framework to put disease prevention into action. The prevention focus is a key concept of community-based nursing. Different preventive strategies are found at three levels of prevention. The public health nursing Intervention Wheel and its 17 corresponding nursing interventions outline common actions nurses working in the community may take at the individual, family, and community levels.

What's on the Web?

National Guideline Clearinghouse (NGC)
INTERNET ADDRESS: **http://www.guideline.gov**
   The NGC is a comprehensive database of evidence-based clinical practice guidelines and related documents. NGC is an initiative of the Agency for Healthcare Research and Quality (AHRQ), U.S. Department of Health and Human Services. NGC was originally created by AHRQ in partnership with the American Medical Association and the American Association of Health Plans (now America's Health Insurance Plans [AHIP]). The NGC's mission is to provide physicians, nurses, and other health professionals, health care providers, health plans, integrated delivery systems, purchasers, and others an accessible mechanism for obtaining objective, detailed information on clinical practice guidelines and to further their dissemination, implementation, and use.

Agency for Healthcare Research and Quality
INTERNET ADDRESS: **https http://www.ahrq.gov/**
   The mission of AHRQ is to improve the quality, safety, efficiency, and effectiveness of health care for all Americans. This site provides numerous resources for clients and nurses to use evidence-based information to make informed treatment decisions.

Nursing Research at the Agency for Health Care Research and Quality
INTERNET ADDRESS: **http://www.ahrq.gov/about/nursing/**
   This site provides evidence-based information on nursing-related topics through research articles; evidence-based reports, testimony, and speeches; as well as links to other related resources and tools. An online newsletter is another source of current research as well as a section on research funding for nursing-related topics.

Wheel of Public Health Nursing Interventions
INTERNET ADDRESS: **http://www.people.vcu.edu/~elmiles/interventions/**
   This interactive site is a great way to expand your understanding of the public health nursing interventions and it is fun to use.

Healthy People 2020
INTERNET ADDRESS: **http://www.healthypeople.gov/2020/default.aspx**

Healthy People provides science-based, 10-year national objectives for promoting health and preventing disease. Since 1979, Healthy People has set and monitored national health objectives to meet a broad range of health needs, encourage collaborations across sectors, guide individuals toward making informed health decisions, and measure the impact of our prevention activity. Currently, Healthy People 2020 is leading the way to achieve increased quality and years of healthy life and the elimination of health disparities. There are numerous resources on this site for nurses working in community-based settings.

References

Centers for Disease Control and Prevention. (2006). *Chronic disease prevention: Chronic disease overview.* Retrieved from http://www.cdc.gov/nccdphp/overview.htm

Centers for Disease Prevention and Health Promotion. Chronic Diseases and Health Promotion. (2009). *Chronic disease overview.* Retrieved from http://www.cdc.gov/chronicdisease/overview/index.htm

Center for Disease Prevention and Health Promotion. (2010) *Heart disease and stroke prevention: addressing the nation's leading killers: At a glance 2010.* Retrieved from http://www.cdc.gov/chronicdisease/resources/publications/aag/dhdsp.htm

Chenoweth, D., & Leutzinger, J. (2006). The economic cost of physical inactivity and excess weight in American adults. *Journal of Physical Activity and Health, 3*(2), 148–163.

Chronic Disease Prevention and Health Promotion. (2010a). *Chronic diseases the power to prevent, the call to control: At a glance 2009.* Retrieved from http://www.cdc.gov/chronicdisease/resources/publications/AAG/chronic.htm

Coffield, A. (2006). Preventive services a good investment for health. *The Nation's Health, 36*(6), 2.

Federal Interagency Forum on Child and Family Statistics. (2009). *America's children: Key national indicators of well being, 2009.* Washington, DC: U.S. Government Printing Office.

Hakim, R., & Ronsaville, D. (2002). Effect of compliance with health supervision guidelines among U.S. infants on emergency department visits. *Archives of Pediatric & Adolescent Medicine, 156*(10), 1015–1020.

Kaiser Family Foundation & Harvard School of Public Health. (2006). *Healthcare costs survey.* Washington, DC: Author. (Doc # 7371). Retrieved from http://www.kff.org/newsmedia/upload/7371.pdf

Keller, L, Strohschein, S, Lia-Hoagberg, B, & Schaffer, M. (1998). Population-based public health nursing interventions: A model from practice. *Public Health Nursing, 15*(3), 207–215.

Kvaavike, G., Batty, D., Ursin, G., Huxley, R., & Gale, C. (2010). Influence of individual and combined health behaviors on total and cause-specific mortality in men and women: The United Kingdom health and lifestyle survey. *Archives of Internal Medicine, 170*(8): 711–718 DOI: http://archinte.ama-assn.org/cgi/content/short/170/8/711

Lasser, K., Himmelstein, K., & Woolhandler, S. (2006). Access to care, health status, and health disparities in the United States and Canada: Results of a cross-national population-based survey. *American Journal of Public Health, 96*(5), 1300–1307.

MacDorman, M. & Mathews, T. (2009). *Behind international rankings of infant mortality; How the United States compares with Europe.* National Center for Health Statistics Data Brief, 23. United States Department of Health and Human Services. http://www.cdc.gov/nchs/data/databriefs/db23.htm

Minnesota Department of Health. Division of Community Health Services. Public Health Nursing Section. (2001). *Public health nursing interventions: Application for public health nursing practice.* Minneapolis, MN: Author.

Mokdad, A. H., Marks, J. S., Stroup, D. F., Gerberding, J. L. (2004). Actual causes of death in the United States, 2000. *Journal of the American Medical Association, 10*(291),1238–1245.

O'Donnell, (1989). Dimensions of optimal health. *American Journal of Health Promotion, 3*(3).3–5.

Orsi, J., Margellos-Anast, H., & Whitman, S. (2010). Black-White health disparities in the United States and Chicago: a 15-year progress analysis. *American Journal of Public Health, 100*(2), 349–356. doi:10.2105/AJPH.2009.165407.

Rajaratnam, J., Alison, J. R., Levin-Rector, L., Chalupka, A. N., Wong, H., Dwyer. L., et al. (2010). Worldwide mortality in men and women aged 15—59 years from 1970 to 2010: a systematic analysis. *Lancet, 375*(9727), 1704–1720. doi:10.1016/S0140-6736(10)60517-X

Sondik, E. J., Huang, D. T, Klein, R. J., & Satcher, D. (2010). Progress toward the Healthy People 2010 goals and objectives. *Annual Review Public Health, 31*, 271–281.

U.S. Department of Health and Human Services, National Center for Health Statistics. (2010). *Health, United States, 2010*. Washington, DC: U.S. Department of Health and Human Services. Retrieved from http://healthypeople.gov/Default.htm

U.S. Department of Health and Human Services. (2009) *National Center for Health Statistics. Health, United States, 2009*. Washington, DC: U.S. Department of Health and Human Services. http://www.cdc.gov/nchs/data/hus/hus09.pdf#executivesummary

World Health Organization. (1986). *Twelve yardsticks for health*. New York: WHO.

World Health Organization. (2008). *The determinants of health*. Retrieved from http://www.who.int/hia/evidence/doh/en/index.html

World Health Organization. (2010). Closing the gap in a generation: health equity through action on the social determinants of health. Report from the Commission on Social Determinants of Health. Geneva, Switzerland: WHO; 2008. Available from: URL: http://www.who.int/social_determinants/thecommission/finalreport/en/index.html

LEARNING ACTIVITIES

JOURNALING ACTIVITY 2-1

1. Think back to your clinical experiences so far and try to remember one of your patients or clients where your nursing care focused on that individual's health rather than on illness, disease process, or recovery from a medical procedure.

2. Discuss how this situation required a way of thinking or responding that was different from what you previously thought of as your role as a nurse.

3. How does this observation affect your impression of the role of the nurse in the community?

4. In your clinical journal, identify issues you have observed in your clinical experiences that relate to Healthy People 2020's goals. For instance, have you taken care of someone who did not have health insurance? (Objectives related to Access to Health Care) Or have you talked to someone about secondary prevention for cervical or breast cancer? (Objective 9, Cancer, Increase provider counseling about cancer prevention regarding mammograms or Pap tests)

5. What do you as a nurse intend to do to impact these health issues?

CLIENT CARE 2-2

1. Levels of prevention determine the primary nursing role(s) and interventions for each of the following clients.

   Jack. Jack is a 43-year-old man with a colostomy. He has evidence of early skin breakdown around the stoma site despite the fact that he has followed the established protocol. The clinic nurse notes the problem at Jack's first visit to the clinic after his surgery. She teaches him about a new product that may interrupt the skin breakdown.

   a. Determine the possible nursing intervention.

   b. Identify the level of prevention the nurse is using.

   Stephen. Stephen is a 12-year-old boy with a neurologic condition that requires self-catheterization every 2 hours. He has had three bladder infections in the past 2 months. The school nurse has taught Stephen about the infectious cycle and the importance of hand washing and has watched Stephen self-catheterize in an attempt to identify the reason for the frequent infections.

   a. Determine the primary nursing intervention.

   b. Identify the level of prevention the nurse is using.

PRACTICAL APPLICATION 2-3

You have been asked to start a support and education group for people in your community who have had strokes.

1. Describe how you will decide who in the community should participate in the group.
2. What would be the objectives for the sessions?
3. Discuss how the components of community-based nursing apply to these problems:
   a. Self-care
   b. Preventive care
   c. Care within the context of the community
   d. Continuity of care
   e. Collaborative care
4. Identify levels of prevention on which you will focus. Determine if there are levels you will not include.
5. State two likely basic or physical needs at each level of prevention.
6. List two behavioral outcomes and nursing interventions for the basic or physical needs you have chosen.
7. State two likely psychosocial needs at each level of prevention.
8. List two client outcomes and nursing interventions for the psychosocial needs at each level of prevention.

PRACTICAL APPLICATION 2-4

You work in an emergency department. An older woman and her husband enter. The woman is loud and combative, and her blood alcohol level is elevated.

a. Identify the level of prevention on which you will focus.
b. Determine if any level of prevention will not be included at all.
c. List the reasons for focusing on tertiary prevention in home health care.

PRACTICAL APPLICATION 2-5

Read the following examples and identify the nursing intervention from the definitions of the public health nursing interventions found at the end of this chapter.

1. Parents of premature infants participate in a program that identifies children from birth to 5 years of age who are at risk for developing health or developmental issues. At discharge, the child is assessed and the parents are asked if they are interested in participating in the program. Every 4 months for the first 2 years and every 6 months after 2 years of age, the parents are asked to complete a mailed questionnaire about the child's development and are contacted if any delays are noted.
2. Every 6 months, nursing students and their instructor administer the Ages and Stages Questionnaire to children at a preschool for homeless families. Students screen the children with the parents present and discuss the results of the screening with parents. Children found to have delays are referred to programs for early intervention.

Chapter 3

Cultural Care

JOAN BRANDT AND PAULA SWIGGUM

Learning Objectives

1. Define culture, cultural care, transcultural nursing, ethnocentrism, cultural blindness, acculturation, assimilation, lifeways, and emic and etic care.

2. Describe the history of transcultural care in nursing.

3. Examine how culture influences worldview, communication, time orientation, family, society, and health.

4. Recognize the components of a cultural assessment.

5. Discuss transcultural nursing skills and competencies in community settings.

6. Explain the nursing role as advocate for clients from diverse cultures.

7. Examine the relationship between diversity of health care providers and health outcomes.

8. Identify transcultural nursing resources.

Key Terms

acculturation	emic care
assimilation	ethnocentrism
cultural assessment	etic
cultural awareness	health belief systems
cultural blindness	lifeways
cultural encounter	racism
cultural humility	stereotypes
cultural knowledge	stereotyping
cultural skill	transcultural nursing

Chapter Topics

Historical Perspectives

Cultural Awareness

Cultural Knowledge

Cultural Skill

Cultural Encounter

Conclusions

The Nursing Student Speaks

When truly embracing the vision of community health, one can't help but realize that what we experience changes us forever. My experiences with community health nursing during my RN to BSN completion altered not only my nursing practice but also my fundamental perception of the world. What affects one of us affects all of us. Health is not just an individual issue; it is a societal issue. We are all connected. People are not separate novels; they are chapters in a book. Take one out, and the story is incomplete. In a sense, this has also become my view of individuals within community. I may deal with individuals, but they are all part of the larger community, and the community is incomplete without each one of them. Getting to know these people as individuals shattered the artificial distance between "them" and "us." Something inside of me shifted as I realized that there are no "them" and "us"; there is only "we."

My personal definition of caring as a nurse continues to evolve but has been changed even more dramatically through my community health experiences. I now truly believe that caring as a nurse is demonstrated by entering into genuine relationships with others rather than "doing to" or "doing for" others. The interaction inherently has value; it is a goal in and of itself. I demonstrate caring by acknowledging another's worth and dignity by being present with them in a nonjudgmental way and accompanying them along their journey for as long as circumstances allow. I will endeavor to keep this as the center of each interaction I have with others as a nurse.

Elizabeth Stockton, RN, BSN
Augsburg College

The face of the United States is changing every day. One needs only to walk the streets of urban areas and farming communities to notice the increasing diversity of people. Recent immigrants have come from the far reaches of the world, primarily Southeast Asia, East Africa, and Latin America. While minorities currently comprise one third of the population, it is anticipated that they will become the majority by 2042 (U.S. Census Bureau, 2008). Nearly one third of the U.S. population was identified as part of a racial or ethnic minority group in 2005 (Kaiser Family Foundation [KFF], 2007). By 2050, this number is expected to reach nearly one half of the population (KFF, 2007; U.S. Census Bureau, 2008). However, limitations in census data collection and the continual influx from secondary migration make it difficult to obtain an exact count of immigrants and refugees to the United States (Schuchman & McDonald, 2004). New groups bring with them a variety of languages, customs, modes of dress, and other cultural practices. Nurses in the 21st century are challenged to provide care to persons whose customs are unfamiliar. Because culture influences health and well-being in a myriad of ways, the professional nurse must understand what that means for each client encountered.

Nursing encompasses caring for the whole person, including the physical, emotional, psychological, spiritual, social, and developmental dimensions. With the shifting U.S. population, it becomes essential for nurses to understand the cultural dimension of health (and illness) as well. Culture encompasses language, thoughts, communication, actions, customs, beliefs, and values shared by a group of people and handed down from generation to generation (Office of Minority Health, 2005).

Healthy People 2020 calls for the achievement of health equity, the elimination of health disparities, and the improvement of health for all groups (U.S. Department of Health and Human Services [DHHS], 2010). Since 1994, the Office of Minority Health has been mandated by Congress to address barriers that exist within health care for limited English-proficient people through the development of models of care that ameliorate health risk factors for minority populations (Office of Minority Health, 2007). People of color are more likely to live in poverty, which has implications for their health and insurance status (KFF, 2007). The 2003 Institute of Medicine report, *Unequal Treatment*, identified that racial and ethnic minorities receive lower quality health care, even when their income and insurance are equal to nonminority populations (Smedley, Stith, & Nelson, 2003). The most significant barrier to health services and ultimately reducing health disparities for minority women and other vulnerable populations is access to culturally appropriate health care resources (Andrews, Felton, Wewers, & Heath, 2004; Cooper, Hill, & Powe, 2002). In the most recent Agency for Healthcare Research and Quality (2010) report on health care disparities, it was again found that racial and ethnic minorities have worse access to and receive poorer quality care across the board than whites. While the cause of health disparities is complex, stereotyping and biases by health care providers contribute to the disparities (Smedley et al., 2003).

Information about the disparity of health outcomes for minority groups is essential for nurses who plan and carry out nursing interventions in community settings. For example, life expectancy is shorter for most ethnic minority groups; African American male life expectancy is 6 years less than that for white males (National Center for Health Statistics, 2010), and American Indians and Alaska Native peoples live 2.4 years less than all other U.S. races (Indian Health Services [IHS], 2006]. At 13.6 deaths per 1,000 live births, the African American infant mortality rate is twice that of Whites (National Center for Health Statistics, 2010). Figure 3-1 shows infant mortality rates by race of the mother.

"American Indians and Alaska Natives die at higher rates than other Americans from tuberculosis, alcoholism, motor vehicle crashes, diabetes, unintentional injuries, homicide, and suicide" (IHS, 2006). *Healthy People 2020* objectives address the importance of increasing the number of local health departments that have established "culturally appropriate and linguistically competent community health promotion and disease prevention programs" (DHHS, 2010). In order to meet these objectives and to address health disparities, community-based nurses are called to learn about cultural and other factors that influence the health status of the communities in which they practice.

Not only is the client population changing, but the face of the health care team is changing as well. Between 2001 and 2008, one third of the growth that occurred in nursing occurred with nurses who are internationally born. With this growing population of internationally born nurses, clearly, nurses will encounter team members who have varied

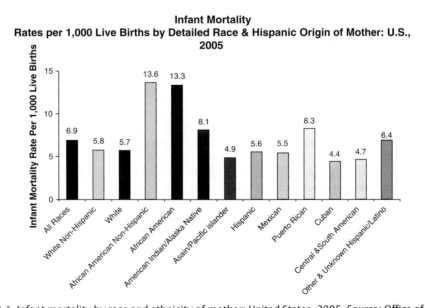

Figure 3-1 Infant mortality by race and ethnicity of mother: United States, 2005. Source: Office of Minority Health. (2008). *Office of Minority Health and health disparities: An overview.* Retrieved April 6, 2010, from http://www.cdc.gov/omhd/About/PDFs/OMHDPresentation.ppt.

experiences and cultures than their own (Buerhaus, Auerbach, & Staiger, 2009). Included in *Healthy People 2020* are objectives that address the importance of increasing diversity among all health care professionals (DHHS, 2010). There is growing evidence that increasing diversity among health care professionals is one way to address growing health disparities (Smedley, Stith, Butler, & Bristow, 2004). Individuals are more comfortable receiving health care from providers who look like them. As we consider the increasing diversity within our work and community settings, **transcultural nursing** knowledge is essential to facilitate attainment of the goals of understanding and improving health.

This chapter discusses transcultural nursing and its historical beginnings. In addition, key concepts are explored related to cultural care, **cultural awareness**, and culturally appropriate nursing competencies involving assessment and intervention. Because there is such a multitude of cultural groups and practices, it is impossible to have knowledge of each and every one. Instead, a culturally sensitive approach are explored, one that incorporates how to discover important cultural beliefs affecting health and wellness and the available resources.

Historical Perspectives

Discussions of cultural competence in nursing are not new. In fact, the field of transcultural nursing had its roots in the early 1900s, when public health nurses cared for immigrants from Europe who came from a wide range of cultural backgrounds and had diverse health care practices. Since the late 1940s, Madeleine Leininger has been a nurse pioneer in establishing the theory and research in transcultural nursing. Leininger believes that care is the essence of nursing or what makes nursing what it is or could be in healing, well-being, and to help people face disabilities and dying (Leininger & McFarland, 2006, p. 3). Over the last five decades, she has seen the importance of nursing care that is based on the client's culture, that is, his or her unique values, beliefs, practices, and **lifeways** passed down from one generation to the next. The idea that culture and care are inextricably linked led her to study other cultures, and she became the first nurse to obtain a PhD in anthropology. Transcultural nursing (a term coined by Leininger) is a body of knowledge and practice for caring for persons from other cultures.

Since those early days, the theory of cultural care diversity and universality, developed by Dr. Leininger, has generated substantive knowledge for the discipline of nursing. The world has been on a fast track to multiculturalism, and nurses have not had the knowledge to provide care that was culturally appropriate. Having this knowledge is a moral and ethical obligation for nurses as they strive to provide the best care possible to all their clients. Community nurses have been particularly interested in this field because they work directly with individuals and families in their own settings and see the need firsthand.

Although the large groups of immigrants came to the United States primarily from Europe in the early 1900s, the recent wave of immigrants to the United States has come from all over the world, including Latin America, Asia, Africa, and other areas. By 2007, 80% of the internationally born population came from countries in Latin America and Asia (Grieco, 2009). Figure 3-2 depicts the country of origin for immigrants from 1850 to 2000.

Today, both urban and rural communities have significant numbers of members whose country of origin is not the United States. Figure 3-3 demonstrates the changes in the origins of the internationally born population in the United States since 1960. The Native American population has significant numbers who live off the reservation and contribute to the multicultural makeup in cities and towns.

Many nurse leaders and educators have embraced the need for culture-specific care, and various approaches to gaining this knowledge have been developed. Dr. Josepha Campinha-Bacote, a Cape Verde native who now lives and works in the United States, developed one such model. Her model involves the components of cultural awareness, **cultural knowledge**, **cultural skill**, and **cultural encounter** (Campinha-Bacote, 2003). It is used here as a framework to help nurses learn the concepts necessary to gain cultural competence working within the community setting.

Percent distribution. For 1960-90, resident population. For 2000, civilian noninstitutional population plus Armed Forces living off post or with their families on post.

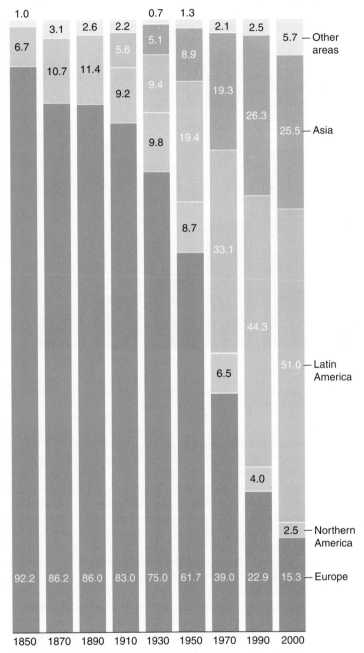

Figure 3-2 Foreign-born population by region of birth: Selected years 1850 to 2000. Source: U.S. Census Bureau (2008). *Press release*. Retrieved April 6, 2010, from http://www.census.gov/Press- Release/www/releases/archives/population/012496.html

Cultural Awareness

Before nurses can intervene appropriately with clients and enter into a community from another culture, they must first understand their own, that is, have a self-awareness of their own cultural background, influences, and biases. Only with this cultural awareness can they appreciate and

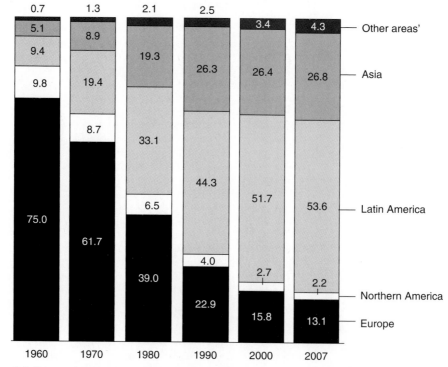

Percent Distribution of Foreign-Born Population by Region of Birth: 1960 to 2007
(Data based on sample. For information on confidentially protection, sampling eror, non sampling error, and definitions, see *www.census.gov/acs/www/*)

Figure 3-3 Race and Hispanic origin of the foreign-born population in the United States: 2007. Source: U.S. Census Bureau, Census of Population, 1960 to 2000, and 2007 American Community Survey, as cited by Shin, H. B., and Kominski, R. A. (2010). *Language use in the United States: 2007* (p. 1). American Community Survey Reports, ACS-12. Washington, DC: U.S. Census Bureau.

be sensitive to the values, beliefs, lifeways, practices, and problem-solving methods of a client's culture. With self-awareness, a commitment to lifelong self-evaluation, and through engaging in mutually respectful relationships with openness to learning in cross-cultural interactions, nurses begin to understand the importance of **cultural humility**. "Building culturally sensitive relationships of mutual respect and trust is essential before becoming immersed in collaborative planning and decision making related to community initiatives" (Racher & Annis, 2007, p. 267).

One exercise that can be illuminating for nurses is to respond to a "cultural tree" in which one's own cultural heritage is evaluated in terms of the various components that make up a culture. Figure 3-4 depicts the components of a cultural tree. By considering specific examples and anecdotes about family traditions and beliefs, one becomes aware of beliefs and practices that are highly influenced by one's cultural background. There can be amazing diversity, even within a group that outwardly appears very much alike.

This new awareness of one's own cultural influences helps the nurse avoid attitudes that can be detrimental to the nurse–client relationship. **Cultural blindness** occurs when the nurse does not recognize his or her own beliefs and practices, nor the beliefs and practices of others. **Ethnocentrism** refers to the idea that one's own ways are the only way or the best way to behave, believe, or do things. For example, a dominant cultural value in the United States is planning for the future. Calendars are kept religiously, goals are set, events are planned weeks and months in advance, and money is saved for retirement. In some cultures, value is placed on the present, and there is a belief that life is preordained, so there is no point in planning or trying to change the future. Future-oriented individuals may feel that this is the only correct way to live and may be disdainful of those with another time orientation. This is ethnocentrism. Ethnocentrism can lead to stereotyping. **Stereotyping** is generalizing

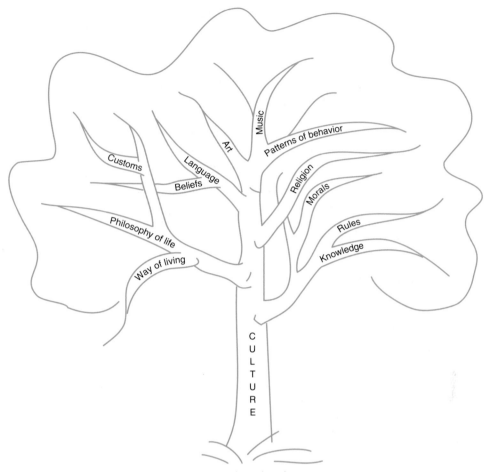

Figure 3-4 The cultural tree.

and oversimplifying information about others. Using **stereotypes** to make assumptions about others has a way of depersonalizing the interaction, as one enters into the relationship thinking that they "know" how the other will be or behave. As with ethnocentrism, stereotypes are not supported by evidence and perpetuate prejudice. This way of thinking and being in the world can lead to **racism**. Believing that individuals who are culturally, ethnically, or racially different from oneself are inferior is racism. When nurses act on these beliefs, recognizing the uniqueness of each individual is replaced by placing people in a hierarchy. These behaviors perpetuate inequality and privilege and contribute to health disparities (Racher & Annis, 2007).

A concept in mainstream U.S. culture that is taken for granted as normal is the concept of time. Individuals tend to live by the clock, make time, waste time, kill time, want to know what time, and worry about having enough time. However, in many communities around the world, one's daily activities take place as the need arises without regard to a prescribed time of day. For members of these cultures, "being on time" for an appointment may have a range of several hours and this understanding of time does not necessarily change upon arrival in the United States. The community nurse must be aware of these views and accommodate them accordingly.

The reliance on self is another dominant cultural value in the United States. There are more than 100 words in the English language that begin with the word "self." In many languages there is no translation for the word "self." Individual needs are secondary to the needs of the group. This has strong implications for the concept of self-care. Mainstream U.S. culture places high value on taking care of one's self. People are reluctant to have someone do for them what they think they can do for themselves. This is not so for all cultures.

CLIENT SITUATIONS IN PRACTICE

The Meaning of Self-Care

Maria, a Mexican American woman, gave birth 2 days ago. For a period of time called "la cuarentena" or "la dieta," specific rules apply regarding the postpartum woman's activity and diet (Andrews & Boyle, 2007). During this time, she is not to do any heavy lifting, exercise, or housework. Family and community members take over the chores of the household, including child care and meal preparation. Jane, a community nurse visiting during this postpartum period, is aware of this cultural practice and provides teaching according to her client's values, which are different than the more active approach to a mother's recovery from childbirth practiced in her own culture.

Because nurses working in the community are frequently visiting postpartum mothers and their newborns, it is essential that they understand how strongly culture influences postpartum self-care and how much that may vary from Western practices.

The way that health decisions are made is culturally based. These decisions are private and individual for some, while others wouldn't think of making a treatment decision without first consulting their extended families.

CLIENT SITUATIONS IN PRACTICE

Client's Right to Know

Karen is the hospice nurse assigned to an Ethiopian woman who has end-stage kidney disease. As the primary decision maker for the family, the son requested that his mother not be told of her terminal condition. Respectful of cultural mores, she would be obligated not to divulge the serious nature of the client's terminal illness. Within Ethiopian culture, the wishes of the family are dominant over an individual. Protecting the client from the prognosis is viewed as caring and a way to offer hope (Barclay, Blackhall, & Tulsky, 2007; Calloway, 2009; Johnstone & Kanitsaki, 2009).

Just as cultural norms dictate much of our daily behavior, attitudes, and values, it is not surprising that culture influences the individual's response to pain. Pain is the second most common reason people seek health care and has significant socioeconomic, health, and quality-of-life implications. Racial and ethnic minorities tend to be undertreated for pain when compared to non-Hispanic Whites (Research in Community-Based Nursing Care 3-1). In two separate systematic reviews of the literature, the majority of studies found that racial and ethnic disparities exist in access to effective pain treatment (Cintron & Morrison, 2006; Ezenway, Ameringer, Ward, & Serlin, 2006).

It is important that nurses develop an understanding of the interaction between culture and the expression of pain (Giger & Davidhizar, 2004; Maier-Lorentz, 2008). Some people come from backgrounds where stoicism is the norm and pain is not expressed, while others have the view that openly verbalizing pain is expected. It is important for the nurse to be knowledgeable about possible cultural variations and the cultural influences on pain tolerance, expression of pain, and alternative practices used to manage pain. At the same time, it is important to consider individual differences and use caution not to make assumptions or have stereotypes about pain expressions.

CLIENT SITUATIONS IN PRACTICE

Pain Expression

Julie, the school nurse, is caring for Marcus, a 15-year-old African American male with sickle cell disease. Marcus has missed multiple days of school this month. He is in school today but has come to her office in obvious pain. When she asks him about it, he states that during a visit to the emergency department last night, one of the staff told him he was "just medication seeking" and he overheard someone else refer to him as "one of the frequent fliers." He reports that they discharged him without treating his pain. He is upset and discouraged. Julie knows that sickle cell causes pain that is severe and sporadic. She spends

RESEARCH IN COMMUNITY-BASED NURSING CARE 3-1

Research Informs Practice

The purpose of this study was to examine the research to date on racial and ethnic disparities in pain management. The authors conducted a systematic review of the literature in order to examine the relationship between race or ethnicity and adequacy of pain management. While the authors found that the definitions of race, ethnicity, and minority are unclear and inconsistently used, it is clear that non-Whites in the United States are at higher risk for "suffering from the complications of inadequate pain treatment" (p. 232). Based on their findings, it is clear that despite recent advances in pain management, disparities do exist. Factors such as racism, stereotyping by health care providers, differences in understanding how to report pain and the use of palliative measures, as well as the lack of access to opioids in minority neighborhoods all impact the ability to manage pain effectively in nonwhite populations. The authors call for health care providers to increase their understanding and attentiveness as they care for racial and ethnically diverse people in order to effectively address this issue and improve palliative care for these populations.

From Ezenway, M. O., Ameringer, S. E., Ward, R. C., & Serlin. (2006). Racial and ethnic disparities in pain management in the U.S. *Journal of Nursing Scholarship, 38*(3), 225–233.

time talking with Marcus, assesses his pain, and then calls his mother and his physician to arrange to be seen today (Andrews & Boyle, 2007).

Cultural self-awareness is essential to help the nurse recognize and value the right of others to follow their cultural beliefs and practices. Awareness of one's own cultural values, beliefs, and practices opens the nurse's mind to the possibility that the client's values, beliefs, and practices may vary in ways that are very different from his or her own, which can significantly impact the provision of care. The effective nurse will recognize other cultural beliefs and practices as valid and accommodate the client's ways in providing care. The nurse should ask, "How will knowing these things about my client influence my care?"

Cultural Knowledge

Once nurses are more sensitive and aware of their own cultures and biases, they are ready to discover the culture and lifeways of the community within which they work. Cultural knowledge encompasses the familiarity of the worldview, beliefs, practices, and problem-solving strategies of groups that are ethnically or culturally diverse (Campinha-Bacote, 2003).

Community-based nursing practice requires that the nurse has cultural humility as she enters a new community, where she can seek cultural knowledge and gain understanding of the community. This knowledge allows the nurse to use a preventive approach and facilitate self-care according to the client's particular culture. Collaboration and continuity are also enhanced when the nurse has an understanding of the cultural community in which he or she is working with the client. Having cultural knowledge about the community will influence what is seen, leading to a more thorough and appropriate assessment and intervention. Lack of cultural knowledge and cultural humility stands in the way of cultural competence. Nurses can have wonderful intentions and be sensitive and caring, but if there is a lack of specific knowledge or willingness to learn about the client's culture, then mistakes are bound to be made.

CLIENT SITUATIONS IN PRACTICE

Breast-feeding

Kate is a public health nurse visiting Adika, who emigrated from Ghana. During a recent home visit, she observed that Adika was breast-feeding her 2.5-year-old son. She immediately began to question Adika as to why she was still breast-feeding her son. Kate wasn't being cruel, but her lack of awareness of the culture meant that she was unaware that mothers in Ghana often breast-feed their children until age 3. A simple question such as; "What cultural practices are important to you?" would have alleviated the trauma to this young mother.

✳ CLIENT SITUATIONS IN PRACTICE

Diabetic Care

Mohammed is a new immigrant to the United States from Iran. He makes a visit to the clinic for a follow-up visit to check his blood sugar. On this visit, Kris noted that his blood sugar was particularly low and she expressed concern. Being aware of the practice of fasting during Ramadan, Kris offered suggestions to Mohammed as to how he might avoid such a drop in his blood sugar.

The physician wasn't being cruel, but he was ignorant of cultural knowledge related to the practice of fasting during Ramadan.

GENERIC AND PROFESSIONAL KNOWLEDGE

Dr. Madeleine Leininger uses the terms "emic" and "etic" to describe types of care (Leininger & McFarland, 2006). **Emic** refers to the local or insider's views and values about a phenomenon. **Etic** refers to the professional or outsider's views and values about a phenomenon. The community-based nurse uses both these types of care knowledge and verifies with the client and family those areas that are meaningful and acceptable to them (Fig. 3-5). Discovering how generic (emic) and professional (etic) systems are alike or different assists the nurse in providing culturally congruent care to individuals or groups.

In many cultures, there are several levels of healers. For example, in Mexican American culture, there are several levels of healers within the *curanderismo* folklore system. At one level is a *curandero*, or folk healer, who is believed to have God-given gifts of healing. This folk healer may treat those with a wide range of physical and psychological problems, ranging from back pain and gastrointestinal distress to irritability or fatigue. After a diagnosis is made, the *curandero* may use treatments such as massage, diet, rest, indigenous herbs, prayers, magic, or supernatural rituals (Andrews & Boyle, 2007). The nurse working in a Mexican American community should know about the levels of folk healers used by her clients and inquire as to the consultation and treatment already rendered.

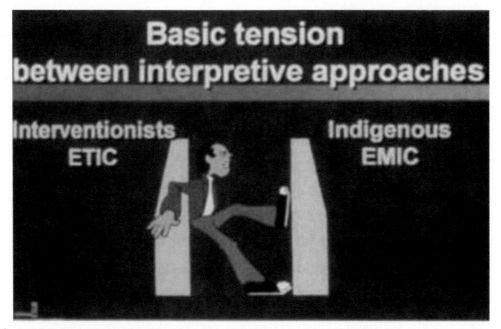

Figure 3-5 Basic tension between the emic and the etic. Source: Andrews, M., & Boyle, J. (2007). *Transcultural concepts in nursing care* (5th ed., p. 252). Philadelphia, PA: Lippincott Williams & Wilkins.

Using this emic understanding of the client's beliefs about health issues, the community nurse can coordinate that care with professional (etic) care that would be acceptable to the client. If massage or a specific diet treatment has been successful, then those interventions can be incorporated into a plan of care. When cultural practices are acknowledged and respected by the professional nurse, clients are more willing to incorporate Western medicine that may augment and enhance the response to treatment.

COMPONENTS OF CULTURAL ASSESSMENT

Six phenomena related to a **cultural assessment** are discussed in this section (Assessment Tools 3-1).

Communication

Because the community-based nurse spends much of his or her time teaching and communicating roles, knowledge of communication styles and meanings is essential. Verbal and nonverbal behavior, space between persons talking, family member roles, eye contact, salutations, and intergender communication patterns vary significantly among cultures. For example, lack of eye contact to Western cultures is seen as impolite and may indicate indifference or no interest. In Native American and Southeast Asian cultures, on the other hand, lack of eye contact is a gesture of respect. In conversations, European Americans tend to answer quickly, often before the person speaking has finished; however, Native Americans use silence before answering to carefully absorb what the other has said and to formulate their own response. For individuals from the Middle East, it can be important to engage in lighter, personal conversation before moving to the business of the appointment. A nurse working within this community must be aware of this and allow time for these interactions.

In many Eastern cultures, agreeing by nodding or saying "yes" is considered polite, whether or not the individual really agrees or understands what has been asked. Interpersonal harmony is important in Asian cultures; therefore, a nod or smile may not reflect agreement at all. Rather, in the desire to be respectful, the expression of true feelings may be withheld. In situations such as this, it is important to tell the client (or coworker) that an open discussion is welcome and it is okay to disagree.

Assessment Tools 3-1
Six Phenomena of Cultural Assessment

- *Communication.* A continuous process by which one person may affect another through written or oral language, gestures, facial expressions, body language, space, or other symbols.
- *Space.* The area around a person's body that includes the individual, body, surrounding environment, and objects within that environment.
- *Social organization.* The family and other groups within a society that dictate culturally accepted role behaviors of different members of the society and rules for behavior. Behaviors are prescribed for significant life events, such as birth, death, childbearing, child rearing, and illness.
- *Time.* The meaning and influence of time from a cultural perspective. Time orientation refers to an individual's focus on the past, the present, or the future. Most cultures combine all three time orientations, but one orientation is more likely to dominate.
- *Environmental control.* The ability or perceived ability of an individual or persons from a particular cultural group to plan activities that control nature, such as illness causation and treatment.
- *Biologic variations.* The biologic differences among racial and ethnic groups. It can include physical characteristics, such as skin color; physiologic variations, such as lactose intolerance; or susceptibility to specific disease processes.

From Giger, J. N., & Davidhizar, R. E. (1991). *Trans-cultural nursing: Assessment and intervention.* St. Louis MO: Mosby Year Book.

CLIENT SITUATIONS IN PRACTICE

Nilofar brings her infant daughter to the Child Health Clinic at the local health department. Susan, the public health nurse, begins the conversation by admiring how cute the baby is. Because she knows that within Middle Eastern culture it is important to take some time to "warm up" before moving into business, they briefly exchange informal conversation about recent books they've both read. She then tells Nilofar that her own daughter is a new mom and that her grandchild seems to be a bit "fussy" and how she's been working with her daughter on finding ways to calm the baby. This then leads Susan to begin a conversation with Nilofar about her baby's temperament and the business of the appointment begins.

CLIENT SITUATIONS IN PRACTICE

Teaching

John, a community health nurse, is making a home visit with Bao, a community health worker, to a Hmong family who recently immigrated. Lacking knowledge of Hmong culture, he is unaware that nodding and smiling after beginning to give direction does not mean agreement or understanding; rather it indicates respect. This lack of awareness compromises the nurse's ability to provide appropriate care to the family. Through observation, John becomes aware that Bao did not fully understand his instructions. On his next visit to this family, he asked Bao what foods she might teach this family how to make.

Space and Physical Contact

The concept of space is another important dimension of cultural knowledge. How close people stand by each other in conversation, overt expressions of affection or caring with touch, and rules relating to personal space and privacy vary greatly among cultures. For example, in Italian and Mexican cultures, physical presence and touching is valued and expected. Family members of both genders embrace, kiss, and link arms when walking. In Middle Eastern cultures, close face-to-face conversations where one can almost feel the breath of the other person is the norm, whereas in the United States, the normal space for conversation between persons is an arm's length. In Muslim cultures, it is inappropriate for males and females to even shake hands before marriage. It would be highly improper and distressing for a female Somali client to be assessed by a male nurse.

CLIENT SITUATIONS IN PRACTICE

Physical Contact

Within the Muslim community, physical contact between unrelated genders is strictly forbidden and females are required to wear loose fitting clothing that covers their entire body, from head to toe. Because of this, women are limited in the physical activity that they may comfortably engage in. This has resulted in isolation and obesity for many of the women in the Somali community of Seattle. In response, the Seattle Public Health Department, in cooperation with several community partners, including the Seattle Parks and Recreation and the Seattle Department of Neighborhoods, came together to develop and implement a gender-specific swim program at two of the city's public pools (Moore, Ali, Graham, & Quan, 2010).

This is an example of a creative, culturally sensitive, community-based response to the unique needs of this cultural group.

Time

The Western orientation to time and its value was discussed previously. Because the concept of time has such different meanings in various cultures, it is important for the nurse to know of this dimension within the cultural group receiving care. Implications for making appointments, follow-up care, and proper medication administration need to be considered. For example, a physician may prescribe a medication to be taken three times a day with meals. Three meals a day is the norm for most Americans, but this is not so in all other cultures. The nurse should find out when the family has a meal and how much time there is between meals to determine how to explain the regimen within this client's normal patterns of eating.

When scheduling a home visit, 2 PM is an exact time to a nurse accustomed to Western orientation to time, but it may mean "sometime in the afternoon" to a person who doesn't share that value of exactness to clock time. Clarifying with the client and family what is meant by a designation of an appointment time saves frustration for both parties.

Another aspect of time is that of past, present, or future orientation. As described already, traditional American culture is future oriented. Calendars and plans for the future are a part of everyday American life. In contrast, Native American cultures tend to be past oriented, with a focus on ancestors and traditions. African American culture tends to focus on the present, with an emphasis on "now" and day-to-day activities. Persons without a future orientation need a different approach when discussing preventive care.

CLIENT SITUATIONS IN PRACTICE

Sean is a community health nurse who works for the Indian Health Service on Pine Ridge Indian Reservation. Knowing that diabetes is an epidemic among native people (Andrews & Boyle, 2007), Sean would like to work to develop a community-based intervention that will decrease the incidence of diabetes within the local community. He approaches the local elders of the community and asks, "How can we work together to help individuals avoid this disease in the future?"

Social Organization

The community-based nurse must understand the family or kinship patterns of the groups within the community being served. The family is the basic unit of society, but the nurse must recognize that there are multiple meanings of "family." Cultural values can determine communication within the family group, the norm for family size, and the roles of specific family members (Taylor, Lillis, & LeMone, 2006). The client's meaning of family may differ from the nurse's understanding; therefore, in order to avoid misunderstanding and miscommunication, it is important to ask, "Who is in your family?" or "Tell me about your family." Among Pacific Islanders, it is appropriate to ask "Who are your people?" (McGrath & Edwards, 2009). The use of a genogram or a similar tool for collecting information about family relationships and health history can facilitate a discussion on who the client identifies as his or her family (LeahyW & Svavarsdottir, 2009; Limb & Hodge, 2010; McGrath & Edwards, 2009).

Nurses should consider, learn about, and assess for the following:

- What is the definition of family in this cultural group; does it include primarily the nuclear family or is the extended family considered the basic unit?
- Are there gender or age roles that affect the choice of whom the nurse should address when entering the home or in consultation about a client's health?
- What are the traditional roles within the family that affect caregiving?
- What value is placed on children and the elderly, and how does that affect health care decision making within the family?
- What is the status of females within the culture, and how does that affect the acceptability of a health care provider?
- What is the expected family involvement in health care decisions, and who is the primary decision maker within the family?
- How is information regarding the health of a family member shared with others in the community?
- What role does religion play in health care practices and decision making within the culture and the family unit?

Biologic Variations

To perform a thorough assessment and provide culturally congruent care, the community-based nurse who knows biologic variations specific to his or her clients will be most effective. Although some biologic variations are obvious (e.g., skin color, hair texture, facial features, stature, and body markings), others require knowledge based on medical information and research. For example, Africans and African American persons have a much higher incidence of sickle cell disease than other groups. Many children of African, Asian, and Latin descent are born with Mongolian spots. These spots occur on the sacral and gluteal areas of the body and are bluish in color, which has been mistaken as bruising, resulting in erroneous reports of child abuse and unnecessary anxiety for parents. Much of the world's population (many Asians, Africans, Hispanics, and Native Americans) is lactose intolerant or unable to digest milk sugars. To provide health teaching related to a diet that includes milk and milk products to people in these groups is ethnocentric. Native Americans have a high incidence of diabetes mellitus. Health assessment by community-based nurses working with this population should include screening for high blood sugar levels and culturally appropriate preventative teaching.

The action, absorption, excretion, and dose parameters of many pharmacologic agents also vary among ethnic groups. Genetic differences, structural variation in binding receptor sites, and environmental conditions may affect the drug action in different groups of people. Blood pressure medications, analgesics, and psychotropic drug doses may be significantly different, depending on the ethnic group requiring the medication (Andrews & Boyle, 2007). Adult doses for many medications are not determined by weight as for pediatric doses; instead, body mass should be considered for groups of small stature, such as people of Japanese and Korean descent. The nurse should also ask about herbal remedies that the client might be taking that could affect the action or metabolism of certain medications.

Environmental Control

The meaning of health and illness is greatly influenced by a group's cultural belief system, which in turn influences the health attitudes, beliefs, and practices. There are three predominant **health belief systems**: magicoreligious, scientific, and holistic. The magicoreligious view sees illness as having a supernatural force; that is, malevolent or evil spirits cause disease, or illness is a punishment from God. People from Hispanic and Caribbean cultures may have this health belief system. Because the belief is that a supernatural influence (rather than organic) caused the health problem, people with this perspective will look for a supernatural counterforce to rid them of the problem. People with this belief will seek a voodoo priestess or spiritualist who has the powers to remove "spells" from a variety of sources. Although Western medicine has classified voodoo illness as a psychiatric disorder, nurses who practice cultural care will understand this view of illness and intervene accordingly.

In the scientific or biomedical view, disease and illness are believed to be caused by microorganisms or a malfunction of the body. Historically, the scientific paradigm has rejected any connection to religious or holistic practice; however, more recently, integrative therapies have been more inclusive of practices beyond biomedical. People with this health view generally look to medicines, medical treatment, or surgery to cure their illness.

The holistic health belief looks for a balance or harmony with nature. Disease and illness is understood as an imbalance or disharmony between human, geophysical, and metaphysical forces of the universe. Health is viewed in a broader context than biologic or physical, and is influenced by environmental, sociocultural, and behavioral factors. Florence Nightingale viewed health as holistic.

Many cultures reflect a holistic belief system. Many Eastern cultures ascribe to the theory of yin and yang being opposite forces that must be kept in balance. Imbalance results in illness or disease. The hot and cold theory of many Latino, Asian, Arab, and Caribbean cultures is similar. This is based in an ancient Greek understanding of the four body humors: yellow bile, black bile, phlegm, and blood. Health is the balance of these four humors. The treatment of disease becomes the process of restoring the body's humoral balance through the addition or subtraction of substances that affect each of these humors. Foods, beverages, herbs, and other drugs are classified as hot or cold based on the effect they have on the body.

The healthy body is characterized by evenly distributed warmth and that illness results when the body is attacked by an increase of either hot or cold (Andrews & Boyle, 2007).

✻ CLIENT SITUATIONS IN PRACTICE

Holistic Health Theory

To the Chinese, childbirth is seen as an experience in which the body loses heat balance that must be restored. Mrs. Yiu, a postpartum Chinese woman, will refuse ice water and will accept only foods that are seen as "warm," such as chicken and rice. Bathing would contribute to the loss of body warmth and would be refused for a period of time after childbirth. The nurse visiting this client in a community setting would be sensitive to these practices and provide care accordingly.

Many variations exist among cultural groups as to how health care is managed and decisions are made. It is important to also keep in mind that individual families may have their own roles, beliefs, and practices that differ from the larger cultural group. This may reflect the degree to which the family has been acculturated to Western cultural patterns and beliefs, or it may be a regional or familial variation. Professional nurses who desire to provide effective care that is culturally congruent to the beliefs of the client are aware of the potential for variations and know what questions to ask. While it is helpful to have a holding knowledge (i.e., knowledge of a group learned from transcultural nursing texts, literature, and previous encounters) of cultural groups, the nurse must always verify with each client which beliefs and practices are personally relevant to him or her. In this way, cultural sensitivity and humility are conveyed even when the nurse is not well versed in the lifeways of a particular group.

Acculturation and Assimilation

Two other concepts are important for nurses to keep in mind as they learn about the culture of particular groups. Individuals within a group may adhere to the traditional culture to varying degrees; this variation may result from **acculturation** or **assimilation**.

As new groups enter a different society, acculturation may occur as they learn the ways to exist in a new culture. This may include learning to drive, going to school, negotiating public transportation, getting a job, and interacting in an environment unlike that of the home country. As these activities become more comfortable, individuals become more acculturated to the dominant society, yet they may retain much of their own cultural traditions within their communities. For example, a young Somali girl may continue to wear her traditional Muslim attire (*hijab*) and retain the tradition of gender roles while going to an American high school and getting a job at a fast-food restaurant on weekends.

Assimilation takes place when individuals or groups identify more strongly with the dominant culture in values, activities, and daily living. This usually occurs over longer periods of time, sometimes generations. These assimilations are important for the nurse to keep in mind as there may be a wide variation in how cultural traditions are carried out, even within the same family. The parents may have emigrated from another country, but the children have been raised surrounded by the dominant culture and have, therefore, assimilated more aspects of the dominant culture.

Cultural Skill

Campinha-Bacote describes cultural skill as the ability to collect relevant cultural data regarding the client's health history. Up to this point, we have discussed the need for nurses to examine their own cultural traditions, beliefs, values, and practices to increase awareness of how influential their culture is on their view of the world and to open their mind to the valid variations in worldviews of varying cultures. This helps to avoid cultural blindness, cultural imposition, ethnocentrism, and stereotyping. It is then the nurse's responsibility to learn as much as possible about the ethnic or cultural groups encountered in the community where the nursing care is being delivered. A holding knowledge of the emic or folk care practices along with the etic or professional care practices gives the community nurse a basis from which to individualize care that is culturally sensitive to the client as an individual or as a family. Practices within cultural groups or families may vary significantly from general descriptions; therefore, knowing the questions to ask for culturally specific care is essential to avoid stereotyping. Having cultural skill is essential to that process. One area of important cultural knowledge is mental health. Box 3-1 describes recent research related to culture and mental health.

Leininger defines a cultural assessment as a "systematic identification and documentation of culture care, beliefs, meanings, values, symbols and practices of individuals or groups with a holistic perspective" (Leininger & McFarland, 2002, p. 117). Community-based nurses focus on preventive care. These nurses assess the health risks of a particular group and consider cultural practices and beliefs to plan teaching and activities to prevent disease or health risks (primary prevention). Using culturally based knowledge of generic or folk health care practices in the group, community-based nurses then incorporate their **etic** and **emic care** knowledge to diagnose and treat threats to health and wellness (secondary prevention). Tertiary prevention in the community seeks to rehabilitate or prevent recurrence of health problems. Through a skillful cultural assessment, the community nurse has listened to the clients' perception of the health problem and compared it to his or her own perception, explaining and acknowledging the similarities and differences. Involving members of the community, the nurse then negotiates a treatment plan that will be seen as beneficial to the community.

BOX 3-1 **Research Related to Culture and Mental Health**

The purpose of this study was to examine five ethnic communities' (Latin American, Mandarin-speaking Chinese, Polish, Punjabi Sikh, and Somali) perspectives on mental health, mental illness, and mental health care. Through key informant interviews, focus groups, case studies, surveys, and a literature review, the researchers found that the meaning and understanding of mental health is clearly linked to culture. Participants indicated that mental health was not necessarily a concept that they discussed within the countries they came from. Each group offered distinct understandings of mental health. For Somali participants, mental health was reflective of spiritual and religious strength. For Latino participants, the importance of family and a healthy childhood was connected to one's mental well-being. For Chinese participants, mental health related to one's individual strength and ability to overcome hardships. However, within their present context, mental health reflected their ability to adapt and to cope with their current, new life circumstances, as well as to meet family and work responsibilities, and to maintain financial stability. Each group saw their ability to adapt to their new life in a new country as particularly important for mental health.

Participants initially described mental illness in negative terms, such as crazy, insane, perverted, abnormal, hysterical, and deranged. However, as conversations progressed, participants identified depression, a feeling of hopelessness, insecurity, and failure as signs of mental illness. Each of the cultures indicated that there is a great deal of shame and stigma attached to mental illness within their communities, and therefore, discussion about it is usually avoided or hidden. Significant differences were identified in how individuals with mental distress or mental illness were managed within their homelands. The importance of a shared cultural understanding for treatment and recovery was key. For example, Polish participants discussed how treatment within Poland was holistic, emphasizing body, mind, *and* spirit as part of becoming well. They described treatment as including massage, relaxation techniques, proper nutrition, and exercise.

Recommendations for transcultural mental health care include

- Education for both providers and consumers, providing an understanding of both culture and mental health within health care organizations and within ethnic communities. An interactive discussion between providers and community members would provide an opportunity for increased understanding between the two
- Community health workers from within the community who specialize in mental health
- Health care providers increase their understanding of cultural values and strengths, as well as improve understanding of the systemic barriers to culturally appropriate mental health care

Source: Simich, L., Maiter, S., Moorlag, E., & Ochoka, J. (2009). Taking culture seriously: Ethnolinguistic community perspectives on mental health. *Psychiatric Rehabilitation Journal, 32*(3), 208–214.

Numerous models for cultural assessment have been developed by various authors in the field of transcultural nursing (Andrews & Boyle, 2007; Giger & Davidhizar, 2004; Leininger & McFarland, 2006) and health care (Purnell & Paulanka, 2008). Each organizes assessment data in a different manner, and individual nurses will determine which model works best within their scope of practice and the community served. A cross-cultural assessment tool (Assessment Tools 3-2) can be useful with any client (Andrew & Boyle, 2007; Kemp, 2005; Maier-Lorentz, 2008). The questions are open-ended and provide the opportunity for the client to describe his or her perception of the health problem. For example, in response to the second question, "How would you describe this problem you have?" The parents of a Hmong child with epilepsy might respond, "The spirit catches you and you fall down" (Fadiman, 1997).

Assessment Tools 3-2
Cross-Cultural Assessment

What is the client's greatest concern?

How does the client perceive the nurse can be helpful?

Communication:
- What is the client's primary language? What language does the client prefer to communicate with you in?
- Who is the primary decision maker in the family? Do decisions involve individuals or people beyond the family (i.e., elders or religious leaders in the community)?
- Are questions answered freely and openly? Is there an atmosphere of trust between the client and the health care provider?
- Does the client have a stoic or expressive manner?
- What are the styles of nonverbal communication of the client? Between family members?

Space
- Is family closeness important?

Time
- What time orientation does the client tend toward: past, present, or future?

Environmental Control
- Who does the client believe has control over the future?
- Does the client have an internal or external locus of control? (i.e., Do they believe they have the power to change or that the power is beyond their control? Is the outcome dependent on a higher power, or fate, or luck?)

Social Organization
- Who does the client consider family?
- What are the roles within the family? What is the client's role in the family?
- What is the function of the family?
- What are the client's spiritual beliefs?

Biological Variations
- What is the current health status of the client?
- Is pain expressed freely or only when asked?
- How does the client perceive pain? Is it something to be tolerated?

Adapted from Giger, J. N., Davidhizar, R. E., & Fordham, P. (2006). Multi-cultural and multi-ethnic considerations and advanced directives: Developing cultural competency. *Journal of Cultural Diversity*, *13*(1), 3–9.

The cultural assessment gives the nurse good information with cultural implications to use as a basis for planning teaching and treatment plans. All clients have a right to have their values, beliefs, and practices considered, respected, and incorporated into the plan of care.

Cultural Encounter

The cultural encounter is the opportunity for the nurse to engage in direct contact with the members of cultural communities. Through frequent contact with numerous members of a cultural group, the nurse keeps in mind that variations will exist within the community and stereotypical expectations are to be avoided. Trust builds over time between the caregiving nurse and members of the community, and it is essential to the well-being of both.

Using knowledge of etic and emic care practices and having completed a cultural assessment, the nurse now uses the skills and competencies necessary to effect healthful outcomes for the clients in the community. Leininger has identified three modalities that "guide nursing judgments, decisions or actions so as to provide cultural congruent care that is beneficial, satisfying and meaningful to people nurses serve" (Leininger & McFarland, 2006, p. 8). These three modalities are defined in Table 3-1.

CULTURAL CARE PRESERVATION

The first of the modalities is cultural care preservation and/or maintenance. After careful assessment and observation, the nurse identifies those cultural care practices that are helpful to the client. The nurse then assists, supports, facilitates, or enables the client and family to preserve those actions or behaviors. For example, in the Amish community, the extended family, neighborhood, and church expect to assist and care for members within the community. The nurse working in this community encourages and supports ways to enlist the help of the extended community and facilitates ways to let the care needs be known.

CULTURAL CARE ACCOMMODATION

The second mode of cultural care accommodation or negotiation refers to those nursing actions and decisions that assist or enable the client and family to continue with practices that are meaningful to them but may be altered due to circumstances. For example, the

Table 3-1 Leininger's Guidelines for Providing Culturally Congruent Care

Modality	Definition
Cultural care preservation and/or maintenance	Refers to those assistive, supporting, facilitative, or enabling professional actions and decisions that help people of a particular culture to retain and/or preserve relevant care values so that they can maintain their well-being, recover from illness, or face handicaps and/or death
Cultural care accommodation or negotiation	Refers to those assistive, supporting, facilitative, or enabling creative professional actions and decisions that help people of a designated culture (or subculture) adapt to or negotiate with others for a beneficial or satisfying health outcome with professional care providers
Cultural care repatterning or restructuring	Refers to those assistive, supporting, facilitative, or enabling professional actions and decisions that help a client reorder, change, or greatly modify lifeways for new, different, and beneficial health care patterns while respecting the client's cultural values and beliefs and still providing beneficial or healthier lifeways than before the changes were coestablished with the client(s)

Source: Leininger, M. N., & McFarland, M. (2002). *Transcultural nursing concepts, theories, research, practice* (p. 84). New York: McGraw-Hill.

nurse in the community may be setting up a referral for a client to be seen in a clinic for follow-up care. The client is Muslim and must adhere to the practice of praying five times a day. The nurse will negotiate with the client as to times of day that would provide enough time between prayers for an appointment or assist in helping the client find a place within or near the clinic where these prayers may be said.

In another example, the community-based nurse is doing a follow-up visit to a Jewish child recently diagnosed with type 1 diabetes. Knowing the Jewish restriction of pork products, the nurse might intervene to ask the physician to prescribe a nonporcine insulin product.

In addition to assisting the client in carrying out his or her religious practices, the respect and care shown by the nurse toward these clients enhances trust and feelings of caring support.

CULTURAL CARE REPATTERNING

The third way in which nurses make decisions or intervene is cultural care repatterning or restructuring. When the nurse assesses the client, family, and community and finds practices that may be detrimental to health and well-being, he or she will work with the client to change behaviors that are harmful.

CLIENT SITUATIONS IN PRACTICE

Dietary Repatterning

Donna is working within the Latino community, where members observe the practice of making and eating tortillas fried in fat as a staple for every meal. Knowing that this much fat soaked into the tortilla is detrimental to a community at risk for heart disease, Donna works with the women to explore ways to decrease the amount of fat in frying the tortilla. Together they may decide that placing the tortilla vertically or on paper towels before serving may decrease the amount of fat as it drips off before eating. Because the nurse works with the client(s) to diminish risks to health, the changes are more likely to take effect.

Box 3-2 presents research that led nurses to provide culturally responsive care using three modes of action in an ambulatory care setting. Note how knowing the culture and learning the emic care can lead to simple but important nursing actions and decisions that will be perceived by the clients as cultural care.

Whether the nurse is validating and supporting helpful existing practices, helping clients to negotiate ways to maintain their health care practices, or working to identify and change harmful behaviors, it is essential that he or she work with the community as a partner. Because optimum health care for all clients is the goal of nursing, these three modes of nursing actions and decisions, in close cooperation with the clients, can be enormously beneficial and satisfying to both the community and the nurse.

CLIENT SITUATIONS IN PRACTICE

Planning for a Cultural Encounter

Sarah is a home health care nurse assigned to visit Awa for a postpartum visit. This Somali family consists of Awa, her husband, a 3-year-old daughter, and the new baby. The family has been in the United States for 4 months, after spending 5 years in a refugee camp in Kenya. Both Adam and Awa were residents of Mogadishu before the civil war and were from well-educated, middle-class, traditional Somali families. Both speak English, although not fluently. Prenatal history indicates the baby was born by C-section after a reported uneventful pregnancy, notable only for the fact that Awa's first prenatal visit to a physician was 1 week prior to the child's birth. She experienced false labor and was brought to the physician's office by her neighbor.

BOX
3-2 **Research Related to Community-Based Nursing Care**

CULTURAL CARE MODALITIES FOR THE PUERTO RICAN CLIENT IN AN AMBULATORY CARE SETTING

The purpose of this study was to examine the cultural beliefs and practices of Puerto Rican families that influence feeding practices and affect the nutritional status of infants and young children. The goal of the study was to outline strategies that would enable nurses to provide culturally congruent care for this population. Resulting cultural care modalities are listed below.

Cultural Care Preservation Modalities

Reinforce family caring values of nurturance and succorance.

Respect and understand use of religious symbols and protective care symbols.

Touch the infant or child and say "God bless you" if complimenting the child.

Treat the family with respect, use professional demeanor, and maintain eye contact.

Promote continuity of care.

Cultural Care Accommodation Modalities

Use the Spanish language to include the grandmother; reinforce intergenerational caregiving.

Promote respeto (respect) and confianza (confidence, trust) by accommodation (or deference) to family and community values.

Encourage introduction of traditional, healthy foods—rice, beans, and eggs—at the appropriate time, linking their use with green vegetables and meat.

Encourage the generic folk practice of Ponche as needed, with additional health considerations.

Develop a comprehensive bilingual feeding assessment guide to improve anticipatory guidance.

Cultural Care Repatterning Modalities

Include grandmother and kin in a collaborative participatory approach to feeding.

Emphasize the cultural ideology and beliefs. Explain how a new approach will contribute to a big, healthy baby.

Anticipatory guidance about overfeeding formula should begin at 2–4 weeks.

Anticipatory guidance about not adding solids to the bottle should be given at 4–8 weeks before the practice is initiated. Stress the ease of feeding solids by mouth at 4–6 months of age.

Develop Spanish-language pamphlets linking emic and etic feeding practices.

Provide nutrition and cooking demonstration classes with a cultural theme, linking emic and etic foods for mothers, fathers, and grandmothers.

Advertise classes on Spanish-speaking radio and TV stations.

Develop a nutritional outreach program including bilingual Puerto Rican mothers who are interested in nutrition and health.

Source: Higgins, B. (2000). Puerto Rican cultural beliefs: Influence on infant feeding practices in western New York. *Journal of Transcultural Nursing, 11*(1), 19–30.

What considerations does Sarah need to think about as she prepares to make her first visit to Awa and her baby?

Sarah should consider the traditional Somali practice of female circumcision and her own cultural beliefs related to that practice. She cannot assume Awa is circumcised or to what degree, but the decision to have a C-section may have been a result of this possibility (although circumcised women can give birth vaginally as well).

Sarah knows that most Somalis are Muslims. Where can she find out some basic beliefs and practices of those who practice Islam?

Sarah can review current literature and transcultural nursing books as well as access information online related to Muslim religious practices. She notes that 99% of Somalis are

Sunni Muslims. She knows this will be an important question to ask as culture and religion are highly intertwined in Somalia.

What basic cultural practices are important for Sarah to know prior to visiting this Somali family?

Gender roles are quite specifically defined in traditional Somali culture. Sarah will know that she must not offer to shake hands with Adam, as physical contact with a woman other than a close family member is forbidden. She will also know that female modesty is a high priority when assessing Awa's incision.

Sarah plans to discuss family planning. What is important for her to know in providing culturally sensitive care?

In the Muslim religion, children are seen as gifts from Allah and many children are considered a blessing. Preventing conception is not acceptable, but to assure sufficient time for the mother to regain her strength, to allow for the adequate provision of all children in the family, and to preserve family tranquility, child "spacing" is considered an acceptable method of family planning (Burkland, 2008; Degni, Pöntinen, & Mölsä, 2006).

As in any cultural encounter, Sarah must proceed slowly, aware of her own cultural beliefs and values and how this may impact her practice. If she familiarizes herself with some basic cultural practices and beliefs she is likely to encounter and uses cultural sensitivity and respect, Sarah is likely to successfully create a climate of trust and understanding.

Conclusions

All nurses, regardless of their own cultural background, are obligated to learn what is important to their clients. "Health and illness states are strongly influenced and often primarily determined by the cultural background of the individual" (Leininger, 1970, p. 22). Cultural awareness of one's own background, beliefs, values, and practices opens the nurse's mind to value and support the diversity of others. Cultural knowledge learned from books, formal coursework, and discussions with community members gives the nurse a background or framework in which to understand the cultural health care beliefs of a group. This information can then be validated or altered based on individual interactions. Cultural skill is the ability to conduct a cultural assessment that will guide nursing actions and decisions. In the cultural encounter, the nurse reinforces, negotiates, or assists clients to repattern care practices for optimum health care.

An attitude of sensitivity, acceptance, and sincere desire to work with culturally diverse clients results in continuity and collaborative care and promotes a trusting relationship with the client. Nurses in the community setting must establish a bond based on trust with the home health care client to provide excellent care and do so cost-effectively (Heineken & McCoy, 2000). Using knowledge of the generic or emic care practices of the cultural community and integrating these with professional or etic knowledge, the nurse assists in self-care by encouraging existing healthy behaviors and establishing preventive measures that are culturally congruent and acceptable in creating a healthy future for each community served.

What's on the Web

Cultural Competency and Health Literacy for Health Care Providers (Health Resources and Services Administration)
INTERNET ADDRESS: http://www.hrsa.gov/culturalcompetence/#assessment
This Web site of the Department of Health and Human Services Health Resources and Services Administration provides links to multiple tools and educational modules related to cultural assessment, health literacy, and the development of cultural sensitivity in health professionals.

Office of Minority Health
INTERNET ADDRESS: http://minorityhealth.hhs.gov
The Office of Minority Health is dedicated to eliminating health disparities through the development of programs and policies that improve and protect the health of racial and ethnic populations in the United States. This Web site provides a link to resources specific to the development of linguistic and cultural competence in health care. Specifically, the site offers a link to a free online educational program for nurses.

INTERNET ADDRESS: **http://www.thinkculturalhealth.hhs.gov**

This Web site is maintained by the Department of Health and Human Services Office of Minority Health as a link to continuing education programs for health care providers, and more specifically nursing, as a way to bridge the gap between health care providers and the increasing diverse population they serve. Through this case-based curriculum, aimed at developing cultural competency skills, nurses will better understand the cultural and linguistic needs of the individuals they care for. This site also provides links to multiple consumer advocacy groups for health care.

Office of Minority Health (Centers for Disease Control)
INTERNET ADDRESS: **http://www.cdc.gov/omhd/**

The mission of the Office of Minority Health and Health Disparities (Centers for Disease Control and Prevention) is to improve the health of the U.S. population and address health disparities for vulnerable populations. Multiple resources that relate eliminating health disparities and improving health care through the provision of culturally sensitive care by health care providers are provided.

Center for Cross-Cultural Health
INTERNET ADDRESS: **http://www.crosshealth.com**

The mission of the Center for Cross Cultural Health is "to integrate the role of culture in improving health." The vision of this organization is increased health and well-being for all through cross-cultural understanding. To achieve this goal, the center promotes the education and training of health and human service providers and organizations as well as a research and information resource. Through information sharing, training, organizational assessments, and research, the center works to develop culturally responsive individuals, organizations, systems, and societies.

Center for Healthy Families and Cultural Diversity
INTERNET ADDRESS: **http://www2.umdnj.edu/fmedweb/chfcd/index.htm**

The Center for Healthy Families and Cultural Diversity is dedicated to leadership, advocacy, and excellence in promoting culturally responsive, quality health care for diverse populations. It began as a program focused primarily on multicultural education and training for health professionals but has grown to an expanded resource for technical assistance, consultation, and research/evaluation services.

Ethnomed
INTERNET ADDRESS: **http://www.ethnomed.org**

This Web site, through the University of Washington, offers excellent information on a wide range of cultures.

National Center for Cultural Competence (NCCC)
INTERNET ADDRESS: **http://nccc.georgetown.edu/index.html**

The mission of the National Center for Cultural Competence (NCCC) is to increase the capacity of health and mental health programs to design, implement, and evaluate culturally and linguistically responsive service delivery systems.

Transcultural Nursing Society
INTERNET ADDRESS: **http://www.tcns.org**

This is an excellent Web site, with links to other resources, information about membership in the Transcultural Nursing Society, and transcultural nursing workshops, courses, and certifications. The site also provides an online index for all articles published in the Journal of Transcultural Nursing since 1989.

References and Bibliography

Agency for Healthcare Research and Quality. (2010). *National healthcare disparities report.* Retrieved May 20, 2010, from http://www.ahrq.gov/qual/nhdr09/nhdr09.htm

Andrews, J. O., Felton, G., Wewers, M. E., Heath, J. (2004). Use of community health workers in research with ethnic minority women. *Journal of Nursing Scholarship, 36*(4), 358–365.

Andrews, M., & Boyle, J. (1999). *Transcultural concepts in nursing care.* Philadelphia, PA: Lippincott Williams & Wilkins.

Andrews, M., & Boyle, J. (2007). *Transcultural concepts in nursing care* (5th ed.). Philadelphia, PA: Lippincott Williams & Wilkins.

Barclay, J. S., Blackhall, L. J., & Tulsky, J. A. (2007). Communication strategies and cultural issues in the delivery of bad news. *Journal of Palliative Medicine, 10*(4), 958–977.

Buerhaus, P., Auerbach, D., & Staiger, D. (2009). The recent surge in nurse employment: Causes and implications. *Health Affairs, 28*(4), w657–w668.

Burkland, H. (2008). *Somali perspectives on child spacing*. Minnesota International Health Volunteers (MIHV). Retrieved June 20, 2010, from http://www.health.state.mn.us/divs/idepc/refugee/metrotf/childspacing.pdf

Calloway, S. J. (2009). The effect of culture on beliefs related to autonomy and informed consent. *Journal of Cultural Diversity, 16*(2), 68–70.

Campinha-Bacote, J. (2003). Many faces: Addressing diversity in health care. *Online Journal of Issues in Nursing, 8*(1), 3. Retrieved July 3, 2006, from http://nursingworld.org/ MainMenuCategories/ ANAMarketplace/ANAPerodicals/OJIN/TableofContents/Volume   82003/Num1Jan31_2003/ AddressingDiversityinHealthCare.aspx

Cintron, A., & Morrison, R. S. (2006). Pain and ethnicity in the United States: A systematic review. *Journal of Palliative Medicine, 9*(6), 1454–1473.

Cooper, L., Hill, M., & Powe, N. (2002). Designing and evaluating interventions to eliminate racial and ethnic disparities in health care. *Journal of General Internal Medicine, 17,* 477–486.

Degni, F., Pontinen, S., & Molsa, M. (2006). Somali parents' experiences of bringing up children in Finland: Exploring social–cultural change within migrant households. *Forum: Qualitative Social Research, 7*(3), 298–303. Retrieved June 20, 2010, from http://www.qualitative-research.net/fqs-texte/3-06/06-3-8-e.pdf

Ezenway, M. O., Ameringer, S, Ward, S. E., Serlin, R. C. (2006). Racial and ethnic disparities in pain management in the U.S. *Journal of Nursing Scholarship, 38*(3), 225–233.

Fadiman, A. (1997). *The spirit catches you and you fall down*. New York, NY: Noonday Press.

Giger, J. N., & Davidhizar, R. E. (1991). *Trans-cultural nursing: Assessment and intervention*. St. Louis, MO: Mosby-Year Book.

Giger, J. N., & Davidhizar, R. E. (2004). *Trans-cultural nursing: Assessment and intervention* (4th ed.). St. Louis, MO: C. V. Mosby.

Giger, J. N., Davidhizar, R. E., & Fordham, P. (2006). Multi-cultural and multi-ethnic considerations and advanced directives: Developing cultural competency. *Journal of Cultural Diversity, 13*(1), 3–9.

Grieco, E. M. (2009). *Race and Hispanic origin of the foreign-born population in the United States: 2007*. American Community Survey Reports, ACS-11. Washington, DC: U.S. Census Bureau.

Heineken, J., & McCoy, N. (2000). Establishing a bond with clients of different cultures. *Home Healthcare Nurse, 18*(1), 45–51.

Higgins, B. (2000). Puerto Rican cultural beliefs: Influence on infant feeding practices in western New York. *Journal of Trans-cultural Nursing, 11*(1), 19–30.

Indian Health Services. (2006). *Facts on Indian health disparities*. Retrieved April 16, 2010, from http://info.ihs.gov/Files/DisparitiesFacts-Jan2006.pdf

Johnstone, M., & Kanitsaki, O. (2009). Ethics and advance care planning in a culturally diverse society. *Journal of Transcultural Nursing, 20*(4), 405–416.

Kaiser Family Foundation. (2007). *Key facts: Race, ethnicity and medical care*. Retrieved June 15, 2010, from http://www.kff.org/minorityhealth/upload/6069–02.pdf

Kemp, C. (2005). Cultural issues in palliative care. *Seminars in Oncology Nursing, 21*(1), 44–52.

Leahy, M., & Svavarsdottir, E. K. (2009). Implementing family nursing: How do we translate knowledge into clinical practice? *Journal of Family Nursing, 15*(4), 445–460.

Leininger, M. M. (1970). *Nursing and anthropology: Two worlds to blend*. Columbus, OH: Greyden Press.

Leininger, M. M., & McFarland, M. (2002). *Transcultural nursing concepts, theories, research, practice*. New York, NY: McGraw Hill.

Leininger, M. M., & McFarland, M. (2006). *Culture care diversity and universality: A worldwide nursing theory*. Boston, MA: Jones & Bartlett.

Limb, G. E., & Hodge, D. R. (2010). Helping child welfare workers improve cultural competence by utilizing spiritual genograms with Native American families and children. *Children and Youth Services Review, 32*(2), 239–245.

Maier-Lorentz, M. M. (2008). Transcultural nursing: Its importance in nursing practice. *Journal of Cultural Diversity, 15*(1), 37–43.

McGrath, B. B., & Edwards, K. L. (2009). When family means more (or less) than genetics: The intersection of culture, family and genomics. *Journal of Transcultural Nursing, 20*(3), 270–277.

Moore, E., Ali, M., Graham, E., & Quan, L. (2010). Responding to a request: Gender-exclusive swims in a Somali community. *Public Health Reports, 125S*(3), 63–70.

National Center for Health Statistics. (2010). *Health, United States, 2009: With special feature on medical technology*. Hyattsville, MD: Author.

Office of Minority Health. (2005). *What is cultural competency*. Retrieved April 6, 2010, from http://minorityhealth.hhs.gov/templates/browse.aspx?lvl=2&lvlID=11

Office of Minority Health. (2007). *About the center of cultural and linguistic competence in health care*. Retrieved April 6, 2010, from http://minorityhealth.hhs.gov/templates/browse. aspx?lvl=2&lvlid=16

Purnell, L., & Paulanka, B. J. (2008). *Transcultural health care: A culturally competent approach*. Philadelphia, PA: F.A. Davis.

Racher, F. E., & Annis, R. C. (2007). Respecting culture and honoring diversity in community Practice. *Research and Theory for Nursing Practice, 21*(4), 255–270.

Schuchman, D. M., & McDonald, C. (2004). Somali mental health. *Bildhaan: An International Journal of Somali Studies, 4*(8). Retrieved April 6, 2010, from http://digitalcommons.macalester. edu/bildhaan/vol4/iss1/8

Simich, L., Maiter, S., Moorlag, E., & Ochoka, J. (2009). Taking culture seriously: Ethnolinguistic community perspectives on mental health. *Psychiatric RehabilitationJournal, 32*(3), 208–214.

Smedley, B. D., Stith-Butler, A., & Bristow, L. R. (Eds.). (2004). *In the nations' compelling interest: Ensuring diversity in the health care workforce*. Washington, DC: The National Academies Press.

Smedley, B. D., Stith, A. Y., & Nelson, A. R. (Eds.). (2003). *Unequal treatment: Confronting racial and ethnic disparities in health care*. Washington, DC: The National Academies Press.

Taylor, C., Lillis C., & LeMone, P. (2006). *Fundamentals of nursing: The art and science of nursing care*. Philadelphia, PA: Lippincott Williams & Wilkins.

U.S. Census bureau. (2008). *Press release*. Retrieved April 6, 2010, from http://www.census.gov/ Press- Release/www/releases/archives/population/012496.html

U.S. Department of Health and Human Services. (2010). *Healthy people 2020: The road ahead*. Washington, DC: U.S. Government Printing Office.

LEARNING ACTIVITIES

JOURNALING ACTIVITY 3-1

1. In your clinical journal, write about your own culture, including your values and beliefs about health and health care? Use the cultural tree (Fig. 3-4) to guide your thinking.

Consider:

   a. What cultural, racial, ethnic, and/or religious group do you identify with?

   b. What was the primary language spoken in your home as you grew up?

   c. What cultural practices or customs did your family engage in (i.e., specific foods, holidays or special celebrations, etc.)?

   d. What music did your family listen to? What type of art did you have in your home?

   e. What rules did your family have? How were those rules communicated?

   f. As a child, what special foods or medicines were you given when you were ill? Do you still use them?

   g. How do you decide when to seek health care, when you are sick, for preventive care?

   h. What causes you to become ill (viruses or bacteria, stress, life imbalance, spiritual issues, etc.)?

   i. Who helps you make health care decisions (your spouse or partner, your health care provider, an elder, a spiritual leader, extended family members, health insurer, etc.)?

   j. Have you ever experienced being in a place where no one else spoke your language or looked like you? What was it like? How did you feel? What did you do? What resources did you use?

2. Now partner with someone from another culture, race, or ethnicity than your own and discuss the questions from question 1.

   a. What are the similarities between your culture and theirs?

   b. What are the differences?

c. What did you find surprising?

d. How will this encounter inform your future practice?

3. Attend a church service, visit a community center or market, or dine at a restaurant in a cultural, racial, or ethnic community different than yours. Write about this encounter, where you are different from the "other" either ethnically, racially, or from life experience.

a. What previous experience have you had with someone from this cultural, racial, or ethnic group?

b. What assumptions or beliefs did you have as you entered into this experience?

c. Describe what the experience was like for you. How did you respond in the situation?

d. Were your assumptions accurate? (i.e., Was this experience what you expected? How was this experience similar or different to what you expected?)

e. What did you learn about yourself in this situation?

f. What would you do differently next time?

g. How did this encounter change your thinking about transcultural nursing?

LEARNING ACTIVITY 3-2

Watch the news and/or prime time television and read the newspaper and/or popular magazines over the course of a few weeks. In your clinical journal, write about your observations about how racial and ethnic individuals/groups/communities are portrayed. What stories make the news? What are the images that you see portrayed? How does the media influence our beliefs about cultural, racial, and/or ethnic individuals/groups?

LEARNING ACTIVITY 3-3

Make a list of various ethnic and minority or cultural groups (e.g., Native Americans, Asians, the elderly, Latinos, WASPs [White Anglo-Saxon Protestants], Jews) and write a stereotype you have or have heard about each group.

1. How does knowing these stereotypes exist make you more sensitive to clients about potential barriers in daily living and access to health care?

2. In what way can nurses break through stereotypes to deliver the best possible care?

LEARNING ACTIVITY 3-4

Consider the following Western cultural values and reflect on how these values may vary with other cultural groups:
Future orientation
Prevention
Time is money
Staying on schedule
Hard work
Achievement
Individualism
Assertiveness
Directness and openness
Openness of affection
Competition
Free market
Importance of training and education
Independence

Self sufficiency

Youth, being young

Follow these instructions in your clinical journal:

1. What other values and beliefs are prevalent in U.S. culture?

2. How are these values reflected in your everyday life?

3. How might these values influence your nursing practice?

4. How do those values differ from other cultural groups within your community?

5. Knowing that significant value orientation differences may exist between you and your clients in the community, what specific actions might you take that reflect culturally sensitive care?

LEARNING ACTIVITY 3-5

Choose a cultural group within your community and examine the health data for your community. What data are available for the cultural group of interest? What are the differences in morbidity and mortality rates for whites and members of the community you're interested in? What factors influence the health outcomes for the group of interest?

LEARNING ACTIVITY 3-6

Using the cultural assessment guide referenced in the chapter, conduct a cultural assessment with a client from a cultural group that differs from your own. What specific information did you learn that will guide your nursing actions related to (1) cultural preservation, (2) cultural accommodation, and (3) cultural repatterning?

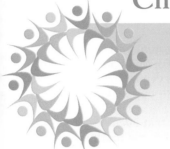

Chapter 4

Family Care

ROBERTA HUNT

Learning Objectives

1. Recognize the relationships among family structure, family roles, family functions, and culture.
2. Differentiate between the concept of the care of the family as the client and the care of the client in the context of the family.
3. Identify family developmental tasks throughout the life span.
4. Describe characteristics of healthy family functioning.
5. Discuss the health–illness continuum and family needs during illness.
6. Describe the role of the nurse in family assessment.
7. Identify the steps of planning, implementing, and evaluating family-focused community-based nursing.
8. Identify community agencies for family interventions at each level of prevention.

Key Terms

affective interventions
behavioral interventions
cognitive interventions
culturagram
developmental assessment
family developmental tasks
family functions
family health
family role

family structure
family systems theory
functional assessment
genogram
healthy family functioning
role conflict
structural family assessment
vulnerable populations

Chapter Topics

Significance of Family Care

Facilitating Family Coping

Families from Vulnerable Populations

Nursing Competencies and Skills in Family Care

Conclusions

The Nurse Speaks

For many years, the nursing students at our college had the opportunity to see patients in a pediatric primary care clinic. To meet the needs of working parents, this clinic was open during the week from 5:00 to 9:00 PM. One evening, one of my students completed the initial assessment with Ty, a 3-year-old boy. Ty was accompanied by his mother and father and two younger siblings.

Ty had a history of frequent otitis media and was being seen that evening for ear drainage, ear pain, and a low-grade fever. Ty was accustomed to the routine and allowed the student to do the initial assessment as he sat on his mother's lap.

The pediatrician did her evaluation and diagnosed otitis media of the right ear. Because the pediatrician was familiar with the family, she asked if they had kept the referral appointment she had made for Ty to see an ear, nose, and throat (ENT) specialist the month before. The mother, who spoke very little English, shook her head no.

After leaving the room, the pediatrician voiced her concern with us because she noted hearing impairment as a result of the otitis media. Next, she wrote a prescription for an oral antibiotic, which was filled at the clinic, and found a sample bottle of oral analgesic. The nursing student and I went back to see the family and to review the home care instructions. I encouraged the student to have the mother and father administer the first dose of antibiotic and analgesic before the family left the clinic. The student questioned why she would need to observe this as Ty had a long history of otitis media. I again encouraged her to observe the mother and father administer the medications. The student asked the parents to administer the first dose of medications while at the clinic. The parents agreed, so Ty's mother washed her hands, read each medication bottle, and precisely measured the exact amount to be administered. Next, Ty's mother placed him across her lap and attempted to administer the oral antibiotic into his right ear. In utter surprise, the nursing student stopped the mother before she was able to place the medication into Ty's ear. The student politely explained how the medications worked and the need to administer both medications orally. At this point, a staff person who could serve as an interpreter was able to visit with the family, and it was discovered that the parents had routinely given the oral medications into whichever ear was affected.

Through the assistance of the interpreter, the student reviewed the home care instructions with the parents. The parents verbalized their understanding of the route of administration, and each medication was correctly administered by the mother before leaving the clinic. The parents agreed to a follow-up by a community health nurse and the ENT specialist.

We all learned an important lesson that evening in the midst of a very busy pediatric clinic—that is, the value of making time for discharge teaching along with a return demonstration, especially when administering medications to children.

Susan O'Conner-Von, DNSc, RNC,
Associate Professor, School of Nursing
University of Minnesota, Minneapolis, Minnesota

Not only is the family the basic social unit in American society but it is also the most influential and dynamic entity. It has been the primary focus of nursing care in the community since the establishment of public health nursing in the late 19th century. The family performs a variety of key functions and has a central role in promoting and maintaining the health of its members.

What is a family? The definition of a family varies by culture and geographic regions of the world. In the United States, Canada, and some European countries, family is often defined as the nuclear family, while in most of the rest of the world, it includes extended family. In the last decade, the more traditional definition of family has been challenged. For the purposes of community-based care, family is defined by the individual and family receiving care. Nurses should ask clients to identify who they consider to be members of their family and, with the client's permission, include those persons in health care planning. In this way, families are empowered to define family as it applies to them and their situation. This approach sets the stage for a collaborative process of planning care.

Family health has numerous definitions. In this text, family health is defined as "a dynamic changing state of well-being, which includes the biological, psychological, spiritual, sociological, and cultural factors of individual members and the whole family system" (Kaakinen, Gedaly, Coehlo, & Hanson, 2010, p. 5). Understanding **family structure**, roles, and functions lays a foundation for comprehensive nursing care. Knowledge of **healthy family functioning** allows the nurse to identify family health needs and take appropriate actions when deemed necessary. In the current health care climate, the nurse must be cognizant of the needs, feelings, problems, and views of the family when collaborating with the family and other health care professionals to provide care.

Numerous models depict the relationship between nursing care and the family. Four approaches are often cited to illustrate ways to consider the family as it relates to the provision of nursing care. *Family as context is when the nurse plans the care of the individual in the context of the family.* This point of view considers the family as it relates to the recovery of the individual client. Consequently, the client is the focus, and the context is the family. Assessment, planning, implementation, and evaluation of care revolve around the care of the individual client considering the context of the family.

When the focus is on the family's potential impact on the recovery of the client, this determines how need for care is assessed, planned, implemented, and evaluated. This approach emphasizes how family structure, function, development stage, and interpersonal interactions influence the recovery of the client. While care focuses on improving the health status of the individual client, the nurse may target some care planning to address issues and strengths exhibited by the family.

When the family is seen as the client, the nurse focuses care on the family's collective health. This method centers on the family as a system as well as the unit of service. The nurse assesses the family, determines the family's strengths and health needs, and develops goals with the family that is intended to improve its collective health. The individual and family are concentrated on simultaneously with the emphasis on the interaction between family members.

If family is viewed as a component of society, the nurse considers the family as a basic or primary unit of society as well as a part of the larger community. This point of view allows the family to be seen as one of many institutions or social systems in the community that interacts with other institutions to receive, exchange, or give services. This perspective focuses on the interface between families and community agencies, which are a crucial aspect of community-based care.

This book incorporates concepts from all four models to guide nursing care to families that are presented in this chapter. However, family health will be considered primarily in the context of the impact of the family on the health of the individual. Nursing process skills will center on the health of the family as it relates to the recovery and maximizing the health potential of the individual client.

Significance of Family Care

Regardless of the approach to family care, it is evident the health status of the individual and that of the family are closely interrelated. The individual's health affects the family, and the family's health affects the client. The *Healthy People 2020* document, referred to in previous chapters, also includes information for the nurse on the significance of family care to individual health.

Healthy People provides a road map to improve the health of individuals, families, and communities in the United States. The goals of this initiative also apply to family health. The goals are

1. Attain higher quality, longer lives free of preventable disease, disability, injury, and premature death.
2. Achieve health equity, eliminate disparities and improve the health of all groups.
3. Create social and physical environments that promote good health for all.
4. Promote quality of life, healthy development, and healthy behaviors across all life stages.

Nurses working in community-based settings are well positioned to use the principles of family nursing to work toward these goals. Some Objectives of *Healthy People 2020* relates specifically to families or homes (Box 4-1).

CONCEPTS

Definitions of family have evolved over the past several decades as have the concepts of family structure, roles, and function.

Family Structure

Traditionally, the family has been defined as a nuclear family, with a mother, father, and two or more children. In fact, many different family structures exist. Table 4-1 lists the various family structures and their components; Figure 4-1 depicts different family structures.

Everyday life is stressful for many families in the United States. For example, the poverty rate is on the rise. In 2008, 19% of all children aged 0 to 17 (14.1 million) lived in poverty, an increase from 18% in 2007 and the highest rate since 1998. Racial disparity is seen in poverty rates among children in that 1 in 10 White, non-Hispanic children (11%);

BOX 4-1   Healthy People 2020: Family Implications

Increase the proportion of persons with hemoglobinopathies who receive care in a patient-/family-centered medical home.

Increase the proportion of elementary, middle, and senior high schools that have health education goals or objectives that address the knowledge and skills articulated in the National Health Education Standards (high school, middle, elementary).

Increase the proportion of children with special health care needs who receive their care in family-centered, comprehensive, coordinated systems.

Reduce the proportion of persons aged 18–44 years who have impaired fecundity (i.e., a physical barrier preventing pregnancy or carrying a pregnancy to term).

Increase the proportion of women with a family history of breast and/or ovarian cancer who receive genetic counseling.

Reduce the proportion of married couples whose ability to conceive or maintain a pregnancy is impaired.

Increase the proportion of sexually active women who received reproductive health services in the last 12 months.

Increase the number of states that set the income eligibility level for Medicaid-covered family planning services to at least the same level used to determine eligibility for Medicaid-covered, pregnancy-related care.

Increase the percentage of women in need of publicly supported contraceptive services and supplies who receive those services and supplies.

Source: U.S. Department of Health and Human Services, National Center for Health Statistics. (2010). *Health, United States, 2010*. Washington, DC: Author. Retrieved from http://healthypeople.gov/Default.htm.

Table 4-1 Family Structures	
Structure	**Participants**
Nuclear family	Married couple with children Unmarried, heterosexual, or same-sex couples with children
Nuclear dyad	Couple, married or unmarried; heterosexual or same sex
Single-parent family	One adult with children (separated, divorced, widowed, or never married)
Single adult	One adult
Multigenerational family	Any combination of the first four family structures
Kin network	Two or more reciprocal households (related by birth or marriage)

more than 1 in 3 Black children (35%); and nearly 1 in 3 Hispanic children (31%) live in poverty. Although most children who are living in poverty are White and not Hispanic or Black, the proportion of African American or Hispanic children in poverty is much higher than the proportion of White, non-Hispanic children.

Marked differences in income are apparent among the different family structures. Children in married-couple families are much less likely to be living in poverty than children living only with one parent, usually their mother. In 2008, 10% of children in married-couple families were living in poverty, compared with 42% in female-householder families.

Some trends in family health are encouraging. In 2008, 90% of children had health insurance coverage for at least some time during the year, up from 89% in 2007. The number of children without coverage at any time during the year was 7.3 million or 10% of all children. The percentage of children with public health insurance increased from 31% in 2007 to 33% in 2008 (Federal Interagency Forum on Children and Family Statistics, 2010).

Disparity is seen in health care coverage. In 2008, Hispanic children were less likely to have health insurance, compared with White, non-Hispanic, and Black children. Specifically, 83% of Hispanic children were covered by health insurance at some time during the year, compared with 93% of White, non-Hispanic children and 89% of Black children (Federal Interagency Forum on Children and Family Statistics, 2010). These statistics are important because poverty impacts the level of health and the quality of health care. Those living in poverty, and consequently receiving poor health care, represent a large number of families in the United States.

Family Roles

A **family role** is an expected set of behaviors associated with a particular family position. Family roles associated with a spouse/partner or parent include a wide variety of functions often influenced by culture. Roles can be formal or informal. Formal roles are defined by cultural expectations associated with the roles, such as partner, wife, husband, mother, father, or child. Examples of formal roles include breadwinner, housekeeper, child caretaker, financial manager, or cook. Informal roles are those that are casually acquired within a family. An example of an informal role would be the family member who plans the social schedule or who takes out the garbage.

Sick role is another role that may be seen in family members. Individuals learn health and illness behaviors in their family of origin and cultural affiliation, whether related to primary, secondary, or tertiary prevention of disease or injury; health promotion; or actions to reduce the effect of chronic disease. Each family, depending on family processes and learned behaviors related to illness, understand and act out the sick role differently.

Role conflict may occur when the demands of one role conflict with or contradict another. This may also transpire when one family member's expectations conflict with another's expectations. Role overload arises when an individual is confronted with too many role responsibilities at one time. Role strain or role overload stems from difficulties in defining and enacting family roles. Flexibility with family roles becomes particularly important in times of crises. Exacerbation of chronic conditions or hospitalization often requires shifts in family roles as the ill family member is unable to fulfill usual household tasks

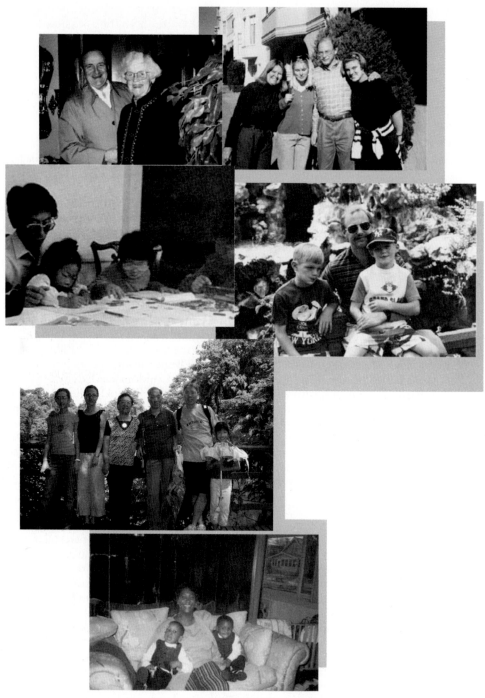

Figure 4-1 Various family structures.

and other family members have to assume new roles temporarily or permanently. In some situations, this may mean that a child takes responsibility for a parental role in the event that a parent becomes ill or is hospitalized. During illness, various family members' ability or willingness to take on different roles facilitates the family's adaptation or return to homeostasis. Role flexibility allows the family to provide support to a family member who is recovering from an illness or injury. Similarly, role flexibility may allow the ill family member to be more comfortable with giving up roles, which may, in some situations, facilitate recovery.

Family Functions

Family functions are defined as outcomes, or consequences, of family structure. They are the reason families exist. Functions are divided into several categories: affective, socialization, reproductive, economic, and health care, as shown in Figure 4-2.

The affective function of the family is defined as the family's ability to meet the psychological needs of family members. These needs include affection, understanding, and support, which rely on the ways family members relate to one another and to those outside of the immediate family boundaries. Families promote a sense of belonging and identity to their members, a purpose vitally important throughout the entire life cycle.

Socialization is the process of learning to adapt to life within the norms of a family and a community. This involves helping children become accustomed to the norms of the community and become productive members of society. This socialization process is built into all cultures. Specific functions include a variety of day-to-day family and social experiences that prepare children to assume adult roles such as learning the customs of dress, hygiene, and preparing and eating food. However, there is wide variability in the ways that families attend to physical, emotional, and economic needs of children, and these patterns are influenced by the historical point in time and larger society.

The reproductive function is procreation. In the past, it was thought of as the family's provision of recruits for society to ensure the continuity of the intergenerational community. However, as cultural prescriptions change, families change. Families now have more means to control reproduction, both to prevent conception and through reproductive technology to facilitate or create conception. In addition, adoption, both international and

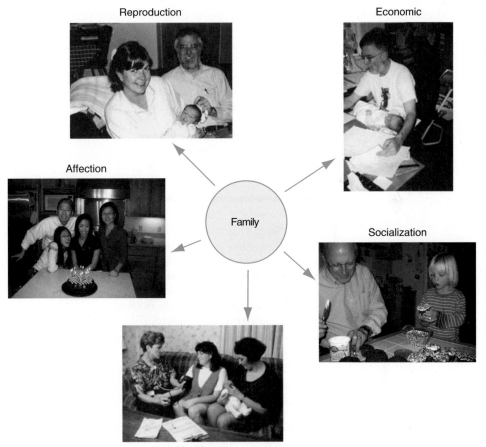

Figure 4-2 Basic family functions.

domestic, has become a more accepted means of becoming a parent. This transformation creates numerous roles and issues for families, which are of concern to nurses working in community-based settings.

Economic functions encompass the allocation of adequate resources for family members. This entails the provision of sufficient income to provide for basic necessities as well as the allocation of these resources to all family members, especially those unable to provide for themselves. During the end of the 20th century, the most observable changes in family function related to economics. In the last three decades, a lower mean wage that has come from a shift from an industrial to a service economy requires dual earners in most families to keep pace with the rising cost of living. For many families, financial vulnerability and bankruptcy have increased even in the middle class. Social pressures may impact many families' ability to adequately meet their economic needs. Add the costs that occur with chronic conditions or hospitalization to those already at risk, and the extent to which families may experience profound stress is obvious.

Providing for health care and physical necessities is the final family function. Physical care is the provision of material necessities, such as food, clothing, and shelter. Family health care includes health and lifestyle practices, such as nutrition, chemical use and abuse, recreation, and exercise and sleep practices. As the cost of health care has risen beyond the reach of many Americans, many families are unable to fulfill the function of providing access to care. With the Affordability Care Act of 2010, it is hoped that more families will have access to care. In Canada and all other large industrialized countries, all citizens have access to health care through government-provided services.

Family functions can also be viewed in relation to Maslow's hierarchy of needs (Fig. 4-3). According to Maslow, the family must first meet physiologic needs (e.g., food, fluids, shelter, sleep) before members can consider any other opportunities in life. Maslow's

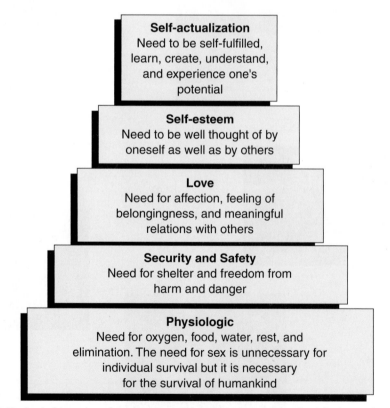

Figure 4-3 Maslow's hierarchy of needs. According to Maslow, basic physiologic needs must be met before the person can move on to higher-level needs. Adapted from Maslow, A. H. (1954). *Motivation and personality.* New York: Harper & Row.

theory is a very important concept when working with families in the community. For example, following a family assessment, the nurse may conclude that the family's need is to learn more about parenting, which falls into the category of safety needs and love and belonging. When the nurse asks the family if they are interested in learning about the importance of reading to their child and the parent appears not to be interested, the nurse may want to assess if the family has unmet physiological needs. If the nurse asks the family what is their number one concern, they may state "worry about whether or not there will be enough money to purchase food for the rest of the month." When physiologic needs remain unmet, families are unlikely to see higher needs as a priority.

Safety needs include both the physiologic and the psychological safety of family members. This is seen as a young child experiences safety in the family when the environment is sufficiently structured to protect the child from harm. Similarly, adolescents feel safe in an environment that allows freedom and provides responsibility and structure, while for adults, physical safety includes living in a safe community. Psychological safety originates from living in an environment without threat of verbal or physical abuse. There are always numerous safety needs at each stage of the family life cycle.

Another family function is meeting needs for love and belonging, which aligns with Maslow's level 3. Every human being needs meaningful relationships with other people. In classic research by Spitz (1945), two groups of infants and children were studied. Both groups received excellent physical care, but the members of the first group were talked to, held, and caressed. The second group received little demonstrative affection. There was a higher mortality rate as well as impaired development among the infants and children of the second group who received no physical affection. Although there have been numerous studies since this research that have demonstrated the relationship between affection and love and physical vitality, this simple study elegantly illustrates this point.

The fulfillment of esteem needs is also a family function, which is also found in Maslow's hierarchy. Self-esteem comes from feeling that we are valued by those around us. Family members may assist one another to feel good about themselves through acceptance and approval. Self-actualization is being "true to oneself," to fulfill one's potential. It is not about what one chooses to do in life but how one feels about that choice. To joyfully do in life what one wants and is suited to do is self-actualization.

Family Systems Theory

The identification of the family as the unit of care is an emerging trend in **family systems theory**. Family systems theory is considered the most influential of all family social science frameworks. It defines family as a collection of people who are integrated, interacting, and interdependent where the actions of one member influence the actions of other members. The family system has a boundary that is selectively permeable according to the family's wishes, so items such as material goods, people, and information are allowed in or out according to the perceived needs of the family. Families with closed boundaries in one area may, for instance, be reluctant to use community resources. When family boundaries are semipermeable and rules are flexible, families will have a greater capacity to periodically seek and receive assistance during times of crisis.

After a crisis or during a transition from one developmental stage to another, the family system may experience disequilibrium. This imbalance causes a large amount of energy to be expended by individual family members in an attempt to cope with the discomfort typical of the transitions from one stage to another. System theory states that systems tend to move to a state of equilibrium, so it follows that families generally attempt to return to the state of equilibrium prior to the crisis. Knowledge about family systems theory allows the nurse to assist the family to return to their normal state of functioning. In some cases, the family may be moved to a higher level of health following a crisis.

The nurse considers the actions of family members as they apply to the health of the individual client. Family boundaries can be assessed to determine the likelihood that the family will use needed services. Similarly, disequilibrium of the family system as it pertains to the client can also be assessed with strategies developed to return the family to normalcy.

FAMILY HEALTH

The Health–Illness Continuum

The family's structure, roles, ability to fulfill family functions, culture, and developmental tasks all affect the way the family functions. Adaptation depends on each of these areas when a family member is ill or injured, whether associated with physical, mental, or social well-being. An individual's place on the wellness–illness continuum affects all members of the family and all interactions within the family.

Family structure also affects the health recovery of an individual. In a family with two adult members, recovery may be different from that in a family headed by one adult. In some families, there may be two adult members but neither are competent to fulfill all the role functions. Certainly, when an individual lives alone, there is always a greater need to tap extended family and friends for support and assistance than when the family has at least one other competent adult member.

The capacity for members of a family to fulfill the requirement of roles may have an impact on the health recovery of the individual, as the health of the individual often influences one's ability to carry out family roles. When a family member is hospitalized or acutely ill, it may be difficult to find the energy to address the family's basic physical necessities and care. Examples include the inability to grocery shop, provide meals, maintain a regular bedtime, or wash laundry.

Several variables impact the amount of disruption to a family when there is illness or injury. First is the timing of the illness or injury in the life cycle. This may be considered from the point of view of the individual developmental stage of the impaired family member and all other family members as well as the developmental stage of the family. If several persons in the family are in transition from one individual developmental stage to another, it may be even more difficult for the family to deal with an illness or injury. Likewise, a family may experience more disruption from illness or hospitalization if they are currently moving from one family developmental stage to another.

The nature and extent of the illness or injury is another variable that impacts the amount of disruption to the family. An incapacitating injury such as a major head trauma or a spinal cord injury would have more influence on family functioning compared to hip replacement. The roles of the ill family member predict the amount of family disruption. If the sole breadwinner of a family sustains a major head injury and is never able to return to the workforce, the consequences for the family are likely to be more dire than those from a head injury to a person retired from work and living in a long-term care facility.

Family Needs Before and During Illness and at End of Life

Attending to family needs during and after illness or serious injury have been recognized for some time as an important role for nurses. Regardless of the setting, studies show that nurses are often in the best position to meet families' needs during these times (Browning & Warren, 2006). The following section outlines various ways nurses can assess and intervene with families before, during, and following illness or injury or at the end of life.

There are some practical steps that every family can take to be prepared prior to the serious illness or injury of a family member. The nurse can coach families to consider these suggestions. First, families should pay attention to the health insurance plan and choose one that offers (1) a deductible they can afford to spend, (2) a home care provision, (3) a medication plan, and (4) doctors and hospitals they can trust. Second, during an annual exam, family members should talk to their primary physician to establish rapport and sign an advance directive. Next, the family's legal affairs should be in order including a will, power of attorney, 401 Ks, individual retirement accounts (IRAs), life insurance, care titles, and house titles (Wagner-Cox, 2005).

Nurses in each setting along the continuum of care have important responsibilities to provide family-centered care. When families have loved ones on the medical–surgical units, nurses have numerous opportunities to provide family-centered care. This begins with the simple intervention of listening to the patient and family members' concerns. Nurses should respect and support family coping mechanisms and caregiving behaviors while recognizing the uniqueness of each family. Families benefit from information about options and assistance with decision making but also need time to visit privately with one another. Nurses may also facilitate family conferences. Information should be clarified and resources appropriate for the needs the family has identified. Positive nurse–family relationships are necessary throughout all phases of care (Kaakinen et al., 2010).

For decades, the needs of family members with a loved one in the intensive care unit (ICU) have been studied, but progress to create more family-centered care in adult critical care and medical–surgical units has been slow (Latour & Haines, 2007). The classic research on this topic by Molter in 1974 identified that families need hope, health care providers who care about the patient, a place to wait, daily and ongoing updates on change of status and prognosis, questions answered honestly, explanations in understandable terms, and to see the loved one frequently.

Intensive-care nurses also facilitate family-centered care by providing information to family members and allowing families to see their loved ones frequently. It is also important to provide reassurance to family members and assist them to address their own self-care needs (Browning & Warren, 2006). Other family intervention strategies that are underutilized in supporting families with loved ones in the ICU include facilitating shared decision making, ICU family rounds, family conferences, family progress journals, as well as having a family ICU nurse specialist on the unit (Kaakinen et al., 2010).

In cases where the client's condition is terminal, the nurse can guide families to appreciate the importance of preparing emotionally and psychologically for death and dying by talking about the client's and family's preferences. This preparation is best accomplished through a series of conversations between spouses or partners, siblings, parents, and adult children. Creating a thoughtful plan requires more than one frantic discussion.

Family Needs for Chronic Conditions

Families require assistance from nursing staff across the continuum of care during the course of a lifelong chronic condition. Most of the needs discussed in the last section along with the suggested interventions also apply to chronic conditions. However, there are some needs and interventions that are particularly pertinent for families with a member with a chronic condition. Obviously, these needs vary by the nature of the illness. For example, the needs, preferences, and knowledge base of family members of an adult with chronic mental illness may be varied. Families benefit from ongoing teaching and support tailored to meet the needs of individual members. There are numerous barriers associated with chronic mental illness including stigma. These issues may require continued effort on the part of the nurse to understand and address family needs and potential barriers to participation in family services (Drapalski et al., 2008).

Culture and ethnicity is another variable that influences family needs during the course of a chronic condition. Culture and ethnicity is the lens through which families see and experience the world as well as view health, so it follows that family needs and appropriate nursing interventions are influenced by the family's cultural values. This is seen in research findings that, among African American parents with chronically ill children, there is a significant relationship between positive parental coping patterns and spirituality. It is important for nurses to recognize the ethnic and cultural aspects of coping and spirituality among parents of children with chronic health conditions (Allen & Marshall, 2010).

In any setting, it is essential, when a family member experiences an acute or chronic illness or injury, that the nurse assists the rest of the family to mobilize their support system. These resources may be friends and extended family that can be counted on to listen, assist them to face their fears, and encourage them to be kind to themselves and the rest of the family. Each individual family member will have his or her own manner of coping and benefits from employing healthy coping mechanisms.

Facilitating Family Coping

Although the nursing profession's attention to understanding family needs has increased, over the last decade, it remains important to identify and tailor strategies to assist all families to cope throughout a course of illness and recovery (Paul & Rattray, 2008). Nurses play a critical role in facilitating family coping.

Healthy coping is achieved by assisting family members to become more resilient by interacting in ways that optimize each family member's abilities and strengths. Hope seems to be a prerequisite for coping during a critical illness or injury, and instilling hope may have an empowering effect on a family's coping ability. Important hope-inspiring strategies are set in motion from religious and/or spiritual activities, support from significant others, positive relationships with caregivers, devotion to the patient, optimism, proximity to the patient, talking to others, and distraction (Paul & Rattray, 2008). Hope for the future fosters resilience (Black & Lobo, 2008).

Over the last decade, an increasingly important realm of family nursing practice is the identification, enhancement, and promotion of family resiliency. Successful coping of family members in crisis enables them to flourish with warmth, support, and cohesion and is a sign of family resilience. A review of recent research by Black and Lobo (2008) identified recurrent and prominent attributes among resilient, healthy families. These include a positive outlook, spirituality, family member accord, flexibility, communication, financial management, time together, mutual recreational interests, routines and rituals, and social support. When caring for families in community settings, nurses can use these attributes of healthy families to promote resilience. This approach is based on the belief that all families have inherent strengths and the potential for growth. In all assessment, planning, and intervention, if nurses focus on family strengths, these can become the foundation for continued growth and positive change in a family and a society. By first looking to family strengths, capabilities, previous successful coping mechanisms, and current responses to stress, the nurse lays the foundation for planning interventions to facilitate resilience in families.

Families From Vulnerable Populations

Some families may have specific needs beyond those seen in the situations discussed so far in this chapter. Sometimes these families are referred to as at risk or **vulnerable populations** because they have unique needs often inadequately met in current health care systems. These include, but are not limited to, families without permanent housing, caregivers, the elderly, adolescents, and racially and ethnically diverse populations. Recently active duty service members and their families may also be considered vulnerable. To meet the particular needs of these groups, nurses need additional clinical experience and continuing education. In subsequent chapters in this text, there is additional information on providing nursing care for vulnerable populations.

Nursing Competencies and Skills in Family Care

As nursing has moved away from a task orientation, it has adopted a more holistic view of clients as individuals with a life beyond their illness, injury, and hospitalization. A holistic perspective allows the nurse to address the cadre of needs families experience across the continuum of care when lives have been irrevocably changed by the illness of one member. Providing nursing care to families is a logical development of the holistic approach to the care of the client and is an important cornerstone of nursing practice.

The essential considerations when caring for individuals in the context of their families are as follows:

- One part of the family cannot be understood in isolation from the rest of the system.
- A family's structure and organization cannot be understood in isolation from the rest of the system.
  - A change in one part of a family system affects change in other parts.
- Communication patterns between family members are essential in the functioning of the family.

Competence in using the nursing process with families requires different skills and knowledge as compared to the care of the individual client.

FAMILY NURSING PROCESS

Assessment, as it applies to the client within the context of the family in community-based nursing, strives to determine the client and family needs and strengths to plan and intervene. When the nurse uses an approach that considers the family's impact on the recovery of the client, he or she will assess, plan, implement, and evaluate care that centers on all individual family members as the foreground with the individual as the background. Influences that family structure, function, development stage, and interpersonal interactions have on the recovery of the client must be considered. While assessment, planning, implementation, and evaluation of care focuses on improving the health status of the individual client, the nurse may target some care planning on incorporating strengths exhibited by the family. The intent of these actions is to improve the health status of the individual client through a collaborative process. Assessment begins with the family interview.

FAMILY ASSESSMENT

The Family Interview

The same principles used when interviewing an individual client apply to a family interview. Effective communication begins by establishing a trusting relationship with the family. A short period of informal conversation at the start of the interview may put those present at ease. It is helpful to have all the family members present and create a comfortable environment to encourage participation from everyone.

Numerous family assessment tools are available. A short family assessment form is shown in Assessment Tools 4-1. Many agencies have a standard form intended for a family interview.

Assessment Tools 4-1
Family Assessment Guide

Family Members

Member	Birth Date	Sex	Marital Status	Education

Genogram

Ecomap

Assessment of Family Strengths

What strengths does your family have?

_____

_____

What special abilities or capabilities do you have as a family?

_____

_____

Discuss what your family has done in the past to cope with difficult times.

_____

_____

Talk about how you are currently coping with the situation your family is facing.

_____

_____

Identify how your family shows signs of resilience. (Show Table 4-2 to the family.)

_____

Development Assessment

What is this family's developmental stage?

_____

Discuss how the family is meeting the tasks at this stage.

_____

_____

_____

Does, or will, the client's health problem interrupt the family's ability to meet the developmental tasks? If yes, describe how it interrupts it.

_____

_____

_____

Functional Assessment

Discuss how the family is or is not meeting the individual member's need for affection, love, and understanding.

_____

_____

_____

Discuss how the family is or is not meeting the member's need for physical necessities and care.

_____

_____

_____

_____

Describe the family's economic resources or lack of the economic resources necessary to provide for the basic needs of the family.

_____

_____

_____

Describe how the family is or is not meeting the function of reproduction as defined by the family.

_____

Discuss how the family is meeting the family function of socialization.

_____

Describe how the family is fulfilling the function to socialize children to become productive members of society.

_____

_____

_____

Describe how the family attempts to actively cope with problems.

_____

_____

_____

_____

Assessment of Presence of Characteristics of a Healthy Family

Explain how communication between members is or is not open, direct, and honest. Discuss how feelings and needs are shared.

_____

_____

_____

Give examples of how family members express self-worth with integrity, responsibility, compassion, and love to and for one another.

_____

_____

_____

Discuss what leads you to believe that family rules are known to all members.

_____

_____

_____

Describe if and how the family makes rules clear and flexible. Give an example of why you think that the family allows or does not allow individual members freedom.

_____

_____

_____

Give examples of how the family has regular links to society that demonstrate trust and friendship.

_____

_____

_____

Provide examples of various groups and clubs the family belongs to.

_____

_____

An assessment may determine if a family's response to the current situation indicates that they are adapting to the stressors of the situation. This permits the nurse to identify problem areas and the need for additional assessment and referral. For example, after a family interview, the nurse may encourage family members to share their individual concerns with the entire family, and one family member may share his or her concerns about family communication. With the entire family present, the nurse may invite each member to share observations about how the family is communicating. Based on this discussion, the nurse may then suggest that the family explore this topic with a nurse practitioner, social worker, public health nurse, physician, clergy member, or counselor. Family needs and strengths identified from the family interview provide a basis for an intervention. This

Table 4-2 Factors and Characteristics of Resilience in Families and Potential Nursing Interventions

Resilience Factor	Family Characteristic	Potential Nursing Interventions
Positive outlook	Confidence and optimism; repertoire of approaches; sense of humor	Counseling • Acknowledge present behaviors that demonstrate positive outlook • Model confidence, optimism, and humor Health teaching • Use family's positive outlook, confidence, and sense of humor as the need for health teaching is assessed, planned, implemented, and evaluated Referral • Refer family to services that accentuate the positive qualities of families, such as teaching relationship patterns, interpersonal skills, and competencies
Spirituality	Shared value system that gives meaning to stressors	Counseling • Encourage identification of shared values and ways to tap into resources related to these values Health teaching • Use family strengths in spirituality as the need for health teaching is assessed, planned, implemented, and evaluated Referral • Provide information about community resources that may allow for expression of stated values
Family member accord	Cohesion; nurturance; authoritative discipline; avoidance of hostile parental conflict	Counseling • Encourage identification of nurturance and cohesiveness and ways to tap into related resources Health teaching • Build teaching on family strengths of nurturance and conflict management • Use family strengths of cohesiveness and nurturance as the need for health teaching is assessed, planned, implemented, and evaluated Referral • Refer family to services that accentuate the positive qualities of families to enhance cohesiveness, healthy relationship patterns, parenting
Flexibility	Stable family roles with situational and developmental adjustments	Counseling • Encourage identification of present behaviors that demonstrate flexibility and ways to use this trait • Model flexibility Health teaching • Build teaching on family strengths of flexibility • Use family strengths of flexibility as health teaching is assessed, planned, implemented and evaluated Referral • Refer family to services that accentuate the positive qualities of families to enhance stable family roles and flexibility

Resilience Factor	Family Characteristic	Potential Nursing Interventions
Table 4-2 Factors and Characteristics of Resilience in Families and Potential Nursing Interventions *(Continued)*		
Family communication	Clarity; open emotional expression; and collaborative problem solving	Counseling • Acknowledge present behaviors that demonstrate clear, open expression of emotions and collaborative problem solving • Model clear, open communication acceptance of the expression of emotion and collaborative problem solving Health teaching • Use family strengths in communication as the need for health teaching is assessed, planned, implemented, and evaluated Referral • Refer family to services that accentuate the positive qualities of families, such as collaborative problem solving, open expression of emotions, and interpersonal skills and competencies
Financial management	Sound money management; family warmth despite financial problems	Counseling • Encourage identification of family strengths related to sound money management Health teaching • Use family strengths in sound money management as the need for health teaching is assessed, planned, implemented, and evaluated • Build teaching on family strengths related to sound money management Referral • Refer family to services that accentuate the positive qualities of families to enhance sound money management
Family time	Makes the most of togetherness with daily tasks	Counseling • Encourage the identification, planning, and resource allocation that make the most of family time Health teaching • Use family strengths in making the most of togetherness with daily tasks as the need for health teaching is assessed, planned, implemented, and evaluated • Build teaching on family strengths related to completing daily tasks Referral • Refer family to services that value and emphasize families spending time together
Shared recreation	Develops children's social and cognitive skills; cohesion and adaptability	Counseling • Encourage identification, planning, and resource allocation of recreation that family enjoys doing together Health teaching • Use family strengths in developing child social and cognitive skills, cohesion, and adaptability as the need for health teaching is assessed, planned, implemented, and evaluated

Continued on following page

Table 4-2 Factors and Characteristics of Resilience in Families and Potential Nursing Interventions *(Continued)*		
Resilience Factor	**Family Characteristic**	**Potential Nursing Interventions**
		• Build teaching on family strengths related to shared recreational time Referral • Refer family to services that accentuate the positive qualities of families to enhance skills in developing child social and cognitive skills, cohesion, and adaptability
Routines and rituals	Embedded activities that promote close family relationships; maintenance even during family crisis	Counseling • Encourage the identification of activities that promote close family relationship and ways to maintain these routines and rituals through illness or crisis Health teaching • Build teaching on family strengths of routines and rituals • Use family strengths in routines and rituals as the need for health teaching is assessed, planned, implemented, and evaluated Referral • Refer family to services that accentuate the positive qualities of families to develop and enhance the use of routine and rituals
Support network	Individual, familial, and community networks to share resources; particularly important for families in poverty	Counseling • Encourage the identification of a support network and ways to tap into related resources Health teaching • Build teaching on family strengths of support networks • Use family strengths in support networks as the need for health teaching is assessed, planned, implemented, and evaluated Referral • Refer family to services that accentuate the positive qualities of families to enhance the use of support networks

Adapted from Black, K., & Lobo, M. (2008). A conceptual review of family resilience factors. *Journal of Family Nursing, 14*(1), 33–55. Retrieved from CINAHL Plus with Full Text database.

could include a referral to a family therapist or social worker with special expertise in family therapy.

The type of family assessment used depends on the focus of the treatment provided by the agency employing the nurse and the knowledge level of the care provider, as illustrated in Figure 4-4. Family members are asked questions regarding the client and the client's condition.

The first step is to assist families to identify what they see as their family's strengths. Families may be encouraged to make a list of family strengths and put the list in a visible place in their home. Strengths may be considered in light of how they may enhance family resilience. When assessing the family as the client, the goal is to determine the family's potential impact on the recovery of the client. Although this is especially a priority when the family's functioning is clearly impeding the recovery, it is always essential to

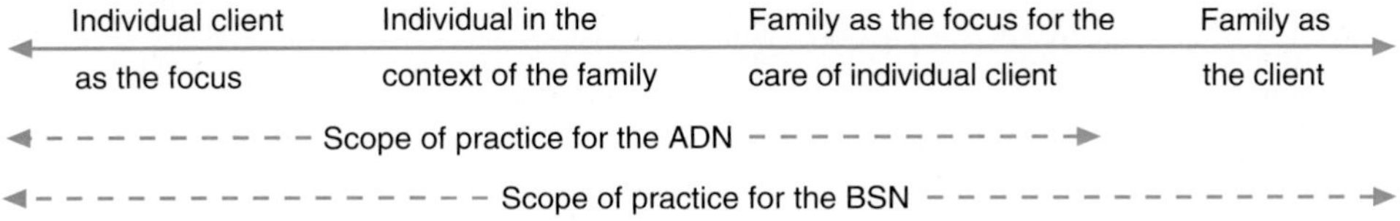

Individual client	Individual in the	Family as the focus for the	Family as
as the focus	context of the family	care of individual client	the client

◄ – – – – – – – – – Scope of practice for the ADN – – – – – – – – – – ►

◄ – – – – – – – – – – – – – – Scope of practice for the BSN – – – – – – – – – – – – – – ►

Figure 4-4 Focus of nursing care for individuals and families.

family-centered care. Figure 4-5 illustrates the levels that are necessary in a comprehensive family assessment. Overall, the intent of assessing the family is to analyze the client's potential for recovery and self-care, given the familial conditions. To facilitate the client's return to the highest level of wellness, the circumstances in which the client lives must be considered.

Models of Family Assessment

Developmental Assessment

Possible trouble spots for family functioning during a health crisis may be considered by completing a family **developmental assessment** focusing on normal **family developmental tasks**. As individuals have development stages that they must go through to move to the next stage of development, so do families. Duvall (1977) developed a commonly used theory of development stages of family life as it relates to nursing care. According to Duvall, there are predictable stages within the life cycle of every family; each stage includes distinct family developmental tasks (Table 4-3). Stages of the family life are useful when implementing care for families as roles, developmental stages, and tasks change over time. This model can be used as a guide to assessment by following these steps:

1. Determine the family's developmental stage. This can be done by determining the age of the oldest child in the family and correlating it with the level in Table 4-3.
2. Consider the family members' health problems in the context of the tasks in their developmental stage. Is it likely that health conditions will interrupt the family's developmental tasks?
3. Determine if family members are meeting the tasks at their levels of development.
4. Identify the nursing interventions that would assist the family in meeting these developmental tasks.

Because of the wide variety of family structures, this model has been criticized because not all families fit neatly into this family stage theory. For individuals who do not marry, remain childless, divorce, and remarry to form a blended family or are in same-sex unions, the stages are viewed differently. In families in which the stages of the family life cycle are

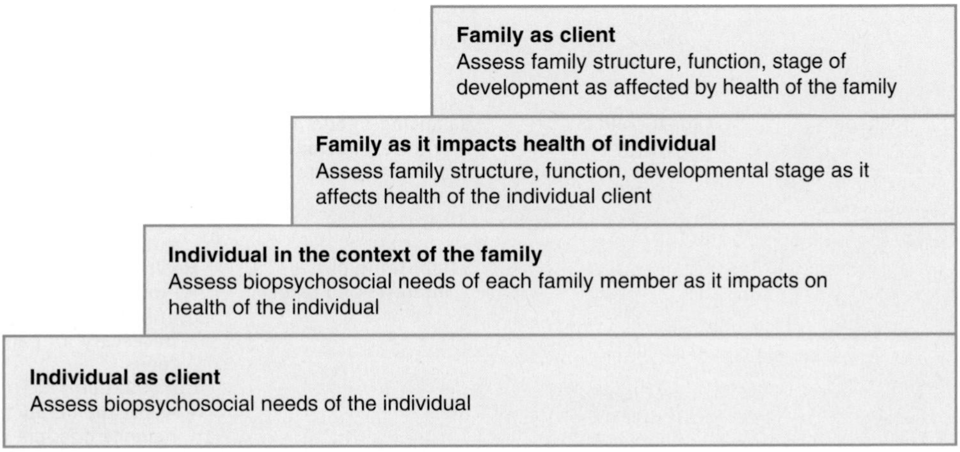

Family as client
Assess family structure, function, stage of development as affected by health of the family

Family as it impacts health of individual
Assess family structure, function, developmental stage as it affects health of the individual client

Individual in the context of the family
Assess biopsychosocial needs of each family member as it impacts on health of the individual

Individual as client
Assess biopsychosocial needs of the individual

Figure 4-5 Levels of a comprehensive family assessment.

Table 4-3 Stages of the Family Life Cycle

Stage of Family Life Cycle	Scope of the Stage	Stage Critical Developmental Tasks	Nursing Interventions
Forming a partnership	Couple makes commitment to one another	Establishing a mutually satisfying marriage Fitting into the kin network	Counseling ■ Identification of family strengths ■ Identification of family stressors to enhance capacity for self-care and coping ■ Assist in developing a strong relationship
Childbearing	Pregnancy of first child to child who is 30 mos old	Adjusting to infants and encouraging their development Establishing a satisfying family life for both child and parent	Counseling ■ Anticipatory guidance before the birth of the infant ■ Increase capacity for self-care and coping with the birth of the first child Health teaching ■ Provide information to enhance knowledge base necessary for new role responsibilities
Preschool	Oldest child is 2½–6 y	Adapting to the needs of preschool children in growth-producing ways Coping with lack of privacy and energy	Counseling ■ Anticipatory guidance as the child goes through developmental stages ■ Increase capacity for self-care and coping as the child develops ■ Encourage partners to make time for each other Health teaching ■ Provide information to enhance knowledge base necessary for new role responsibilities
School age	Oldest child is 7–12 y	Fitting into age-appropriate community activities Encouraging the children's achievement	Counseling ■ Anticipatory guidance as the child moves through developmental landmarks ■ Increase capacity for self-care and coping Health teaching ■ Provide information to enhance knowledge base necessary for new role responsibilities
Teenage	Oldest child is 13–20 y	Balancing freedom with responsibility as teens mature and emancipate Establishing outside interests and career	Counseling ■ Anticipatory guidance ■ Increase capacity for self-care and coping as the child becomes more autonomous Health teaching ■ Provide information to enhance knowledge base necessary for parents of teens Consultation ■ Assist the family to balance freedom with responsibility as teens mature and emancipate

Table 4-3 Stages of the Family Life Cycle *(Continued)*

Stage of Family Life Cycle	Scope of the Stage	Stage Critical Developmental Tasks	Nursing Interventions
Launching center	First child leaving home to last child leaving home	Assisting young adults to work, attend school or military, marry, with appropriate rituals	Counseling • Increase capacity for self-care and coping as the child leaves home and the couple relationship changes Health education • Provide information to enhance knowledge base necessary to successfully launch children
Middle-aged parents	Empty nest to retirement	Rebuilding marital bond Cultivating kin ties with younger and older family	Counseling • Increase capacity for coping as the couple rebuilds the relationship and identifies mutual interests
Aging family	Retirement to moving out of family home	Coping with loss and living alone Adapting to retirement and aging	Counseling • Increase capacity for coping with loss of health status, friends, sibling, and partner and living alone Health teaching • Provide information on options in the community for resources and recreation and alternative living options

disrupted, the emotional processes and issues relating to transition and development also differ from those set out in Duvall's stages.

Disruption of the family cycle because of a divorce requires additional steps to be taken to restabilize the family. In the postdivorce phase, a single custodial parent experiences a different emotional process and transition than does a noncustodial parent. The developmental issues differ as well (Table 4-4). There is now evidence that, postdivorce, many women experience financial stress, which, in turn, has a negative effect on physical health and morbidity (Coleman & Glenn, 2010). Further, the stress of divorce directly influences children, with a minority reporting negative longer term outcomes such as socioeconomic disadvantage, behavioral problems, poor educational achievement, and physical and emotional health problems. Family assessment must regard the impact that divorce may have on families over time. These families may have needs for disease prevention and health promotion interventions that differ from other families.

In families where there is a remarriage, emotional transitions or developmental issues may be experienced (Table 4-5). Emotional transitions include attaining an adequate emotional separation from the previous marriage and accepting and dealing with fears about forming a new family. When beginning a blended family, members must find the time and patience necessary to permit another emotional adjustment. Resolving the feelings of attachment to a previous spouse and accepting the new family model require transitions as developmental issues are also seen in each phase of the new marriage. The needs of the individual family members, family developmental tasks, and family functions must mesh.

Meeting family developmental tasks is not necessarily easy for families under normal circumstances with predictable day-to-day stressors. The conflict that often occurs in families with adolescents illustrates this point. Typically, adolescents are attempting to break away from parents and spend more time with friends than family. Yet, parents may wish

Table 4-4 When Families Divorce

Phase	Emotional Responses	Transitional Issues
1. Stressors leading to marital differences	Reveal the fact that the marriage has major problems	Acknowledge the fact that the marriage has major problems
2. Decision to divorce	Recognize the inability to resolve marital differences	Admit one's own contribution to the failed marriage
3. Planning the dissolution of the family system	Negotiate viable arrangements for all family members	Cooperate on custody, visitation, and financial issues Inform and deal with extended family members and friends' responses
4. Separation	Mourn losses associated with separating family Work on resolving attachment to spouse	Develop coparental arrangements/relationships Monitor children's adjustment to new living arrangements Restructure living arrangements Adapt to living apart Realign relationship with extended family and friends Begin to rebuild own social network
5. Divorce	Continue working on emotional recovery by overcoming hurt, anger, or guilt	Give up fantasies of reunion Stay connected with extended families Rebuild and strengthen own social network
6. Postdivorce	Separate feelings about ex-spouse from parenting role Prepare for the possibility of changes in custody as children get older; be open to their needs	Create flexible and generous visitation arrangements for children and noncustodial parent and extended family members Be open to possibilities of changing custody arrangements as children get older

Adapted from Allender, J. A., Rector, C., & Warner, K. D. (2010). *Community health nursing: Concepts and practice* (7th ed., p. 490). Philadelphia, PA: Lippincott Williams & Wilkins.

for the adolescent to participate as more of an adult in family activities. This conflict may be compounded, for instance, when family members need adequate rest regularly to provide health care to an ill family member, but the adolescent's need is to stay out late and get support and approval from peers.

Structural Family Assessment

Structural family assessment considers family composition. A structural assessment defines the immediate family members, their names, ages, and the relationship among those who live together. **Genograms** and ecomaps are valuable tools to actively engage families in their own care while providing caregivers with visual diagrams of the current family situation. A genogram is constructed to clarify the relationship and information about each member of the family. Symbols often used for the genogram are shown in Figure 4-6.

Genograms can be helpful to nurses in many settings. A nurse working in a clinic or hospital can quickly sketch a genogram and identify family members; this helps to define which family members should be involved in the collaboration of planning care, including being present at care conferences with professional staff. Genograms may also be used in discharge planning by identifying the need for support and assistance when the client returns home. Genograms may help the home care nurse clarify the dynamics of the family in relation to the recovery of the client.

Ecomaps seek information about systems outside the immediate nuclear family that are sources of social support or are stressors for the family. It is a visual representation of

Table 4-5 Remarriage and Blending Families

Phases	Emotional Responses	Developmental Issues
1. Meeting new people	Being open to the possibility of developing a new intimate relationship	Accepting children's and ex-family members' reactions to a parent dating
2. Entering a new relationship	Completing an "emotional recovery" from past divorce and loss of marriage Accepting one's fears about developing a new relationship Adopting an optimistic attitude to what the future may bring	Recovery from loss of marriage Determining what you want from a new relationship Being open to a new relationship
3. Planning a new marriage	Accepting one's fears about the ambiguity and complexity of entering a new relationship with such issues as: New roles and responsibilities Boundaries: space, time, and authority Affective issues: guilt, loyalty, conflicts, unresolvable past hurts	Committing to marriage and forming a new family unit Developing healthy relationships with stepchildren as custodial or noncustodial parent Maintaining coparental relationships with ex-spouses Assisting children to deal with fears, loyalty conflicts, and membership in two systems Realigning relationships with ex-family to include new spouse and children Restructuring family boundaries to allow for new spouse or stepparent
4. Remarriage and blending of families	Forming a final resolution of attachment to previous spouse Accepting of new family unit with different boundaries	Realigning relationships to allow intermingling of systems Expanding relationships to include all new family members Sharing family memories and histories to enrich members' lives

Adapted from Allender, J. A., Rector, C., & Warner, K. D. (2010). *Community health nursing: Concepts and practice* (7th ed., p. 490). Philadelphia, PA: Lippincott Williams & Wilkins.

the family in relation to the larger community. Symbols commonly used for the ecomap are shown in Figure 4-7. Ecomaps are useful for ensuring continuity between settings through comprehensive discharge planning as well as continuity over time. For the nurse providing home visiting care, an ecomap provides a valuable visual tool that is easy to use to identify support when planning care. Further, the nurse gains increased understanding of social networks as a context for caregiving (Rempel, Neufeld, & Kushner, 2007).

Both the ecomap and the genogram are valuable tools for planning care. Further, completing these structural family assessments offers an opportunity for an interactive process that allows nurses and families to establish a foundation of mutual trust and respect. As trust develops between the nurse and the family, there will be more opportunities to explore sensitive questions and be actively involved with families in the health care management process. Families often enjoy completing the genogram and ecomap and may ask for a copy once completed. This may empower and inspire ongoing self-care.

Functional Assessment

Six family functions are considered during **functional assessment**: affective, health care and physical necessities, economics, reproduction, socialization and placement, and family coping. Through interviews, the nurse collects information about the family members' perceptions of how well the family is fulfilling basic functions. Sample questions that address each family function are as follows:

- Is the family meeting the individual member's need for affection, love, and understanding?

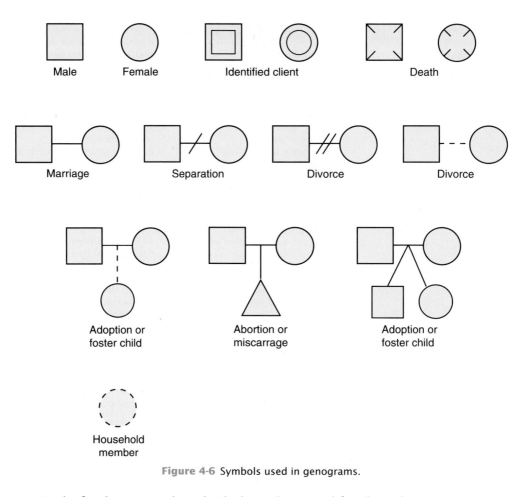

Figure 4-6 Symbols used in genograms.

- Is the family meeting the individual member's need for physical care?
- Does the family have the economic resources required to provide for basic needs of the family?
- Is the family meeting the function of reproduction, as defined by the family?
- Is the family meeting the family function of socialization? Is the family fulfilling the function of socialization of its children to prepare them to become productive members of society?
- Does the family attempt to actively cope with problems?

Using Characteristics of a Healthy Family for Assessment

The characteristics of a healthy family can be used as the construct for a simple family assessment. Family health depends on the ability of family members to share and to understand the feelings, needs, and behavior patterns of each individual (Satir, 1972). Healthy families demonstrate the following characteristics, and the nurse can look for the presence or absence while working with the family:

- There is a facilitative process of interaction among family members.
- The family enhances the development of its individual members.
- Role relationships are structured effectively.
- The family actively attempts to cope with problems.
- The family has a healthy home environment and lifestyle.
- The family establishes regular links with the broader community.

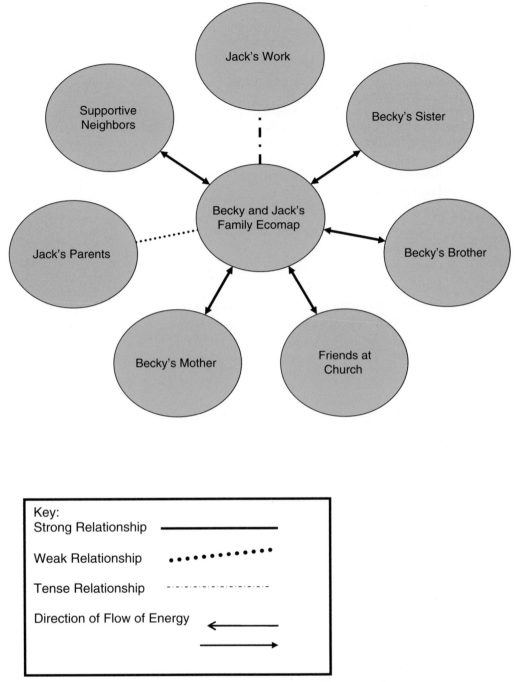

Figure 4-7 Symbols used in an ecomap.

In addition, interactions in a healthy family display the following qualities:

- Communication among members is open, direct, and honest, with shared feelings.
- Family members express self-worth with integrity, responsibility, compassion, and love to, and for, one another.
- All members know the family rules. Rules are clear and flexible and allow individual members their freedom.

* Family has regular links with society, which demonstrate trust and friendship.
* Family members belong to various groups and clubs.

CULTURAGRAM AS A FAMILY ASSESSMENT TOOL

The **culturagram** is a family assessment tool that attempts to individualize care according to the context of the culture or the ethnicity of the family. Completing a culturagram of a family enables a better understanding of the sociocultural context of the family. It also identifies appropriate interventions for the family. Administered in a manner similar to an ecomap or genogram, the culturagram examines the following areas (Congress & Kung, 2005):

* Reasons for relocation (if family has recently relocated)
* Legal status
* Time in the community
* Language spoken at home and in the community
* Health beliefs
* Crisis events in the last year
* Holidays and special events
* Contact with cultural and religious institutions
* Values about education and work
* Values about family structure (power, hierarchy, rules, subsystems, and boundaries)

An example of a culturagram is seen in Figure 4-8.

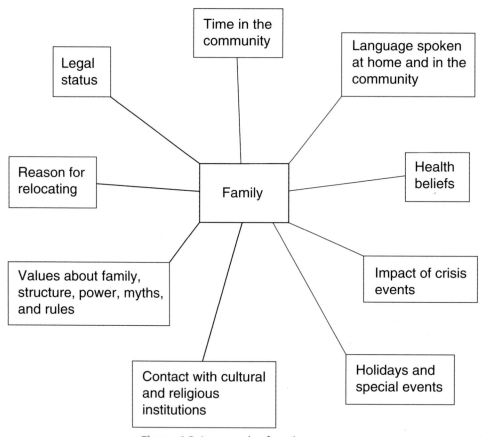

Figure 4-8 An example of a culturagram.

NURSING DIAGNOSIS: IDENTIFYING FAMILY NEEDS AND STRENGTHS

Upon completion of the family interview, assessment data are analyzed allowing the nurse to identify family strengths and needs. By first looking to family strengths, capabilities, previous successful coping mechanisms, and current responses to stress, the nurse lays the foundation for planning interventions. Again, the primary focus of this process as presented in this text is directed to the care of the client. Assessment and identification of the needs of the family is a collaborative process considering the family's potential influence on the care, recovery, and health status of the client.

The process of identifying the needs of the family follows the same steps as those used for the care of the client. By comparing data about the family with defining characteristics of the North American Nursing Diagnosis Association (NANDA) diagnosis, the nurse can arrive at the appropriate diagnosis for the client in the context of the family. Box 4-2 presents NANDA nursing diagnoses relevant to family nursing. Maslow's model may guide in individualizing and prioritizing care for clients in the context of the family. Again, food and shelter, the most basic family needs, must be met first after which the priority of care can shift to safety and then up the hierarchy of needs. The priorities of the family can change as the circumstances of the family vary.

PLANNING: GOALS

In many ways, planning care for families mirrors the process for an individual. But there are differences. Although the family may benefit from the goals, the primary aim is to enhance the health of the individual client. Goal setting is a mutual process that has the potential to have a positive effect on the health care provider's interactions with families. Further, through family interactions, participation, and accountability with the planning of care, families are much more likely to work toward goals they have chosen and support. Examples of goals for family interventions are listed in Box 4-3.

NURSING INTERVENTIONS

Nursing interventions appropriate for families in community-based settings are similar to those discussed for individuals (Table 4-6). Interventions fall into three types: cognitive,

---

BOX 4-2 NANDA Family Diagnoses Relevant to Family Nursing

- Caregiver role strain
- Risk for caregiver role strain
- Parental role conflict
- Compromised family coping
- Disabled family coping
- Readiness of enhanced family coping
- Dysfunctional family processes: alcoholism
- Readiness for enhanced family processes
- Interrupted family processes
- Readiness for enhanced parenting
- Impaired parenting
- Risk for impaired parenting
- Relocation stress syndrome
- Ineffective role performance
- Ineffective family therapeutic regimen management

Source: Carpenito, L. (2010). *Handbook of nursing diagnosis* (13th ed.). Philadelphia, PA: Lippincott Williams & Wilkins.

BOX
4-3

Examples of Goals for Commonly Used Nursing Diagnoses

Caregiver role strain: The caregiver will report a plan to decrease his or her burden.

Decisional conflict: The client or family will make an informed choice.

Anticipatory grieving: The client and/or family will express grief.

Complicated grieving: The client and/or family will verbalize intent to seek professional assistance.

Parental role conflict: The parents will demonstrate control over decision making regarding the child and collaborate with health professionals in making decisions about the health/illness care of the child.

Risk for loneliness: The client and/or caregiver will report decreased feelings of loneliness.

Risk for violence: The client or family will have no or fewer violent responses.

Readiness for enhanced family coping: The family will engage in effective problem solving.

Ineffective coping: The client and/or family will make decisions and follow through with appropriate actions to change provocative situations in personal environment.

Disabled family coping: The client and/or family will set long- and short-term goals for change.

Interrupted family process: The family will maintain functional system of mutual support for one another.

Dysfunctional family process: Alcoholism. The family will acknowledge the alcoholism in the family.

Relocation stress syndrome: The client and/or family member will report adjustment to the new environment without physiologic and/or psychological disturbances.

Adapted from Carpenito, L. (2010). *Handbook of nursing diagnosis* (13th ed.). Philadelphia, PA: Lippincott Williams & Wilkins.

affective, and behavioral. **Cognitive interventions** involve the act of knowing, perceiving, or understanding. An example is teaching a client or family member about the exchange system for a diabetic diet. Many aspects of health teaching involve a cognitive component. **Affective interventions** have to do with feelings, attitudes, and values. Helping family members to understand their fears about a loved one's diagnosis of diabetes is an illustration of an affective intervention. Another would be to discuss concerns about drawing up and injecting insulin. These two examples are counseling interventions. **Behavioral interventions** are those that have to do with skills and behaviors. Teaching clients and family members about giving insulin injections is one example of a behavioral intervention. Another is a group exercise program for newly diagnosed diabetic clients. Both of these interventions are health teaching. Many interventions have a cognitive, affective, and behavioral component.

Basing and planning care on family strengths may be accomplished by using family resilience factors as a foundation for formulating nursing interventions. For instance, if a family has a positive outlook, the nurse may develop a nursing intervention capitalizing on the families' ability to be confident, optimistic, and have a sense of humor when counseling, developing health teaching, or making a referral. Table 4-2 provides a list of attributes, typical family characteristics, and possible nursing interventions to promote resilience.

Nursing interventions serve the function of providing specific directions and a consistent, individualized approach to the client's care. They are written as instructions for others to follow. Interventions in community-based care require the active involvement in a mutual process among the client, family, and nurse to determine appropriate interventions. This emphasis is crucial because the client or family will be responsible for implementing the interventions at home. As with goal setting, the plan of care is more likely to be successful if it is formulated through an active process. Examples of goals and nursing interventions appear in Table 4-6.

Nursing interventions for families may be crafted to address primary, secondary, or tertiary prevention. Primary prevention encompasses nursing interventions that obviate the

Table 4-6 Examples of Goals and Nursing Interventions for Commonly Used Nursing Diagnoses for Family Intervention

Nursing Diagnosis	Goals	Nursing Intervention
Decisional conflict	The client and family will make an informed choice	Counseling establishes an interpersonal relationship with the family by establishing a trusting and meaningful relationship that promotes mutual understanding and caring Acknowledge strengths of the family when appropriate Facilitate a logical decision-making process
Parental role conflict	The parents will demonstrate control over decision making regarding the child and collaborate with health professionals in making decisions about the health/ illness care of the child	Counseling establishes an interpersonal relationship with a family to increase or enhance their capacity for self-care and coping. Allow parents to share frustrations Acknowledge strengths of the family when appropriate Refer for counseling for management of stressors and role, if indicated
Disabled family coping	The client and/or family will set long- and short-term goals for change	Counseling establishes an interpersonal relationship with a family intended to increase or enhance their capacity for self-care and coping Be direct and nonjudgmental. Encourage a realistic appraisal of the situation; dispel guilt and myths Acknowledge strengths of the family when appropriate
Interrupted family process	The family members will maintain a functional system of mutual support for each other	Counseling establishes an interpersonal relationship with a family intended to increase or enhance their capacity for self-care and coping Assist the family with appraisal of the situation Acknowledge strengths of the family when appropriate

Adapted from Carpenito, L. (2010). *Handbook of nursing diagnosis* (13th ed.). Philadelphia, PA: Lippincott Williams & Wilkins.

initial occurrence of a disease or condition. When attempting to implement interventions for individual clients, it is often necessary to involve family members because they are affected as well. An example of primary prevention where it may be necessary to involve other family members is family planning. This decision varies by culture in that in some cultures, partners make decisions together about birth control and the spacing of children, while in others, the female or male partner decides independently of the other about family planning. Tertiary prevention is seen in support programs for families with a family member with dementia (see Research in Community-Based Nursing Care 4-1).

CLIENT SITUATIONS IN PRACTICE

Intervention at the Primary Prevention Level

Pam works in a clinic that serves many clients from Southeast Asia. When she first began teaching female clients about family planning, Pam met individually with the women and did not include the husband or significant other. Over time, she discovered that most of the women she was meeting with were not using family planning as they requested and

RESEARCH IN COMMUNITY-BASED NURSING CARE 4-1

Family Care as Collaboration: Effectiveness of Multicomponent Support Program for Elderly Couples with Dementia

The objective of this research was to determine whether community care of people with dementia can be prolonged with a 2-year multicomponent intervention program and to analyze effects of the intervention on total usage and expenses of social and health care services. Community-dwelling couples with one spouse caring for the other spouse with dementia were randomly assigned to an intervention or control group. Intervention couples were provided with an intervention program with a family care coordinator, a geriatrician, support groups for caregivers, and individualized services. The use of services and service expenditure of couples were measured after 1.6 and 2 years. At 1.6 years, a statistically significant larger proportion of those in the control group than the intervention group were in long-term care. After 2 years, the proportion remained larger but was not statistically significant. Although the intervention did not result in a significant difference in the need for institutional care after 2 years, individualizing services and collaborating with families was found to reduce the use and expenditures of government services.

Eloniemi-Sulkava, U., Saarenheimo, M., Laakkonen, M., Pietilä, M., Savikko, N., Kautiainen, H., et al. (2009). Family care as collaboration: Effectiveness of a multicomponent support program for elderly couples with dementia. Randomized controlled intervention study. *Journal of the American Geriatrics Society, 57*(12), 2200--2208. doi:10.1111/j.1532--5415.2009.02564.x.

indicated interest in it during the clinic visits. Upon further exploration, she learned that the use of birth control, for many of her clients, was decided by the male partner. Pam began involving the male partner in choosing a method of birth control and teaching the couple about its use and found the couples were more likely to follow the plan of care.

Secondary prevention is the early detection and treatment of a condition. In some families, lack of information may be a barrier to seeking services related to secondary prevention.

CLIENT SITUATIONS IN PRACTICE

Intervention at the Secondary Prevention Level

Tom works in a day care center for older adults. One of the clients, Irene, is having problems with her eyesight and has a family history of glaucoma. Tom has been encouraging her to have her eyes tested. Although Irene has severe arthritis, she is alert and cognitively intact. Irene tells Tom that she does not want to ask her son to take her to anymore clinic visits. Tom learns that the son is unaware of his mother's vision problems. Tom learns that only by involving another family member (Irene's son) will the secondary prevention strategy (vision screening) occur.

Tertiary prevention is seeking treatment and rehabilitation for maximizing recovery and health. In some situations, the family is motivated to follow the treatment plan but is not aware of resources in the community that may support the plan. By simply assessing family knowledge about community resources and making a referral, the nurse assists the family to take steps to engage in tertiary prevention.

CLIENT SITUATIONS IN PRACTICE

Intervention at the Tertiary Prevention Level

Kristi is a staff nurse in charge of discharge planning for Barb who has had a fusion of four cervical vertebrae and will leave the hospital in 3 days. Barb lives alone; however, her daughter (the mother of five children) lives an hour's drive from Barb's home. After discharge, Barb will need assistance with activities of daily living for at least 2 weeks at home. She will not be permitted to drive for 6 weeks and will receive physical therapy four times a week, starting 2 weeks after discharge. Kristi, Barb, and Barb's daughter sit down together to plan for the care and assistance Barb will need once home. They also discuss the community services that are available to transport Barb to physical therapy until she is permitted to drive.

CLIENT SITUATIONS IN PRACTICE

Intervention at the Tertiary Prevention Level

Justin works as a nurse on an ortho unit in a hospital and is in charge of discharge planning for Damien, a 30-year-old gentleman who was in a motor vehicle accident and broke both his legs and his pelvis. Damien lives with his wife and two preschool children in an apartment. In doing a quick family assessment the first day he meets Damien, Justin learns that he just moved to the region. Damien mentions that he was in the army for the last decade and was deployed overseas for active duty on three separate occasions. Over the course of Damien's hospitalization, Justin attempts to continuously assess Damien's needs upon discharge. Justin reads that the night staff charts every night that Damien is not sleeping well, noting two episodes when Damien's loud cursing and shouting during a dream could be heard in the hall outside his room. When asked about the dreams, Damien states that he has had difficulty sleeping and is experiencing violent dreams since returning from active duty. When asked if he has spoken to his doctor about these episodes, he replies that he has not. Justin encourages Damien to talk to his physician about the dreams and puts a note in the chart about the conversation. The day before Damien is to be discharged, Justin suggests that he considers making an appointment at the Veterans Administration (VA) clinic for his sleep disturbances. With Damien's consent, Justin contacts the VA clinic and makes an appointment for him for the next week as a part of the discharge plan.

EVALUATION

Evaluation is a joint effort of the indiviual, nurse, family, and other caregivers. As is true in an acute care setting, it is in the evaluation of care that the nurse discovers if the plan of care is a success or needs refinement. This analysis leads to more assessment or refinement of the goals set out in the care plan and results in the identification of additional diagnoses, goals, or interventions.

The following questions for reflection may be useful during evaluation of the family care plan:

- What additional data are required to evaluate progress?
- Did the nursing diagnosis focus on the most important problem for this family as it relates to the potential for the client to do self-care?
- What other needs are seen with this family and client?
- What other strengths are apparent in this family?
- Were the diagnosis, goals, and interventions realistic and appropriate for this client and family?
- Were the family strengths considered when the goals and interventions were defined? If not, how could these strengths be used to enhance the outcome?
- Are the nurse, client, and family satisfied with the outcome? If not, what do each indicate would enhance satisfaction?

The nursing process continues in an ongoing, circular, and dynamic manner. Information gained from asking the questions above is used to define a new problem and new strengths and identify new or additional goals and interventions as the ongoing process of providing care and evaluating its effect continues.

DOCUMENTATION

Complete and accurate information is an essential element of quality nursing care of the client or family. This includes documentation of the client and family's strengths and ongoing needs. Creating a clear account of what the nurse saw and did related to the family's care provides a record of that care, thereby enhancing other professional caregivers' ability to collaborate and improve continuity care. Charting is also used to determine eligibility for care needed and for reimbursement for care provided.

✳ CLIENT SITUATIONS IN PRACTICE

The Family and Nursing Process

Tamesha, a home health care nurse, is assigned to care for Becky, a 30-year-old homemaker who is the mother of three preschool children (Joe, age 4; Kevin, age 2; and Michael, age 2 months). Becky has been diagnosed with liver cancer. Jack, Becky's husband, is a 32-year-old accountant with his own accounting firm. Jack's parents are in good health and live in another city. Ila, Becky's mother, lives in the same neighborhood as Jack and Becky. Becky's father died 10 years ago, and Ila remarried Stephen last year. Ila has severe arthritis. Becky also has a sister and brother who both live out of state.

As Becky's home care nurse, Tamesha completes a family assessment during the first visit. She begins the family interview by getting acquainted with all of the family members. Joe shows her the new toy his grandmother gave him for his birthday; Kevin is very shy and sits in Becky's lap during the home visit. Jack holds the baby. Tamesha hopes to be able to identify from this family assessment how much support the family will be able to provide to Becky. She is also interested in identifying family strengths and any needs requiring intervention. Assessment Tools 4-2 reflects the information gleaned from the interview.

Identification of the Nursing Diagnosis

Tamesha reviews the family assessment as well as Becky and Jack's responses. She identifies these family strengths:

- *The family and a large number of supportive friends are willing to assist with the care of the children and the home.*
- *A strong marital bond between Becky and her husband is apparent; they show mutual support and love and use humor in a kind, nurturing way.*
- *The family has a stable financial status.*

She identifies these family needs:

- *They are finding it difficult to keep up with both home management and child care of three preschool children. This was evident when Becky stated she needed help managing the family's daily needs. Tamesha also observed that the house was very cluttered.*
- *There is the potential for ineffective family coping. This was evident when Becky and Jack were unable to be honest and open when discussing Becky's illness and prognosis.*

Setting Priorities

To identify the priority of family needs, Tamesha uses Maslow's hierarchy of needs. Recognizing that the family and client must have their basic needs addressed first, she concentrates on the family's difficulty in managing the home and child care.

As a result, Tamesha believes that this is Becky and Jack's priority problem:

- *Impaired home maintenance management related to Becky's complex care regimen as evidenced by a disorderly home environment and Becky's statement, "I can only care for the kids a few minutes at a time. I am too tired to make the meals and clean up afterwards. We need help."*

Planning

At the second home visit, Tamesha, Becky, and Jack discuss the family assessment. Tamesha shares her conclusion about their primary need. She asks Becky and Jack for their impressions, and they agree that the major concern is the care of the home and the children. Becky adds, "I am concerned about being able to continue to provide care for the kids. I'm also worried about Jack and me having time together and being able to talk."

Through the intervention of counseling, Tamesha assists the family to enhance their capacity for self-care. The three decide to address the problems about home management and save the discussion about communication for the third visit. Tamesha suggests that if some of the issues regarding care of the home and family are addressed, Becky may have more energy for the children.

Goals

Tamesha, Becky, and her husband define the following goals that address impaired home maintenance. The goal is to accomplish them by the third visit:

1. Becky and Jack will identify home maintenance tasks that need to be done daily and weekly.
2. Becky and Jack will compile a list of family members and friends who are able and willing to assist with these tasks.
3. Becky and Jack will match the list of tasks with the list of people and contact them within the next 3 days.
4. Becky will call Tamesha with the list of tasks that their family and friends can do.
5. Jack will contact the list of community agencies that Tamesha gave him to see what assistance they can provide.

Nursing Implementation

Tamesha lists the specific nursing interventions she has identified for the plan of care:

1. Through counseling, Tamesha will assist the family in determining a realistic plan for both health care and home maintenance.
2. Through the intervention of referral, Tamesha will identify resources in the community that can assist with the tasks that the family and friends cannot do. She will contact Jack and give him the list of resources and telephone numbers.
3. Tamesha will use case management and schedule periodic home visits to evaluate the effectiveness of the plan and identify any changes that occur in Becky's condition that may need intervention.

Evaluation

At the third home visit, Tamesha uses the nursing intervention of case management as she assists Becky and Jack to evaluate the plan to date. The first four goals were met; however, Jack did not contact the community agencies. He will contact them next week. Tamesha and the family agree on the plan and the method for evaluating the plan. Tamesha also reviews the list of community resources with Becky and Jack. They all agree on which ones to contact. They agree to discuss Becky's concern about caring for her children at the next visit.

Assessment Tools 4-2
Family Assessment

Family Members

Member	Birth Date	Sex	Marital Status	Education
Becky	7/15/83	F	Married	College grad
Jack	11/10/81	M	Married	College grad
Joe	9/18/09	M		
Kevin	2/15/11	M		
Michael	2/22/13	M		

Culturagram

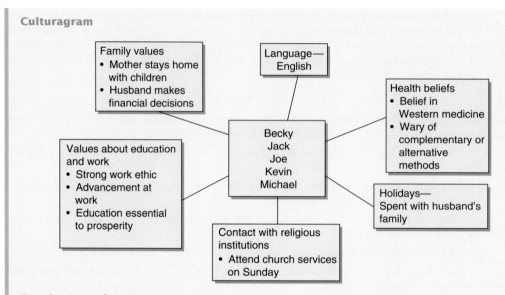

Family values
• Mother stays home with children
• Husband makes financial decisions

Language— English

Health beliefs
• Belief in Western medicine
• Wary of complementary or alternative methods

Becky
Jack
Joe
Kevin
Michael

Values about education and work
• Strong work ethic
• Advancement at work
• Education essential to prosperity

Holidays— Spent with husband's family

Contact with religious institutions
• Attend church services on Sunday

Developmental Assessment

What is this family's developmental stage?

Preschool age stage

Is the family meeting the tasks of its stage?

No, the added energy depletion of Becky's illness has caused profound exhaustion for all membersof the family.

Does, or will, the client's health problem interrupt the family's ability to meet the developmental tasks? If yes, how does it interrupt it?

Becky's illness has interrupted the family's ability to meet the developmental tasks. Becky and Jack state they are "unable to keep up with the demands of the kids, the baby, and rigors of dailyliving."

State nursing interventions to assist family members in meeting their developmental tasks.

1. Through the intervention of counseling and health teaching:
2. Identify specific parental roles that Becky and Jack want to retain.
3. Identify parental responsibilities that they are willing to give up to someone else.
4. Identify possible support persons who could assist more with child care.
5. Through the intervention of case management:

Determine other household tasks that can be assumed by family members or community services.

Functional Assessment

Does the family meet the individual's need for affection, love, and understanding?

Both Becky and Jack continue to be very affectionate and loving to each other and their children. This is evident in the way they interact with each other and with the children, hold the children, explain things to them, and comfort them. The children are in turn affectionate to Becky. Becky states, "My sister has provided me with a lot of emotional support. We talk on the phone everyday."

Does the family meet the individual's need for physical necessities and care?

Jack is able to continue working, and he still has the opportunity to take some time off if necessary.Becky is unable to fulfill her prior role responsibilities as homemaker, which included cooking, cleaning, marketing, and most of the child care. Becky states that she is "exhausted and able to participate only in a limited manner in the care of the children and the work of running the household." Becky states, "I want to be able to bathe the kids and read them their bedtime story. I also want to continue to give Michael his bottles." Note disorderly surroundings with the children's toys, dirty clothes, and dirty dishes scattered in all of the rooms. The children are cranky, and the baby cries most of the visit.

Does the family have the economic resources necessary to provide for the basic needs of the family?

Jack states, "My job is very secure. I have been lucky that I have a job which allows me to provide so well for my family. I have a lot of vacation time saved up, because we were going to take a big family vacation next summer."

Is the family meeting the function of reproduction as defined by the family?

Yes

Is the family meeting the family function of socialization? Is the family fulfilling the function to socialize children to become productive members of society?

Becky states, "It is very hard to provide guidance and discipline for Joe because I am so tired. He wears me down. Maybe he should be in day care a few days a week. There is a day care at our church, which is only a few blocks away."

Does the family attempt to actively cope with problems?

Becky says, "Jack does not want to talk about the future and what the doctor has said about my prognosis. He believes that I will be better by summer. He has been so angry since the diagnosis." Jack says, "I believe that Becky will be better by summer. She has the best doctor in the Midwest, and people survive from cancer all the time."

Assessment of Presence of Characteristics of a Healthy Family

Is communication between members open, direct, and honest, and are feelings and needs shared?

Becky says, "It is hard for Jack to share his feelings with me. I think he talks to his dad but not to me. Sometimes his dad tells me what he has said. It's hard for me to tell him what I really think because it seems like then I am giving up." Jack says, "I have a close relationship with my dad. It is so hard for me to talk to Becky about my fears because I want to be upbeat and hopeful; I don't want her to have to comfort me."

Do family members express self-worth with integrity, responsibility, compassion, and love to and for one another?

Both Becky and Jack express love and concern for each other. They are so concerned about each other that Becky states, "Our concern for each other gets in the way of open communication."

Are family rules known to all members?

Becky and Jack describe the family in precisely the same way—"Becky is responsible for the care of the children and the home, and Jack is the breadwinner."

Are rules clear and flexible, and do they allow individual members freedom?

Both state that before Joe was born, Becky worked full time and the home maintenance was shared. Becky says that since she became ill, Jack has assumed many of the responsibilities at home. Becky states, "He is working too hard and is exhausted. We need help!"

Does the family have regular links to society that demonstrate trust and friendship?

During the home visit, three neighbors came over with food, and two people called. There were many plants, cards, and flower arrangements in the house. Becky stated, "Our friends have been wonderful. They have offered to take the kids, brought food, and visited."

Do family members belong to various groups and clubs?

The family is active in a church, and Jack is involved in an environmental group. Becky has many friends in the neighborhood.

CLIENT SITUATIONS IN PRACTICE

Jane, a home care nurse, is assigned to care for Maria, a 64-year-old mother of six children. Five of her adult children live in the neighborhood and one resides in Mexico. Maria has been diagnosed with stage four ovarian cancer. She was recently hospitalized with severe dehydration and malnutrition. A central line was placed in during outpatient surgery. Jane is making her first visit to Maria's home for infusion therapy.

As Maria's home care nurse, Jane completes a family assessment during the first visit. She begins the family interview by getting acquainted with all of the family members. Juan, her husband, died five years ago from lung cancer. Her children are Philippe, Jose, Miguel, Roberto, Rose, and Eliana and range in age from 44 to 30 years. Since Juan's death, Maria has been living with Rose.

Jane hopes to be able to identify how much support the family will be able to provide to Maria from this family assessment. She is also interested in identifying any problem areas where intervention is needed. Jane learns that Maria worked as a field worker until she became ill. The family does not have insurance. Maria is a devout Catholic and goes to daily mass. Maria consults the local curandero for minor ailments. Maria has the equivalent of a sixth-grade education and speaks only Spanish. She is an undocumented worker and relocated to the United States 15 years ago. They live in a rural area in a mobile home community. The completed family assessment is shown in Assessment Tools 4-3.

Identification of the Nursing Diagnosis

Jane reviews the data from the family assessment as well as comments from the family. She identifies these family strengths or assets as

1. Committed to supporting Maria financially and emotionally.
2. Large network of support in the community.
3. Maria has enjoyed good health up to this point.
4. The extended family is close and sees each other on a weekly basis.
5. Family wants to care for their mother at home, which is a cultural norm for the community.

She notes family needs as

1. Family communication as family does not want their mother to know that her condition is terminal.
2. Maria is resistant to having surgery.
3. Maria does not have insurance.

Jane is concerned about the burden that may result from the family caring for Maria without the support of other community services. She also wonders about Maria refusing surgery. She wonders whether Maria and the family have all the information they need to make decisions about what treatment to pursue. She thinks that the issue may be a knowledge deficit.

In order to collect more information, she calls Maria about her concerns. Maria refuses to answer Jane's questions directly and keeps referring to Philippe. Maria suggests that Jane call Philippe. Jane states that if Maria prefers that she speaks to Philippe, she will do so but must have her sign a release permitting her to speak to Philippe about Maria's health.

Jane is puzzled by her conversation with Maria. She talks to Josefina, one of the agency nurses who is from Mexico, about her concerns. Josefina explains that, in Mexican culture, a hysterectomy, even in postmenopausal women, is seen by some as a threat to a woman's femininity. Although one of the most successful treatments for this type of cancer is surgery, Maria's cultural values may impact her openness to life-extending surgery. Josefina further states that it is a common reaction in Maria's culture not to tell a family member of a terminal diagnosis. Josefina also explains that often the oldest son is considered the decision maker. This is why Philippe is the family decision maker in this patriarchal family system and probably why Maria requested that Jane speak to Philippe. Based on Josefina's recommendations, Jane calls Philippe to schedule a meeting with Maria and her children the next day.

To identify the priority of family needs, Jane uses Maslow's hierarchy of needs.

What do you think Jane identifies as a priority for this family?

State two nursing diagnoses based on the data collected so far that Jane might propose for this family.

List several goals for each nursing diagnosis.

State two indicators that the goals are met.

Identify two possible nursing interventions for each goal.

Assessment Tools 4-3
Family Assessment

Family Members

Member	Birth Date	Sex	Marital Status	Education
Maria	11/30/51	F	Widow	4th grade
Philippe	8/8/71	M	Married	8th grade
Jose	5/7/73	M	Married	6th grade
Miguel	5/15/75	M	Married	10th grade
Roberto	10/4/77	M	Married	10th grade
Rose	1/24/79	F	Married	12th grade
Eliana	11/6/81	F	Married	12th grade

Completed Culturagram

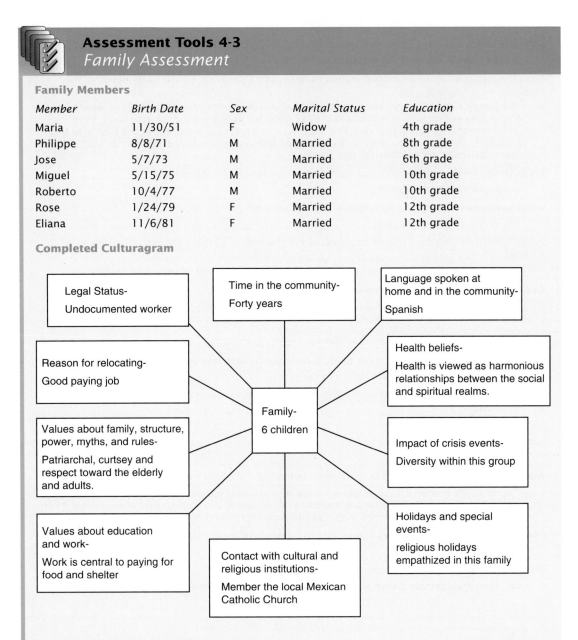

Legal Status-
Undocumented worker

Time in the community-
Forty years

Language spoken at home and in the community-
Spanish

Reason for relocating-
Good paying job

Health beliefs-
Health is viewed as harmonious relationships between the social and spiritual realms.

Family-
6 children

Values about family, structure, power, myths, and rules-
Patriarchal, curtsey and respect toward the elderly and adults.

Impact of crisis events-
Diversity within this group

Values about education and work-
Work is central to paying for food and shelter

Contact with cultural and religious institutions-
Member the local Mexican Catholic Church

Holidays and special events-
religious holidays empathized in this family

Developmental Assessment

What is this family's developmental stage?

Aging family: tasks of coping with loss, adapting to aging, accepting shifts and changes in parent–child roles, and preparing for death.

Is the family meeting the tasks of its stage?

Yes.

Does, or will, the client's health problem interrupt the family's ability to meet the developmental tasks? If yes, how does it interrupt it?

No interruption seen at this time.

Functional Assessment

Does the family meet the individual's need for affection, love, and understanding?

Yes.

Does the family meet the individual's need for physical necessities and care?

Yes, but the family may need assistance as the client's needs change.

Does the family have the economic resources necessary to provide for the basic needs of the family?

The family has limited economic resources but has adequate resources for basic needs. Maria does not have health insurance. Over time, the family may need assistance from some community resources, and Jane may need to assess the openness of the family to this possibility. Jane may also need to explore what resources exist in the community that may be more culturally appropriate for this family.

Is the family meeting the function of reproduction as defined by the family?

Not applicable to this family.

Is the family meeting the family function of socialization?

Yes, this is a family strength.

Is the family fulfilling the function to socialize the children to become productive members of society?

Not applicable to this family as children are already productive members of society.

Does the family attempt to actively cope with problems?

Yes, but the family coping must be considered within the family's cultural values. The family coping is less explicit and more defined by the family value of patriarchal decision makers.

Assessment of Presence of Characteristics of a Healthy Family

Is communication between members open, direct, and honest, and are feelings and needs shared?

Yes, according to the cultural values of the family.

Do family members express self-worth with integrity, responsibility, compassion, and love to and for one another?

Yes.

Are family rules known to all members?

Yes.

Are rules clear and flexible, and do they allow individual members freedom?

The rules are not flexible by American cultural standards but closely follow those of the older siblings in the family. The younger members of the family are women who are expected to be the caregivers, yet they are not a part of the decision-making process.

Does the family have regular links to society that demonstrate trust and friendship?

Yes.

Do family members belong to various groups and clubs?

Yes, they are active in parish activities and within the community.

Conclusions

The family is the basic social unit of American society and has long been the primary focus of nursing care in the community. Understanding family structure, roles, and functions is essential in providing comprehensive nursing care both in the acute care and community-based setting. Knowledge of healthy family functioning permits the nurse to identify unhealthy functioning and take appropriate action, including referrals to community resources. Often, families with an ill family member are in crisis and require nursing intervention or referrals.

Today, more than ever, the nurse must be cognizant of the needs, feelings, problems, and views of the family when providing care for the individual client. Community-based nursing requires the nurse to provide care in the context of the client's family to enhance self-care. This is accomplished by assessing the client in the context of the family.

To provide continuous care with a preventive focus, the nurse must consider the family's ability and needs. The care of the client in the context of the family is enhanced by following the principles of community-based care.

What's on the Web

Bright Futures for Families
INTERNET ADDRESS: http://www.brightfutures.org
This Web site is supported by the Maternal and Child Health Bureau of the U.S. Department of Health and Human Services and has numerous family resources.

Using Family History to Promote Health
INTERNET ADDRESS: http://www.childwelfare.gov/can/factors/resilience.cfm
This Web site provides fact sheets, case studies, tools, presentations, and other resources that may be used with family histories to promote health. Very informative resource.

Family Resilience
INTERNET ADDRESS: http://www.childwelfare.gov/can/factors/resilience.cfm
This site provides numerous resources for nurses who want to help families become more resilient.

The Road to Resilience
INTERNET ADDRESS: http://www.apa.org/helpcenter/road-resilience.aspx
This site is intended to provide information that describes resilience and some factors that affect how people deal with hardship. Much of the site focuses on developing and using a personal strategy for enhancing resilience.

Centers for Disease Control and Prevention: National Office of Public Health Genomics
INTERNET ADDRESS: http://www.cdc.gov/genomics/default.htm
This site provides updated information on how human genomic discoveries can be used to improve health and prevent disease. It also provides links to CDC-wide activities in public health genomics.

National Center for Cultural Competence
INTERNET ADDRESS: http://www11.georgetown.edu/research/gucchd/nccc/resources/publicationstitle.html or http://www11.georgetown.edu/research/gucchd/nccc/documents/fcclcguide.pdf
The mission of the National Center for Cultural Competence is to increase the capacity of health care and mental health care providers to design, implement, and evaluate culturally and linguistically competent service delivery systems to address growing diversity, persistent disparities, and to promote health and mental health equity. There are numerous guides for using family-centered and culturally competent care with families.

National Resource Directory for Family and Caregiver Support
INTERNET ADDRESS:http://www.nationalresourcedirectory.gov/health
The National Resource Directory for Family and Caregiver Support provides numerous resources to learn about health-related issues, treatment options, the locations of medical facilities, health insurance programs, and tips on staying healthy for members or former members of the armed services as well as support for family members.

After Deployment from Active Duty in the Military
INTERNET ADDRESS: www.afterdeployment.org
This site offers comprehensive information on a variety of topics, including physical and emotional health; relationship with families, friends, and children; and substance abuse. Online assessments and workshops are offered, as well as online videos of military members and families dealing with similar issues.

References

Allen, D., & Marshall, E. (2010). Spirituality as a coping resource for African American parents of chronically ill children. *MCN: The American Journal of Maternal Child Nursing, 35*(4), 232–237. Retrieved from CINAHL Plus with Full Text database.

Allender, J. A., Rector, C., & Warner, K. D. (2010). *Community health nursing: Concepts and practice* (7th ed.). Philadelphia, PA: Lippincott Williams & Wilkins.

Black, K., & Lobo, M. (2008). A conceptual review of family resilience factors. *Journal of Family Nursing, 14*(1), 33–55. Retrieved from CINAHL Plus with Full Text database.

Browning, G., & Warren, N. (2006). Unmet needs of family members in the medical intensive care writing room. *Critical Care Nursing Quarterly, 29*(1), 86–95.

Carpenito, L. (2010). *Handbook of nursing diagnosis* (13th ed.). Philadelphia, PA: Lippincott Williams & Wilkins.

Coleman, L., & Glenn, F. (2010). The varied impact of couple relationship breakdown on children: Implications for practice and policy. *Children & Society, 24*(3), 238–249.

Congress, E. P., & Kung, W. W. (2005). Using the culturagram to assess and empower culturally diverse families. In E. P. Congress & M. J. Gonzales (Eds.), *Multicultural perspectives in working with families* (pp. 4–21). New York, NY: Springer.

Drapalski, A., Marshall, T., Seybolt, D., Medoff, D., Peer, J., Leith, J., et al. (2008). Unmet needs of families of adults with mental illness and preferences regarding family services. *Psychiatric Services, 59*(6), 655–662. Retrieved from CINAHL Plus with Full Text database.

Duvall, E.M. (1977). *Marriage and family development* (4th ed.). Philadelphia: Lippincott.

Eloniemi-Sulkava, U., Saarenheimo, M., Laakkonen, M., Pietilä, M., Savikko, N., Kautiainen, H., et al. (2009). Family care as collaboration: Effectiveness of a multicomponent support program for elderly couples with dementia. Randomized controlled intervention study. *Journal of the American Geriatrics Society, 57*(12), 2200–2208. doi:10.1111/j.1532-5415.2009.02564.x.

Federal Interagency Forum on Children and Family Statistics. (2010). *American's children: Key national indicators of well-being, 2010.* Washington, DC: U.S. Government Printing Office. Retrieved from www.http://childstats.gov

Kaakinen, J., Gedaly Duff, V., Coehlo, D., & Hanson, S. (2010). *Family health nursing care: Theory, practice and research* (4th ed.). Philadelphia, PA: F.A. Davis.

Latour, J., & Haines, C. (2007). Families in the ICU: Do we truly consider their needs, experiences, and satisfaction? *Nursing in Critical Care, 12*(4), 173–174.

Maslow, A. H. (1954). *Motivation and personality.* New York, NY: Harper & Row.

Paul, F., & Rattray, J. (2008). Short- and long-term impact of critical illness on relatives: Literature review. *Journal of Advanced Nursing, 62*(3), 276–292. Retrieved from CINAHL Plus with Full Text database.

Rempel, G., Neufeld, A., & Kushner, K. (2007). Interactive use of genograms and ecomaps in family care giving research. *Journal of Family Nursing, 13*(4), 403–419. Retrieved from CINAHL Plus with Full Text database.

Satir, V. (1972). *People making.* Palo Alto, CA: Science and Behavioral Books.

Spitz, R. A. (1945). Hospitalism: An inquiry into the genesis of psychiatric conditions in early childhood. *Psychoanalytic Study of the Child, 1*, 53–74.

U.S. Department of Health and Human Services, National Center for Health Statistics. (2010). Health, United States, 2010. Washington, DC: U.S. Department of Health and Human services. Retrieved from http://healthypeople.gov/Default.htm

Wagner-Cox, P. (2005). Lessons learned: From the other side of the nurse-patient family relationship. *Homecare Nurses, 23*(4), 218–223.

LEARNING ACTIVITIES

LEARNING ACTIVITY 4-1

You are working in a chemical dependency day treatment unit for adolescents. Your client is Chris, a 16-year-old boy, admitted yesterday. His father, Michael, and his stepmother, Joanna, brought Chris into your facility after he was picked up by the police for violation of curfew and underage drinking. Michael says that Chris' grades in school have been on a downhill slide since his sophomore year began 6 months ago. Both parents have noticed that Chris' behavior has changed as he is spending more time in his room; his appearance has become disheveled; and he is increasingly more listless, fatigued, hostile, and erratic. Michael describes his son as a cheerful, focused boy—until this year.

Chris has a 13-year-old brother, and both boys live for a week with their mother, Lori, and a week with their father, Michael, and his second wife, Joanna. Lori and Michael have been divorced for 4 years. Michael and his new wife have a 1-year-old daughter. Lori visited Chris this morning. While at the treatment center, she mentions that she is suing Michael for money he owes her. After lunch, you are visiting with Michael, and he relates to you that two of Lori's brothers are lawyers, and the family is always engaged in some sort of litigation. Last year, he alleges that Lori claimed that she had lupus and collected disability payments until the insurance company discovered it was a fraudulent claim.

During the initial family intake interview, Lori blames Michael for Chris's problems, maintaining that Michael has suffered from depression over the past years. Michael talks about his feelings that the ongoing battle between him and Lori is stressful for their children. He wants the conflict to end.

1. Construct a genogram and an ecomap for this family.
2. What is Chris's position in the family?
3. Discuss the nature of the illness
4. Describe additional information you will need to plan care. Identify family strengths.
5. Identify the developmental stage of each member of the family. Explain how you will use this information.
6. Identify the developmental stage of each family. Explain how you will use this information when planning care for Chris.
7. Detect which family functions are not being met.
8. Develop goals you hope to see with this family.
9. Propose referrals you could initiate.

LEARNING ACTIVITY 4-2

Complete a family assessment on the family of a client you are caring for in clinical who has a nontraditional family structure. Use the family assessment tool in the text of this chapter (Assessment Tools 4-1) to collect basic information on the family. After you have completed the family assessment, respond to the following questions.

1. Identify the family problem or need that may interfere with the client's recovery.
2. Identify the family problem or need that may interfere with the client's ability to maximize his or her functioning within the limitations of his or her health condition.
3. Identify the family strengths, and discuss how you will use these to enhance the client's recovery.
4. What client or family goals do you hope to see based on the family's needs stated in the first question?
5. List nursing interventions that will help you, the client, and the family achieve the goals you have identified.
6. Describe ways you will evaluate your nursing plan for the family.

LEARNING ACTIVITY 4-3

Identify an agency in your community that provides family-centered health services. Look at the agency Web site and answer the following questions about these agencies:

- What is the mission of the agency?
- Does the agency have a definition of family-centered care? If so, what is it?
- Describe some family needs or strengths that could be well addressed by the agency.

LEARNING ACTIVITY 4-4

1. Providing services for family members of veterans is an important role of the nurse in the community. Locate resources in your region that have specific services for veterans and their families.
   - State the mission of the agency.
   - Describe specific services that are offered through the agency.
   - Discuss what is offered at the nearest VA clinic for veterans needing health care.
2. Look at the Web site for the National Resource Directory for Family and Caregiver Support at http://www.nationalresourcedirectory.gov/health.
   - Identify an article or resource on this site that would be helpful for a veteran experiencing mental health concerns.
   - Describe what you found on the topic you explored.
   - Discuss how this information could be used to provide care to a family member of a veteran.

LEARNING ACTIVITY 4-5

Locate a local, state, or federal program that assists families. Call the state or county department of health in your community or the public health or public health nursing division for suggestions. Common federal programs for families are Headstart; the Women, Infants, and Children Program; and immunization programs. These all have Web sites and are administered through county or state agencies. What are the goals of the program you contacted? Do you think the program creates benefits for families? What are the benefits for society? Is there evidence that these programs are cost effective? (This can be a program in your own community, such as an after-school program for children, or a federal program such as Headstart.)

LEARNING ACTIVITY 4-6

1. In your clinical journal, create a genogram of your family showing three generations.
   - As you analyze your own genogram, what patterns do you see regarding health issues?
   - Determine which developmental stage your family is in by using Table 4-3, Table 4-4, or Table 4-5. Examine whether your family members are meeting the developmental tasks of the stage. If not, analyze what is preventing this from occurring.
   - What was the most important thing you learned from doing this activity?
2. In your clinical journal, discuss a situation you have observed or served as the caregiver in whom the family enhanced or interrupted the client's self-care or return to maximum functioning. What was the family doing to influence the client's health? What other things could they have done? Use theory from this chapter to support your ideas.
   - What did you do (or would you have done) as a nurse to facilitate family involvement in this situation? What did you learn from this experience? What would you do differently next time? Use a theory from this chapter to support your ideas.

Community-Based Nursing Across the Life Span

Now that you understand the concepts of community-based nursing, including the importance of a healthy community, cultural surroundings, and care of the family, you are ready to explore how you can develop skills in applying your knowledge. Skills in assessment, teaching, case management, and continuity of care are all important in community-based nursing. Although you probably have studied these concepts previously, they are discussed in this unit in the context of their specific relationship to community-based health care. Nursing interventions directed to the care of individuals, families, and communities or populations in community-based care are emphasized. This chapter is only intended to be an introduction to using nursing process in community-based settings. Chapters 8, 9, and 10 discuss in more depth the topics of health promotion, disease prevention, and the corresponding nursing interventions across the life span for community-based care.

Chapter 5 opens with a discussion of the use of nursing process including assessment, planning, intervention, and evaluation of the individual client, family, and community in community-based care. An evolving case study illustrates the principles and concepts of nursing process related to the care of the client and family in community settings. Population-based care highlights community assessment including concepts, methods, and applications.

The importance of client teaching along with teaching theory and developmental considerations in Chapter 6 leads to a discussion of the relationship of the nursing process to the teaching process.

Chapter 7 addresses continuity of care and the role of the case manager in community-based settings. It is all too common for clients and families to experience gaps in care as they move from one setting to another. It is the responsibility of the nurse to work in collaboration with the client, family, and other professionals to build bridges between settings, caregivers, and other resources. Entering and exiting the various agencies and providers along with the skills and competencies involved in continuity of care are covered.

Chapter 5

Assessment of Individuals, Families, and Communities for Population-Based Care

ROBERTA HUNT

Learning Objectives

1. Identify components essential to assessment of the client, family, and communities in community-based settings.

2. Discuss health needs common to community-based settings.

3. Identify the components of the 15-minute family interview.

4. Discuss the value of population-based care.

5. Utilize nursing interventions designed for community-focused population-based care.

6. Describe assessment, planning, intervention, and evaluation of community-focused population-based care.

7. Explain ways in which the concept of epidemiology can be used in community-based nursing.

8. Discuss methods for collecting community data.

9. Apply nursing process to situations including the care of the client, the family, and the community.

Key Terms

activities of daily living (ADL)
assessment
community assessment
community health need
constructed surveys
demographics
environmental assessment
epidemic
epidemiologist
epidemiology
functional assessment
holistic assessment

informant interviews
instrumental activities of daily living (IADL)
mortality
morbidity
participant observations
power systems
existing data
social system
spiritual assessment
windshield survey
vital statistics

Chapter Topics

The Nurse Speaks

While working as a staff nurse in a children's hospital, I had the opportunity to care for a 13-year-old young man on his day of discharge. Josh was an "old pro" when it came to the hospital environment, as he had endured 12 reconstructive surgeries on his right ear since birth. When I entered his room, Josh was lying in bed with the head of the bed slightly elevated. He was alone in the room and had turned off the radio and TV. He had a large dressing over his right ear and a bandage wrapped around his head to hold the dressing in place. On assessing his vital signs, I noted that he was afebrile; however, his blood pressure and pulse were slightly elevated. After assessing his vital signs, I asked Josh to rate his pain on a numeric scale of 0 to 10. Without hesitation, Josh replied a 9. I was quite concerned about his pain intensity level as the surgeons had already examined his ear and decided that he was ready to go home. In addition, they recommended over-the-counter analgesics for postoperative ear pain.

Before consulting with his physicians, I continued with my pain assessment. I asked Josh about the quality and duration of his pain, along with analgesic effectiveness. Then I asked Josh what the color of pain was, and he replied, "red." Lastly, I asked Josh to use my red pen to mark on a body outline pain tool the exact location of the pain. Much to my surprise, when Josh handed the pain tool back to me, there was a large red mark on his left leg, the donor site for his ear grafting!

When I inquired about the pain in his right ear, he replied, "What pain? My ear feels fine." Josh taught me an important lesson about the subjectivity of pain.

Although the obvious site of pain was his right ear, as a nurse, I cannot assume the obvious. I needed to be holistic in my pain assessment and remember to assess the location(s) of pain. Based on the valuable information from Josh, I was able to consult with his physicians and arrange for an effective analgesic to cover the pain at his donor site that would allow him to have pain control once he was home.

Susan O'Conner-Von, DNSc, RNC,
Associate Professor
School of Nursing University of Minnesota
Minneapolis, Minnesota

Nursing Process in Community-Based Settings

There are similarities and differences in the way that nursing process is used in community-based settings as compared with the acute care setting. It is important that nurses in community settings emphasize that it is a deliberate, adaptable, cyclic, client focused, and interactive process. Further, in community settings, nursing process has wider application to guide care of individuals, families, and populations or communities.

Whatever the setting, the basic construct is the same: **assessment**, diagnosis, outcomes, planning/intervention, and evaluation.

History of Nursing Process in Community Settings

Nurses have long understood the significance of the community in the health of the individual and family. Florence Nightingale was involved in assessing and intervening in community health in the middle of the 19th century. Her analysis of 1861 census data became the foundation of England's sanitary reform act, which is an excellent example of the use of nursing process to identify a community diagnosis (Woodham-Smith, 1950). Nightingale focused on assessment of the physical and social environment and its role in causing or contributing to illness. She also identified how sanitation, nutrition, and rest contribute to successful recovery from injury and illness as well as determined the relationship among adequate housing, recreation, employment, and health. From this data, she identified community-wide problems (diagnosis), determined what changes needed to be made (outcomes), formulated plans to address the problem through the sanitary reform act (intervention), and evaluated the results. Nightingale is often referred to as the first nurse **epidemiologist**.

Nursing Process for the Care of the Individual Client in Community Settings

Assessment, the first step in the nursing process, is a dynamic, ongoing method that uses observations and interactions to collect information, recognize changes, analyze needs, and plan care. Physicians primarily use assessment to determine pathology. Hospital-based nurses use assessment as the first step in the nursing process for ongoing monitoring of acute conditions and as an essential component in ensuring continuity with discharge planning. In community-based settings, assessment provides baseline information to help evaluate physiologic and psychological normality and functional capacity and to identify environmental factors that may enhance or impair the individual's health status. Because the community-based nurse sees clients only periodically and the status of conditions varies over time, thorough assessment is the cornerstone of quality community care.

To perform an accurate assessment, the nurse must communicate effectively, observe systematically, and interpret the collected data accurately (Carpenito, 2010). Typically, the health assessment consists of the interview and health history. The focus and parameters of the assessment depend on the scope of the service provided by the agency and the role of the nurse in that service. However, the first contact is always extremely important because it acts as the foundation for the nurse–client relationship. Establishing trust begins with the first contact with the individual, family, or community.

Community care differs from nursing care provided in hospital settings. Because the client and family are in charge of nearly all aspects of care the majority of the time, the nurse is primarily a facilitator of self-care rather than solely a care provider. Thus, the assessment process is intended to assess the client, whether it is the individual client, family, or community, and to identify needs and strengths and proceed accordingly. It is a continuous process that occurs in the context in which the response occurs. Thus, delivery of care must be considered within the environment, whether it be family, culture, immediate physical environment, or community environment. A **holistic assessment** often requires the collaboration of many professionals. This approach expands the usual definition of holistic assessment—body, mind, and spirit—to an even broader view.

This comprehensive view is used across the life span. The nurse in community-based settings is always diligent to complete a comprehensive assessment but is particularly attentive when caring for vulnerable populations. Thus, when assessing a newborn during a home visit, the nurse will bear in mind that a holistic assessment of the physical and psychological condition of the newborn, the immediate environment, and the skill of the primary caregivers are all essential to the infant's normal growth and development and protection from harm. The newborn is unable to speak on his or her behalf, and so a thorough assessment is the primary way the nurse advocates for the infant. Comprehensive assessment is essential to injury and disease prevention as well as health promotion and maintenance.

The assessment process is never an isolated course of action; rather information is continuously collected to be used for an immediate intervention or as a foundation for additional assessment at a later time. For example, a nurse visits the home of a family following the birth of an infant and notices that the infant's weight is not tracking within the norms of the growth chart for infants of the same age and race. This deviation from a typical finding would lead the nurse to additional assessment, which may include

- What are the infant's feeding patterns, including when and how much it consumed?
- What methods of feeding are used (formula or breast-feeding)?
- What is the size and type of the bottle and nipple?
- Does the family have access to potable water?
- What type of formula is being used? Ask the mother to explain how the ratio of water to formula is calculated.
- Observe the mother feeding the infant to see the caregiver's comfort in feeding the infant.
  - Does the mother hold the infant or prop the bottle?
  - Does the mother watch the infant's face during the feeding to gauge how the process is progressing for the infant?
- If using formula, does the family have the resources to purchase formula?

If the family has adequate supplies, information, and resources for formula, the nurse and the mother of the infant may devise a feeding plan and determine how much weight they would like the infant to gain before the next visit. At the next visit, if the outcomes are reached, the nurse and the mother may continue with the same plan. Alternatively, if the infant does not gain weight, the nurse may assess for other problems or refer for additional assessment by a nurse practitioner or physician. This exemplifies the role of the nurse in the community using assessment to plan the care of the individual client.

INFANTS AND CHILDREN

When assessing the infant and toddler, the nurse should begin by interviewing the primary caregiver. Typically, nutrition, growth and development, and vision and hearing are included.

Monitoring growth and development is easily done by weighing the infant, measuring length and head circumference, and plotting the results on a growth grid (National Center for Health Statistics, 2010, @www.cdc.gov/growthcharts/). Psychological status along with development of the infant, toddler, and preschooler should also be assessed by using a screening tool. Evidence-based screening tools that incorporate parent reports (e.g., Ages and Stages Questionnaire, the Parent's Evaluation of Developmental Status, and Child Development Inventories) can facilitate structured communication between parents and providers so as to elicit parent concerns, increase parent and provider observations of the child's development, and increase parent awareness (see Fig. 5-1).

Once variations from normal development are identified, the nurse and parent(s) determine possible outcomes and interventions to enhance further development.

Vision disorders are the fourth most common disability among children in the United States and the leading cause of impaired conditions in childhood (American Academy of Pediatrics [AAP], 2010). This is troubling because insufficient vision can affect a child's cognitive, emotional, neurological, and physical development by potentially limiting the type and amount of information to which the child is exposed. Infants and toddlers are not routinely screened for vision until 3 years of age (AAP, 2010). Recent studies estimate that only 21% of all preschool children are screened for vision problems and only 14% receive a comprehensive vision exam. However, a parent's observations may indicate the possible

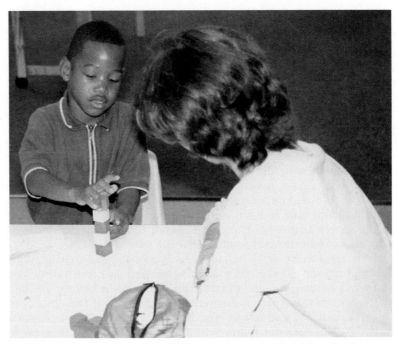

Figure 5-1 Developmental screening uses a series of tasks to screen children for developmental delays.

presence of vision and hearing problems. For a simple assessment of the vision of infants and toddlers, the nurse can ask the parent the questions found in Assessment Tools 5-1.

Hearing loss is the most common congenital condition in the United States, according to the AAP (2010). Infants at high risk for hearing impairment should be screened at birth. These include infants with the following:

- Family history of childhood hearing impairment
- Perinatal infection (e.g., cytomegalovirus, rubella, herpes, toxoplasmosis)
- Anatomic malformations of the head or neck
- Low birth weight (<1,500 g)
- Hyperbilirubinemia exceeding indications for exchange transfusion

Assessment Tools 5-1

Assessment questions related to the vision of infants older than 6 weeks:
- Does the infant return your smile?
- Do the infant's eyes follow you as you walk past or move around the room?
- Do you have any concerns that the infant is unable to see?

Assessment questions for evidence of the need to screen the vision of toddlers:
- Does the child cover one eye when looking at objects?
- Does the child tilt his or her head to look at things?
- Does the child hold toys, books, or other objects very close or very far away to look at them?
- Does the child rub his or her eyes, squint, frown, or blink frequently?

If the parent responds affirmatively to one or more of these questions, the nurse may use the intervention of referral to an eye doctor so that the child has additional assessment.

- Bacterial meningitis
- Birth asphyxia, infants with an Apgar score of 0 to 3, failure to breathe spontaneously in 10 minutes, or hypotonia of 2 hours past birth

Infants and toddlers are not routinely screened for hearing until 3 years of age (AAP, 2010). However, a parent's observations may indicate the possible presence of vision and hearing problems. And even if an infant's hearing has already been tested, the parents should be aware of signs that hearing is intact. During the first year, most babies react to loud noises, imitate sounds, and begin to respond to their name. By the age of 2 years, most children play with their voice, imitate simple words, and enjoy games like peek-a-boo and pat-a-cake. They may also use two-word sentences to talk about and ask for things. To determine if a toddler should be screened for hearing impairment, ask if the child has had frequent ear infections or has the same risk factors listed previously for infant screening.

Speech should also be assessed as hearing impairments often become apparent when the child begins to talk and are evidenced by the child's difficulty with pronunciation, resulting in speech that is hard to comprehend. If there are deficits in any of these areas, the infant should be referred for additional assessment.

Periodic assessment of preschool- and school-age children includes a health history and physical and developmental evaluation as well as home safety assessment. As with the infant and toddler, height, weight, and head circumference are important indicators of growth. Not only do these measurements determine if the child is following a normal growth curve, but they also reflect whether the child's weight is proportional to his or her height. If the child does not follow within the parameters of the growth chart, referral to a pediatric nurse practitioner, pediatrician, or other physician is necessary. Injuries are a leading cause of death among toddler, preschool children, and school-age children. The best strategy to assess for home safety is by using a home safety checklist. Several Web sites listed in What's on the Web contain this type of assessment tool. In addition to assessing normal growth using standardized growth charts, it is important to assess and intervene in the area of nutrition when caring for infants, children, and adolescents. Screening tools for infants, children, and adolescents are found in Appendix B. Childhood obesity has more than tripled in the past 30 years. The prevalence of obesity among children aged 6 to 11 years increased from 6.5% in 1980 to 19.6% in 2008, while among adolescents aged 12 to 19 years, obesity increased from 5.0% to 18.1% (Centers for Disease Control and Prevention, National Center for Health Statistics, 2010a). Because obesity substantially increases the risk of chronic illness from high blood pressure, high cholesterol, type 2 diabetes, heart disease and stroke, arthritis, sleep disturbances, and cancer (breast, prostate, and colon), it is important to identify overweight children early to allow for timely intervention.

ADULTS AND ELDERLY ADULTS

Increasingly, the caseload of nurses working in community-based settings will reflect the rapid growth of the population aged 65 and older, which is the most demographically influential trend in the United States and globally. Starting in 2011, when the first wave of baby boomers turns 65, elderly people will represent an even larger percentage of the total population than was seen in the past. Between 2010 and 2030, the number of people aged 65 or older will grow by more than 30%, while total population growth will be between 8% and 9% per decade (Population Reference Bureau, 2010). The fastest growing segment of the elderly population will continue to be individuals over 85 years of age. Because contact with the nurse is intermittent in community-based settings, it is essential that nursing care be holistic, addressing environmental, cultural, spiritual, and nutritional factors, as well as functional and physical aspects of the client.

Assessing and Intervening With Functional Status

Functional assessment requires the nurse to determine whether there are environmental, cognitive, neurologic, or behavioral barriers to independent function and self-care. Societal and cultural factors may also create barriers. The primary consideration of the functional assessment is whether the client needs the assistance of another person for daily function. The client's ability to conceptualize an activity is just as important as the client's physical ability to perform the activity. Once functional status is assessed with the needs and strengths or assets of the client identified, then planning begins by determining desired outcomes and possible nursing interventions.

Functional capacity is evaluated through an **environmental assessment** of the client's home and neighborhood. The client may be physically, cognitively, or emotionally disabled yet able to function independently except for the limitations created by barriers in the home. The next areas assessed are neurological status, cognitive and emotional status, integumentary status, and respiratory status. Last, the individual's abilities to complete **activities of daily living (ADL)** and **instrumental activities of daily living (IADL)** should be assessed. Analyzing a client's ADL is a standard method for evaluating the ability to perform the activities that are essential for independent living. They include grooming, dressing, bathing, toileting, transferring, walking, and feeding or eating. IADL involve planning and preparing light meals, traveling, doing laundry, housekeeping, shopping, and using the telephone. Assessment Tools 5-2 presents an example of a common functional assessment.

Assessment Tools 5-2
Functional Assessment

Environmental Assessment

Structural Barriers

Do stairs in the home limit the client's independent mobility to reach the bathroom, kitchen, and bedroom?
Check for the presence of the following:

Handrails on stairs and in the bathroom and tub.

Narrow doorways.

Unsafe flooring or floor-covering materials. material.

Inadequate lighting.

Safe gas and electrical appliances.

Improperly stored hazardous material.

Neurologic Status

Perceptual Function

Is the client able to perceive his or her immediate environment?

Sensory Function

Does the client have impaired vision?

Does the client have impaired hearing and ability to understand spoken language?

Is the client able to participate in an appropriate conversation 10 to 15 minutes long?

Is the client experiencing chronic pain?

Cognitive and Emotional Status

Does the client make eye contact with the visitor, greet the visitor, and appear to be well groomed or have made an attempt to be?

Assess if the client is oriented to person, place, and time. Work these questions into the conversation.

Ask the client to perform a simple task such as getting the nurse a glass of water (but without putting the client on the spot or acting as if this is a test).

Integumentary Status

If the client is unable to perform ADL or IADL because of a wound, dressing, or pain, then the wound impairs the client's functional ability.

Respiratory Status

Respiratory status is impaired if the client's respiratory status, typically shortness of breath or dyspnea, prevents functioning. Here are some indications:

If the client stops or slows down the activity before it is completed.

If the client sits down midway through or after the activity.

If the client complains of chest tightness or pain or breathes in quick shallow breaths.

Adapted from Neal, L. J. (1998). Functional assessment of the home health client. *Home Healthcare Nurse, 16*(10), 670–677; Hunt, R. (Ed.). (2000). *Readings in community-based nursing* (pp. 168–177). Philadelphia, PA: Lippincott Williams & Wilkins.

CLIENT SITUATIONS IN PRACTICE

Richard, a 63-year-old widower who has just had a hip replacement, is going home from the hospital tomorrow. Richard is 5′ 9″ tall and weighs 216 lb. Both extensive rheumatoid arthritis and brittle type I diabetes make it difficult for him to manage self-care at home. When the nurse assesses ADL/IADLs and asks him about how he will manage when he is home, he says, "With trying to move about with the walker and the trouble I have with my hands, I am not sure how I will be able to dress myself, take a bath, or prepare food let alone go to the grocery store." When the nurse asks Richard about his typical diet in a normal day, he states, "I live a block from a bakery and I like to walk down there at 5:00 PM every day to buy the day old doughnuts, cookies, and pies. I have a sweet tooth." This simple functional assessment indicates Richard may have the potential for ineffective therapeutic regimen management. When the nurse assesses the neighborhood, she learns that Richard can seek services through the Block Nurse program in his neighborhood with the goal that Richard will have resources to improve his nutritional status to enhance recovery from surgery. A nurse from the Block Nurse program is scheduled to visit him the day after he is discharged from the hospital. Through the nursing interventions of counseling, case management, and referral and follow-up, Richard begins to use services through the Block Nurse program in his neighborhood. (This program is discussed in Chapter 11.)

Nutrition

Nutrition screening is an important part of providing care for clients across the life span in community-based settings. An example of a nutrition screening tool for adults is found in Assessment Tools 5-3. After assessing the client's nutritional risk, the nurse, client, and family will devise a plan together to address the identified needs. If the client requires additional assessment, a nurse specially trained in nutrition or a dietitian assesses the client.

Assessing Medication Knowledge

Assessing medication knowledge and practice is an important aspect of comprehensive assessment. Polypharmacy, the use of multiple medications, is common among anyone with a chronic condition but particularly in older people. Fifty percent of individuals over the age of 65 have multiple chronic conditions requiring an average of two to six prescribed medications routinely. The prevalence of polypharmacy among nursing home residents is approximately 40%. Advanced age, white race, comorbid conditions, and female gender have been found in previous research to be among the risk factors for polypharmacy (Dwyer, Han, Woodwell, & Rechtsteiner, 2010). Polypharmacy, itself, is a well-known risk factor for adverse outcomes such as hospitalizations and falls (Flaherty, Perry, & Lynchard, 2000; Ziere et al., 2006). Polypharmacy also has been associated with higher **mortality** in elderly persons (Jyrkkä, Enlund, Korhonen, Sulkava, & Hartikainen, 2009). However, the correct use of medication is a concern across the life span. The tool in Assessment Tools 5-4 can be used in a community-based setting to assess a client's medication use.

Assessment Tools 5-3
Mini Nutritional Assessment Tool for the Elderly

Nestlé Nutrition INSTITUTE

Mini Nutritional Assessment
MNA®

Last name: First name:

Sex: Age: Weight, kg: Height, cm: Date:

Complete the screen by filling in the boxes with the appropriate numbers. Total the numbers for the final screening score.

Screening

A   Has food intake declined over the past 3 months due to loss of appetite, digestive problems, chewing or swallowing difficulties?
0 = severe decrease in food intake
1 = moderate decrease in food intake
2 = no decrease in food intake   ☐

B   Weight loss during the last 3 months
0 = weight loss greater than 3 kg (6.6 lbs)
1 = does not know
2 = weight loss between 1 and 3 kg (2.2 and 6.6 lbs)
3 = no weight loss   ☐

C   Mobility
0 = bed or chair bound
1 = able to get out of bed / chair but does not go out
2 = goes out   ☐

D   Has suffered psychological stress or acute disease in the past 3 months?
0 = yes   2 = no   ☐

E   Neuropsychological problems
0 = severe dementia or depression
1 = mild dementia
2 = no psychological problems   ☐

F1 Body Mass Index (BMI) (weight in kg) / (height in m^2)
0 = BMI less than 19
1 = BMI 19 to less than 21
2 = BMI 21 to less than 23
3 = BMI 23 or greater   ☐

IF BMI IS NOT AVAILABLE, REPLACE QUESTION F1 WITH QUESTION F2.
DO NOT ANSWER QUESTION F2 IF QUESTION F1 IS ALREADY COMPLETED.

F2 Calf circumference (CC) in cm
0 = CC less than 31
3 = CC 31 or greater   ☐

Screening score
(max. 14 points)   ☐☐

12-14 points: Normal nutritional status
8-11 points: At risk of malnutrition
0-7 points: Malnourished

Source: Nestle Nutrition Institute. (2010). Mini nutritional assessment. Retrieved from http://www.mna-elderly.com. Used with permission.

Assessment Tools 5-4
Medication Assessment

The sequence of the interview is intended as a guideline when using the interview. All topics should be included in the assessment, but it is acceptable to reword statements or change the format to better meet the needs of the individual.

Who is the respondent? ☐ Client ☐ Spouse ☐ Other (list) _____

Please Check the Appropriate Response

We will be reviewing all of your medications. Please show me those you take every day and those you take occasionally. This includes eye drops, insulin, laxatives, vitamins, antacids, ointments, or any over-the-counter drugs or supplements you sometimes use. Are there any other medications that you regularly take that are not here today?

I. Medication Administration and Storage

☐ Yes ☐ No   Can client open a pill bottle? (Have client demonstrate.)

☐ Yes ☐ No   Can client break a pill in half? (Have client demonstrate. Omit if not applicable.)

☐ Yes ☐ No   Does someone help you take your medicine?

☐ Yes ☐ No   Do you use any type of system to help you take your pills, such as a pillbox or a calendar?
                     List: _____

☐ Yes ☐ No   Do you have problems swallowing your pills?
                     Where do you store your medicines? _____

II. Medication Purchasing Habits

What drugstore do you use? _____

☐ Yes ☐ No   Does the drugstore you use deliver the medications to your home?
                     If no, then how do you get your medications? _____

☐ Yes ☐ No   Do you always use the same drugstore? If no, explain: _____

☐ Yes ☐ No   Do financial difficulties ever prevent you from buying your medications?

III. Attitudes

☐ Excellent ☐ Good ☐ Fair ☐ Poor How would you describe your health? _____
What do you see as your health needs? _____

☐ Yes ☐ No   Does taking your medications upset your daily routine? If yes, explain: _____

☐ Yes ☐ No   Do side effects from your medications upset your daily routine?

☐ Yes ☐ No ☐ Don't know   Do your medications help you?

☐ Yes ☐ No   Do you ever share your medications with anyone else?

IV. Lifestyle Habits

How many times a week do you
_____ drink coffee, tea, or colas, or eat chocolate.
_____ use cigarettes, snuff, or tobacco products.
_____ consume beer, wine, or liquor.
_____ use recreational drugs, such as marijuana.

V. Home/Environment

Please list the name, relationship, and age of anyone who lives with you.

_____

_____

If someone else lives in your home, does that person participate in your health care? _____

VI. Medication Profile

Record each medication separately on the following form: (Attach additional sheets as necessary.) _____

_____

_____

_____

_____

_____

_____

(Medicine name, dosage, route, expiration date exactly as printed on label)

☐ Yes ☐ No   Can you read the name, dosage, and expiration date of this medicine? Why do you take the medication? _____

                                   _____

                                   How long have you taken this dosage? _____

                                   When do you take the medicine and how many do you take?

                                   _____

                                   Do you know what the side effects are? List: _____

                                   _____

☐ Yes ☐ No   Does the medicine cause you any problems or side effects?

                                   _____

                                   What do you do if you experience side effects? (Stop the pills, call the doctor, etc.) _____

Adapted from DeBrew, J. K., Barba, B. E., & Tesh, A. S. (1998). Assessing medication knowledge and practice in older adults. *Home Healthcare Nurse, 16*(10), 686–692.

After assessing the client's knowledge base, the nurse and client then devise an education program to address identified learning needs. Interventions to address medication safety range from teaching the individual client about safe ways to self administer medications to developing a teaching program for a group of clients with CHF related to the safe use of medications to creating a hospital policy that requires comprehensive medication teaching prior to discharge (see Research in Community-Based Nursing Care 5-1).

RESEARCH IN COMMUNITY-BASED NURSING CARE 5-1

Frail Elderly Patients in Primary Care—Their Medication Knowledge and Beliefs About Prescribed Medicines

The purpose of this study was to describe elderly patients' knowledge and attitudes toward their medicines. Patients 65 years old or older seeking services in primary care who had multiple chronic illnesses were recruited to participate in the study. A questionnaire measuring knowledge about indications and possible adverse effects for each medication and the Beliefs about Medicine Questionnaire, which measured attitudes, were used. Generally, at least 75% of medications were known to 71% of patients. However, patients with polypharmacy and multidose drugs had significantly less knowledge, with 84% reporting no knowledge about possible adverse effects or synergistic drug interactions. For 93% of the patients, the benefits of the medication outweighed the concerns. The researchers concluded that knowledge about possible adverse effects was poor, but patients had strong faith in the benefits of the medication they were taking.

Source: Modig, S., Kristensson, J., Ekwall, A., Hallberg, I., & Midlöv, P. (2009). Frail elderly patients in primary care—Their medication knowledge and beliefs about prescribed medicines. *European Journal of Clinical Pharmacology, 65*(2), 151–155. Retrieved from CINAHL Plus with Full Text database.

✳ CLIENT SITUATIONS IN PRACTICE

Marge, the nurse from the Block Nurse program, visits Richard the day after his morning discharge from the hospital. He is sitting in a chair in the living room but is unshaven and looks like he has slept in his clothes. When he stands up, he says he is weak, in pain, and has not eaten since yesterday. He reports he has not taken his medication today. Pain and medication assessment indicates Richard has need for nursing intervention due to ineffective therapeutic regimen management. First, Marge asks him what makes it difficult for him to take the medication. He states he wants to take his medication but is neither able to open the new bottle of medication that he received the day before nor does he understand when he is to take which of the pills. He does not have a family member or friend to help him take his medications. Marge's goal is that Richard will regularly take his medication to promote postoperative healing. Using the intervention of health teaching, Marge puts his medication in an egg carton and labels the time and day they are to be taken. On her next visit, she will bring a plastic medication case. Marge knows the services in the neighborhood, so through the nursing interventions of case finding, care management, and referral, Marge calls Meals on Wheels to deliver a meal that day and for a neighbor to purchase and deliver some groceries for him for the next few days. The goal is that Richard will have access to adequate nutrition to recover from his surgery and facilitate incision healing. Richard states he is embarrassed by the way he looks and that his other main concern now is to be able to have a bath twice a week. Using the nursing intervention of case management and referral, Marge calls and arranges for a home health aide to come in to assist him in taking a shower twice a week. She and Richard then discuss how often he would like her to visit him in the next few weeks and other help that he believes he needs.

Psychosocial Factors and Culture

Culture and the impact culture have on health and health beliefs are discussed in Chapters 3 and 4. A cultural assessment is always a part of the health history as it is imperative to incorporate the client's understanding of health-related issues, the family's cultural perspective, and the various cultural viewpoints within neighborhoods, communities, and regions into all health care planning. A comprehensive cultural assessment guide is seen in Assessment Tools 5-5. Additional cultural assessment tools are found in Chapter 3. After the

---

Assessment Tools 5-5
Cultural Assessment Guide

Client _____

Cultural/ethnic identity _____

Religion _____ Spiritual rituals _____

Primary language _____ Speaks English?   Yes No

Language resources _____

Health beliefs_____

Client's explanation of health problem _____

Traditional healer_____

Contact information _____

Traditional treatments _____

Where obtained and prepared _____

Do cultural health practices conflict with current medical practice?
If so, how? _____
Expectations of nurse/care providers _____

Pain Assessment
Cultural patterns/client's perception of pain response _____

Nutrition Assessment
Ethnic preferences _____
Religious prohibitions and preferences _____
Sick foods _____
_____
Food intolerances/taboos _____

Medication Assessment
Client's perceptions of medications _____
_____
Possible pharmacogenetic variations _____
_____

Psychosocial Assessment
Family structure and decision-making patterns _____
_____
Sick role behavior _____
_____
Cultural/ethnic/religious resources/supportive systems _____
_____

assessment is complete, the nurse, client, and family devise a plan of care, which is built around the identified cultural considerations.

Further, a psychosocial assessment in tandem with the cultural assessment will enable the nurse to understand the client in the context of family, as defined by the client's culture. This may involve exploring the topics of family decision maker, sick role behavior, language barriers, and community resources as they relate to the client's culture. This assessment may simply address the following issues:

- Who is the decision maker in the family?
- What are the characteristics of the sick role in the client's culture?
- Do any language barriers exist?
- What resources are available in the community that are sensitive to the client's culture?

Assessing Environment

An environmental assessment is an essential aspect of any assessment across the life span and across settings. Figure 5-2 and Assessment Tools 5-6 are useful when completing an environmental assessment.

The primary consideration of any environmental assessment is to identify safety concerns. Again, vulnerable populations, the very young and very old, and those with serious chronic conditions are most at risk for safety issues. Many communities have home safety check kits available through the Red Cross or local fire department to assess for unsafe conditions in the home.

Environmental Assessment Checklist

Patient _____ Patient Number _____ Team/Person Completing Form _____

Date and initial as each assessment area is addressed. Describe unsafe/unmet needs. Suggest modifications.

Assessment Areas	Safe/Meets Client's Needs	Unsafe/Needs Adaptation	Recommended Modifications and Possible Referral
Physiologic and Survival Needs Food/Fluids/Eating			
Elimination/Toileting			
Hygiene/Bathing/Grooming			
Clothing/Dressing			
Rest/Sleeping			
Medication			
Shelter			
Safety and Security Mobility and Fall Prevention			
Fire/Burn Prevention			
Crime/Injury Prevention			
Love and Belonging Caregiver			
Communication			
Family/Friends/Pets			
Self-Esteem, Self-Actualization Enjoyable/Meaningful Activities			

Figure 5-2 Environmental assessment checklist (see Assessment Tools 5-5 for questions for each category). Adapted from Narayan, M. C., & Tennant, J. (1997). Environmental assessment. *Home Healthcare Nurse, 15*(11), 799–805.

Assessing Spirituality

Numerous studies show that spiritual or religious practice is correlated with greater health and longer life. Assessing spiritual health and intervening according to the client's values may be one of the most important areas to address in community-based care. A **spiritual assessment** allows the nurse to determine the presence of spiritual distress or identify other spiritual needs. Illness often triggers spiritual discord in addition to emotional, mental, and physical pain. Spiritual care is an integral part of holistic care. The health care team must be comfortable with and receptive to these needs for them to emerge and be addressed.

Assessment Tools 5-6
Questions to Complete: Environmental Assessment Checklist

Physiologic and Survival Needs
Food and Fluids/Eating

What are the client's plans for getting groceries? Who will prepare the food?

Is there food in the home? Who will do the grocery shopping?

Are there opportunities for food storage? Is there water potable?

Does the kitchen have barriers to the client actually preparing the food?

Elimination/Toileting

Can the client get to the bathroom? Is the pathway clear? Is a bedside commode needed? Is a raised toilet indicated?

Will the client be able to wash hands? Able to turn water off and on?

Will the client have a hard time getting up and down from the commode? Are there grab bars? (Towel racks, if used for steadying, can pull away from the wall.)

Hygiene/Bathing/Grooming

What is the plan for bathing? Does the client need assistance?

Is there hot and cold running water? Is the water temperature 120° or less?

Are there grab bars next to the tub and shower?

Are there nonskid tiles/strips/appliqués/rubber mats on tub bottom and shower floor?

Are the bathroom and fixtures clean? What provisions are there for mouth care? Hair care?

Clothing/Dressing

Does the client have shoes or slippers that are easy to put on and fit properly with nonskid soles?

Will the client be able to change clothes? Are the clothes so baggy that they could trip the client?

Are there clean clothes? How will the laundry be washed?

Rest/Sleeping

Where will the client sleep? Would the client benefit from a hospital bed? A trapeze?

How far is the bed from the floor? Can the client get in and out of the bed? How far is the bed from the bathroom? From other family members?

How much time will the client spend in bed? Does the client need a special mattress?

Medications

Does the client have a plan for taking the right medications at the right time?

Is there a secure place to store the medications? Are they safe from children and the cognitively impaired? Can the client reach the medications needed? Open the container? Read the label? Is there adequate lighting where the client will be preparing medications?

Is there a safe way to dispose of syringes? Medical supplies?

Shelter

Is the house clean and comfortable for the client? Who will do the housework?

Are the plumbing and sewage systems working? Is there adequate ventilation?

Is there a safe heat source? Are space heaters safe? Are the electrical cords in good condition?

Is the house infested with roaches, other insects, or rodents?

Safety and Security
Mobility/Fall Prevention

Is the client able to get around the home? Does the client have good balance? Steady gait?

Is the caregiver thinking of using restraints? What sort of restraints? Are they necessary?

Does the client use assistive devices (walkers, canes) correctly? Are they the right height?

Do the devices fit through the pathways without catching on furnishings?

Are the pathways, hallways, and stairways clear? Are there throw rugs?

Are there sturdy handrails on the stairs? Are the first and last steps clearly marked?

Is there adequate lighting in hallways and stairways? Is the path to the bathroom well lighted at night?

Are the floors slippery? (Floors should not have a high gloss or be highly waxed.)

Are there uneven floor surfaces?

Are the carpets in good repair without buckles or tears that could cause tripping?

Can the client walk steadily on the carpets? (Thick-pile carpets can cause tripping if the client has a shuffling gait.)

Are the chairs the client uses sturdy? Are they stable if the client uses them to prevent a fall?

Does the client use furniture or counters for balance when walking? Are these sturdy enough to withstand the pressure?

Are there cords or wires that could cause the client to trip?

Fire/Burn Prevention

Is there a smoke detector on each level of the home? Is there a fire extinguisher?

Is there an escape plan for the client to get out of the house in case of fire?

Is the client using heating pads and space heaters safely?

Are wires and plugs in good repair?

If the client smokes, are there plans to make sure the client smokes safely?

Are there signs of cigarette burns? Burns in the kitchen?

Are oxygen tanks stored away from flames and heat sources?

Crime/Injury Prevention

Are there locks on the doors and the windows?

Can the client make an emergency call? Is the telephone handy?

Are emergency numbers clearly marked?

Are firearms securely stored in a locked box? Is the ammunition stored and locked away separately?

Is there evidence of criminal activity?

Love and Belonging
Caregiver

Is there a caregiver? Is the caregiver competent? Willing? Supportive?

Does the caregiver need support?

Can the caregiver hear the client? Should there be additional communication device such as a baby monitor or hand bell?

Communication

Is the telephone easily accessible?

Should the telephone have an illuminated dial? Oversized numbers? Memory feature? Audio enhancer?

Is there a daily safety check system? Should there be an alert system like Lifeline?

How will the client obtain mail?

Family/Friends/Pets
Are there supportive neighbors?

Does the client have family, friends, or church/synagogue/mosque members to help and visit?

Is the client able to take proper care of any pets? Are pets well behaved?

Self-Esteem and Self-Actualization

What kind of activities does the client enjoy? Are there creative ways that these activities can be brought to the client?

Does the client have access to meaningful activities? Listening to music/book tapes? Interactive activities?

Adapted from Narayan, M. C., & Tennant, J. (1997). Environmental assessment. *Home Healthcare Nurse,* *15*(11), 799–805.

Through the intervention of presence, the health care provider is available and listens in a meaningful way to the client and family. This intervention, a component of counseling, also necessitates being aware that not only is it a privilege to be invited into another person's life in this way, it is also an ethical responsibility.

Questions that could begin the process of a spiritual needs assessment are shown in Assessment Tools 5-7. The nurse, client, and family may in a mutual process use the information from this assessment to identify spiritual issues and incorporate them in the plan of care. Since 2006, the Joint Commission on Accreditation of Healthcare Organizations (JCAHO) requires that all clients cared for by accredited health care organizations must have a spiritual assessment (JCAHO, 2010).

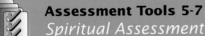

Assessment Tools 5-7
Spiritual Assessment

Examples of elements that could be but are not required in a spiritual assessment include the following questions directed to the patient or his/her family:

- Who or what provides the patient with strength and hope?
- Does the patient use prayer in his or her life?
- How does the patient express their spirituality?
- How would the patient describe their philosophy of life?
- What type of spiritual/religious support does the patient desire?
- What is the name of the patient's clergy, minister, chaplain, pastor, rabbi, or imam?
- What does suffering mean to the patient?
- What does dying mean to the patient?
- What are the patient's spiritual goals?
- Is there a role of church/synagogue/mosque in the patient's life?
- How does faith help the patient cope with illness?
- How does the patient keep going day after day?
- What helps the patient get through this health care experience?
- How has illness affected the patient and his or her family?

Source: Joint Commission. (2008). *Provision of care, treatment, and services: Spiritual assessment.* Retrieved from http://www.jointcommission.org/AccreditationPrograms/HomeCare/Standards/ 09_FAQs/PC/Spiritual_Assessment.htm

CLIENT SITUATIONS IN PRACTICE

Marge has been seeing Richard for 3 weeks. At the last visit, his incision was healing well, and with Marge setting up his medications, he was taking them every day. He was able to do his ADLs and his IADLs except grocery shopping. Today, when Marge knocks and walks into the house, Richard is sitting on the sofa with his head in his hands. When he looks up, his eyes are red and teary. Marge says, "Richard, what is wrong?" He says, "I am so lonely. Maryanne and I used to go to Mass every day together. I have missed that so much." Marge immediately recognizes that Richard is experiencing spiritual distress. Marge problem solves with Richard and helps him to identify a local parish that provides rides to Mass for people otherwise homebound. Her goal is that Richard will be able to attend Mass, and her nursing intervention is counseling and case management. She completes her assessment and learns that his incision is healed, and he continues to take his medication. His nutritional status is stable, but his blood sugars continue to be labile. They schedule the next visit for the following week when his daughter is visiting from another state.

As discussed in Chapter 4, assessment of the family's ability to provide caregiving that may keep the client at home and out of the hospital or nursing home is often imperative.

A simple family assessment, completed in 15 minutes or less, may actually save the nurse time, allowing the nurse to identify issues early and prevent problems later. The key ingredients to a simple family interview are speaking politely and respectfully, using therapeutic communication, constructing a family genogram, asking therapeutic questions, and commending the family and individual on their strengths (Wright & Leahey, 1999). For complete details on these items, reread Chapter 4.

Some of the most basic suggestions include the following:

- Invite families to accompany the client to the unit/clinic/hospital.
- Involve families in the admission procedure or interview.
- Encourage families to ask questions during the client orientation or first visit.
- Acknowledge the client and family's expertise in self-care or assisting in self-care.
- Ask about routines at home and incorporate them in the plan of care.
- Encourage the clients to practice interactions that may come up in the future related to health regimens (e.g., have a parent practice telling a diabetic child that she may not eat ice cream at a birthday party).
- Consult with clients and family about their ideas for treatment and discharge. (Adapted from Wright & Leahey, 1999, p. 264)

CLIENT SITUATIONS IN PRACTICE

When Marge arrived for the visit the next week, Richard answered the door and invited her into the living room. As Marge and Richard sat down, Marge heard someone doing dishes in the kitchen. She asked Richard, "Did your daughter arrive?" "Yes, she is in the kitchen," Richard replied. Marge went into the kitchen and invited his daughter to join the conversation. After Richard's daughter Kathy sat down, Marge introduced herself, told her that she was a nurse working for the Block Nurse program, and explained that she had been visiting Richard since the day after he was discharged from the hospital. She asked if Kathy had any questions, and Kathy indicated she did not. Marge went on to praise Richard for how he had managed his own care after his surgery and summarized his progress for Kathy. Marge then asked Richard if he had anything to add, and he indicated he did not. She asked Kathy what she would like to know about Richard's health care needs. Kathy replied that because she had been transferred back to the area and had purchased a house two blocks from her father, she expected that she would be as involved with her father's care as he desired. Richard stated that he was having a lot of trouble regulating his diet, blood sugars, and insulin and needed help with this. Marge then suggested that they start by talking about his usual routine and how his diet and diabetes regulation could follow that routine. She then asked what Kathy and Richard knew about diabetes and what they wanted to know. Marge's intervention of health teaching began based on what Kathy and Richard already knew and wanted to know about diabetes. Kathy, Richard, and Marge decided that they would meet the next week. Their goal next week would be to talk about the diabetic diet and recipes that were appropriate for the diabetic diet.

A genogram and ecomap are essential elements of the quick family interview. See Chapter 4 for detailed information on completing a genogram or ecomap. Asking therapeutic questions is also important to the family interview. Numerous examples are found in Chapter 4.

The last aspect of the simple family interview is to focus on strengths rather than on needs and problems. Strength-based nursing validates the client and family's assets. In every encounter with a family, the acknowledgment of the resources, competencies, and efforts observed allows the family and client to realize their assets and develop new perspectives of themselves and their abilities.

In summary, this framework recommends the following steps:

1. Use good manners to engage or reengage the client's family; introduce yourself by offering your name and role and orienting family members to the purpose of a brief family interview.
2. Assess key areas of internal and external structure and function; obtain genogram information and key external support data.
3. Ask three key questions to family members.
4. Commend the family on two strengths.
5. Evaluate the usefulness of the interview and conclude (Wright & Leahey, 1999).

Population-Based Care: Assessment of the Community

All nurses have a role in **community assessment** and a contribution to make to population-based care. These activities may include conducting a simple community assessment to determine available, accessible, and appropriate community resources for the referral of an individual client or a family in a given community. Or when a nurse notes an increase in the number of cases of a particular disease or injury in her agency or community, this may lead to an exploration of demographic **morbidity** data from that community to establish if there is an increase from previous years or seasons. This type of community assessment might lead to an attempt to address this need through a new educational program or service. In population-based care, medication safety may be addressed by involving state or federal entities in developing regulations regarding medication safety.

As discussed earlier in this chapter, childhood obesity rates have more than tripled in the past 30 years. Population-based care of communities is seen when a school nurse recognizes that many children are overweight within a particular neighborhood. He or she may lead a group of citizens to encourage the local school to reinstate recess and lunch playtime on the playground. Or the group may ask the school board to add physical education to the school curricula. An example of a population-based community-wide program that a nurse might be involved in to reduce obesity through a school-based program is seen in Research in Community-Based Nursing 5-2. To address childhood obesity, this school-based program offers more nutritious meals and snacks in the cafeterias, increases physical activity, and improves education about health.

Public health nurses typically use community assessment to determine needs for particular services or programs in a given geographic area or neighborhood. This is seen, for example, when a community health nurse uses community assessment to determine the need for flu shot clinics in a neighborhood. A more complex example is the use of community assessment in influencing public policy. The nurse with a graduate degree, or a nurse statistician or epidemiologist, may be contracted by a state or local government to do a community assessment to determine the number and percentage of citizens in a particular geographic area who are uninsured or underinsured.

Through community assessment, the nurse determines how a community influences the health of its residents. Community assessment is a technique that may be used to determine the health status, resources, or needs of a group of individuals and is the first step in population-based care. Similar to assessment in nursing process, community assessment collects information about the physiological, psychological, sociocultural, and spiritual health of the community. It allows the nurse to explore the relationship between a variety of community variables and the health of its citizens. Professionals from a number of

RESEARCH IN COMMUNITY-BASED NURSING CARE 5-2

A School-Based Intervention for Diabetes Risk Reduction

School-based programs to improve nutrition and education about healthy living that also offer more opportunities for exercise for at-risk children have been shown to be effective in helping children maintain a weight within normal range. A total of 4,603 children in 42 schools participated in community-based research that randomly assigned schools to either a multicomponent school-based intervention or to an assessment-only school (control group). Children in the intervention group were offered healthier food choices in school through the cafeteria, at the snack bar, in vending machines, and during class events. Longer, more intense periods of physical activity for the children were built into the school day as well as activities to promote healthy living. Researchers reported that children who were already obese at the start of the program lost a significant amount of weight, indicated by a reduction in waist size resulting in a 21% lower risk of being obese by the end of the eighth grade. This translates into reducing the risk for the development of type 2 diabetes in children. The researchers concluded that school-based programs can make a difference in the obesity rate of children.

Source: Singhal, N., & Misra, A. (2010). A school-based intervention for diabetes risk reduction. *New England Journal of Medicine, 363*(5), 443–453. doi:10.1056/NEJMoa1001933.

disciplines may participate in community assessment activities. These professionals include nurses, social workers, therapists, community health workers, public health nurses, physicians, epidemiologists, statisticians, and public policy makers.

COMPONENTS OF COMMUNITY ASSESSMENT

Chapter 1 describes the community as an entity made up of people, a place, and **social systems**, and it discusses the characteristics of a healthy community. Community assessment reflects a problem-solving process similar to the nursing process and uses steps similar to those used to assess the individual client or family. All three dimensions of the community are assessed: the people, the place, and the social systems.

People

A community can be assessed by analyzing the characteristics of the people in that community. These characteristics are defined through the **demographics** of the community, which include the number, composition by age, rate of growth and decline, social class, and mobility of the people in the community. Other **vital statistics** include the birth rate, overall death rate (mortality), mortality by cause and by age, and infant mortality rate. Of these, the infant mortality rate is considered to be the most important statistical indicator regarding the level of maternal–infant health in a community. Vital statistics also include the morbidity or rate of a particular disease within a community. These vital statistics are the "vital signs" of the community. They tell a very important story about the health of a community or population.

Place

Place or location is where the community is geographically located and its boundaries. It may include the type of community, such as rural or urban; location of health services; and climate, flora, fauna, and topography. Assessment of location is important because it determines what services are accessible and available to the people living within that area. Place also impacts well-being and, in turn, mortality and morbidity in certain conditions. For instance, the rates of Lyme disease are considered as an **epidemic** in some parts of the country, such as sections of Wisconsin and Connecticut. Similarly, deaths from hypothermia or severe frostbite are more common in regions of the United States where there may be temperatures below 0°F for long periods of time.

Every year, the Gallup Healthway Well-Being Index publishes the Healthiest Cities, which ranks U.S. cities in terms of chronic disease prevalence. In addition, the report

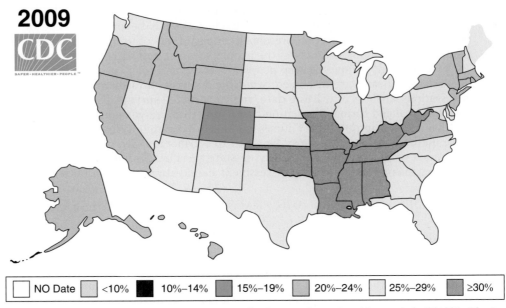

Figure 5-3 Obesity rates by state. From Centers for Disease Control and Prevention. (2010b). *Obesity trends*. Retrieved from http://www.cdc.gov/obesity/data/trends.html

describes the degree to which these cities take steps to promote preventive health behaviors, ensure access to health care, and support physical activity (2010). The impact place has on health is also seen in the wide range of rates of obesity from state to state in the United States as seen in Figure 5-3.

Social Systems

Social systems are assessed as economic, educational, religious, political, and legal systems. Further, human services, opportunities for recreation, and communication systems are components of a community's social systems. **Power systems** within a community must also be assessed as part of the overall social system—how power is distributed throughout a particular social system. Determining how decisions are made and how change occurs is essential in planning. Power systems impact health and health care. There are wide disparities in the rates of those without health insurance by state, which is mostly a result of the existence or quality of the social systems. For example, in Minnesota, the percentage of poor children who do not have health insurance is 4.4% and in Texas 13.4% (U.S. Census Bureau, 2008).

Social Determinants of Health

Where people live, learn, work, and play affect how long they will live and how healthy they will be. Thus, the people, place, and social systems of a community all contribute to the health of those living in that community and must be addressed as a part of community assessment and the population intervention that may follow. The wide variation in the "health" of cities, counties, and states across the United States predicts the health of the people living in that city, county, or state. This is seen in how the rates of obesity vary by state and region. A national study of 448 metropolitan counties found that people living in sprawling, low-density counties walk less, weigh more, and are more likely to be obese or have hypertension (Ewing et al., 2003).

DATA SOURCES FOR POPULATION HEALTH ASSESSMENT

Many methods can be used to collect data for a community assessment. **Epidemiology** offers nurses working in community settings a way of thinking about the health of populations and provides a frame of reference for investigating and improving health in any setting. Epidemiology "is the study of the distribution and determinants of health-related states or events in specified populations, and the application of this study to the control of health problems" (Last, 1988). A complete discussion of epidemiology is beyond the scope of this book. However, the following section presents a simplistic way of using some of the foundational elements of epidemiology to assess the people, location, and social systems of a community.

Five methods of investigating people, location, and social systems of a community as they relate to health are discussed: **windshield survey**, **informant interviews**, **participant observations**, analysis of **existing data**, and **constructed surveys**. These assessments seen in both informal and formal population-based initiatives are within the domain of the public health nurse. It is important for nurses working in a community-based setting to understand these methods because they may be asked to collaborate with more complex community assessment conducted by city, county, or state agencies. As with the care of the family or individual in community settings, assessment should always look for both needs and assets.

CLIENT SITUATIONS IN PRACTICE: COMMUNITY ASSESSMENT

A formal population-based assessment is seen when a school nurse observes from the daily log of student visits to the office an increasing number of children at the school with symptoms of cough and fever that lasts for more than a week (existing data). This leads the nurse to call some of the parents of these children to ask two or three questions to learn more about the symptoms the children have been having with the lingering cough (constructed survey and participant observation). With this information in hand, the nurse calls the county health department wondering if there may be cases of pertussis in the county (informant interviews). Upon learning that there have been several cases of pertussis in a bordering school district, the nurse goes to the state department of health Web site wondering if pertussis is a reportable condition (disease and health event investigation). Because the nurse has been in the school for some time, he or she knows that parents of children in the school are highly motivated to improve the health status of their children but some lack basic health literacy. Based on this information, the nurse contacts families of the children he or she knows to have symptoms, provides information about pertussis, and connects them to appropriate community resources (health education, referral, and case finding). In collaboration with the school district communications department, the nurse uses the sample health education sheet on pertussis from the state department of health Web site to develop a flyer to be distributed to all parents in the district (collaboration, health teaching, outreach, case finding).

Windshield Survey

A common method of community assessment is a windshield survey. The windshield survey is the motorized equivalent of a simple head-to-toe assessment employing the public health intervention of surveillance. The observer drives through a chosen neighborhood and uses the five senses and powers of observation to conduct a general assessment of that neighborhood. Conclusions from a windshield survey show common characteristics about the way people live, where they live, and the type of housing that exists in a given neighborhood. An example of a windshield survey is seen in Assessment Tools 5-8.

Assessment Tools 5-8
Windshield Survey

This assessment has been designed to assist the nurse traveling around the neighborhood to identify objective data related to people, places, and social systems that help define the community. This information may help identify trends, stability, and changes that may affect the health of the individual living in the community.

People

Who is on the street (e.g., women, children, men)?

How are they dressed?

What are they doing?

Are the people African American, White, Asian?

How are the different racial groups residentially located?

How would you categorize the residents: upper, upper middle, middle, lower class? How did you come to this conclusion?

Is there any evidence of communicable diseases, alcoholism, drug abuse, mental illness? How did you come to this conclusion?

Are there animals on the street? What kind?

Place

Boundaries

Where is the community located?

What are its political boundaries?

Natural boundaries?

Human-made boundaries?

Location of Health Services

Where are the major health institutions located?

What health institutions may be necessary for a community of this size but are not located in the community (e.g., a large community with few or no acute care or ambulatory care facilities)?

Are there geographic features that may pose a threat or impediment?

What plants or animals could pose a threat to health?

Human-Made Environment

Do you see major industrial areas with heavy industrial plants?

Do the roads allow easy access to health institutions? Are those roads marked by easily seen and understandable signs?

Housing

What is the quality of the housing?

How old are the houses?

Are there single or multifamily dwellings?

Are there signs of disrepair and decay? If so, explain.

Are there vacant dwellings? If so, explain.

Social Systems

Are there schools in the area? Are they in good repair?

Are there parks and outdoor recreation opportunities?

What churches, synagogues, and mosques are located in the community?

What schools, community centers, clinics, or other services for the community are provided by the churches, synagogues, and mosques?

Does the community have public transportation that provides accessible service?

What supermarkets and stores are available in the neighborhoods?

Is there evidence of police and fire protection in the area?

Are there social agencies, clinics, hospitals, dentists, or other health care providers?

Informant Interviews

Informant interviews involve community residents who are either key informants or members of the general public. Key informants are individuals in positions of power or influence in the community, such as leaders in local government, schools, and the religious or business community. General public interviews may include random telephone or person-on-the-street interviews. Interviews are typically unstructured and are conducted to collect general information.

Nurses working in acute care settings use the equivalent of informant interviews to elicit information from the client, family members, social workers, and spiritual counselors. In a more informal way, nurses may use this technique as they explore with other nurses, social workers, or discharge planners the potential community resources that may be appropriate for referral purposes. If the hospital or agency uses follow-up telephone calls after discharge, informant information about referral sources is elicited.

Participant Observations

The third method of data collection is participant observations where the nurse observes formal and informal community activities to determine significant events and occurrences. This leads to conclusions about what is happening in selected settings, providing information about community values, norms, and priorities. Formal gatherings include government, city council, county board, and school board meetings, while informal gatherings occur at the local coffee shop or cafe, barbershop, or school. Participant observations can be effective in determining the values, norms, and concerns of a community while offering an opportunity to identify the power systems within the community. Recognizing how power is distributed throughout the community social system and how decisions are made provides important insight into how change occurs in a community.

Nurses in in-patient settings use participant observation when they watch a client in physical therapy, occupational therapy, or as they interact with family members. These observations may tell the staff nurse something about the client's values and behavior. Home visits, conducted with clients after discharge from the acute-care setting to assess their ongoing needs or before admission to an acute-care setting, are examples of participant observation. During the home visit, the nurse collects information about the client in the context of the family and the community.

Existing Data

Sources of existing data include records, documents, and other previously collected information often related to vital statistics, census data, and reportable diseases. Existing data can be used to assess people, place, or social systems. Depending on the community, an abundance of demographic data may be available to describe the health status of its members by neighborhood, city, county, state, and nation. These may include databases from schools, departments of health at the city and state levels, county data, private foundations, and state universities. Health data kept by the state may be thought of as the health records of the citizens of that state. Basic health status of a population is reflected in vital statistics such as birth rates, death rates, death rates by age, gender, race, ethnicity and cause, morbidity and mortality data for specific diseases to mention a few. Geographic Information Systems enables retrieval of computerized health status data and social system data by geographic location (Scotch, Parmanto, & Monaco, 2008). Existing data provide the statistical information about a neighborhood, county, state, or country that are the vital signs of the community.

An example of existing data may be seen in a clinic setting. Last week, you noticed that many of the adults seen in the clinic where you work were admitted with the diagnosis of bronchitis. You calculate that within the last week 30 of 100 clients who came to the clinic had bronchitis. You wonder if this is an epidemic. To determine if it is, you look at the clinic statistics for the year before and find that during the same week last year, 20 of 60 adults were admitted for bronchitis. Are you seeing an epidemic this year? Nurses in acute care and clinics use existing data when they consult old charts and past notes, vital signs, orders, and other indicators of client progress documented in client charts.

Another source of data is found in hospitals, medical centers, and other health systems that use digital dashboard technology to assist in their performance monitoring and quality improvement processes. In these facilities, data trends are displayed for health care workers to see and compare.

Constructed Surveys

Constructed surveys may be used to collect information about communities. This method of data collection is typically time consuming and expensive. A random sample of a targeted population asks a list of specific questions. Data collected are analyzed for patterns and trends. This type of assessment is beyond the scope of this book but is an important aspect of the role of the nurse with a graduate degree working in community-based settings. However, armed with the knowledge from a program evaluation or research evaluation course, any nurse can develop a simple survey tool to solicit information on a topic pertinent to the health of the community.

NURSING PROCESS AND POPULATION-BASED CARE

Population-based community care occurs through partnerships among constituents just as nursing care of the individual and family is a mutually formulated process. In many ways, partnerships in community-based care are similar to interprofessional teams. Partnerships form to serve a specific purpose and develop agreed-upon mission, values, goals, measurable outcomes, and accountability for the partnership. The relationship between partners is characterized by mutual trust, respect, genuineness, and commitment, built upon identified strengths and assets. The partnership balances power among partners and enables resources among partners to be shared (Campus-Community Partnerships for Health, 2010). Partnership requires ongoing dialogue in a reciprocal relationship between all stakeholders. For instance, a school nurse and a nurse working in a community clinic may build a coalition with a group of social workers at a transitional housing facility serving homeless families located in the same neighborhood. After a few meetings, data collected show that only 10% of the children in the transitional housing facility receive recommended well-child visits and immunizations. The group develops a goal to enhance the coordination of well-child services and immunizations for school children living in the transitional housing. The group invites interested parents from the housing facility to join the coalition. For 2 years they work together in an attempt to promote the coalition's goals. The evaluation of the project reveals that after 2 years 90% of the children in the housing facility receive all recommended well-child services and immunizations. Population-based community care is not something that the nurse does "for" a community rather "with" a community.

Community assessment may begin by using any one, or a combination, of the methods just discussed. These methods are applied to the three dimensions of community: people, place, and social systems. Another method of assessment could be based on the recommendations from the Robert Wood Johnson Foundation Commission to build a healthier America (Fig. 5-4). Every nurse in community-based settings would find at least one or two of these recommendations pertinent to the population with whom he or she works and an area to assess.

POPULATION-BASED COMMUNITY-FOCUSED SITUATIONS IN PRACTICE

You are a nurse who just moved from South Dakota to Washington County, located in another state. You notice that there seem to be many more children who have asthma in the clinic where you now work as a pediatric nurse compared to what you saw in South Dakota. In your new community, you see young children on the street using inhalers much more frequently compared to what you have seen in other communities. You ask a friend who is a school nurse, and he tells you that in the last decade, the number of children with asthma has increased dramatically in the school district where he works. He says that some of the community members believe that the problem is a contaminated waste dump near the oil refinery on the outskirts of town. He also mentions that according to the newspapers, the oil refinery plans to expand the size of the facility to double current capacity.

You do a Web search and compare your state statistics with those from other states and notice a higher rate of asthma in the state where you are now living with an average of 13 per 100 children, aged 0 to 17, diagnosed with asthma. You find that the emergency department visit rate for children aged 0 to 17 is five in your state and is nearly twice the *Healthy People 2020* goal. There is disparity in which children are diagnosed with asthma. Male children are significantly more likely to be told that they have asthma with a rate of 15.1% for boys compared with 11.5% of girls. African American children are the most likely to be diagnosed; nearly one fifth (19.5%) are reported to have asthma, a significantly higher percentage compared to white children. In comparison, 12.2% of Whites, 9.5% of Asians, and 16.0% of Hispanic children are reported to have asthma. The school nurse tells you that she thinks that in her school, the rate is around 30 per 100 in children aged 5 to 12. Further, you learn from www.countyhealthrankings.org that Washington County has the highest rate of asthma in children in the state. You also learn that your county has three times the rate of high pollution days as compared to the national average. You wonder if the oil refinery located nearby could contribute to the high rate of asthma.

Your community has many strengths. Most of the individuals and families you have worked with report positive support systems and the ability to perform self-care once they have the information they need. Self-efficacy as a community strength is evident in how a

Recommendations From the Robert Wood Johnson Foundation Commission to Build a Healthier America

1. **Ensure that *all* children have high-quality early developmental support (child care, education and other services). This will require committing substantial additional resources to meet the early developmental needs particularly of children in low-income families.**	Children who do not receive high-quality care, services and education begin life with a distinct disadvantage and a higher risk of becoming less healthy adults, and evidence is overwhelming that too many children are facing a lifetime of poorer health as a result. Helping every child reach full health potential requires strong support from parents and communities, and must be a top priority for the nation. New resources must be directed to this goal, even at the expense of other national priorities, and must be tied to greater measurement and accountability for impact of new and existing early childhood programs.
2. **Fund and design WIC and SNAP (Food Stamps) programs to meet the needs of hungry families for nutritiousfood.**	These federal programs must have adequate support to meet the nutritional requirements of all American families in need. More than one in every 10 American households do not have reliable access to enough food, and the foods many families can afford may not add up to a nutritious diet. Nutritious food is a basic need to start and support an active, healthy and productive life
3. **Create public-private partnerships to open and sustain full-service grocery stores in communities without access to healthful foods**	Many inner city and rural families have no access to healthful foods: for example, Detroit, a city of 139 square miles has just 5 grocery stores. Maintaining a nutritious diet is impossible if healthy foods are not available; and it is not realistic to expect food retailers to address the problem without community support and investment. Communities should act now to assess needs to improve access to healthy foods and develop action plans to address deficiencies identified in their assessments.
4. **Feed children only healthy foods in schools**	Federal funds should be used exclusively for healthy meals. Schools should eliminate the sale of "junk" food and federal school breakfast and lunch funds should be linked to demonstrated improvements in children's school diets.
5. **Require all schools (K-12) to include time for all children to be physically active every day.**	One in five children will be obese by 2010. Children should be active at least one hour each day; only one-third of high-school students currently meet this

	goal. Schools can help meet this physical activity goal, through physical education programs, active recess, after-school and other recreational activities. Education funding should be linked to all children achieving at least half of their daily recommended physical activity at school, and over time should be linked to reductions in childhood obesity rates.
6. Become a smoke-free nation. Eliminating smoking remains one of the most important contributions to longer, healthier lives	Progress on many fronts—smoke-free workplaces, clean indoor air ordinances, tobacco tax increases, and effective, affordable quit assistance— demonstrates that this goal is achievable with broad public and private sector support.
7. Create "healthy community" demonstrations to evaluate the effects of a full complement of health-promoting policies and programs.	Demonstrations should integrate and develop successful models that can be widely implemented and that include multiple program approaches and sources of financial support. Each "healthy community" demonstration must bring together leaders and stakeholders from business, government, health care and nonprofit sectors to work together to plan, implement and show the impact of the project on the health of the community.
8. Develop a "health impact" rating for housing and infrastructure projects that reflects the projected effects on community health and provides incentives for projects that earn the rating.	All homes, workplaces and neighborhoods should be safe and free from health hazards. Communities should mobilize to correct severe physical deficiencies in housing, and health should be built into all efforts to improve housing, particularly in low-income neighborhoods. New federal housing investments should be held accountable to demonstrate a health impact.
9. Integrate safety and wellness into every aspect of community life.	While much remains to be done to create safe and health-promoting environments, many schools, workplaces, and communities have shown the way, with education and incentives for individuals, employers, and institutions and by fostering support for safety and health in schools, workplaces and neighborhoods. Funding should go only to organizations and communities that implement successful approaches and are willing to be held accountable for achieving measurable improvements in health
10. Ensure that decision-makers in all sectors have the evidence they need to build health into public and private policies and practices.	Decision-makers at national, state and local levels must have reliable data on health status, disparities, and the effects of social determinants of health. Approaches to monitor these data at the local level must be developed by, for example, adapting ongoing tracking systems. Funding must be available to promote research to understand these health effects and to promote the application of findings to decision-makers.

Figure 5-4 Recommendations from the Robert Wood Johnson Foundation Commission to build a healthier America. From Robert Wood Johnson Foundation. (2009). *Beyond health care: New directions to a healthier America.* (pp. 6–7). Retrieved from www.commissionon health.org. Copyright 2009 Robert Wood Johnson Foundation Commission to Build a Healthier America. Used with permission.

health issue was handled when two children were killed 3 weeks apart on the same busy intersection. A group brought a concern for the placement of a stoplight at the intersection, which was quickly approved and completed.

Source: Environmental Protection Agency (2010). *Report on the environment: Asthma prevalence.* Retrieved from http://cfpub.epa.gov/eroe/index.cfm?fuseaction=detail. viewind&lv=list.listbyalpha&r=201583&subtop=381

NURSING DIAGNOSIS FOR POPULATION-BASED COMMUNITY-FOCUSED CARE

Common nursing diagnoses for community care include ineffective community coping, readiness for enhanced community coping, community contamination/risk for community contamination, and ineffective community self-health management. One way to state a nursing diagnosis for a community would be community contamination as manifested by an unexpected increase in the rate of asthma among children over three decades (Carpenito, 2010). In the real world, the diagnosis is more likely to be stated as a problem statement rather than a nursing diagnosis. Formatting statements of the community's health concerns or problems, as well as its assets, concludes the assessment phase. It is important to document the data that support the problem and the overall processes used for the identification of the problem.

PLANNING/GOALS AND OUTCOMES

Planning follows the formulation of the nursing diagnosis for the community. Recommendations from the Robert Wood Johnson Foundation Commission to build a healthier America (previously mentioned in Chapter 1) are national goals but could be used to develop population-based goals or outcomes (Fig. 5-4). For instance, if a school nurse sees an increase in obesity among children in a school or school district, recommendations 4 or 5 (Fig. 5-4) provide possible goals for a population-based initiative. Planning involves prioritizing the community needs, establishing goals and objectives, and determining an action plan.

POPULATION-BASED COMMUNITY-FOCUSED SITUATIONS IN PRACTICE

You decide that the nursing diagnosis for the need you have identified in your community is contamination related to the high number of pollution alert days and possibly related to the oil refinery located in the region, as manifested by the high rate of asthma among children aged 5 to 12 years compared to national rates. This may also be stated as a problem statement: In Washington County in 2011, compared to the national average, there are twice as many pollution alert days and three times the rate of asthma among children aged 5 to 12 years.

INTERVENTIONS

Nursing interventions in population-based care include community organizing, collaboration, advocacy, social marketing, policy development and enforcement, and coalition building. Coalition building promotes and develops alliances among organizations or constituencies for a common purpose by building linkages, solving problems, and enhancing local leadership to address health concerns. Through community organizing, the nurse assists community groups to identify common problems or goals, mobilize resources, and develop and implement strategies for reaching these goals. In this case, you are organizing and building coalitions to build awareness of the issue and investigate the causes of the high rate of asthma among children in your community. Coalition building and community organizing may be accomplished by using an asset-based community development model seen in Box 5-1.

Expected outcomes are compared with outcomes achieved at the end of the established timeframe. Some questions that may be asked when evaluating a population-based community assessment include

1. Were all the key stakeholders satisfied with the program? Why or why not?
2. What additional data do we need to collect to evaluate the program?
3. Did the problem statement focus on the most important problems for the individuals living in the community? If not, what has emerged as the most important problem?

> **BOX 5-1**
>
> ## Asset-Based Community Development
>
> Asset-based community development is a process that focuses on the strengths of a community in order to mobilize assets for community improvement. Each community has unique assets upon which to work toward a better future. The following are suggested steps to facilitate community building:
>
> 1. Map the capacities and assets of individuals, citizens' associations, and local institutions that exist and that can be approached for participation in the community initiative.
> 2. Build and strengthen the existing partnership among local assets for mutually beneficial problem solving within the community.
> 3. Mobilize the community's assets appropriate for sharing information and economic development.
> 4. Convene a broadly representative group to craft a community vision and plan.
> 5. Leverage activities, investments, and resources from outside the community to support asset-based, locally defined development.
>
> Adapted from Kretzmann, J., & McKnight, J. (1993). *Building communities from the inside out: A path toward finding and mobilizing a community's assets.* Evanston, IL: Institute for Policy Research. Retrieved from http://www.northwestern.edu/ipr/publications/community/introd-building.html

4. What community strengths were missed and should be used as the project moves forward?

5. Were the problem statement, expected outcome, and interventions realistic and appropriate for this community? If not, what should be included in the next phase of the project? If so, which should be expanded or revised?

6. Are all stakeholders in the community satisfied with the outcome? If so, why? If not, how can the project be redesigned to increase satisfaction?

Similar to the nursing process, community assessment is cyclical and continuous. Evaluation is not an end point. It begins again with the assessment step of the next phase of the population-based initiative.

POPULATION-BASED COMMUNITY-FOCUSED SITUATIONS IN PRACTICE

In Washington County, you have enlisted several other nurses and parents interested in this issue. The group meets in your living room and determines that the priority need is to form a task force of representatives from various constituencies (e.g., local department of public health, school districts, parents of children with asthma, nurses and physicians from the local hospital and clinic, individuals from the local industries and business communities). The goal or outcome is for the task force to study the issue and, if deemed necessary, develop recommendations to be presented to the county department of health. Priorities of the initiative are to block the plans to expand the refinery but also to create pressure to reduce emissions. Within the framework of the task force, your main interventions will be to promote and develop alliances among the constituents as well as build linkages and enhance local leadership to address the concern of the increased rate of asthma. Further, through community organizing, you plan to mobilize resources and develop and implement strategies for reaching the goals the task force sets. Six months later, the study and recommendations are completed and presented to the Department of Health and County Board. After the presentation, the Department of Health and County Board suggests that the task force proceeds with a public health assessment (PHA) (Box 5-2) as well as initiates a health impact assessment (HIA). An HIA establishes the potential effects of a policy, program, or project on the health of a population (Department of Health and Human Services, 2007). Additional information about HIA is found in What's on the Web.

BOX 5-2 Public Health Assessment

A PHA examines hazardous substances, health outcomes, and community concerns at a hazardous waste site to determine whether people could be harmed from coming into contact with those substances. The Agency for Toxic Substances and Disease Registry conducts a PHA at each of the sites on the EPA National Priorities List. The aim of these evaluations is to find out if people are being exposed to hazardous substances and, if so, whether that exposure is harmful and should be stopped or reduced. This agency also conducts PHAs when petitioned by concerned individuals. The process is that a health assessor is called in from the federal government to review site-related environmental data and general information about toxic substances at the site. The assessor estimates the dose of the substance to which people in the community might be exposed and compares this with regulatory standards. A PHA can be compared to a clinical evaluation of a community because the relationship between actual exposures to contaminants is compared to the subsequent signs of disease and illness. The conclusions report the likelihood that those living near a site were exposed, are being exposed, or might be exposed at some future time to harmful levels of hazardous substances from the site. Community input is valued as community members may have useful information about the community history, the site history, and human activities and land use near the site. Information from members of the community can improve estimates of exposure, risks, and health threats.

Source: Centers for Disease Control and Prevention. (2009). *Agency for Toxic Substances and Disease Registry. Public health assessment and health consultation.* Retrieved from http://www.atsdr.cdc.gov/hac/pha/pha_foreword.asp#HE or http://www.atsdr.cdc.gov/hac/pha/index.asp

CLIENT SITUATIONS IN PRACTICE

Addressing Community Needs in the School

Maria is the school nurse for Harmony High School, which has an enrollment of 2,300 students. To determine the health needs of the students attending Harmony, she is conducting an assessment of the school community. She has collected the following information about the school district and the students at Harmony High.

Windshield Survey

Maria began her assessment of the community by spending time traveling around the school district, completing a windshield survey. This is what she discovered:

Most of the people on the street during the day are women and small children. Based on the way they are dressed and the cars they are driving, they appear to be middle class.

Most of the people are Mexican American or White. There is no evidence of drug abuse or blatant sale of drugs on the street observed and no problems with communicable diseases, as may be evidenced by people with hacking coughs or a wasted appearance.

Harmony is a community of 20,000 people located at the outer suburban ring of Metropolitan City, which has a population of 3,000,000; it is a predominantly suburban community with 10% of the citizens in rural areas. The racial mix is 20% Hispanic, 30% African American, and 50% White. There is little pollution of any type in the area. There are no hospitals or clinics in the community. The houses are primarily well-kept, single-family dwellings between 5 and 20 years old.

In evaluating the social systems, Maria found that there are primary, secondary, and tertiary health care services nearby. However, because there is no public transportation, it is difficult for students to gain access to these services. In addition, none of the health services offers services for adolescents. For instance, 100% of the participants in the prenatal classes offered at the closest hospital are suburban, middle-class couples. The closest facility in which adolescents can receive confidential pregnancy testing, prenatal care, or prenatal classes is 45 minutes away by car. There is no public transportation available to this clinic.

Informant Interviews

Maria then interviews some of the key informants in the community. She asks them what they think are the primary health issues among high school students in their community. The county public health nurses, counselor, principal of the high school, and parish nurse all mention that many pregnant adolescents do not receive prenatal care. The fire chief and mayor believe there is a need for more emergency medical services.

Participant Observations

Based on the students who come to her office for care, Maria has identified two categories of students who frequently need health care. One group consists of students with somatic complaints related to personal or family stress. The second group consists of students who have questions about sexuality or who are pregnant and need information about available services. The girls who are pregnant have a great deal of difficulty getting early prenatal care.

Maria attends the school board meetings where issues of health are occasionally discussed. All of the school board members are concerned about cost containment, and two members are particularly sensitive about including sexuality in the school's curriculum. The superintendent is committed to curricula sensitive to community values and reluctant to consider curricula that may include sexuality if the board members' concerns are representative of the community.

Existing Data

Maria collects existing data on the community from the state health department. She discovers demographic facts about Harmony and compares them with data on all the high school students in the state. Harmony has a lower rate of prenatal care among adolescents and a higher infant mortality and rate of low birth weight newborns for students of color.

Community Health Need or Problem Statement

Maria decides that the **community health need** in Harmony High School is early identification of pregnancy and provision of prenatal care for pregnant adolescent girls. The community problem is Harmony High students have a lower rate of prenatal care and a higher infant mortality rate and rate of low birth weight newborns for students of color as compared to the state statistics due to lack of early identification of pregnancy and access to prenatal care.

Outcome and Interventions

Maria defines the outcomes and interventions for the project to the school board and public health nurses, teachers, counselors, and other community stakeholders.

Outcome After 6 Months

Establish a task force made up of a teacher, a counselor, a public health nurse, and a member of the school board to determine how the school and community can address this need.

Interventions for the Next Year

1. Establish and convene a task force once a month for six months to conduct a community assessment.
2. Present a summary of the results of the community assessment to the school board, public health nurses, teachers, and counselors.
3. Keep the key players apprised of the progress of the task force.

After 1 year, the task force presents the results to the school board, public health nurses, teachers, and counselors. The task force recommends that the school offer a prenatal course to all pregnant students at the high school. They recommend the following outcomes after 1 year:

1. Develop a method for referring all pregnant adolescents seen by school and community personnel to the school's prenatal program.
2. Develop a prenatal course to be offered in the school.

3. Develop a list of community referral sources for prenatal adolescents.

4. Develop a mechanism for follow-up after birth.

5. Ask for input and involvement of all key players.

Once the method for referral process, prenatal course, list of community referrals sources, and follow-up process is complete, they report back to the school board and other key stakeholders. The task force recommends and the school board agrees to the following interventions for the next year:

1. Begin the program.

2. Evaluate the prenatal program, including the number and percentage of pregnant students attending the classes, satisfaction with the program, total percent now receiving prenatal care, infant mortality rate, and rate of low birth weight infants compared to the data preceding initiation of the program.

3. Increase community awareness about the importance of prenatal care.

Evaluation

Are the outcomes met?

1. Yes: Continue with the interventions.

2. No: Revise the interventions: Reconvene the task force; reassess the community.

Reassessment

To reassess the community, Maria determines if the key constituents are satisfied with the program. She explores whether there is additional information necessary in order to evaluate the program. Maria affirms that the problem statement focused on the most important problems for the individuals living in the community. She asks if there were other problems important to this community. She establishes that the problem statement, expected outcome, and interventions were realistic and appropriate for this community. Last, Maria explores whether there were other members of the community who were satisfied with the outcome.

Population-based community-focused care is an important aspect of community-based nursing. It utilizes nursing process to direct interventions toward entire populations within a community to change community norms, attitudes, awareness, practices, and behaviors.

SITUATIONS IN PRACTICE

Examples of nursing process applied to planning the care of the individual, family, or community are seen below.

Statement of a Concern or Problem and Goals

From the problem statement, the nurse defines goals or expected outcomes. These outcome statements are specific and based on measurable criteria. Examples with possible outcomes follow.

Example 1: When the Individual is the Client
Nursing diagnosis: Ineffective airway clearance related to asthma as manifested by a respiratory rate of 28 breaths/minute and wheezes in all lung fields.

Goals: The client will demonstrate a respiratory rate of 16 breaths/minute and cessation of wheezes in all lung fields.

Example 2: When the Community of the School District is the Client
Problem statement: The number of children between the ages of 5 and 18 years with asthma in the school district of Rosie Mountain increased from 50/1,000 in March 1990 to 100/1,000 in March 2010.

Expected outcome: Reduce the number of children between the ages of 5 and 18 years in Rosie Mountain with the diagnosis of asthma from 100/1,000 in 2010 to 50/1,000 by the year 2020.

Example 3: When the Community of the County is the Client

Community problem: The infant mortality rate for Normaldale County was 14/1,000 births in 2015, compared with the state infant mortality rate of 8/1,000 and the national rate of 7/1,000.

Expected outcome: Reduce the infant mortality rate for Normaldale County to 9/1,000 births by 2020.

Example 4: When the Community of the Hospital is the Client

Community problem: In March 2015, at Normaldale County Hospital, 65% of the nursing staff washed their hands between clients. The recommended percentage is 90%.

Expected outcome: By March 2020, 90% of the nursing staff will wash their hands between clients.

Public Policy

Public policy may appear, at first glance, to evolve primarily from the government, but policy makers consider many sources when developing public policy. Nurses are valued professionals whose opinions and input are often sought by those who participate in the policy-making process. The nurse may participate in a variety of ways from calling or sending a letter to a city, state, or federal lawmaker to testifying at a public hearing to informing a client about proposed changes in the law related to health care. Often, through public education and social marketing, the nurse may influence public opinion and, in turn, public policy. It is a professional responsibility of the graduate nurse to stay current on health care issues and to share that expertise with other members of the community.

Evidence of public opinion affecting public policy is seen in maternal care (Fig. 5-5). Until the late 1970s, third-party payers allowed a postpartum woman to stay in the hospital from 3 to 5 days. Gradually, reimbursement reduced the length of stay to 2 to 4 days and, eventually, to 24 hours to 3 days. As the negative consequences of early discharge on the mother and newborn became common knowledge through the medical and nursing community's disapproval and advocacy for longer stays, this policy was changed. By the late 1990s, many states by law or regulation extended the 24-hour stay to 48 hours.

Numerous issues offer nurses the opportunity to act as advocates for individuals, families, and communities. Through advocacy, social marketing, and education, the nurse may influence public opinion and health care public policy.

Conclusions

Assessment in community settings has long been a part of nursing practice. Assessment is directed toward individual clients across the life span, families, and communities. Holistic assessment considers not only physical and psychosocial factors but also cultural, functional, nutritional, environmental, and spiritual aspects of the client. Nursing process is a tool that

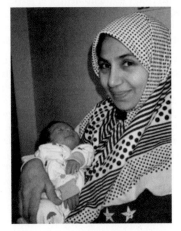

Figure 5-5 Public opinion and advocacy led to increased postpartum care.

can be used to determine how people, place, and social systems influence health. Community assessment helps the nurse become aware of problems in the community that directly or indirectly affect the lives of clients and their families. Although nurses infrequently conduct a formal large-scale community assessment alone, they may, along with other health care professionals, participate in some aspect of community assessment to inform population-based care. As the nursing profession continues to shift to a more community-based emphasis, the role of the nurse in community assessment will remain important to the health of communities.

What's on the Web

Developmental Screening of Children
INTERNET ADDRESS: http://www.cdc.gov/ncbddd/child/devtool.htm
This site provides information about the importance of developmental screening, the Centers for Disease Control and Prevention recommendations for developmental screening tools, as well as what is happening state by state related to developmental screening.

Home Safety Council
INTERNET ADDRESS: http://www.homesafetycouncil.org/
The Home Safety Council (HSC) is the only national nonprofit organization solely dedicated to preventing home-related injuries that result in nearly 20,000 deaths and 21 million medical visits on average each year. Through national programs, partnerships, and the support of volunteers, HSC educates people of all ages to be safer in and around their homes. This site has an interactive safety checklist to allow individuals across the life span to determine safety needs.

American Red Cross
INTERNET ADDRESS: http://www.redcross.org/
The American Red Cross has numerous resources related to safety including home, fire, flood, water, and many other topics. Use the search box to look for your topic of interest.

Mayo Clinic/Make Weight Loss a Family Affair
INTERNET ADDRESS: http://www.mayoclinic.com/health/childhood-obesity/FL00058
This page on the Mayo Clinic Web site has slide shows, tools including a child and adolescent body mass index (BMI) calculator, and teaching materials for weight control. There are also numerous links to information on nutrition and activity.

The Community Tool Box
INTERNET ADDRESS: http://ctb.ku.edu/
The Tool Box for population-based community-focused care includes practical guidance for the different tasks necessary to promote community health and development. Sections include leadership, strategic planning, community assessment, grant writing, and evaluation to give just a few examples of what is found on this Web site. Each section includes a description of the task, advantages of doing it, step-by-step guidelines, examples, checklists of points to review, and training materials.

MAP-IT: A Guide to Using Healthy People 2020 in Your Community
INTERNET ADDRESS: http://www.healthypeople.gov/2020/implementing/default.aspx
Healthy People 2020 establishes national health objectives that provide data and tools to enable states, cities, communities, and individuals across the country to combine their efforts to achieve them. This guide provides information for building community coalitions, creating a vision, measuring results, and creating partnerships dedicated to improving the health of a community.

Centers for Disease Control and Prevention/Health Impact Assessment
INTERNET ADDRESS: http://www.cdc.gov/healthyplaces/hia.htm
This site describes an innovative process for addressing the potential impact projects that effect land use or expansion of existing industries could have on the health of communities. HIA can be used to evaluate objectively the potential health effects of a project or policy before it is built or implemented. It can provide recommendations to increase positive health outcomes and minimize adverse health outcomes. A major benefit of the HIA process is that it brings public health issues to the attention of persons who make decisions about areas that fall outside of traditional public health arenas, such as transportation or land use. This process has been used extensively in Europe, Canada, and Australia and is beginning to be used in the United States.

Obesity Rates by State over Time

INTERNET ADDRESS: **http://www.cdc.gov/obesity/data/trends.html**

Obesity trends by state, 1985 to the present.

Obesity is defined as a BMI of 30 or greater. BMI is calculated from a person's weight and height and provides a reasonable indicator of body fat and weight categories that may lead to health problems. Obesity is a major risk factor for cardiovascular disease, certain types of cancer, and type 2 diabetes. During the past 30 years, there has been a dramatic increase in obesity in the United States. Thirty-three states had prevalence ≥25%; nine of these states (Alabama, Arkansas, Kentucky, Louisiana, Mississippi, Missouri, Oklahoma, Tennessee, and West Virginia) had a prevalence of obesity ≥30%. In 2009, only Colorado and the District of Columbia had a prevalence of obesity <20%. The animated map in this site shows the United States' obesity prevalence from 1985 through the present. There are also maps that can be downloaded: The prevalence of obesity is depicted in a PowerPoint slide presentation format (30 slides total, PPT-2.9Mb). This is also available as a text-only Acrobat file (PDF-472k).

County Health Rankings

INTERNET ADDRESS: **http://www.countyhealthrankings.org/about-project**

According to this Web site, the County Health Rankings show that where we live matters to our health. The health of a community depends on many different factors—ranging from individual health behaviors, education, and jobs to quality of health care to the environment. This first-of-its-kind collection of 50 reports—one per state—helps community leaders see that where we live, learn, work, and play influences how healthy we are and how long we live. This Web site is a valuable tool for any nurse looking for community assessment baseline data for counties for use with population-based initiatives.

References and Bibliography

American Academy of Pediatrics. (2010). *Children's health topics: Hearing and vision screening.* Retrieved from http://www.aap.org/healthtopics/visionhearing.cfm

Campus-Community Partnerships for Health. (2010). *About us: Our mission and values.* Retrieved from http://depts.washington.edu/ccph/principles.html#principles

Carpenito, L. (2010). *Handbook of nursing diagnosis* (13th ed.). Philadelphia, PA: Lippincott Williams & Wilkins.

Centers for Disease Control and Prevention. (2009). *Agency for Toxic Substances and Disease Registry. Public health assessment and health consultation.* Retrieved from http://www.atsdr.cdc.gov/hac/pha/pha_foreword.asp#HE OR http://www.atsdr.cdc.gov/hac/pha/index.asp

Centers for Disease Control and Prevention, National Center for Health Statistics. (2010a). *Health topic: Childhood obesity.* Retrieved from http://www.cdc.gov/HealthyYouth/obesity/

Centers for Disease Control and Prevention. (2010b). *Obesity trends.* Retrieved from http://www.cdc.gov/obesity/data/trends.html

DeBrew, J. K., Barba, B. E., & Tesh, A. S. (1998). Assessing medication knowledge and practices of older adults. *Home Healthcare Nurse, 16*(10), 686–692.

Department of Health and Human Services, Centers for Disease Control and Prevention. (2007). *Health impact assessment fact sheet.* Retrieved from http://www.cdc.gov/healthyplaces/publications/Health_Impact_Assessment2.pdf

Dwyer, L., Han, B., Woodwell, D., & Rechtsteiner, E. (2010). Polypharmacy in nursing home residents in the United States: Results of the 2004 National Nursing Home Survey. *American Journal of Geriatric Pharmacotherapy, 8*(1), 63–72. Retrieved from CINAHL Plus with Full Text database.

Environmental Protection Agency. (2010). *Report on the environment: Asthma prevalence.* Retrieved from http://cfpub.epa.gov/eroe/index.cfm?fuseaction=detail.viewind&lv=list.listbyalpha&r=201583&subtop=381

Ewing, R., Schmid, T., Killingsworth, R., Zlot, A., & Raudenbush, S. (2003). Relationship between urban sprawl and physical activity, obesity, and morbidity. *American Journal of Health Promotion, 18*(1), 47–57.

Fieldsmith, R., Van Sell, S., & Kindred, C. (2009). Home assessment. *RN, 72*(3), 26–29. Retrieved from CINAHL Plus with Full Text database.

Flaherty, J., Perry, H., Lynchard, G., & Morley, J. (2000). Polypharmacy and hospitalization among older home care patients. *Journals of Gerontology Series A: Biological Sciences & Medical Sciences, 55A*(10), M554–M559. Retrieved from CINAHL Plus with Full Text database.

Gallup-Healthways Well-Being Index. (2010). *Healthiest cities.* Retrieved from http://www.well-beingindex.com/stateCongresDistrictRank.asp

Hollar, D., Messiah, S., Lopez-Mitnik, G., Hollar, T., Almon, M., & Agatston, A. (2010). Effect of a two-year obesity intervention on percentile changes in body mass index and academic performance in low-income elementary school children. *American Journal of Public Health, 100*(4), 646–653. Retrieved from Academic Search Premier database.

Hunt, R. (Ed.). (2000). *Readings in community-based nursing* (pp. 168–177). Philadelphia, PA: Lippincott Williams & Wilkins.

Joint Commission on Accreditation of Healthcare Organizations (JCAHO). (2010). *Spiritual assessment*. Retrieved from http://www.jointcommission.org/

Jyrkkä, J., Enlund, H., Korhonen, M., Sulkava, R., & Hartikainen, S. (2009). Polypharmacy status as an indicator of mortality in an elderly population. *Drugs and Aging, 26*(12), 1039–1048.

Kretzmann, J., & McKnight, J. (1993). *Building communities from the inside out: A path toward finding and mobilizing a community's assets*. Evanston, IL: Institute for Policy Research. Retrieved from http://www.northwestern.edu/ipr/publications/community/introd-building.html

Last, J. (Ed.). (1988). *Dictionary of epidemiology* (2 ed., p. 42). New York, NY: Oxford University Press.

Mackenzie, L., Byles, J., & D'Este, C. (2009). Longitudinal study of the home falls and accidents screening tool in identifying older people at increased risk of falls. *Australian Journal on Ageing, 28*(2), 64–69. Retrieved from CINAHL Plus with Full Text database.

McConnell, R., Islam, T., Shankardass, K., Jerrett, M., Lurmann, F., Gilliland, F., et al. (2010). Childhood incident asthma and traffic-related air pollution at home and school. *Environmental Health Perspectives, 118*(7), 1021–1026. doi:10.1289/ehp.0901232.

McKnight J., & Kretzmann, J. (2006). *Tip sheet: Asset-based community development*. Retrieved on September 14, 2007, from http://www.health.state.mn.us/communityeng/intro/models.html

Modig, S., Kristensson, J., Ekwall, A., Hallberg, I., & Midlöv, P. (2009). Frail elderly patients in primary care–Their medication knowledge and beliefs about prescribed medicines. *European Journal of Clinical Pharmacology, 65*(2), 151–155. Retrieved from CINAHL Plus with Full Text database.

Narayan, M. C., & Tennant, J. (1997). Environmental assessment. *Home Healthcare Nurse, 15*(11), 799–805.

National Center for Health Statistics. (2010). *Growth Charts*. Retrieved from www.cdc.gov/growthcharts/

Neal, L. J. (1998). Functional assessment of the home health client. *Home Healthcare Nurse, 16*(10), 670–677.

Nestle Nutrition Institute. (2010). *Mini nutritional assessment*. Retrieved from http://www.mna-elderly.com/

Ohio Department of Health. (2009). *The burden of asthma in Ohio*. Retrieved from http://www.odh.ohio.gov/odhPrograms/eh/asthma/asthdata/data.aspx

Population Reference Bureau. (2010). *The state of metropolitan American*. Retrieved from http://www.prb.org/Articles/2010/usmetropolitanchanges.aspx?p=1

Satcher, D. (2010). Include social determinants of health approach to reduce health inequities. *Public Health Reports*, (Suppl. 4), 125. Retrieved from http://www.publichealthreports.org/archives/issueopen.cfm?articleID=2476

Scotch, M., Parmanto, B., & Monaco, V. (2008). Evaluation of SOVAT: An OLAP-GIS decision support system for community health assessment data analysis. *BMC Medical Informatics & Decision Making, 8*, 1–12.

Singhal, N., & Misra, A. (2010). A school-based intervention for diabetes risk reduction. *New England Journal of Medicine, 363*(5), 443–453.

U.S. Census Bureau. (2008). Health insurance data: Low income uninsured children by state. Retrieved from http://www.census.gov/hhes/www/hlthins/data/children/uninsured/liuc08.html

Woodham-Smith, C. (1950). *Florence Nightingale, 1820–1910*. London: Constable.

Wright, L., & Leahey, M. (1999). Maximizing time, minimizing suffering: The 15-minute (or less) family interview. *Journal of Family Nursing, 5*(3), 259–274.

Ziere, G., Dieleman, J., Hofman, A., Pols, H., van der Cammen, T., & Stricker, B. (2006). Polypharmacy and falls in the middle age and elderly population. *British Journal of Clinical Pharmacology, 61*(2), 218–223.

LEARNING ACTIVITIES

LEARNING ACTIVITY 5-1

Nhu is a home care nurse who is making a home visit to Marion, an 85-year-old woman who has just been discharged from a transitional hospital after a hip replacement. After completing the agency admission intake interview, Nhu takes a few minutes to assess Marion's functional capacity.

What areas will Nhu assess?

Nhu learns that Marion is able to perform all ADL, her home environment is basically safe, her sensory and perceptual function is intact, and her cognitive, emotional, integumentary, and respiratory status are all within normal limits and sufficient to allow her to live independently. However, as Nhu is assessing function, Marion tells her, "I was doing fine until the physician changed my medication for high blood pressure. Now I am dizzy all the time."

What does Nhu assess next?

LEARNING ACTIVITY 5-2

Conduct a windshield survey of your community. Consider people, place, and social system using Assessment Tools 5-8.

What community needs and assets did you identify?

What would you identify as the priority need or community problem?

What goals or outcomes would you suggest for this problem?

LEARNING ACTIVITY 5-3

Complete a functional assessment (see Assessment Tools 5-2) for a vulnerable client in his or her home or apartment or as a part of discharge planning. Determine one or more appropriate nursing diagnoses, goals and outcomes, and nursing interventions. Identify interventions from the public health intervention wheel. Summarize the safety concerns you identified for this client as well as the client's strengths or assets. Identify resources in the community that provide safety devices, such as the safety council. Share all of the information with the client and his or her family and suggest that he or she share it with the appropriate community providers, such as the client's physician, nurse practitioner, or public health nurse.

LEARNING ACTIVITY 5-4

Individual Client Assessment

In your clinical journal, describe a situation in which you used an assessment guide from this chapter to assess a client in a community-based setting:

What were the client's needs and strengths?

What was your nursing diagnosis?

What were the outcomes and nursing interventions?

What benefit do you think you created for your client?

What did you do that didn't work?

What did you learn from this activity?

What will you do differently next time?

Family Assessment

In your clinical journal, describe a situation in which you used an assessment guide from this chapter to assess a family in a community-based setting.

What family needs and strengths did you identify?

What was your nursing diagnosis?

What were the outcomes and nursing interventions?

What did you learn from this activity?

What benefit do you think you created for the family?

What did you do that didn't work?

What will you do differently next time?

Community Assessment

In your clinical journal, describe a situation in which you used an assessment guide from this chapter to assess a community.

What community needs and assets did you identify?

What was your nursing diagnosis?

What were the outcomes and nursing interventions?

What did you learn from this activity?

What benefit do you think you created for the community or could create for the community?

What did you do that didn't work?

What will you do differently next time?

LEARNING ACTIVITY 5-5

Look at Figure 5-3 Obesity Rates by State and respond to the following questions.

- Find your state on the map.
  - What is the rate of obesity for your state?
  - How does it compare to bordering states?
  - Why do you think your state has a higher or lower rate of obesity?

Find Colorado on the map.

- What is the obesity rate?
- Why do you think this is the case?

Find West Virginia on the map

- What is the obesity rate?
- Why do you think this is the case?

Why do you think that some states have high obesity rates while others have low ones? What population, location, social systems, and social determinants of health might impact obesity rates?

What can nurses do to impact the rate of obesity in their own states?

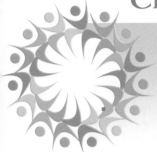

Chapter 6

Health Teaching

ROBERTA HUNT

Learning Objectives

1. Discuss teaching and learning theory, learning domains, and successful teaching techniques as related to community-based nursing.

2. Define health teaching.

3. Discuss assessment, planning, and teaching methods required in determining learning needs.

4. Summarize Medicare reimbursement guidelines for teaching.

5. Identify barriers to successful teaching.

6. Explore the characteristics of successful teaching.

7. State methods used in teaching the client who is not adhering to the treatment plan.

8. Discuss specific teaching techniques for each level of prevention.

Key Terms

affective learning
cognitive learning
health literacy
health teaching
learning domains
learning needs

learning objective
need to learn
psychomotor learning
readiness to learn
reimbursement requirements

Chapter Topics

Health Teaching in the 21st Century
Teaching and Learning Theory
Learning Domains
Developmental Considerations
Teaching and Levels of Prevention
Nursing Competencies and Skills in the Teaching Process
Teaching the Challenging Client
Conclusions

The Nursing Student Speaks

In one of my senior-level nursing courses, students were asked to complete an extensive community-based nursing rotation wherein they would provide ongoing care to a vulnerable family that had recently experienced a crisis. I was asked to visit a family who had recently experienced homelessness, but I had been provided with relatively little information beyond that. In my initial visit with the family, I was focused on getting to know each family member, building trust and rapport, and learning what needs, preferences, and goals the family was interested in working on during my visits. I learned that the father of the family was a decorated Gulf War veteran who had been diagnosed with posttraumatic stress disorder (PTSD) upon returning from the war; unfortunately, he had not received treatment for his PTSD for over a decade. I asked him whether he would be interested in pursuing treatment for his PTSD, recognizing that this may be negatively impacting his ability to function in his multiple roles of father, employee, husband, brother, and son. His initial response was "absolutely not." He then explained that he had a very negative experience when he first sought treatment and, therefore, had been resistant to pursue services for his PTSD since his initial diagnosis. Respecting his decision to not pursue treatment for his PTSD, I steered the conversation to a less-threatening topic.

At our next visit, I gave the father a packet of information on PTSD and briefly reviewed the signs and symptoms of the disorder. The father was interested to learn that it is very common for veterans to resist seeking services for this particular disorder. We continued to work on other health topics, focusing on meeting the family's basic needs of good nutrition, safe housing, and sleep hygiene.

By the time of the third visit, the father mentioned to me that he might be interested in pursuing treatment for his PTSD after all. He described an incident that had occurred at work the previous week in which he had "nearly lost my cool," and he stated that it had reminded him of what he had learned at our last visit: that severe irritability, overwhelming anxiety, and persistent avoidance of talking about the traumatic event are common in PTSD.

From my work with this family, I learned many important lessons that I will carry forward into my professional nursing practice. Above all, I learned that actively listening to a client and responding to the client's unique needs and preferences are essential elements in the formation of a therapeutic alliance. Recognizing when a teachable moment presents itself can allow the nurse to intervene with health teaching when the client is most receptive to it. Informing the client that many veterans with PTSD are resistant to seeking treatment caught his attention and gave me an excellent opportunity to provide health teaching on this disorder. Once the client had been exposed to this information, he began recognizing the symptoms that he had been struggling with for over a decade. More importantly, he began to realize that the symptoms he was experiencing were negatively impacting him not only in what he described as his "secret life," but also in his role as "employee," "father," and "husband." In my role as registered nurse, I will need to continuously assess my clients for a readiness for enhanced knowledge and intervene accordingly.

Justin Robinson
Student in a postbaccalaureate program completing a major in nursing
St. Catherine University, St. Paul, Minnesota

At no other time in history has client teaching been so important. Owing to the decreased length of stay in all acute care settings and increased amount of care provided in community settings, teaching is a central role for nurses in all settings. At the same time, there is a low rate of health literacy that acts as a barrier to self-care. Lack of health literacy affects both health and health care and has significant economic implications. **Health literacy** is the degree to which individuals have the capacity to obtain, process, and understand information and services needed to make appropriate health decisions (U.S. Department of Health and Human Services, 2010). Health literacy is important because it allows one to navigate complex health systems and better manage self-care. The consequences of inadequate health literacy include poorer health status, lack of knowledge about medical conditions and care for the conditions, lack of understanding and use of preventive services, low level of self-reported health, inadequate compliance rates with treatment modalities, increased hospitalizations, and increased health care costs. Low health literacy has negative psychological effects on those with limited health literacy skills reporting a sense of shame about their lack of skill that may result in not revealing reading or vocabulary difficulties to maintain their dignity.

One consequence of inadequate health literacy is seen in the use of potentially inappropriate medications prevalent in ambulatory care, home care, hospital care, and long-term care (Molony, 2009). Studies show that 16% to 22% of clients discharged from hospitals do not even fill their prescriptions (Karter et al., 2009). One study reported that individuals who take medications as ordered for congestive heart failure (CHF) are less likely to have a hospitalization (4%), have fewer hospitalizations (13%) and inpatient days (25%), are less likely to have an emergency department (ED) visit (3%), and have fewer ED visits (10%) compared to those who do not take medications as ordered (Esposito, Bagchi, Verdier, Bencio, & Kim, 2009). Total health care costs are 23% less per year for those who take medication as ordered compared with patients who do not. The researchers concluded that health care costs among Medicaid beneficiaries with CHF would be lower if more patients were adherent to prescribed medication regimens. This research highlights the need for comprehensive teaching as a cost containment measure as well as improving quality of life.

In the last decade, management of chronic conditions has become an important health need. Studies repeatedly show that client education prevents up to 50% of medication errors for clients in community settings where they self-administer their medications. As health care is more community based, an illness is primarily managed by clients or family members. Nurses have an important role in promoting quality self-care through health teaching.

This chapter addresses **health teaching**, defined as "communicating facts, ideas, and skill that change knowledge, attitudes, values, beliefs, behaviors, and practices of individuals, families, systems, and/or communities" (Minnesota Department of Health, 2001). The benefits of teaching and strategies for successful health teaching are presented in light of the current health care system. Teaching and learning theory are discussed along with learning domains. A large section of the chapter is devoted to helping the nurse develop skills and competencies in teaching, discussing teaching as it follows the nursing process, and sharing useful teaching techniques. The chapter ends with activities to be used in further developing knowledge and skills in teaching.

Health Teaching in the 21st Century

In the 21st century, care will increasingly be provided outside the acute care setting. In addition to the economic arguments already presented, there are other reasons to support prioritizing health teaching within the health care system. The most important goal of health teaching in community-based care is to assist the client and family in achieving independence through self-care management. When client learning needs are considered within the context of the family, community care is improved, recovery facilitated, and complications reduced. Good teaching improves client and family satisfaction and confidence about discharge and follow-up care. A client's sense of control is enhanced through mutual participation in the teaching process.

Likewise, staff satisfaction improves when teaching results are positive. It is professionally satisfying to prepare a client for discharge and receive subsequent feedback that the discharge was satisfactory. It is professionally satisfying for the home care nurse to prepare a client to successfully manage self-care at home. On the other hand, it is stressful when a nurse sees a client with inadequate preparation trying to manage home care unsuccessfully only to return to the clinic or hospital. Ultimately, clients and families inadequately prepared for discharge and self-care management at home are more likely to be rehospitalized. In the last decade, the most costly consequence of poor preparation for discharge, unnecessary rehospitalization, has been on the rise (O'Daniel & Rosenstein, 2009).

Quality health education paves the way for continuity between settings of care. Providing information about diet, activity, medications, equipment, and follow-up appointments enhances self-care capacity. For over a decade, there has been evidence that it is not only cost-effective to provide health education but that such education also improves quality of life for the client and lay caregivers. Recent research that supports the value of health education in enhancing self-care behavior and improving quality of life is found in Research in Community-Based Nursing Care 6-1. In addition to the financial costs to the client, family, and third-party payers, it is frustrating when teaching has to be repeated several times because it was not done well the first time. Furthermore, concern for cost containment requires that all teaching incorporates prevention strategies, which further allow resources to be used efficiently. Teaching begins at whatever point the client enters the system.

Teaching and Learning Theory

To be a successful teacher in any setting, one must understand and apply basic teaching and learning principles. Learning depends on both the **need to learn** and the **readiness to learn** and is influenced by the individual's life experiences (Knox, 1986).

Learning is facilitated when the client perceives information as needed or relevant for immediate application. For example, a postoperative client is scheduled to go home in 2 hours with a client-controlled analgesia pump. The client learns quickly how to use the pump and administer medication to control postoperative pain. This learning is facilitated by the need for pain relief and the immediate application of learning.

Learning depends on readiness. Readiness involves factors such as emotional state, abilities, and potential. Examples of these are listed in Community-Based Teaching 6-1. An example of lack of learning readiness follows. You are doing preadmission teaching with

---

RESEARCH IN COMMUNITY-BASED NURSING CARE 6-1

Effects of Education on Self-Care Behavior and Quality of Life in Patients With Chronic Health Failure

Improving outpatient management of patients with congestive heart failure (CHF) to positively impact outcomes and control cost is an important challenge. The objective of this study was to determine effects of health education sessions on self-care behaviors and quality of life for 44 patients with CHF. Baseline indicators were recorded and supportive educational programming was provided by an interprofessional team of specialist nurses and an MD. Physical activity, energy, pain, sleep, social isolation, and emotional reactions were evaluated by descriptive statistics. Comparison between the baseline indicators and posteducational programming data showed all parameters were significantly higher following the education sessions. The researchers concluded that systematic and planned health education provided by a specialist cardiologist and nurse specialists led to an increase in patients' self-care behaviors and improved quality of life.

Source: Enç, N., Yigit, Z., & Altiok, M. (2010). Effects of education on self-care behavior and quality of life in patients with chronic heart failure. *CONNECT: The World of Critical Care Nursing*, 7(2), 115–121. Retrieved from CINAHL Plus with Full Text database.

COMMUNITY-BASED TEACHING 6-1

Factors That Affect Readiness to Learn

- Physiologic factors: Age, gender, disease process currently being treated, intactness of senses (hearing, vision, touch, taste), preexisting condition
- Psychosocial factors: Sociocultural circumstances, occupation, economic stability, past experiences with learning, attitude toward learning, spirituality, emotional health, self-concept and body image, sense of responsibility for self
- Cognitive factors: Developmental level, level of education, communication skills, primary language, motivation, reading ability, learning style, problem-solving ability
- Environmental factors: Home environment, safety features, family relationships/problems, caregiver (availability, motivation, abilities), other support systems

a 30-year-old woman, an attorney with a busy law practice who has outpatient surgery scheduled for the next day. She is thinking about the important trial she has beginning the afternoon following surgery. She may not hear you when you tell her she should not drive or make important decisions for a full day after surgery with general anesthesia. Because of her distracted mental state, she is not ready to learn.

Motivation is a strong determinant of learning readiness. Motivation starts with the client's need to know and then provides the drive or incentive to learn. Because so many things can affect motivation, it can change from day to day. For instance, a young woman who drinks alcohol becomes pregnant, and her health care provider tells her alcohol is harmful to the fetus. Because she is concerned for her baby's welfare, she discontinues drinking. The motivation is strong enough to make her stop. However, at a party, her friends insist that she join them in a drink. "One drink won't hurt you," they say. Now the woman may be motivated to drink. Her decision depends on which motivation is stronger.

Both differences and similarities between past and present life experiences influence learning. For example, you are doing discharge planning from a birth center for a multipara who delivered her second child yesterday evening. Her delivery was complicated by a 1,000-mL blood loss and a fourth-degree laceration. She has an 18-month-old toddler at home. Her husband is an accountant. It is tax season, and he presently works 12 or 13 hours a day. Neither set of grandparents nor any other family nor close friends live nearby. Your client is going home this afternoon and insists that she does not need help at home because she did not need help after her first child. The client does not understand the difference between her first delivery and the circumstances complicating the second one.

Learning Domains

Teaching and learning occur in three **learning domains**: cognitive, affective, and psychomotor. Bloom and colleagues originated the measurement of learning outcomes with a detailed taxonomy of educational objectives in 1956. From this taxonomy, educational objectives were classified into one of three domains: cognitive, affective, and psychomotor. Bloom's taxonomy also makes finer distinctions within each domain, and it has received wide acceptance in the educational community (Bolin, Khramtsova, & Saarnio, 2005). All three domains must be considered in all aspects of the teaching and learning process. Thus, the nurse must assess the client's need, readiness, and past experience in the cognitive, affective, and psychomotor domains.

Cognitive learning involves mental storage and recall of new knowledge and information for problem solving. Sometimes this domain is referred to as the *critical thinking* or *knowledge domain*. Cognitive objectives are satisfied when students obtain an appropriate level of knowledge. An example of cognitive learning is seen in the client who has recently been diagnosed with insulin-dependent diabetes. Not only will this client need information about diet, insulin, and exercise, but he or she will also need to use the information to formulate menus and an exercise plan. In addition, as blood sugar levels fluctuate, a client with diabetes must alter food intake and exercise. All this requires cognitive learning.

Affective learning involves feelings, attitudes, values, and emotions that influence learning. This is also referred to as the *attitude domain*. Affective objectives are satisfied when students obtain an appropriate level of internalization or value for the content. In the last decade, the role emotion plays in learning has been speculated to be the most influential of all the domains in impacting motivation, thus the first domain that educators should assess. For example, the client who has just been identified as having diabetes may have to talk about his or her feelings about having diabetes before being ready to learn about insulin. Some of the client's feelings may stem from his or her prior knowledge and preconceived ideas about diabetes.

Psychomotor learning consists of acquired physical skills that can be demonstrated. This may be referred to as the *skill domain*. Psychomotor objectives are very important for health teaching because they are satisfied when an appropriate level of physical skill is demonstrated. For example, the client with newly diagnosed insulin-dependent diabetes must learn to give self-injections, which will require learning the skill of using syringes to draw up and inject correct amounts of insulin.

Developmental Considerations

It is helpful for the nurse to understand various theories of development. Implications for Teaching at Various Developmental Stages (Appendix B) outlines intellectual development as well as other developmental stages and nursing implications related to them. Just as the need to learn will be different at various ages, the ability to use information to problem solve (cognitive domain) will differ, as will life experiences. For example, teaching a 6-year-old girl about insulin administration will require an approach that may vary from that used to teach a 24-year-old woman, which would, in turn, not be identical to teaching a 69-year-old woman. The nurse must consider all of these variables when developing teaching plans.

Affective learning and psychomotor learning depend on developmental stage. The 6-year-old girl will experience learning insulin administration in a different way emotionally than will the 69 -year-old woman. The 6-year-old girl may not have the fine motor skills needed to administer insulin, which may cause frustration and anxiety. On the other hand, the older woman may have arthritis and not have the dexterity needed to fill the syringe or insert the needle in the site. Box 6-1 shows signs and symptoms associated with visual age-related changes and diseases that can interfere with the client's teaching–learning process. Chronologic age does not always indicate maturity. A young child may respond more maturely and with less anxiety to health teaching compared to a 69-year-old client. Much depends on the client's responses to changes and stress in life experiences.

When nurses instruct parents about administering medication to their children, parents may not always understand instructions. Walsh et al. (2010) reported that it is not uncommon to find errors in giving medication to children at home. Even with a high education level among parents, with 37% having bachelor's degrees and 12% holding advanced degrees, mistakes happen often with parents sometimes not using the proper syringe to measure liquid medicine or a pill cutter to cut tablets, resulting in children getting too little pain medicine or chemotherapy.

In the Walsh study, 128 medication errors were discovered, with 73 that could have hurt children and 10 actually causing injury. Parents need help administering complicated drug regimens, even if they're highly educated. Box 6-2 provides tips when teaching parents safe administration of medication to children.

Nurses may need to show adults why they need to learn before the actual teaching can begin. Many adults have not been involved in an educational process for many years. They may show a hesitancy to learn something new, perhaps because they are afraid of failing. In addition, many older clients may have concerns about memory loss.

The nurse should never assume that all clients possess the ability to understand verbal directions or read and write. Illiteracy is found in every walk of life, among all races and cultures, and at all socioeconomic levels. Of older clients, two thirds have inadequate or

<table>
<tr><td>BOX
6-1</td><td>**Signs and Symptoms of Age-Related Changes That Can Interfere With the Client-Teaching Process**</td></tr>
</table>

- Diminished visual acuity
- Distorted central vision
- Blurred or clouded vision
- Loss of visual field
- Loss of central vision
- Loss of peripheral vision
- Reduced accommodation
- Glare
- Decline in depth perception
- Decreased color perception
- Decreased contrast sensitivity
- Decreased light/dark adaptation
- Scotomas
- Reduced night vision
- Slower processing of visual input

Adapted from Barry, C. S. (2000). Teaching the older client in the home: Assessment and adaptation. *Home Healthcare Nurse*, 18(6), 379; Jarvis, C. (1996). *Physical examination of health assessment* (2nd ed., pp. 306, 322). Philadelphia, PA: Saunders.

marginal literacy skills. One study in a public hospital revealed that 81% of clients over 60 years could not read or understand basic materials such as prescription labels. Nor should nurses believe that all the individuals they care for speak or read English as about 5% of Americans are not literate in English. Of these Americans, many are literate in their native language (White, 2008).

<table>
<tr><td>BOX
6-2</td><td>**Tips for Parents Administering Medication to Children**</td></tr>
</table>

Don't rely on your memory. Ask your child's doctor for instructions in writing, including the proper dosage and time of day to give the medicine.

Be inquisitive. Ask for clarification if you don't understand.

Get organized. Select a specific area in which to keep all medications. Keep them in a box or container.

Use the proper equipment. Ask your child's doctor how best to administer the medicine and any specific equipment needed such as a pill splitter or syringe.

Make a list. Keep a running tally of your child's medicines including why and when the medication is taken. Bring this list with you to all doctor's appointments.

Be creative. Use reminders such as a cell phone alarm or computerized calendars or Excel spreadsheets to monitor dates and times medications are taken. Medication containers labeled with the day of the week in order to keep track of a child's medication schedule should be used with caution as they are not childproof.

Don't stop a medication without telling your child's doctor.

Don't let your child take medication on his or her own. Even older children and teenagers still need some oversight.

Source: Payne, J. (2010). *A new study finds that medication errors are common in children.* Retrieved from http://health.usnews.com/health-news/family-health/childrens-health/articles/2010/05/03/8- ways-to-prevent-medication-errors-in-kids.html

The risk of miscommunication and unsafe care is not solely the potential fate of only those who cannot read or speak English. It is a risk for a large segment of the American population that, according to the most recent national literacy study, has basic (29%) to below-basic (14%) prose literacy skills, with about half of the U.S. adult population having difficulty using text to accomplish everyday tasks. These levels of ability may impair individuals from understanding some written instructions related to self-care management. The ability of the average American to use numbers in comparison to literacy skills is even lower—33% have basic and 22% have below-basic quantitative skills. Being unable to use numbers may impair a client's ability to take prescription drugs as ordered (Joint Commission, 2008). Basic literacy skills and command of the English language influence health literacy.

This vulnerable group at risk for the lowest level of health literacy report poorer health, no access to health information over the Internet, having one or more disabilities, no health insurance, taking few preventive health measures and being largely from racial and ethnic minorities, being older adults, or living in prison (White, 2008). Although a risk factor, educational level is not a true determinant of a person's ability to read or write. Health literacy or illiteracy must always be assessed as part of the client's need and readiness to learn.

Teaching and Levels of Prevention

Teaching, whether it is in the acute care or community-based setting, occurs at all levels of prevention. An important goal of teaching is to prevent the initial occurrence of disease or injury through health promotion and prevention activities. Teaching parents and day care providers about the importance of immunization is primary prevention, as is teaching about community resources that provide free or inexpensive immunization. Secondary prevention teaching targets early identification of and intervention in a condition seen when a home care nurse teaches the parents of a ventilator-dependent child about early signs of upper respiratory infection and when to contact the nurse on call. Teaching aimed at tertiary prevention attempts to restore health and facilitate self-care management and coping skills. A home care nurse who provides instruction to clients newly diagnosed with diabetes about the diabetic diet, handling syringes, giving themselves injections, and measuring their blood sugar is an example (Fig. 6-1).

Nursing Competencies and Skills in the Teaching Process

Teaching and learning follows several prescribed steps, similar to those of the nursing process, as shown in Table 6-1. A comprehensive assessment determines the client and/or family members' need and readiness to learn and past life experiences. Learning outcomes, which guide the learning plan and provide outcome criteria, arise from the learning needs. Once the learning objectives or outcomes are defined, the nurse/teacher will determine

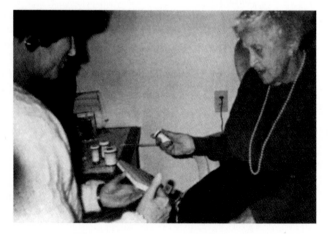

Figure 6-1 Tertiary prevention involves helping restore the client to health. On this visit, the nurse uses a weekly medication container to help an older woman with limited vision devise a plan for compliance in taking her medications.

Table 6-1 Relationship Between Nursing Process and Teaching and Learning

Steps	Nursing Process	Teaching and Learning
Assessment	Assessment of client/family/caregiver determines strengths and need for nursing care	Assessment of client/family/caregiver determines strengths and need for health teaching
Diagnosis	Statement of nursing problem	Statement of learning need
Goals/expected outcome	Goals and expected outcomes for client or family	Learning objectives/goals for the learner
Planning	Nurse and client work together to develop plan of nursing care	Nurse and client work together to develop learning plan
Interventions	A variety of actions can be used to implement the plan	A variety of actions in cognitive, affective, and psychomotor learning are used to augment plan
Evaluation	Nurse and client/family evaluate success of outcomes; nurse and client/family determine why the plan was not successful (if so); nurse and client/family revise and set new objectives and plan	Nurse and client/family evaluate success of outcomes; nurse and client/family determine weakness of plan; new objectives and plan are written

appropriate nursing interventions and teaching strategies or tools and methods appropriate for the learner. After implementation of the plan, an evaluation determines the success of teaching. A diagram of this process is shown in Figure 6-2.

ASSESSMENT

Assessment begins by looking at the learning needs, readiness, and life experiences of the client, family, and caregiver in all three learning domains. Nursing implications for various developmental stages should also be considered and are listed in Appendix B. Successful teaching is positively associated with a nonjudgmental attitude. This is especially true when the nurse's culture is different from the client's. An accommodating attitude develops when the nurse recognizes and accepts differences between the nurse and client and tries to understand the cultural or value basis for the client's expressed needs or behavior. This leads the nurse to listen and learn before initiating the teaching plan and to always empathize with the client regardless of differences in attitudes and values.

A cultural assessment tool assists the nurse to determine how learning need is influenced by culture and is discussed in more depth in Chapters 3 and 5. An assessment guide can be used to assess the learning need of the client. An example is found in Assessment Tools 6-1. After assessing the client, family, and caregiver needs; readiness to learn; and past life experiences, the learning need can be determined.

IDENTIFICATION OF THE LEARNING NEED

The nurse draws inferences based on the information discovered during the assessment (see Table 6-2). A list of client and family strengths and **learning needs** emerges, from which priority needs are identified. When lack of knowledge, motivation, or skill hinders a client's self-care, a nursing diagnosis can be used to name the need or strength.

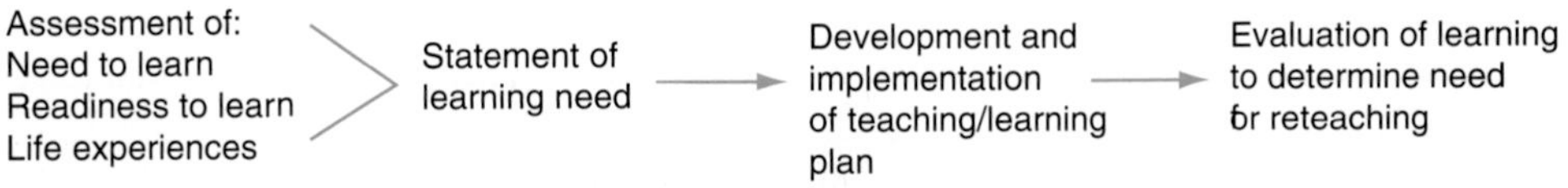

Assessment of:
Need to learn
Readiness to learn
Life experiences
> Statement of learning need → Development and implementation of teaching/learning plan → Evaluation of learning to determine need 6r reteaching

Figure 6-2 Diagram of the teaching process. The nursing process and the teaching process have some similarities.

Client name _____

Health condition requiring health education _____

Primary caregiver _____

Learner _____ Relationship to client_____

Age _____ Gender _____Occupation _____

Developmental stages and implications for learner _____

Psychosocial stage _____

_____

Cognitive stage _____

Language _____

_____

What do the client and family identify as client and family strengths? _____

_____

_____

How does the caregiver or client feel about the responsibilities of self-care? _____

_____

_____

Describe any disabilities or limitations of the learner (including sensory disabilities).

_____

Describe any preexisting health conditions of the learner. _____

_____

List sociocultural factors that may impede learning.

_____

State learner behaviors that indicate motivation to learn. _____

_____

State learner statements that indicate motivation to learn._____

Indications that the learner reads and comprehends at the reading level required by the task?

_____

Indications that the learner possesses ability to problem solve at a level that provides safe care in the home? _____

_____

Describe the home environment. Is it conducive to the learning required by the condition?

_____

_____

If not, what modifications are necessary? _____

_____

If the learner is not able to carry out the care, are other caregivers available for backup support?

_____

If so, please name. _____

Contact information _____

_____

_____

_____

What other support is available for the client and caregiver? _____

_____

Table 6-2 Examples of Inferences Made From Assessment Data

Factors to Consider When Assessing Readiness to Learn

Physiologic Factors	Data	Inference
Age	85 y	Elderly client may have special needs
Gender	Male	Men and women each have special needs
Disease process currently under treatment	Newly diagnosed diabetic	New diabetics have many teaching needs
Intactness of senses—hearing, vision, touch, taste	Hearing and vision are impaired	Teaching must be modified considering sensory deficit
Preexisting conditions	Cataract surgery 2 y ago	Vision may still be partially impaired or may be corrected
Psychosocial Factors		
Sociocultural	Hmong refugee	Teaching must consider diet common to this culture
Occupation	Retired	Does the client have health insurance?
Cognitive Factors		
Motivation	Learner states, "I am interested in learning about ____"	Learner is motivated
Reading ability	Observed reading the newspaper	Shows ability to read
Learning style	Observer, doer, or listener	Tailor teaching to style
Problem-solving ability	Learner can come up with concepts and alternatives	Learner can problem solve
Environmental Factors		
Home environment	Home cluttered with no place to sit or set up teaching	Environment must be modified before teaching
Caregiver		
Availability	Client is a widow or spouse works full time	No caregiver available
Motivation	Caregiver states, "I can't handle hearing about that device"	Caregiver not motivated
Abilities	Caregiver is unable to follow simple instructions or directions	Caregiver has limited ability to provide care
Other support	Client is active in his or her church	Church may be another source of care

The list of the North American Nursing Diagnosis Association International diagnoses can help identify the learning needs of the individual, family member, or caregiver. According to Carpenito (2010), knowledge deficit should be used in a nursing diagnosis as a related factor. Most nursing diagnoses incorporate teaching as a part of the diagnosis. This is illustrated in the following examples:

- Risk for Ineffective Health Maintenance related to lack of knowledge of management, signs, and symptoms of complications of diabetes mellitus
- Decisional Conflict related to lack of knowledge about advantages and disadvantages of infant circumcision

- Risk for Impaired Home Maintenance Management related to lack of knowledge of home care and community resources
- Risk for Injury related to lack of knowledge of bicycle safety

Learning needs can be determined in one, two, or all of the learning domains. Consider the learning domains in the examples below.

CLIENT SITUATIONS IN PRACTICE

Discharge Teaching With Newborn Circumcision

Pat, a primipara, delivered a boy yesterday afternoon. The newborn is to be circumcised this afternoon before Pat and her newborn are discharged. Pat states at the beginning of the teaching session that she knows nothing about circumcision care and needs the information to be able to take "good care" of her baby. Despite the fact that you have gone over the teaching outline about circumcision twice with Pat, she states a second time, "How will the penis look in 3 days?" She is also unable to demonstrate the application of the dressing to the site and states, "Maybe we shouldn't have the baby circumcised if it will hurt the baby."

For this scenario, the following is an example of a learning need in the affective domain:
Anxiety related to lack of knowledge as manifested by the mother's statement, "Maybe we shouldn't have the baby circumcised if it will hurt the baby."

Here is an example of a learning need in the psychomotor domain:
Risk for Impaired Home Maintenance Management related to lack of knowledge and lack of ability to demonstrate dressing change.

The following is an example of a nursing diagnosis in the cognitive domain:
Impaired parenting related to lack of knowledge and inexperience as manifested by the mother's statement, "How will the penis look in 3 days?"

Reimbursement for Teaching in the Home

After the learning need is identified, the nurse determines if the teaching needed by the client is reimbursable. In the example above, teaching is an expected part of the role of the nurse in discharge planning and is a reimbursed activity. However, nursing care in the home that is only focused on teaching is reimbursed only if it meets certain requirements. Medicare, Medicaid, and most other third-party payers reimburse only skilled nursing care that falls within specific parameters. Consequently, referrals for health education needs depend on **reimbursement requirements** of the payer of the services. Most insurance companies, health maintenance organizations, and other third-party payers follow Medicare Guidelines. The specific requirements are defined in the Medicare Guidelines, 30.2.3.3-Teaching and Training Activities (Revision 1, 10-01-03, summarized in Box 6-3).

An example is seen in a client who is newly diagnosed with diabetes. The client's learning needs must meet the requirements seen in Assessment Tools 6-1; otherwise Medicare or the insurance company, depending on the coverage, will not reimburse for the home visit for health teaching. It is imperative that the nurse knows the reimbursement requirements of the various third-party payers as agencies will not receive payment for teaching if the nurse does not follow the requirements specified by the particular payer.

PLANNING

Planning for learning involves developing a teaching plan similar to nursing care plans—both follow the steps of the nursing process. Many agencies use standardized or computerized teaching plans. If standardized plans are used, the plan must always be individualized to the client and his or her needs.

The teaching plan identifies teaching goals and learning objectives that reflect the specifics of the ongoing care at home. Goals of teaching are broad in scope and set down what is expected as the final outcome of the teaching learning process. For example, the goal may be to ensure the client's safety and total reliance on self-care. Planning care is a mutual

| BOX 6-3 | **Medicare Guidelines** |

TEACHING AND TRAINING ACTIVITIES AND QUESTIONABLE SITUATIONS

Teaching and training activities, which require skilled nursing or skilled rehabilitation personnel to teach a patient how to manage their treatment regimen, constitute skilled services. Some examples are

- Teaching self-administration of injectable medications or a complex range of medications
- Teaching a newly diagnosed diabetic to administer insulin injections, to prepare and follow a diabetic diet, and to observe foot-care precautions
- Teaching gait training prosthesis care for a patient who has had a recent leg amputation
- Teaching patients how to care for a recent colostomy or ileostomy
- Teaching patients how to perform self-catheterization and self-administration of gastrostomy feedings
- Teaching patients how to care for and maintain central venous lines, such as Hickman catheters
- Teaching patients the use and care of braces, splints and orthotics and any associated skin care
- Teaching patients the proper care of any specialized dressings or skin treatments

30.2.3-QUESTIONABLE SITUATIONS (REV. 1, 10-01-03).

There must be specific evidence that daily skilled nursing or skilled rehabilitation services are required and received if

- The primary service needed is oral medication *or*

- The patient is capable of independent ambulation, dressing, feeding, and hygiene

From Medicare Benefit Policy Manual. (2008). Medicare guidelines, 30.2.3.3—Teaching and training activities (Revision. 1, 10-01-03). Retrieved from www.cms.gov/manuals/Download/bp102c08.pdf

---

process among the nurse, client, and family caregivers with goals developed using the three learning domains.

- Cognitive objectives: Relate to learning activities that strengthen comprehension regarding the illness and its treatment.

- Affective objectives: Relate to learning activities that enhance the acceptance of and the adjustment to the illness and subsequent treatment.

- Psychomotor objectives: Relate to learning activities that demonstrate skill mastery necessary for the management of the treatment procedures.

A **learning objective** is similar to a client goal or expected outcome used in the nursing process. It is usually short term, specific, and accomplished in one or two sessions. Each objective includes a subject, action verb, performance criteria, target time, and special conditions (Box 6-4).

The following learning objective contains these components:

- Client will state three signs and symptoms of infection by (date) _____ and know which complications require contacting the nurse on call.

- Subject: client
- Action verb: state
- Performance criteria: signs and symptoms of infection
- Target time: (date)
- Special conditions: when to contact the nurse on call

Examples of learning objectives in the three learning domains are as follows:

- Cognitive objectives: Family or caregiver will state three signs and symptoms of infection by (date) _____.

BOX 6-4	Active Verbs for Learning Objectives		

Cognitive Domain	Affective Domain	Psychomotor Domain
categorize	answer	adapt
compare	choose	arrange
compose	defend	assemble
define	discuss	begin
describe	display	change
design	form an opinion	construct
differentiate	express	create
explain	help	manipulate
give example	initiate	move
identify	join	organize
label	justify	rearrange
list	relate	show
name	revise	start
prepare	select	work
plan	share	inject
solve	use	draw up
state		
summarize		
write		

- Affective objectives: Family or caregiver will express feelings about having to be in charge of client's central line care by (date) _____.
- Psychomotor objectives: Family or caregiver will demonstrate aseptic technique when cleaning and flushing sites on vascular access device by (date) _____.

In most situations, the nurse and the client plan a series of small, incremental learning objectives based on the specific needs of the client. The overall goal of planning is to assist the client or family caregiver to have adequate skills and knowledge to be able to provide safe self-care at home. The goal of teaching is to maximize individual potential and quality of life of individuals and families.

INTERVENTION

The nurse carries out the teaching plan according to the client or family caregiver's strengths, and learning needs are accomplished in as many teaching sessions as necessary. Specific approaches for teaching children are shown in Appendix C, and nursing implications for various developmental stages are given in Appendix B. With clients across the life span, the nurse needs to develop rapport and be an honest and open communicator to encourage and give the client self-confidence to learn something new. General principles to guide teaching with older learners are presented in Box 6-5.

EVALUATION

In the last phase, both learning and teaching are evaluated to determine if the learning outcomes were met and if the teaching methods were effective. The plan is then modified as necessary.

General Principles to Guide Community-Based Teaching With the Older Learner

- Meet in a quiet, well-lit room where there is no background noise.
- Face the learner and speak in a low, slow voice so lip-reading is possible.
- With the client's permission, include family members.
- Limit sessions to no more than 20–30 minutes and watch for cues indicating inadequate hearing, lack of attention, or tiredness.
- Relate new information to past experiences if possible. Repeat information frequently; use frequent summaries.
- Encourage autonomous decision making to support ego integrity.
- Provide written materials as reinforcement, when possible with visual aids with large letters and bright colors.
- Compliment the client for accomplishments during and after learning session.

The following questions may be asked by the nurse to assess the level of learning:

- What additional data are needed to evaluate the progress made toward the learning objectives?
- Were the objectives met? If not, why not? What additional objectives are needed in the future?
- Is the nurse, client, and family satisfied with the outcome? If not, what would provide satisfaction?

Evaluation of teaching also appraises the efficacy of the teaching plan and methods. Evaluation of teaching considers the barriers to, and characteristics of, successful teaching. The nurse may ask these questions:

- Did the teaching focus on the most important problem for this family in relation to the potential of the client for self-care? If not, what is the most important problem for the family?
- How was the plan collaborative?
- What reinforcement was used? If applicable, did the learner have the opportunity for hands-on practice?
- Was the home environment appropriate? If not, how was it modified?
- Was the equipment adequate? If not, what additional equipment is needed?
- What teaching methods did the nurse use? What additional methods could be used next time?
- Was the teaching plan realistic? If not, how could it be changed to be realistic?
- If this session were to be repeated, which additional strategies or tools could be used?

Evaluation must always consider what the client and family believe they need to know, as well as what the nurse considers essential. It is also important for the nurse to recognize when the learning needs of the client, family, or caregiver are beyond the educational preparation of the nurse so that a referral to appropriate resources can be made.

DOCUMENTATION

Documentation of teaching is essential (1) as a legal record, (2) as communication of teaching and learning to other health care professionals, and (3) for determination of eligibility for care needed and for reimbursement of care provided. The following parts of the teaching process should be documented:

- Assessment of the learner's readiness, need, and life experiences
- Identification of learning needs and barriers to successful learning

COMMUNITY-BASED NURSING CARE GUIDELINES 6-1

Working With Interpreters

- Determine the language the client speaks at home.
- Use qualified, professional interpreters.
- Avoid using interpreters from rival tribes, states, regions, or nations.
- Use an interpreter of the same gender as the client, if possible. In general, an older interpreter is preferred to a younger interpreter.
- Allow enough time for the interpreted session.
- Look directly at the client, addressing your questions to him or her.
- Speak in a normal tone of voice, clearly and slowly, using words and not just gestures.
- Keep your sentences simple and short; pause often to permit interpretation.
- Ask only one question at a time.
- Give the interpreter freedom to interrupt for clarification.
- Ask the interpreter to take notes if needed when the interview gets too complex.
- Be prepared to repeat instructions several times, use different words and rephrase as necessary for understanding. Be patient.
- Use the simplest vocabulary; avoid slang, jargon, and unfamiliar medical terminology.
- Check to see if the information has been understood. Have the interpreter tell you what the client has said he or she understands. Be direct and expect directness.

Adapted from Andrews, M., & Boyle, J. (2008). *Transcultural concepts in nursing care* (5th ed.). Philadelphia, PA: Lippincott Williams & Wilkins.

- Plan for teaching and learning outcomes
- Content taught
- Teaching techniques used
- Evaluation of teaching and learning, including learner response and recommendations for the next step

Methods of documentation vary, but the trend is toward the use of electronic records that outline teaching needs by diagnosis or procedure and include learning outcomes, content, methods, and strategies for teaching. An additional component of documentation is confidentiality, illustrated in Community-Based Nursing Care Guidelines 6-1.

Barriers to Successful Teaching

It is helpful to be aware of some of the potential obstacles to successful teaching. Conditions and barriers to successful teaching differ between the acute care setting and community setting. Likewise, there may be barriers to successful teaching that differ among community-based settings. In the next section, barriers to successful teaching are presented and followed by characteristics of successful teaching.

Barriers to Discharge Teaching

We have known for over a decade that discharge teaching does not always result in learning. In a questionnaire designed to evaluate the quality of discharge teaching, only one of five family caregivers reported feeling adequately prepared to care for the client at home. Their retention of information may diminish due to the anxiety experienced with the client's homecoming. Time for teaching is now grossly limited in the acute care setting. Barriers to successful discharge teaching are shown in Table 6-3.

A major area of discharge teaching that has been identified as problematic is adherence to medications regime. Fifty percent of individuals over the age of 65 and 86% of individuals over the age of 70 have multiple chronic conditions, with most routinely taking an average of two to six prescribed medications. There is great need for education related to safe and effective use of medication in this age group (Naughton, Bennett, & Feely, 2006). Numerous studies have shown a high rate of nonadherence with the medication regimen

Table 6-3 Combating Barriers to Successful Discharge Teaching

Barriers	Sample Nursing Interventions
Timing is not conducive to learning (client's physical or psychological conditions do not allow learning to occur).	Document client's lack of mastery of the material. Update physician or nurse practitioner on an ongoing basis to plan discharge. Refer for follow-up if learning is not adequate for safe self-care.
Past experiences impede perceived learning readiness or need.	Identify past experiences. Determine and clarify misconceptions. Determine if past experience will interrupt or enhance new learning.
Retention of information impeded by anxiety of going home or leaving security of health care environment.	See interventions for timing. Break learning into small, easily mastered segments. Use positive reinforcement and praise.
Cultural differences between nurse and client or family impede learning or understanding.	Work to build a trusting relationship with client and family. Show respect for the client's culture and incorporate it in discharge planning. Use resources to overcome a language barrier.
Lack of adherence.	Establish trust. Identify reasons for lack of adherence. Clarify misinformation. Use formal and informal contracting.

after discharge from an inpatient setting, resulting in rehospitalization, clinic follow-up, or admission to home care. Comprehensive discharge teaching regarding medication management at home prevents or reduces this problem. Box 6-6 lists strategies to help clients get the full benefit from drug therapy.

Barriers to Successful Teaching in the Home

A number of barriers to successful teaching in the home exist (Table 6-4).

These barriers have the potential to interrupt the coordination of and consistency in teaching and communication with the caregiving team.

Nursing students and novice home care nurses often express dismay over their diminished control of client behavior when providing care in settings other than the acute care setting. Another barrier relates to difficulty in coordinating client teaching among multiple providers. Often, many care providers are involved with the client's care including other nurses, physical therapists, social workers, home health aides, nurse practitioners, and physicians. Each provider may teach the same or a similar procedure, treatment, or process in a different way, confusing the client and family caregiver. The time factor in acute care settings may prohibit teaching, and many home care referrals come from clinics or physicians' offices. As a result, the first teaching, in many cases, may be done in the home. Home care nurses are often pressed for time. It may be difficult for the home care nurse to feel teaching is ever complete or even adequate.

Teaching the Challenging Client

Rather than refer to challenging clients who do not follow treatment regimes as noncompliant, it is more helpful to frame this issue as lack of adherence. Noncompliance suggests a one-sided expectation, while adherence is defined as "being connected or associated by contract, giving support or loyalty to: or a steady or faithful attachment" (Webster, 2010).

When the teaching plan is unsuccessful due to lack of adherence to the treatment plan, special teaching strategies are used. When the nurse and the client are partners in care, they use a mutual process to plan and implement care. These strategies may incorporate the concepts

> **BOX 6-6**
>
> ## AIDES Model for Improving Medication Adherence for Older Adults
>
> **A:** Assessment: Complete a comprehensive medication assessment including
>   - Mental status assessment: Use agency assessment tool to complete mental status assessment.
>   - Brown-bag assessment: Have client bring a bag containing all medications and a list of all medications taken on a regular and PRN basis. Compare the list with the medications. Review the side effects, contraindications, and direction for administration of each drug.
>   - Adherence to prescribed regime: Discuss with the client whether or not he or she takes the medications as ordered or changes the dosage or schedule. Discuss why not and explore what can be done.
>   - Assessment of medication: Evaluate the appropriateness of dose, frequency, and any possible synergistic effects of the combination of medications.
> **I:** Individualization: Partner with clients to ensure individualization of the regiment.
> **D:** Documentation: Choose appropriate documentation to assist with communication between client and provider(s). Provide this written documentation to be shared with the provider at the next office visit. Encourage immediate visit with the providers if necessary based on the findings of the assessment.
> **E:** Education: Provide accurate and ongoing education tailored to the age and needs of the individual.
> **S:** Supervision: Continue supervision of the medication regimen.
>
> Adapted from Bergman-Evans, B. (2006). AIDES to improving medication adherence in older adults. *Geriatric Nursing, 27*(3), 174–182.

of concordance, adherence, and partnering (Huffman, 2005). Concordance is an agreement between the nurse and the client about whether, when, and how treatments occur. Again, this term suggests an agreement that respects the beliefs and wishes of both parties.

It is important to ascertain *why* the client is not following the prescribed treatment. Common reasons clients do not follow treatment regimens stem from lack of information, lack of skill, lack of client value for the treatment, and lack of self-efficacy. The environment may create barriers to adherence. Sometimes the treatment plan itself may be perceived as a barrier. A simple problem-solving technique that can be used is to ask the client about his or her perception of progress made with the teaching plan (concordance). Once the barrier to learning is identified, the nurse and client in partnership can tailor interventions accordingly (partnership). Barriers may come from client factors, home environment, and the teaching plan itself.

CLIENT FACTORS

Client factors may include lack of knowledge, skill, or self-efficacy. Or, in other cases, fear, anxiety, or lack of valuing the treatment plan will produce lack of adherence. It is not uncommon for individuals to not follow a treatment plan because of anxiety or fear. Before any teaching occurs, the nurse must address the anxiety or fear of the learner.

Each factor may require a different approach to resolve the lack of adherence. It is important to first identify the cause as each factor calls for a different approach. Sometimes, nurses may interpret nonadherence as lack of knowledge when the client's behavior simply reflects the values and attitudes of the client and the client's community. Lack of valuing the treatment may require modification of the teaching regimen to better fit the client's value system.

Learning needs stemming from lack of information or skills are easily met by identifying and providing knowledge and opportunities to practice skills. Lack of adherence may stem from the clients' belief about their own self-efficacy, that is, the ability to influence events that affect their life. Self-efficacy has been strongly and positively associated with a number of health indicators including better diabetes control, better functional performance, fewer depressive

Table 6-4 Combating Barriers to Successful Home Teaching

Barriers	Sample Nursing Interventions
Home Environment *Examples:*	
Home setting is nonstructured.	Involve client and family in all stages of planning.
Environment is the client and family's home turf.	Build trusting relationship with client and family, maintaining respect for family's culture and values.
Equipment and setting are inadequate for teaching.	Collaborate with the client and family to adapt the home environment to facilitate learning and compliance.
Nurse Caregiver *Examples:*	
Nurse has less control over the outcomes of the teaching.	Approach the client with a nonjudgmental attitude and embrace a flexible attitude.
Nurse may have inadequate preparation for providing teaching in the home.	Acquire specific knowledge and skill in community-based care.
Nurse must bring all the teaching supplies to the home.	Plan and organize ahead and bring adequate supplies.
Nurse must coordinate client teaching among many providers.	Facilitate communication and documentation among caregivers.
Nurse role shifts from client care manager to health care facilitator.	Focus on enhancing client's autonomy with self-care instead of providing care to the client.
Client/Family/Recipient of Teaching *Examples:*	
Wide variation in family members' ages and cognitive and developmental stages.	Carefully assess learning need, learning readiness, and past learning experiences of all recipients of teaching.
Lack of adherence unless client/family are involved in the teaching plan.	Involve family and client in all stages of planning and teaching.

symptoms, better quality of life, and lower health care utilization (Weng, Dai, Huan, & Chaing, 2010). Health efficacy has positive impact on problem-solving abilities, client–provider partnerships, and self-care management. Clients' self-efficacy can be increased by:

- Setting realistic goals
- Assisting clients to develop problem-solving skills
- Initiating and supporting a partnership model between client, the nurse, and other health care professionals.
- Using gentle persuasion to encourage the client to believe in his or her own ability to achieve goals
- Teaching easy management techniques first
- Using return demonstrations with immediate positive reinforcement
- Pointing out the client's incremental successes
- Supporting the client to recognize perceived threats and fears and manage emotional responses to these concerns

Another strategy that may be helpful to address a specific health behavior involves a collaborative process in which the client chooses a goal, and the nurse and client negotiate a specific action plan to reach the goal. For example, if the client would like to stop smoking, he or she may have an initial action plan of reducing the number of cigarettes consumed in a day from one pack to one half a pack by using nicotine gum. After a week, the next step may be to start using a nicotine patch and only have one cigarette after each meal.

Action plans have been shown clinically as a useful strategy to encourage behavior changes for clients. It is important to remember that no individual is totally compliant with any lifestyle choice. It is prudent to use professional judgment to gauge what level of adherence to treatment is acceptable while remaining open to continuously working with the client to revise the teaching plan.

THE HOME ENVIRONMENT

The home environment may impede or facilitate adherence to treatment regimen. Behaviorally oriented client education, which emphasizes the change of the environment in which the client does self-care, is often a highly successful strategy. Changing the home environment is credited with improving the clinical course of clients instructed in the home. For instance, removing all ashtrays and initiating a rule that no smoking be allowed inside the client's home would create an environment less amenable to smoking. Careful assessment of the home environment allows the nurse to identify and suggest modification of problematic issues to enhance learning outcomes. These interventions may be as simple as providing better light for a teaching session by opening the drapes, moving a lamp, or replacing a burned-out light bulb.

Successful Teaching Approaches

Discharge teaching in both home care and acute care settings must begin at admission. The first and most essential component of successful teaching in community-based settings is building a trusting relationship with the client and family. As trust builds, barriers are removed often resulting in enhanced learning and adherence to the prescribed regimen. Vigilant assessment of the family, its culture, and the community environment creates a foundation for a comprehensive teaching plan. Joint planning leads to better adherence to treatment regimens because this process requires forming a partnership, building an alliance, and working together toward a shared goal.

Frequently, clients and family caregivers may only need reinforcement that the client is progressing normally in the recovery process. In these situations, the focus includes care for the caregiver and the client, as well as focus on client and family strengths.

Anxiety has long been known to be a barrier to learning. When the client is on "home turf" and has more control of the environment and the situation, anxiety may be reduced (Fig. 6-3).

On the other hand, often, the sometimes hurried process of discharge planning in both home care and acute care creates high anxiety for the client and family. As part of the original and ongoing assessment process, the nurse assesses the learner's anxiety level. If the learner exhibits anxiety that is interrupting learning, the learning plan must be modified.

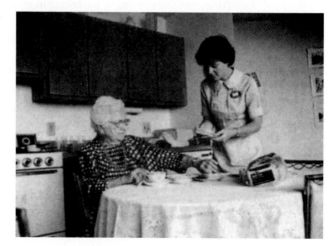

Figure 6-3 A teaching–learning experience in the home often is more successful because the client is in his or her own territory. The nurse is responsible for teaching and coordinating care.

Another way to reduce anxiety is to create lessons that include small "digestible" segments that build on information shared in previous teaching sessions. Reinforcement created by multiple exposures to the content allows for mastery, which, in turn, increases learner confidence and reduces anxiety.

In all settings, teaching is problematic if the nurse does not speak the same language as the client or if the client has sight, comprehension, or retention problems (see Community-Based Nursing Care Guidelines 6-2 and 6-3). There are several community-based guidelines that should be followed when providing health information to a client or family member for whom English is a second language:

- Listen carefully to what the client and family are telling you.

- Discuss one idea at a time, use simple, uncomplicated sentences, and use concrete examples to enhance learning.

- Determine the client's and family members' understanding of the illness being treated and the suggested treatment by using strategies such as return demonstration or questions such as "Tell me why hand washing is important before you change your dressing".

COMMUNITY-BASED NURSING CARE GUIDELINES 6-2

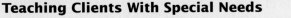

Teaching Clients With Special Needs

Strategies for Visually Impaired Clients
- Speak to the client when approaching and avoid speaking from behind the client.
- Identify yourself by saying your name or gently touching the client to alert him or her to your presence.
- Ask other people in the room to introduce themselves—this allows the client to hear each person's voice.
- Describe the room and the position of furniture to familiarize the client with the surroundings.
- Explain procedures precisely. Inform the client when you are leaving the room; let the client know what you are doing and where you are located at all times.
- Use adaptive devices for the client with low vision such as large-print materials (telephone dials, thermostat dials) and a magnifying glass.

Strategies for Hearing-Impaired Clients
- Provide a well-lit environment; face the client and speak slowly and deliberately.
- When entering a room, place yourself in front of the client so he or she can see you, or lightly touch the client.
- Always ask if the client uses a hearing aid and if it is working properly; ask if the client needs assistance with inserting the hearing aid and if he or she wears the aid.
- Ask the client if he or she desires an auditory amplifier in the telephone, a TDD telecommunications device for the hearing impaired that converts speech to text or text to speech, or a light on the telephone to alert client of a caller.
- Give the client written material that summarizes the information given orally.

Strategies for Clients With Speech and Language Deficits (Aphasia)
- Provide services for communication such as a letter board so the client can spell words, word boards (nurse or client points to word), picture charts (nurse or client points to object), or a computer.
- Be patient; supply needed support when the client falters in communication attempts.
- Provide regular mental stimulation.
- Praise all efforts and encourage practicing what is learned in treatment.

Adapted from Anderson, C. (1990). *Patient teaching and communication in an information age.* Albany, NY: Delmar; Arnold, E., & Boggs, K. (1995). *Interpersonal relationships: Professional communication skills for nurses* (2nd ed.). Philadelphia, PA: Saunders.

COMMUNITY-BASED NURSING CARE GUIDELINES 6-3

Confidentiality

- Maintain confidentiality in consultation, teaching, and writing.
- Ensure privacy before engaging in a discussion of content to be entered into the record.
- Release information only with written consent.
- Use professional judgment regarding confidentiality when the information may be harmful to the client's health or well-being.
- Use professional judgment when deciding how to maintain the privacy of a minor. Be aware of your state's laws and regulations regarding the parent's or guardian's right to know.

- Use materials printed in the client's or family members' first language, when possible. Or use materials written in simple, straightforward English.
- Discuss the client's use of folk medicines and home remedies and bring to the client and family's attention any contraindications for concurrent use of medications and folk medicines.

Some form of follow-up to provide a link between care providers in the community is essential. This may be in the form of a phone call, letter, home visit, or clinic visit. According to numerous studies, these strategies enhance continuity of care. Meticulous documentation is also always an essential component of a successful discharge teaching program.

Behaviorally oriented client education, which emphasizes a change of environment to facilitate client self-care, is the most successful method for improving the clinical course of chronic disease. In addition, behavioral education contributes to care that is more easily managed in the home. For example, when teaching about home safety, rearranging furniture so that it is in the field of vision for a client with hemianopsia is a behavioral-oriented strategy. This strategy encourages ambulation and facilitates self-care while protecting client safety but must be accomplished within the context of the client and family's value system.

Successful Teaching Techniques

The nurse needs to be familiar with a variety of teaching techniques and feel competent to choose which technique is the most suitable for the circumstance. For example, demonstration of a new skill is used to change behavior, whereas videos are used to increase knowledge. DVDs, video, and closed-circuit TV supplement one-on-one and group teaching. Before discharge and once home, the client as well as the family or caregiver may watch programs several times if reinforcement is necessary. Successful teaching strategies include demonstrating and return demonstration of a skill with opportunity for hands-on practice in addition to telling the client about the procedure. Regardless of the setting, much teaching occurs while the nurse is providing client care—taking blood pressure or a temperature, giving a bath, examining a newborn or infant, weighing the client, and changing wound dressings. Client education seldom is the formal process one experiences in a classroom. Weaving teaching into all nursing activities saves time and allows the nurse to repeat the teaching several times.

Actual equipment and objects can be used for effective teaching, including the catheter, tubing, port, monitor, or other devices. Picture cards can be made to illustrate each item in a procedure. Photos can be made of each key step or diagrams can be drawn for the cards. The nurse can design posters with information the client needs to learn. Worksheets can be developed to use with a videotape, DVD or audiotape.

A teaching technique new in the last decade for health education is the use of Web sites on the Internet. Interactive content provides the client with important information without having to leave the home. This method could be used for any type of teaching for clients who are computer literate and have access to a computer at home, school, or the public library. However, as Web-based and Internet use has become the preferred method

BOX 6-7	**Criteria for Evaluating Health Information Web Sites**

CRITERIA	QUESTIONS TO ASK
Purpose of the Web site or mission of the organization	What is the intended use of the site?
Sponsorship	Who funds the site? Why?
Currency	Is the information on the site current? Is the site updated?
Factual information	Is the information opinion or factual? Is there a way to verify from a primary source the information found on the site? Are there links to other credible sites?
Audience	Who is the intended audience? Does the site state clearly whether the information is for the consumer or health professional?
Disclaimer	Is there a statement referring users to health care professionals for diagnosis and treatment?

Adapted from Medical Library Association. (2010). A user's guide to finding and evaluating health information on the web. Retrieved from http://mlanet.org/resources/userguide.html#3; Miller, L., Jones, B., Graves, R., & Sievert, M. (2010). Beyond Google: Finding and evaluating web-based information for community-based nursing practice. *International Journal of Nursing Education Scholarship*, 7(1), article 31. doi:10.2202/1548-923X.1961.

of securing information, the issue of reliability and credibility of the plethora of available information has come to the forefront. Nurses are challenged to find and use reliable and credible information to support evidence-based practice in the community. A tool for evaluating Web sites is found in Box 6-7 (Miller, Jones, Graves, & Sievert, 2010).

Just as it is important when teaching individuals and families in community-based settings to use a collaborative, mutual process, it is necessary when planning group teaching sessions. The Research in Community-Based Nursing Care 6-2 box provides evidence of how collaboration improves learning outcomes for groups of learners.

THE TEACHING PLAN

As previously mentioned, effective teaching requires well-developed interpersonal skills and a nonjudgmental attitude. Concordance is important to effective teaching. The nurse and the client can establish concordance at the first visit and each subsequent visit by contracting at the beginning of a therapeutic relationship about whether, when, and how treatments occur. Concordance may prevent some lack of adherence to the treatment plan from the outset. Most agencies have formal contracts such as a "Bill of Rights" or "Client Responsibilities." Review and implementation of the content of these standards on the first visit is one way to encourage adherence.

CLIENT SITUATIONS IN PRACTICE
Teaching in the Home Setting

Assessment

Allison is the home care nurse assigned to care for Ida, a 76-year-old widow recently diagnosed with insulin-dependent diabetes. On Friday, November 1, Ida visited the clinic with complaints of polyuria, polydipsia, and polyphagia. Her blood sugar was 456 mg/dL. The clinic educator saw her on November 1 and charted the following on the referral form:

Client stated, "I have not slept well for 2 weeks because I have to get up so often to go to the bathroom." After the initial teaching session, which covered the basics of the diabetic

RESEARCH IN COMMUNITY-BASED NURSING CARE 6-2

Teaching so They Hear: Using a Cocreated Diabetes Self-Management Education Approach

The purpose of this study was to develop and evaluate a diabetes self-management education program based on the desires and needs of a group of adults with type 2 diabetes mellitus. A collaborative process between nurses and individuals with diabetes included use of focus groups and the findings from the groups to develop the intervention and cocreated the sessions. Preintervention and postintervention outcomes for participants from the cocreated program were compared to those of participants in two other diabetic education programs at two area, certified diabetes education centers. No significant differences were found between the cocreated and the other two groups with regard to knowledge, adaptation, and program satisfaction. However, diabetes self-care activities significantly improved ($p = 0.02$) for the cocreated group. The researchers stated that a cocreated teaching approach better meets the learning needs of adults with type 2 diabetes mellitus and results in enhanced ability to perform self-care activities required for successful diabetes control. Further, the cocreated program may result in cost savings because better diabetes control reduces visits to monitor and treat complications and the need for repetitive educational sessions. Repetitive sessions may exceed third-party pay limits and extend the time needed for patient encounters.

Source: New, N. (2010). Teaching so they hear: Using a co-created diabetes self-management education approach. *Journal of the American Academy of Nurse Practitioners, 22*(6), 316–325. doi 10.1111/j.1745-7599.2010.00514.

diet and the action of insulin, the client was unable to demonstrate retention of knowledge or skills from any of the topics covered. Client will receive insulin in the clinic until the home visit on Tuesday to teach about injections.

Recommendation to home care: Client requires diabetic teaching in the areas of following a diabetic diet, drawing up insulin, giving injections, and monitoring blood sugar.

Reimbursement: This client requires teaching to manage home treatment of insulin-dependent diabetes diagnosed on November 1. This teaching meets the criteria of *Medicare Guidelines, 30.2.3.3-Teaching and Training Activities (Revision. 1, 10-01-03)*.

On Tuesday, November 5, Allison visits Ida at home. Ida greets Allison at the door with the statement, "When I was at the clinic on Friday, I was so nervous about all of the things they were telling me, but I am more relaxed today. I talked to my friend Richard who is a diabetic and manages really well. When my granddaughter Sommer was a little girl, I gave her shots and got along just fine."

Ida's home is dark, so Allison asks if she can open the drapes and move two chairs closer to the window before they start to talk. They sit down by the window, and Allison begins visiting with Ida in an attempt to help reduce Ida's anxiety and begin developing a trusting relationship. Allison learns that Ida has some knowledge about diabetes from talking to her friend Richard, and Ida has also asked her son Roger, who is a nurse, to pick up some pamphlets about diabetes at the hospital.

Ida states that she learns best by doing. She does not drive but states that her son will be able to pick up her medication and syringes, or she can take the bus to the pharmacy. Allison notices a magnifying glass on the table and a large-print book on a bookshelf. Allison asks Ida about her vision. Ida responds that she has had three cataract surgeries and has difficulty reading, so she frequently uses the magnifying glass.

Allison concludes that Ida perceives a need to learn and is ready to learn. Allison also believes that Ida's past experiences will enhance her learning, not impede it. Concerned about Ida's restricted vision, Allison makes a note to continue to assess this aspect. At this point, Allison completes the learning assessment guide, as shown in Assessment Tools 6-2.

Assessment Tools 6-2
Sample Learning Assessment Guide

Client name *Ida* _____

Health condition requiring health education *Insulin-dependent diabetes diagnosed on November 1, 2012.*

Primary caregiver *Home care nurse, client, and Roger* _____

Learner *Ida*_____Relationship to client_____

Age *76*_____ Gender *Female* _____ Occupation *Retired legal secretary*__

Developmental stages and implications for learner_____

Psychosocial stage *The client is in the integrity versus ego despair stage. She describes her life as follows:* _____

*"I have been blessed. I have 10 wonderful children, 25 grandchildren, and 10 great-grandchildren. I loved my work after my kids grew up. My husband and I had a good relationship."*_____

Cognitive stage *No evidence of cognitive impairment* _____

Language *Speaks English, visual impairment, stated "I was writing a novel about* _____ *Sweden until I started to have problems with my eyes."* _____

How does the caregiver or client feel about the responsibilities of self-care?_____

States she is more relaxed than November 1 when diagnosed. _____

Describe any disabilities or limitations of the learner (including sensory disabilities)_____

Visual impairment and statement "I am afraid that I will not be able to see the numbers on the syringes." _____

Disabilities *Arthritis in left knee and left hip* _____

Describe any preexisting health conditions of the learner

Client has had multiple cataract surgeries and has visual impairment. _____

List sociocultural factors that may impede learning *None*_____

State learner behaviors that indicate motivation to learn

Client stated she was more relaxed about her diagnosis, asked her son to get her information about diabetes, and contacted a friend with diabetes. _____

Can the learner read and comprehend at the reading level required by task?

Yes, but may not have visual acuity to see the calibrations on the syringe. _____

Does the learner show ability to problem solve at a level that provides safe care in the home?_____

*Client managed health problems in her home with her granddaughter's illness 10 years ago.*_____

Is the home environment conducive to the learning required by the care? _____

Home is very dark with poor lighting. _____

If not, what modifications are necessary? *Need better lighting in the kitchen.* _____

If the learner is not able to carry out the care, are other caregivers available for backup support?

If so, please name. *Roger (son), Sommer (granddaughter), Richard (friend)* _____

Phone number *555-5555* _____

Address *3400 Belmont, White Kitty Lake, Pennsylvania* _____

What other support is available for the client and caregiver? *Client has 10 children,* _____ *three of whom live in the area. Client is active in her church, which has a parish nurse and a befriender program.*

*There is a support group for newly diagnosed diabetics, which meets at a hospital near client's home. Client lives on the bus line with service to the clinic, hospital, and church.*_____

Identification of Learning Need

Allison and Ida conclude that Ida's overall learning need for today is as follows:

⬥ *Risk for injury related to lack of knowledge regarding diabetic self-care.*

For this visit, Allison identifies the following priority need:

⬥ *Risk for injury related to client's lack of knowledge and inability to manage diabetes for the next 24 hours until the home visit the next day, as manifested by visual impairment.*

Planning

Allison and Ida decide upon the following learning objectives for today:

1. Cognitive objective: Client will state when insulin is given and how much to draw up by the end of the visit on November 5.
2. Psychomotor objective: Client will identify three sites for subcutaneous injection of insulin and demonstrate proper technique for injection by the end of the visit on November 5.
3. Affective objective: Client will state that she is comfortable injecting insulin by the end of the visit on November 5.

Implementation

1. Cognitive objective: Client will state when insulin is given and how much to draw up by the end of the visit on November 5.

Together, Allison and Ida review the written material on insulin, when it is given, and how much to draw up. Allison proceeds at a slow pace as she teaches, repeats the information frequently, and does not rush Ida. The teaching sheet is on white, nonglossy paper with bold, black print. After the teaching session, Ida states, "Insulin should be given before meals and as the schedule states. I am to give myself insulin according to the schedule." Allison leaves a videotape that covers the information in the teaching session.

2. Psychomotor objective: Client will identify three sites for subcutaneous injection of insulin and demonstrate proper technique for injection by the end of the visit on November 5.

Allison demonstrates injecting the insulin into a model and identifies three sites for subcutaneous injection. Then Ida injects into the model. Allison draws up the insulin as ordered before dinner, and Ida injects herself at 5:00 PM. Ida is unable to see the numbers on the syringe.

Evaluation

Learning objectives 1 and 2 met: Ida identifies three sites for injection and injects herself correctly. Teaching focused on the most important problem for this client, the plan was collaborative, and reinforcement was provided with a videotape. The learner had the opportunity for hands-on practice, and a variety of teaching methods were used.

Implementation

3. Affective objective: Client will state that she is comfortable injecting insulin by the end of the visit on November 5.

Ida discusses her feelings with Allison regarding the teaching session. Allison asks her if she feels comfortable giving herself an injection, and she says, "No, but I think it will come." Allison leaves a short videotape on injecting insulin for Ida to review before the next visit.

Evaluation

Learning objective 3 met at this time.

Teaching: Allison encourages Ida by stating how well she has done the first time handling the syringe. Allison tells Ida specifically what she did well: she did not hesitate before putting in the needle, she found a correct site, and she charted it accurately on the flow sheet. However, she is unable to identify the correct number of units on the syringe. She notes this need and adds an objective to address this issue to the list of the next lesson's objectives.

Assessment and Planning for the Next Teaching Session

Allison noted Ida's problems with her eyesight in the initial assessment, suggesting that Ida might have difficulty drawing up insulin with a syringe. Allison discussed her concern with Ida and asked to come back the next day. She also asked Ida if there was a friend or family member who might be available to assist with her care. Ida responded that her son Roger had indicated that he was willing to help with the injections. Allison requested that Ida contact Roger and ask that he be present at the next home visit.

Identification of Learning Need

Together, Allison and Ida decided on the following learning need for the home visit the next day:

○ *Risk for injury related to client's lack of knowledge and inability to read the cali-brations on the syringe, as manifested by client's statement, "I have to use the mag-nifying glass to see print. I can't see the numbers on the syringes. Is it okay if I just estimate?"*

Planning

Allison and Ida decided that the learning objectives for tomorrow would be as follows:

1. Cognitive objective: Client will state when insulin is given, how much to draw up, and how to use the Magni-Guide syringe.

2. Psychomotor objective: Client will demonstrate how to draw up an accurate amount of insulin with the Magni-Guide syringe.

3. Affective objective: Client will state that she feels confident in her ability to draw up an accurate amount of insulin.

As Allison leaves Ida's home, Ida hugs her and says, "Thanks for all your help today. You have helped me so much!"

Conclusions

In the current health care system, health teaching has become an essential role for the nurse in community-based settings. Client, family, and staff satisfaction is improved if teaching results are positive. Quality instruction leads to more efficient use of resources. Good teaching assists clients and families to achieve independence in self-care. Interpro-fessional communication augment teaching efficacy. Comprehensive assessment of the client and family safeguards accurate identification of learning needs. Collaborative plan-ning preserves successful learning outcomes because clients and families are more likely to learn when they have had input in the process. Learning to avoid or navigate barriers and incorporate characteristics of successful teaching enhances teaching in community-based nursing.

What's on the Web

Medical Library Association: A User's Guide to Finding and Evaluating Health Information on the Web
INTERNET ADDRESS: **http://mlanet.org/resources/userguide.html**
This guide outlines how to find and evaluate health information on the Web. It provides tips on filtering through the plethora of health-related Web pages to find quality electronic finding tools developed by the U.S. government to do an initial screen of Web sites for further exploration. Guidelines for evaluating the content of health-related Web sites are provided. There is also a section of recommended Web sites by health condition.

Public Health and Information Data Tutorial
INTERNET ADDRESS: **http://phpartners.org/tutorial/02-her/index.html**
This site provides information and interactive opportunities to learn to recognize several authoritative, health-related Web sites commonly used for general health information for the public. You will also learn how to find health-related materials written in various languages. The site uses different formats for presenting current, authoritative health information. In addition, there are tools to learn to how to evaluate aspects of a quality health care Web site.

Centers for Disease Control and Prevention (CDC)
INTERNET ADDRESS: **http://www.cdc.gov (home page for CDC)**
This site offers abundant resources about topics related to disease prevention and health promotion.

Health Topics A–Z and CDC Publications
INTERNET ADDRESS: **http://www.cdc.gov/publications.htm; http://www.cdc.gov/az/A.html**
You can find information on any health topic on the Health Topics A–Z site. This CDC site offers an unlimited number of publications, software, and other products for teaching or research.

About CDC
INTERNET ADDRESS: **http://www.cdc.gov/education/ (Education home)**
This site outlines all of the sites to assist you in finding teaching materials. It is intended for health care professionals, teachers, students, parents, and children.

Consumer Health Information Corporation (CHIP)
INTERNET ADDRESS: **http://www.consumer-health.com/**
This site provides patient education on a variety of topics from a variety of perspectives. They provide information for pharmaceutical companies, health care providers, and consumers. The information for health care providers would be of most interest to nurses.

Healthfinders
INTERNET ADDRESS: **http://www.healthfinder.gov/**
This is your guide to reliable health care information with three versions of the site, one for consumers and professional health care providers, one for children, and one in Spanish. Each site includes a health library, health topics, information about health care providers, and a directory of health finder organizations.

Health Literacy
INTERNET ADDRESS: **http://nnlm.gov/outreach/consumer/hlthlit.html**
The national Network of Libraries of Medicine provides this credible site on health literacy. The resources on the site include skills needed for health literacy, research, a list of organizations and programs, and a bibliography and webliography.

Mayo Clinic
INTERNET ADDRESS: **http://www.mayo.edu**
This site has reliable information for a healthier life. You can find information quickly on the A to Z index of various conditions. You can also ask a specialist any questions that you may have about your client's conditions. There are timely topics, as well as slides on various subjects—lots of materials to use as you teach in community-based settings.

References and Bibliography

Anderson, C. (1990). *Patient teaching and communication in an information age.* Albany, NY: Delmar.
Anonymous, (2010). Encouraging patients to take medication as prescribed (2010). *Harvard Mental Health Letter, 26*(7), 4–5. Retrieved from Academic Search Premier database.
Arnold, E., & Boggs, K. (1995). *Interpersonal relationships: Professional communication skills for nurses* (2nd ed). Philadelphia: Saunders.
Barry, C. S. (2000). Teaching the older client in the home: Assessment and adaptation. *Home Healthcare Nurse, 18*(6), 379.
Bergman-Evans, B. (2006). AIDES to improving medication adherence in older adults. *Geriatric Nursing, 27*(3), 174–182.
Bloom, B. S. (Ed.). (1956). *Taxonomy of educational objectives: The classification of educational goals.* New York: McKay.
Bolin, A., Khramtsova, I., & Saarnio, D. (2005). Nursing student journals to stimulate authentic learning: Balancing Bloom's cognitive and affective domains. *Teaching of Psychology, 32*(3), 154–159. doi:10.1207/s15328023top3203_3.

Carpenito, L. J. (2010). *Handbook of nursing diagnosis* (13th ed.). Philadelphia, PA: Lippincott Williams & Wilkins.

Enç, N., Yigit, Z., & Altiok, M. (2010). Effects of education on self-care behaviour and quality of life in patients with chronic heart failure. *CONNECT: The World of Critical Care Nursing, 7*(2), 115–121. Retrieved from CINAHL Plus with Full Text database.

Esposito, D., Bagchi, A., Verdier, J., Bencio, D., & Kim, M. (2009). Medicaid beneficiaries with congestive heart failure: Association of medication adherence with healthcare use and costs. *American Journal of Managed Care, 15*(7), 437–445. Retrieved from Academic Search Premier database

Huffman, M. (2005). Homecare today: A case study in home health disease management. *Home Healthcare Nurse, 23*(10), 636–638.

Jarvis, C. (1996). *Physical examination of health assessment* (2nd ed.). Philadelphia, PA: Saunders.

Joint Commission. (2008). *What did the doctor say? Improving health literacy to protect patient safety*. Retrieved from http://www.jointcommission.org/nr/rdonlyres/d5248b2e-e7e6-4121- 8874-99c7b4888301/0/improving_health_literacy.pdf

Karter, A., Parker, M., Moffet, H., Ahmed, A., Schmittdiel, J., & Selby, J. (2009). New prescription medication gaps: A comprehensive measure of adherence to new prescriptions. *Health Services Research, 44*(5p1), 1640–1661. doi:10.1111/j.1475-6773.2009.00989.x.

Knox, A. B. (1986). *Helping adults learn*. San Francisco, CA: Jossey-Bass.

Lees, L., Price, D., & Andrews, A. (2010). Developing discharge practice through education: Module development, delivery and outcomes. *Nurse Education in Practice, 10*(4), 210–215. doi:10.1016/j.nepr.2009.08.008.

Medical Library Association. (2010). *A user's guide to finding and evaluating health information on the web*. Retrieved from http://mlanet.org/resources/userguide.html#3

Medicare Benefit Policy Manual. (2008). *Medicare guidelines, 30.2.3.3—Teaching and training activities (Revision 1, 10-01-03)*. Retrieved from www.cms.gov/manuals/Download/bp102c08.pdf

Merriam-Webster's online dictionary. (2010). Retrieved from http://www.merriam-webster.com

Milan, J., & White, A. (2010). Impact of a stage-tailored, web-based intervention on folic acid-containing multivitamin use by college women. *American Journal of Health Promotion, 24*(6), 388–395. Retrieved from CINAHL Plus with Full Text database.

Miller, L., Jones, B., Graves, R., & Sievert, M. (2010). Beyond Google: Finding and evaluating web-based information for community-based nursing practice. *International Journal of Nursing Education Scholarship, 7*(1), article 31. doi:10.2202/1548-923X.1961.

Minnesota Department of Health, Division of Community Health Services, Public Health Nursing Section. (2001). *Public health nursing interventions: Application for public health nursing practice*. Minneapolis, MN: Author.

Molony, S. (2009). Monitoring medication use in older adults. *American Journal of Nursing, 109*(1), 68–79. Retrieved from CINAHL Plus with Full Text database.

Naughton, C., Bennett, K., & Feely, J. (2006). Prevalence of chronic disease in the elderly based on a national pharmacy claims database. *Age & Ageing, 35*(6), 633–636. Retrieved from CINAHL Plus with Full Text database.

New, N. (2010). Teaching so they hear: Using a co-created diabetes self-management education approach. *Journal of the American Academy of Nurse Practitioners, 22*(6), 316–325. doi:10.1111/j.1745-7599.2010.00514.

O'Daniel, M., & Rosenstein, A. (2009). Professional communication and team collaboration. In R. G. Hughes (Ed.), *Patient safety and quality: An evidence-based handbook for nurses* (prepared with support from the Robert Wood Johnson Foundation). Rockville, MD: Agency for Healthcare Research and Quality; March 2008. AHRQ publication 08-0043. Retrieved from http://www.ahrq.gov/qual/nurseshdbk/nurseshdbk.pdf

Payne, J. (2010). *A new study finds that medication errors are common in children*. Retrieved from http://health.usnews.com/health-news/family-health/childrens-health/articles/2010/05/03/8-ways-to-prevent-medication-errors-in-kids.html

U.S. Department of Health and Human Services. (2010). *Quick guide to health literacy*. Retrieved from http://www.health.gov/communication/literacy/quickguide/factsliteracy.htm

Walsh, K., Mazor, K., Stille, C., Chysna, K., Moretti, J., Baril, J., et al. (May, 2010). *Pediatrics home medication errors in children with chronic conditions: An opportunity for improvement*. Paper presented at the Pediatric Academic Societies (PAS) annual meeting in Vancouver, British Columbia, Canada. Abstract retrieved from http://www.abstracts2view.com/pas/view.php?nu=PAS10L1_3163&terms

Walsh, K., Stille, C., Mazor, K., & Gurwitz, J. (2008). *Using home visits to understand medication errors in children*. Retrieved from http://www.ahrq.gov/downloads/pub/advances2/vol4/Advances-Walsh_74.pdf

Weng, L., Dai, Y., Huang, H., & Chiang, Y. (2010). Self-efficacy, self-care behaviors and quality of life of kidney transplant recipients. *Journal of Advanced Nursing, 66*(4), 828–838. doi:10.1111/j.1365-2648.2009.05243.x.

White, R. (2008). *Assessing the nation's health literacy.* Retrieved from http://www.ama-assn.org/ama1/pub/upload/mm/367/hl_report_2008.pdf

LEARNING ACTIVITIES

JOURNALING ACTIVITY 6-1

1. In your clinical journal, discuss a situation you observed or in which you were the caretaker for someone who had several teaching needs. Outline the process used to assess, plan, and teach the client and family members.

2. Using theory from this chapter, identify what was successful and what was not successful related to teaching and learning for this client and family.

3. What would you do differently from what was done when you are in a similar situation in the future? From this experience, what did you learn about yourself and teaching clients and families?

CLIENT CARE ACTIVITY 6-2

Jennifer is a nurse working on a postpartum unit. She is caring for Joan, a 35-year-old primipara, who delivered a boy yesterday (normal spontaneous vaginal delivery [NSVD]) and is going home at noon today. Joan states she has been working full time since she graduated from law school. She is the youngest of three siblings. She and her husband Tim took prenatal classes, and she describes him as being very excited about the baby. You observe Tim trying unsuccessfully to diaper the baby when you are in the room doing postpartum checks on Joan.

Jennifer interviewed Joan and Tim to determine their learning needs. They both tell Jennifer that they are wondering about having their baby circumcised. They wonder about the advantages and disadvantages of the procedure; how to take care of the surgical site after the procedure on their son and when they return home; and how to keep the area clean and free from stool. Prior to the teaching session, Joan has had pain medication and placed ice on her perineum. Both parents have good eye contact and relaxed postures as Jennifer interviewed them.

1. Determine the behaviors that show that Joan and Tim are ready to learn.

2. List the factors Jennifer should assess regarding Joan and Tim's readiness to learn.

3. Recognize what indicates to Jennifer that Joan and Tim show a need to learn.

4. Examine Joan and Tim's prior experience and knowledge base related to the topic.

5. Determine the family strengths.

6. Identify Joan and Tim's learning need in each domain: cognitive, affective, and psychomotor.

7. State one learning outcome for Joan and Tim for each learning need.

8. Discuss how the principles of community-based care apply to the learning needs of Joan and Tim.

CLIENT CARE ACTIVITY 6-3

Hazel is a 65-year-old woman whose husband is blind and was recently diagnosed with early signs of dementia. Shannon is doing preadmission teaching with Hazel, who is scheduled for outpatient surgery tomorrow morning. Shannon knows it is important to assess Hazel's readiness to learn. If Hazel is thinking about her husband's care during the presurgery class, she may not hear Shannon tell her that she should not drive or make important decisions for at least 24 hours after receiving general anesthesia.

Explain how Shannon will assess Hazel's readiness to learn. What questions would she ask? What goals and objectives would be feasible for Hazel?

PRACTICAL APPLICATION ACTIVITY 6-4

Volunteer to teach a health-related class at a local elementary, middle, or high school. Ask the school nurse or the class room teacher to recommend a topic, or go to the class and survey the students to find out what topics they would like to learn about. Use the content in this chapter to plan and develop the class. After you teach the students, use some of the following questions to evaluate your class.

- Was the goal met? How did you know that it was achieved? If not, why?
- Were the objectives met? If not, why?
- How do you know that students learned what you planned to teach?
- Did the timing of the teaching impede or enhance learning?
- Were the students satisfied with the outcome? If not, what would increase satisfaction?
- Did the teaching focus on the most important problem or concern of the students?
- Discuss how the teaching plan was collaborative.
- Describe any reinforcement techniques you used.
- Was the environment appropriate? If not, how was it modified?
- Was the equipment adequate? If not, what did you do?
- How would you prepare differently next time?
- Discuss the various teaching methods used.
- Did learners have the opportunity for hands-on practice?
- How was the session structured to reduce anxiety and enhance learning?
- Was the teaching plan realistic? If not, what would you do differently next time?
- If this session were to be repeated what other strategies or tools could be used?

PRACTICAL APPLICATION ACTIVITY 6-5

Monitoring Medication Use in Older Adults

This learning module will provide valuable information on how to complete a medication assessment with an older adult in any setting. Go to http://links.lww.com/A266 to watch a nurse use the Beers criteria to assess medication use in a hospitalized older adult. Then watch the health care team plan interventions. View this video in its entirety and then apply for continuing education credit at www.nursingcenter.com/AJNolderadults; click on the How To Try This series link. All videos are free and in downloadable format, not streaming video, that requires Windows Media Player.

If you have limited Internet access at home, find the following article at the library and complete the module as directed in the journal.

Source: Molony, S. (2009). Monitoring medication use in older adults. *American Journal of Nursing, 109*(1), 68–79. Retrieved from CINAHL Plus with Full Text database.

Chapter 7

Continuity of Care: Discharge Planning and Case Management

ROBERTA HUNT

Learning Objectives

1 Define continuity of care.

2 Define case management.

3 Discuss the implications of admission, discharge, and transfer.

4 Identify the relationships between discharge planning, case management, and continuity of care.

5 Relate community resources and the referral process to continuity of care.

6 Discuss nursing skills and competencies needed in the nurse case manager's and discharge planner's roles in community-based settings.

7 Determine how family, culture, and prevention influence health planning for continuity.

8 List common barriers that interrupt continuity.

Key Terms

case finding	delegation
case management	discharge planning
client advocacy	nursing assistive personnel
collaboration	referral and follow-up
consultation	screening
continuity of care	screening
coordinated care	transferring

Chapter Topics

Significance of Continuity of Care

Entering and Exiting the Health Care System

Discharge Planning

Nurse Case Manager

Nursing Skills and Competencies in Continuity of Care

Barriers to Successful Continuity of Care

Successful Continuity of Care

Conclusions

The Nursing Student Speaks

During my community health nursing rotation, I was asked to visit a family who had recently experienced homelessness and had moved into transitional housing. In my initial visit with the family, I learned that the father of the family was a decorated gulf war veteran who had been diagnosed with posttraumatic stress disorder (PTSD) upon returning from the war; unfortunately, he had not received treatment for his PTSD for over a decade. He explained that he has negative associations with both the healthcare system and many of the health care professionals who work within it and that he has been resistant to pursue services for his PTSD since his initial diagnosis. Respecting his decision to not pursue treatment for his PTSD, I steered the conversation to another topic.

At a later visit, the client mentioned to me that he might be interested in pursuing treatment for his PTSD after all. Immediately after returning home from the visit, I began researching what would be involved in getting the client connected with services to treat his PTSD. A comprehensive mental health intake assessment was the first step. At the next visit, I explained to the client what the mental health intake assessment would entail and asked his permission to schedule an appointment for him to be seen. The client was willing to go through with it, but he asked that I sit in to advocate for him during the assessment. Unfortunately, the next available appointment was over a month away, and my remaining time with the client was becoming very limited.

With the end of the semester rapidly approaching, I began focusing on discharge planning. I realized that the client could benefit from continual support and encouragement as he attempts to navigate the health care system and get the proper treatment for his PTSD. I was concerned that the termination of the relationship was coming, and there was still much work to be done. After reaching out to several resources in the community, I was able to identify a mental health outreach social worker who specializes in helping veterans get connected with services to treat their PTSD. After speaking with this individual by phone, she agreed to meet me and the client to discuss the case. At the meeting, it was discovered that the mental health outreach social worker and the client had a few things in common: they served in the same war, at similar times, and they both suffered from PTSD as a result. Instantly, they began the development of a therapeutic relationship. The mental health outreach social worker eventually accompanied the client to his intake assessment and offered to attend some support group meetings with him. The client continued to use her as an advocate and as a resource for information regarding obtaining veteran's benefits, accessing mental health services, and accessing support groups for combat veterans suffering from PTSD.

The client's distrust of health care professionals and prior negative experiences accessing health care presented a substantial obstacle to connecting the client with the mental health services he so desperately needed; however, in the context of a therapeutic relationship and with proper advocacy efforts, he was able to take positive steps toward health promotion and better management of his PTSD.

Justin Robinson
Student Nurse
St. Catherine University, St. Paul, Minnesota

Continuity of care has always been an important part of the nursing profession going all the way back from the 19th and 20th century to the present. In more recent years, interest in discharge planning was renewed with the concern about escalating medical costs and need for improving continuity of care. About 25% of all U.S. hospital patients are readmitted over a 2-year period for the same conditions that led to their original hospitalization.

Of these, about 42% of Medicare patients experienced multiple hospital admissions and 38% multiple emergency department (ED) visits, while Medicaid patients had multiple hospital visits with 50% visiting the ED more than once during the 2-year period (Agency for Healthcare Research and Quality [AHRQ], 2010). To address this issue, nurses are becoming more involved with continuity of care, both in discharge planning and in case management.

A number of factors contribute to lack of continuity care. Clients are increasingly seen by a large variety of providers in an array of organizations and agencies, often resulting in fragmentation of care. The Affordability Care Act concentrates on improving care continuity and ensuring safe and effective care transitions between settings as well as through the use of inpatient facilities for briefer, more intense encounters. These efforts are all intended to deliver care at the lowest cost with more efficiency. Encouraging routine use of a medical home for care is another attempt to address fragmented care. These strategies are expected to expand community-based care that emphasizes primary, preventive care across the continuum of care. Nurses play an important role in the ongoing development of this reform. Primary care in the Veterans Administration, the largest integrated health system in the United States, is a model that integrates the principles of continuity across the continuum of care (Shear, 2010). Some policy makers and economists support this as one feasible model for designing universal primary care for all citizens in the United States.

Continuity of care requires continuous assessment, planning, and intervention to create a bridge between health care providers and health care settings. The nurse, as the case manager, is often a member of the profession assigned or expected to ascertain the quality of the health plan. In this chapter, continuity of care is presented as essential to facilitating entrance into, exit out of, and transfer within the health care system. Examples are given to show how case management enhances continuity. The concepts of community resources and referral are discussed. The chapter ends with a section on skills and competencies the nurse needs to improve continuity of care, a discussion of barriers to continuity, and examples of programs that have been successful in enhancing continuity.

Significance of Continuity of Care

Continuity of care is described as the coordination of activities involving clients, providers, and payers to promote the delivery of health care. This is the process by which a client's ongoing health care needs are assessed, planned for, coordinated, and met without disruption. Some may view it as a method to control health care cost or ration care, while others may view it as promoting clients' right to make choices about health care services.

Continuity of care is achieved when all appropriate care and treatment interventions are provided by an interprofessional team in a planned, coordinated, and consistent manner. Often continuity of care is accomplished by integrating both formal and informal care. Formal care is what is commonly considered health care by providers such as nurses, nurse aides, physical therapists, occupational therapists, and social workers. Informal care refers to the care that family, neighbors, friends, volunteers, and other nonprofessionals may provide for the individual with a health condition.

Strong organizational structures are necessary to ensure continuity of care and to prevent the client from getting "lost" in the system. Nurses provide leadership in determining how and where the best care can be provided for a client and then ensuring that the client receives that care. This leadership is provided by care coordination through formal and informal nursing case management. For instance, in one large health center, "client navigators" help clients assess, engage, and coordinate their medical, social service, and financial needs and link to appropriate community resources. The navigators coordinate health care services to ensure timely treatment and follow-up, arrange for transportation to and from the center, and provide information about treatment options and preventive behaviors (Commins, 2010). Successful attainment of continuity of care is essential to ensure safe and quality health care and is promoted through successful planning and effective referral.

Entering and Exiting the Health Care System

Typically discharge planning is thought of as occurring between hospital and home, but principles of continuity apply to transitions of care between any community settings. Unlike in the past, when clients typically went from a hospital to home, clients today navigate the health care system in various ways. They may be referred from a clinic visit to home care, from school to a physician's office, from home care to an acute care setting, or from adult day care to an extended care facility. Figure 7-1 illustrates the flow of continuity of care.

Clients may be transferred several times from one community-based setting to another. For example, Juan falls in the bathroom in his home and breaks his hip. He enters the system through the ED and is transferred to the operating room and then to the orthopedic unit in the hospital. After discharge from the hospital, he stays in a transitional facility for follow-up physical therapy and skilled nursing care. Then he is moved to assisted living for 4 months. After being transferred to three different services in the hospital and being discharged from four different agencies, he is back in his own home 6 months after the fall.

ADMISSION

Admission occurs at whatever point an individual enters the health care system, with each new setting requiring a new admission. Each new facility, unit, or agency presents strange surroundings and new people who may increase client and family anxiety levels. What may be a routine admission to the nurse is seldom routine for a client and family. The nurse's confidence, competence, and concern are essential in putting the client and family at ease as the nurse's attitude may exert great influence on the course of care.

Apprehension may be lessened by the following nursing actions:

- Establishing rapport and indicating sincere concern for the client and family
- Defining the purpose and expectations of this admission

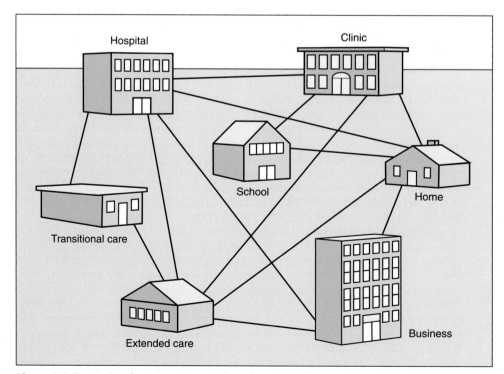

Figure 7-1 Continuity of care in community-based nursing is like a web between and among settings.

Table 7-1 Overview of Admission to Various Health Care Facilities	
Facility	**Possible Admission Procedures**
Acute care setting	Introduction; orientation to room and equipment; complete nursing history, vital signs, and other physical assessment; orientation to room and bathroom
Emergency department	Introduction; ABCs (airway, breathing, and circulation); vital signs; focused assessment for acute problems; orientation to surroundings
Clinic or physician's office	Introduction; reason for seeking medical care and focused assessment of that problem; vital signs
Nursing home	Introduction; review of written or verbal report from transferring agency; nursing history and assessment focusing on functional abilities; orientation to new surroundings
Hospice	Introduction; review of referral; nursing history and assessment focusing on pain control, functional abilities, coping, and support; wishes concerning terminal care and death (e.g., health care directive and power of attorney); orientation to procedures and care
Psychiatric facility	Introduction; mental health evaluation, including history, mood state, suicide risk, use of drugs, support system; orientation to room and unit
Home visit	Introduction; review of referral and client's medical and nursing problems, home environment, caretaker and family support, community resources

Craven, R. F., & Hirnle, C. J. (2009). *Fundamentals of nursing: Human health and function* (6th ed.). Philadelphia, PA: Lippincott Williams & Wilkins.

- Aiding the client in understanding how to participate as fully as possible in care-related decisions
- Clarifying the nursing role in relation to the client's health care needs
- Including the family in explanations, unless the client indicates otherwise
- Explaining equipment and procedures
- Explaining equipment to be used when calling for assistance
- Documenting the admission process

Admission procedures for entering any system share similarities. Examples of admission procedures in various health care facilities are summarized in Table 7-1.

During admission, it is reassuring if the nurse explains to the client and family members how they can participate in decision making and care planning. Admission may be as anxiety provoking for the family as for the client. The nurse supports the family by giving the location of waiting rooms, rest rooms, public telephones, the nurses' station or offices, and other areas of interest, such as vending machines or cafeterias if the client is in an inpatient facility. If the client is being admitted for day surgery, the nurse may explain where the family can wait, who will bring a report, and when they can expect it. In many cases, comforting the family is as important as calming the client. For home care, the nurse will provide the family with information about the purpose of the visits and frequency, what other professionals will be providing additional service such as physical therapy or occupational therapy, and the overall plan of care.

TRANSFER

Sometimes the term discharge is used when client **transfer** is taking place. A transfer typically occurs within the same institution, most often from the ED to the acute care setting or intensive care unit. Another type of transfer is when the client leaves the ED by ambulance to be transferred to another acute care facility or transitional hospital. For example, Nhu is a 60-year-old woman who is admitted to the ED at a small community hospital after a fall in her apartment. After examination, it is discovered that although she has no physical injuries her blood alcohol is 0.28. Her daughter and son confer with the nurse practitioner and decide to transfer her to an inpatient substance abuse program in a nearby community. She is in the inpatient program for 4 weeks and is then discharged to an outpatient substance abuse facility. After 4 months, she returns to her apartment but continues to go to Alcoholics Anonymous meetings in her community twice a week. In community-based health care, clients may be transferred from one setting to another.

Discharge Planning

Discharge planning is an accepted nursing intervention aimed at the prevention of problems after discharge. These problems range from prolonged recovery to rehospitalization, all of which add to the cost of care. Discharge planning ensures continuity of care by a systematic process of coordinating various aspects of care at the time the client is discharged from a facility or program. This planning involves many professionals who make assessments, collaborate with the client and family, plan, and then communicate the critical information to the organization or individual who will assume responsibility for the client's health care needs after discharge. The process, when it works well, is dynamic, interactive, and client centered. However there is a great deal of evidence that continuity through discharge planning is not always adequate.

Over the last three decades discharge planning became a central event as a method to reduce costs, lower hospital readmission rates, and provide the client with posthospital care options. Discharge planning is not limited to the physical transfer of the client, nor does it focus only on physical needs. It is much more. It is a process of early assessment of anticipated, individual client needs centered on concern for the total well-being of the client and family. It involves the client, family, and all caregivers in interactive communication during the entire planning process. It also requires ongoing interprofessional collaboration among many health care providers (Fig. 7-2). This results in mutual agreement and appropriate options for meeting health care needs through an up-to-date review of all of the resource alternatives. This ongoing nursing assessment of future client needs is mandated by accreditation agencies. The Joint Commission, formerly known as the Joint Commission on the Accreditation of Healthcare Organizations, requires that the discharge plan should be initiated at admission as part of the nursing care plan.

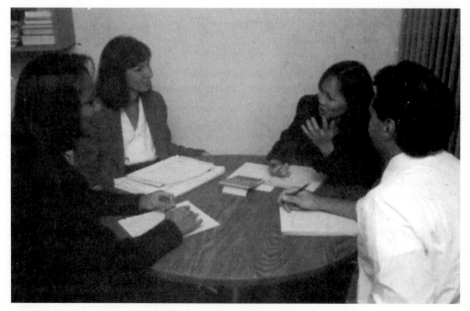

Figure 7-2 The key to successful planning is the exchange of information among those concerned about the client's care.

Discharge planning creates bridges between settings, as shown in Figure 7-1. If the discharge plan is carefully thought out and based on collaboration among the nurse, the physician, other health care providers, the client, and family, then the bridge will be strong and the transition between settings smooth. On the other hand, if the discharge plan is nonexistent or haphazardly thrown together, the transition will be bumpy with resulting complications, readmissions to various care facilities, or unnecessary stress, all interrupting the client's recovery. Consequently, poor continuity of care has the potential to result in disaster for the client and increased cost for the health care system. Nurse-led research directed at improving discharge planning is seen in Research in Community-Based Nursing Care 7-1.

RESEARCH IN COMMUNITY-BASED NURSING CARE 7-1

Discharge Planning: Your Last Chance to Make a Good Impression

Discharge planning is a priority for a 33-bed unit in a large Midwestern teaching hospital. In 2000, leaders from this unit identified a low level of satisfaction among patients and staff members regarding the discharge planning process. As a result nurse managers convened a discharge planning team representing a variety of disciplines. This group designed surveys and audit tools to define the issues and met monthly to review collected data. Four areas were assessed: dismissal summaries, prescription drug acquisition audit, dismissal education, and communication. The audits of these various processes resulted in recommendations for modifications in each area. For the dismissal summaries, it was discovered that the documents were often not complete requiring significant amount of nursing time to follow-up with providers. Many of the providers were residents on 3-month rotations, which suggested a need for regular audit of the dismissal summaries at the midpoint of each quarter. This allowed the physicians to become acquainted with the discharge summary process and review feedback on their work before they completed their rotations. Involving the team's staff physician provided assurance that the resident physicians were educated about this new policy. Data related to dismissal summary indicated that accuracy, completeness, and timeliness increased from 60% in 2000 to 91% in 2007. Prescription acquisition process was modified as a result of the audit to encourage prescribers to write prescriptions the night before the patient was to be discharged. Implementing this modification increased the percentage of prescriptions written the night before discharge from 45% to 88%. This small change in policy dramatically facilitated the discharge process for the patient and family. Dismissal education was revised as a result of the audit process to clarify the roles of the various members of the team. In addition, it was recommended that the discharge process begin several days before actual discharge. Communication issues were identified and addressed through a recommendation to use the dry erase boards in each patient room to note the anticipated dismissal date. This simple change provided a reminder to all team members, family, and patient to plan accordingly. Over the course of 7 years, patient and staff satisfaction was measured. In 2001, the initial staff satisfaction survey of the discharge planning process showed 37% of nursing staff being "completely satisfied" or "satisfied," while in 2007 91% of staff were "completely satisfied" or "satisfied" with the process. Patient satisfaction data collected in 2004 revealed 93% of patients reported their discharge as either "very smooth and organized" or "smooth and organized." In 2007, results showed 100% of patients perceived their discharge process as either "very smooth and organized" or "smooth and organized." This almost decade-long evaluation research reported three lessons learned. Communication is vital to successful discharge planning, interprofessional contributions are essential, and quality improvement is ongoing.

Rose, K., & Haugen, M. (2010). Discharge planning: Your last chance to make a good impression. *MEDSURG Nursing, 19*(1), 47–53. Retrieved from Academic Search Premier database.

Nurse Case Manager

Case management, also known as care management or care coordination, is a complex concept with many definitions. This often leads to confusion about what is the correct or best definition. Case management will be defined in this book as activities that optimize the self-care capacities of clients and families by coordinating services. Although numerous definitions of case management exist, the goals in the last decade have remained constant: to achieve a balance between quality and cost of care. Quality is improved by emphasizing the importance of health promotion and disease prevention and increased continuity of care. Cost of care is decreased through empowering clients and families to maximize self-care. Empowerment prevents unnecessary or lengthy inpatient care. Further, interprofessional collaboration practices enhance **coordinated care**. Note how closely these goals parallel those of community-based nursing. Case management improves outcomes for the client and family. First of all, case management facilitates the provision of information about health benefits, service parameters, the disease process, and plan of treatment for clients and families. Second, successful case management involves the client in the choices, decisions, and actions of self-care. Third, case management allows for realistic evaluation in cases where there is low adherence to treatment plans. Finally, case management facilitates consistency of care across the continuum of care.

There are several case management models used in community-based care. Community-based case management assists clients and families to access appropriate services for independent functioning. This model is used across a wide range of target populations. Individuals with chronic conditions benefit from nurse case management as illustrated in Research in Community-Based Nursing Care 7-2.

Another example is seen in case management for those with chronic and persistent mental illness. Case management may be offered for teenage Hmong girls at risk for dropping out of school, prostitution, drug use, or gang activity. Home health offers care management to those individuals with chronic conditions who qualify for services. Chapter 11 provides numerous examples of this model at work. Similarly, hospice case management coordinates care and comfort of the dying and their families at the end of life.

In some settings, a case manager's only role is to manage a number of individuals or cases, whereas in other settings the nurse has many roles, with case manager being one. For example, a nurse working in an ED may function as a staff nurse and also call clients

---

RESEARCH IN COMMUNITY-BASED NURSING CARE 7-2

Nurse Diabetes Case Management Interventions and Blood Glucose Control: Results of a Meta-Analysis

A meta-analysis of studies reporting diabetes case management interventions was conducted to examine the impact of case management on blood glucose control. Medline, PubMed, Cochran EPOC, CINHAL, and Psycho Info databases were used for the search to identify studies that met the inclusion criteria. Statistical parameters guided analyses. Twenty-nine studies involving 9,397 patients were included in the analysis, which compared patients who received case management with a control group. Demographics of the collective subjects revealed a mean age of 63.2 years; 49% were male and 54% white. Statistical analysis showed a large overall impact on blood glucose in those who received case management compared to those who did not. Researchers concluded that based on a meta-analysis of clinical trials focusing on blood glucose control, nurse-led case management is an effective clinical strategy for those with poorly controlled diabetes.

Welch, G., Garb, J., Zagarins, S., Lendel, I.., & Gabbay, R. (2010). Nurse diabetes case management interventions and blood glucose control: Results of a meta-analysis. *Diabetes Research & Clinical Practice, 88*(1), 1–6. doi:10.1016/j.diabres.2009.12.026.

for follow-up the day after their ED visit. A home care nurse may be the client's case manager responsible for coordinating care, as well as the direct care provider and health educator. The ways the role of case manager is operationalized differ by geographic area, provider, payment restriction, and setting. The role of the case manager is often viewed as that of a gatekeeper or a broker for services. For example, Margaret, an occupational health nurse who served worker's compensation clients, described her role as "interpreting the insurance company's medical information and working with health care providers to find the most efficient means of helping people return to the workplace." Other nurse case managers describe their roles as "assessing and evaluating delivery systems and benefit criteria … making sure that resources are available … stretching the dollar … client advocacy … and making sure the client and family are fully involved in the decision and care."

Thus, case management is a term with many definitions and implementation models. The nurse is often considered the best professional to act as a case manager for clients in all health care settings. In community-based care, case management is the vehicle to care coordination and continuity of care. Case management in community-based settings reflects a commitment to facilitate self-care in the context of the client's family, culture, and community.

Nursing Skills and Competencies in Continuity of Care

Discharge planning and case management are the primary roles for nurses related to continuity of care in community-based care. However, terminology is not consistent and often confusing with titles varying from continuity-of-care nurse, discharge-planning nurse, or case manager given for a position with the same role responsibilities. Even within the same community one agency may use the term continuity-of-care nurse, while another agency will have a role with identical responsibilities and give the title of that position nurse case manager. To add to potential misunderstanding, there is no universal level of educational preparation required for any of these roles. In this chapter the two primary roles of the nurse in continuity care will be discussed as those of discharge planner and case manager/care manager.

THE DISCHARGE PLANNING NURSE

Typically the role of the discharge planning nurse is relatively one dimensional and prescribed in facilitating transition from one setting to another. Discharge planning follows the nursing process, beginning with assessment at the first encounter, as the nurse needs to know the client's plans and expectations for managing care. Planning and setting goals focus on both client and family needs and abilities. Written and verbal instructions about the medication regimen, treatment, and follow-up are provided to the client and family. They also need to be educated about any signs and symptoms that may indicate problems or complications with the condition and who to contact if these should occur. At this point, the client and family must have the opportunity to discuss any concerns or questions regarding care and recovery. The intervention phase of the nursing process involves identifying needed resources and making appropriate referrals. Important telephone numbers, names, and community services should be given in writing to the client and family and explained thoroughly.

THE NURSE CASE MANAGER

The structure and scope of the role of the nurse case manager vary in contrast to the more prescribed role of discharge planner. In some situations case managers function across the continuum of care following and coordinating care whatever service the client and family are receiving. In other situations a case manager's role is provided by each provider service so that a client may have a case manager in the hospital, long-term care facility, home care agency, or hospice service. A case manager may assist with financial arrangements, contact vendors and arrange for equipment, make referrals to home health care agencies, make appointments with health care providers, conduct predischarge teaching, and follow-up with arrangements for additional referrals as indicated.

ASSESSMENT

Generally, the nurse is the first link in the continuity of care through the discharge planning process. In some settings, social workers may have the primary responsibility for discharge planning; however, nurses frequently coordinate and communicate the discharge plan. Assessment of client discharge planning needs must begin on admission to the facility or at preadmission. The nurse uses his or her skills to identify and anticipate the client's specific needs and the services needed after discharge. Assessments may be conducted by different disciplines (e.g., the nurse, someone from the financial department, a physician, a respiratory therapist, a physical therapist, or a social worker) when the client enters the health care environment. In all care coordination ongoing assessment monitors the client's response to treatment; seeks the client and family's input regarding their desires, needs, and resources; and initiates the coordination of the interprofessional team. The essential elements of assessment for a client include health and personal data, client and family knowledge, financial and support needs, and environmental data.

The nurse must concentrate on careful assessment of the client, identifying needs as early as possible. As soon as a client is admitted, the nurse begins to investigate possible discharge needs. With each client encounter, the nurse notes any information that may inform discharge needs and asks the following questions: "When you are discharged ..."

- If you are not able to care for yourself, who is available to be a family or friend caregiver?
- What is the willingness and ability level of your designated caregiver?

The nurse, along with the client and family, is in the best possible position to clearly identify the client's needs related to care coordination. Clients at risk for self-care deficit should be identified early. Carpenito defines self-care deficit as the state in which the "individual experiences an impaired motor function or cognitive function, causing a decreased ability to perform each of the five self-care activities" (2010, p. 377). Self-care activities are defined in a variety of ways, but for this nursing diagnosis they are defined as feeding, bathing, dressing, and toileting and are instrumental aspects of self-care. The information gained about the client's ability to provide self-care after discharge is critical to planning for discharge. Assessing needs, communicating with others, and involving the client and family on an ongoing basis contribute to a realistic strategy for discharge. If the client has special care needs after discharge, the trusting relationship established between the nurse and the client during assessment is essential to the next step of client and family teaching. The nurse can provide answers to the following questions:

- Will the family need changes in routine?
- Will the family be able to provide all of the care needed?
- Do they need home health care assistance?
- What are the family's resources and limitations?

The client's successful recovery and return to optimal health often depend on collecting the right information during the assessment phase of planning. Nurses need to have multiple skills to facilitate this collection of information, interpret, confirm, and plan adequately.

Because elderly clients are more likely to return to inpatient care than any other category of clients, many of the tools designed for this type of assessment are intended for them. Due to the shift in demographics with an increasing percentage of the population being over age 60, the cost–benefit value of best practice was investigated (Bauer, Fitzgerald, Haesler, & Manfrin, 2009). The researchers found that hospital discharge planning for frail older people can be improved through interventions such as family education, communication between nurse and family, interprofessional communication, and ongoing support after discharge. This study is described in detail in Research in Community-Based Nursing Care 7-3 and highlights the need for strategies to improve discharge planning for hospitalized frail elder clients to avoid rehospitalization.

There are few tools that can be easily used in practice to identify individuals at risk for self-care deficits once home. One tool, developed by a nurse over two decades ago, is the

RESEARCH IN COMMUNITY-BASED NURSING CARE 7-3

Hospital Discharge Planning for Frail Older People and their Family: Are We Delivering Best Practice? A Review of the Evidence

An integrative review was designed to examine available evidence related to hospital discharge planning for frail older individual and family caregivers to identify what practices are most beneficial. With increasingly short hospital stays, a rising burden of care is placed on family caregivers who in turn can be linked to adverse outcomes and a higher rate of rehospitalization. Inclusion criteria identified English language literature published after 1995 on hospital discharge of frail older people. The researchers concluded that there are several strategies that could be employed to improve hospital discharge planning for frail older adults. First, early assessment and initiation of family involvement in discharge planning and caregiving are needed when the family member is hospitalized. Next, there must be provision of adequate information and education of the family caregiver during the discharge planning process which is best achieved through effective communication between family caregivers and staff members. The third suggested strategy is proficient interprofessional communication between all health professionals. Last, client and family caregivers benefit from access to ongoing support from community health services, support groups, and counseling.

Bauer, M., Fitzgerald, L., Haesler, E., & Manfrin, M. (2009). Hospital discharge planning for frail older people and their family. Are we delivering best practice? A review of the evidence. *Journal of Clinical Nursing, 18*(18), 2539–2546. Retrieved from CINAHL Plus with Full Text.

Blaylock Risk Assessment Screening Score (BRASS) index. This may be used by the nurse at the bedside to gather comprehensive initial and ongoing data to identify, after hospital admission, elderly clients who are at risk for a prolonged hospital stay. Early identification of those who will have intense discharge needs may prevent or reduce postdischarge problems.

The BRASS index is shown in Figure 7-3. It contains 10 items, each judged by a nurse, using normal diagnostic procedures and questions at admission. The nurse goes through the questions, giving the client a score for every section. The Risk Factor Index at the bottom of the page indicates the client's need for discharge planning and resource planning. Over two decades ago, this tool was established to be a valid and reliable predictor for identifying clients who are not candidates for discharge to home. It also accurately predicts clients who will have problems after discharge (Mistiaen, Duijnhouwer, Prins-Hoekstra, Ros, & Blaylock, 1999). At present, there is no other similar screening tool discussed in the nursing literature.

An example of the role of the nurse in discharge planning and the use of the BRASS index is seen in the following Client Situations in Practice.

CLIENT SITUATIONS IN PRACTICE: DISCHARGE PLANNING

Margret Carolan is a 72-year-old retired woman who lives alone and has no living family members, but she has supportive friends from her church. She does not drive because of her poor vision. She has a history of type 2 diabetes mellitus and congestive heart failure. Currently, she takes insulin, aspirin (ASA), propranolol, potassium (K-Dur), and furosemide (Lasix) every day. Three months ago, Ms. Carolan was seen in the ED for a transient ischemic attack. She was admitted today to ambulatory surgery for arthroscopic surgery on her left knee under general anesthesia. She is instructed not to bear weight on her operative knee for 24 hours and to arrange for physical therapy twice a week for 1 month.

Ms. Carolan's Blaylock Discharge Planning Risk Assessment score is 11 (see Fig. 7-3). She is alert and oriented and depends on assistance for her transportation needs. Her history indicates that because she has complex problems, careful discharge planning

Blaylock Discharge Planning Risk Assessment Screen

Circle all that apply and total. Refer to the Risk Factor Index*

Age
- 0 = 55 years or less
- 1 = 56 to 64 years
- (2) = 65 to 79 years
- 3 = 80 + years

Living Situation/Social Support
- 0 = Lives only with spouse
- 1 = Lives with family
- 2 = Lives alone with family support
- (3) = Lives alone with friends' support
- 4 = Lives alone with no support
- 5 = Nursing home/residential care

Functional Status
- 0 = Independent in activities of daily living and instrumental activities of daily living

Dependent in:
- 1 = Eating/feeding
- 1 = Bathing/grooming
- 1 = Toileting
- 1 = Transferring
- 1 = Incontinent of bowel function
- 1 = Incontinent of bladder function
- 1 = Meal preparation
- 1 = Responsible for own medication administration
- 1 = Handling own finances
- 1 = Grocery shopping
- (1) = Transportation

Cognition
- (0) = Oriented
- 1 = Disoriented to some spheres some of the time†
- 2 = Disoriented to some spheres all of the time
- 3 = Disoriented to all spheres some of the time
- 4 = Disoriented to all spheres all of the time
- 5 = Comatose

Behavior Pattern
- (0) = Appropriate
- 1 = Wandering
- 1 = Agitated
- 1 = Confused
- 1 = Other

Mobility
- 0 = Ambulatory
- (1) = Ambulatory with mechanical assistance
- 2 = Ambulatory with human assistance
- 3 = Nonambulatory

Sensory Deficits
- 0 = None
- (1) = Visual or hearing deficits
- 2 = Visual and hearing deficits

Number of Previous Admissions/Emergency Room Visits
- 0 = None in the last 3 months
- (1) = One in the last 3 months
- 2 = Two in the last 3 months
- 3 = More than two in the last 3 months

Number of Active Medical Problems
- (0) = Three medical problems
- 1 = Three to five medical problems
- 2 = More than five medical problems

Number of Drugs
- 0 = Fewer than three drugs
- 1 = Three to five drugs
- (2) = More than five drugs

Total Score: 11

*Risk Factor Index: Score of 10 = at risk for home care resources; score of 11 to 19 = at risk for extended discharge planning; score greater than 20 = at risk for placement other than home. If the patient's score is 10 or greater, refer the patient to the discharge planning coordinator or discharge planning team.
†Sphere = person, place, time, and self.
Copyright 1991 Ann Blaylock

Figure 7-3 Sample of the Blaylock Discharge Planning Risk Assessment Screen.

is required. The team collects further data on her health, her personal situation including her environment, any teaching she may require for ongoing care, her financial status, and support needs she may require at home.

Ms. Carolan's discharge plan includes teaching her the following: weight-bearing instructions for the first 24 hours, signs and symptoms of infection, wound care, analgesic use, dosage of insulin, and possible increased or decreased dosage need. Referrals for postdischarge physical therapy is completed with transportation to and from the outpatient therapy clinic arranged. No identified needs for home health care are apparent at this time. If complications arise, a home health care agency will be contacted.

When Ms. Carolan leaves the surgery center, the nurse may lose contact with the client. Other members of the interprofessional team assume responsibility for the client's ongoing needs and implementation of the discharge plan.

When Ms. Carolan returns to the orthopedic clinic a month after surgery, she is assessed by a physician and nurse practitioner. They find her completely recovered from her surgery and refer her back to her primary clinic. No more specialist visits are necessary. The orthopedic surgeon sends a report to her primary provider stating all goals were met.

NURSING DIAGNOSIS

Nursing diagnoses provide a record of identified needs and strengths. Methods of need and strength identification are achieved through documentation systems such as clinical pathways or, in the case of home care, the OASIS systems. OASIS is an assessment tool developed over two decades ago to measure outcomes of persons receiving home health care. In 2010, the system was revised to include process measures and renamed OASIS-C. This modified assessment added measures related to administration of vaccinations, standardized pain assessment, pressure ulcer risk assessment, fall risk assessment and depression screen, medication management and education, inclusions of specific best practices in the physician-ordered plan of care, timely notification of the physician in certain circumstances, and implementation of best practices as appropriate to all home care patients (Niewenhous, 2010). With OASIS-C, if the nurse in charge of discharge planning in the hospital identifies Risk for Loneliness as a potential issue for a client, this would guide the clinic nurse on how to direct follow-up. However, in addition to the possible interventions with this nursing diagnosis with the old OASIS, the revised OASIS-C allows the home care nurse to complete a screen for depression when deemed appropriate (Cabin, 2010).

PLANNING

The key to successful planning is the exchange of information between the client, present caregivers (e.g., nurse, physician, social worker, respiratory therapist, physical therapist, occupational therapist, nutritionist, psychologist, speech therapist), and those responsible for the continuing care (e.g., family, support services, and caregivers). Planning is always a mutual process between health care providers, the client, and the family. Improving continuity involves the following:

- Recognizing and using the resources and capacities of the client (and if appropriate) family to enhance continuity
- Educating the client and (if appropriate) family members about the options available and encouraging their participation in the decision-making process related to the continuum of care
- Assisting the client and (if appropriate) family to feel they have control over their own welfare and to identify resources that could help them in this process

Sociocultural factors can influence the planning phase in continuum of care. It is important for the nurse to identify and acknowledge issues that may influence the plan. These may include beliefs about the causes of illness and death and dying, language, nutrition practices, healing practices, and sexual orientation. Likewise, economic factors can influence the planning phase depending on the health insurance status of the client. Those without insurance or those who are underinsured will need more assistance in identifying and accessing community resources compared to clients with comprehensive health insurance. Lack of or inadequate health care insurance remains a common barrier to continuity care.

Frequent communication and coordination among the interprofessional team, client, and client's family facilitates reaching realistic expected outcomes in a well-designed discharge plan. This is accomplished through these actions:

- Consulting between the physician and the social worker or discharge planner
- Determining the client's prognosis
- Setting priorities
- Designing realistic time frames
- Determining responsibility
- Analyzing alternative resources for appropriateness and availability
- Exploring financial resources and burdens
- Involving and educating the family
- Setting appropriate and realistic expected outcomes
- Coordinating community resources

Clear articulation of the expected outcomes helps the interprofessional team know what is expected of the client and what the client expects of the team. When these outcomes have been agreed on by the client and family, all participants know the goals and can evaluate whether they have been met.

IMPLEMENTATION: NURSING INTERVENTIONS TO PROMOTE CONTINUITY

Approaches to promote continuity have remained relatively stable over the last 100 years. Letters of Lillian Wald and Mary Brewster, both nurses who worked in the settlement houses in New York City in the late 19th century, and interviews of nurses currently practicing portray the role of discharge planner or case manager similarly (Rodgers, 2000). Developing the nurse–client relationship and formulating outside connections in the community were described to be central elements to successful care coordination by nurses. These remain essential today.

FORMING THE NURSE–CLIENT RELATIONSHIP

As is true of nursing care in all settings, the nurse–client relationship is the fundamental component in developing continuity of care. According to Rodgers' research, several elements work together to build the nurse–client relationship. In modern day, this process is called *counseling*, as the nurse establishes a trusting relationship with the client and family to engage them at an emotional level in the process of planning (Minnesota Department of Health [MDH], Section of Public Health Nursing, 2001). Counseling may be woven into all aspects of the plan. Initially, counseling is established through the nurse–client relationship that becomes the foundation of care coordination (Fig. 7-4).

> I don't care what color you are, or where you come from or who you are or where you have been in your life, if you are my patient, I am going to do the very best that I can. I have a commitment. It's like when you walk into somebody's home and you form a bond with that person. It's like a pact that I'm going to be there for you until you die, and I'm going to take you through it, we're going to go through it together (Rodgers, 2000, p. 303).

Another essential component in the nurse–client relationship is listening and being present. This concept has been mentioned several times throughout this book and is basic to good therapeutic communication. Sadly, these concepts are often missing between the nurse and the client and bear repeating. Listening allows the nurse to assess the client's most immediate needs and is often a powerful nursing intervention. In some situations, therapeutic presence may be the only intervention that provides comfort.

> Five years ago, my baby daughter died of SIDS. The nurse in the clinic just sat with me and let me cry. That was so helpful. I will always be thankful that she took the time to sit with me (Julie, a nursing student).

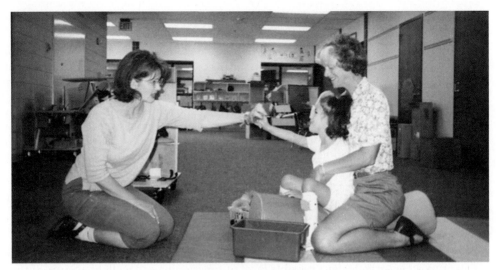

Figure 7-4 A strong and trusting nurse–client relationship is the foundation of coordinated care.

Building trust is another strategy essential to developing the nurse–client and family relationship. Trust is built by

- Cultivating the client and family's trust with the first contact
- Establishing credibility with the client and family
- Using an empathic, nonjudgmental approach
- Guarding the client and family's privacy
- Expecting testing behavior from clients and family
- Learning to trust the client and family
- Persevering with the nurse–client and family relationship

Another aspect of the nurse–client and family relationship related to continuity care is the nurse's willingness to persist in all situations, even those that appear impossible to resolve. This level of perseverance may seem almost impossible with some of the complex individuals and families we care for in community settings. An example is seen in the following.

> George is one of the more difficult clients I have ever taken care of. He is 80 years old with very brittle diabetes. His wife died last year. She was the one who could drive, cook, and check his blood sugar. His daughter said she would help by dropping by with a meal every day. He has refused Meals on Wheels, says that welfare is for old people, and states he will only eat what his daughter brings for him. Now his daughter is in the hospital having a knee replacement, so I don't think he is eating. I am trying to problem solve with him about alternatives, hoping we will be able to uncover an option he is comfortable with before he ends up back in the hospital (Denise, a home health care nurse).

Many individuals have limited or no family or social support. It is not uncommon for family members to become estranged from one another or unable or unwilling to assist one another during illness. In some situations, when an individual has a chronic illness over a long period of time, all sources of support may become completely tapped out from managing the work of the illness. In other cases, estrangement may have persisted for many years. All of these situations call for creative perseverance in problem solving in order to identify appropriate nursing interventions.

> Ernest has no family or social support. He has three children, but they all live on the West Coast. Ernest and his wife separated 15 years ago because of his substance abuse. When we called to see if she would be able to assist with his care, she gave the nurse an earful! His family has been totally unwilling to assist with his care in any capacity. Consequently, his discharge was delayed for a long period of time. Eventually we found a neighbor who was

willing to get groceries for him and accompany him on the bus to his medical appointments. A home care nurse visited him three times a week for 6 months (Phyllis, a home care nurse).

In all situations, the nurse–client relationship remains at the center of all interventions. Likewise, as clients move from one care setting or care provider to another, the relationship remains the consistent element to care. The interprofessional team must plan intervention strategies carefully, considering how the changes affect the client and the family. Clients and family members will probably feel anxious about the change. This is especially true if they have been hurried through the discharge planning process and prohibited from fully participating in a comprehensive plan. Being sensitive to the client's needs during each step in planning care will help to reduce anxiety and increase the client's participation and acceptance of care transitions.

ASSISTING THE INDIVIDUAL AND FAMILY THROUGH NURSING INTERVENTIONS

Some nursing interventions that enhance continuity focus on specific actions that assist the client to achieve the highest possible level of functioning and wellness. Some of these interventions, which help achieve coordinated care, involve screening, counseling, consultation, collaboration, case finding, and health teaching. Before describing each of these, it is important to note that these are not necessarily linear or discrete actions or used alone. Often two or three interventions are used together. Although screening may be used throughout, it is more likely to be used in the early stages of discharge planning while counseling and consultation are commonly used all the way through the planning process yet each intervention contributes to continuity of care.

Screening identifies individuals with unrecognized health risk factors or asymptomatic diseases (MDH, 2001). In discharge planning, one example of screening is using the BRASS index described earlier. Another example of screening could be when a case manager completes a fall risk assessment with a client who is at high risk for falling and is living alone or depression screening for someone at risk for depression due to recent loss or social isolation.

Through **consultation**, the nurse seeks information and generates solutions to problems or issues through interactive problem solving with the client or family to enhance care coordination (MDH, 2001). Consultation is an interactive problem-solving process between the nurse and the client. From a list of alternative options generated by the nurse and client, the client selects those most appropriate for the situation (Box 7-1). As is discussed throughout this book, nursing interventions are mutually determined, implemented, and evaluated in community-based care.

Collaboration commits two or more individuals or agencies to achieve a common goal of promoting and protecting the health of another. The first and foremost collaboration is between the nurse and the client. Fostering or enabling the client to experience more of a sense of control is necessary to forging the nurse–client collaborative relationship. Because discharge planning and case management activities are highly interprofessional endeavors, collaboration is often a part of the process of addressing continuity. From the first chapter, this text has emphasized the use of collaboration in planning, ultimately leading the client to his or her highest achievable level of self-care.

Health teaching communicates information and skills that change knowledge, attitudes, values, beliefs, behaviors, and practices of individuals and families (MDH, 2001). Successful health education depends on the nurse to competently assess the client's ability to manage daily activities in the home, judge the client and family's compliance with the therapeutic regimen, assess the client's knowledge of self-care, and coordinate the team members. Teaching skills are important and may include both prevention and promotion strategies (Fig. 7-5). Health teaching is covered in detail in Chapter 6.

Case finding is a set of activities that nurses working in community settings use to identify clients who are not currently receiving health care but could benefit from such care (MDH, 2001). The nurse, as a member of the interprofessional team, usually has the

> **BOX 7-1**
>
> ## Steps in Consultation
>
> 1. Establish a trusting relationship with the client and family.
> 2. Clarify the client's perception of the problem, causes, and anticipated results.
> 3. Assess all issues in a mutual process with the client.
>   - Determine the impact the issue has on the client's experience.
>   - Identify everyone involved and how they are affected.
>   - Determine how the client and family's attitudes, beliefs, and behaviors may be contributing to the issues.
>   - Explore environmental aspects.
>   - Identify strengths and barriers for the client and family.
>   - Anticipate what may be gained or lost by solving or addressing the issue.
>   - Consider how a solution might affect the client and family.
> 4. Through mutual planning, the nurse and client:
>   - Identify the desired outcome.
>   - Consider the advantages and disadvantages of each.
>   - Support the client as they choose the preferred option.
> 5. Determine support essential to facilitate implementing the plan.
> 6. Evaluate the process and outcome.
>
> Adapted from Minnesota Department of Health, Section of Public Health Nursing. (2001). *Public health nursing interventions II. Basic steps to the consultation intervention*. Minneapolis, MN: Author.

most contact with the client and family. This contact allows the nurse to assess and identify client service needs that, if addressed, would enhance care coordination or case management. In some cases, this may be a simple process, with the nurse making one contact or giving the client one suggested referral. Case finding happens in every setting where care is provided, and it requires an open attitude and skillful assessment by the nurse.

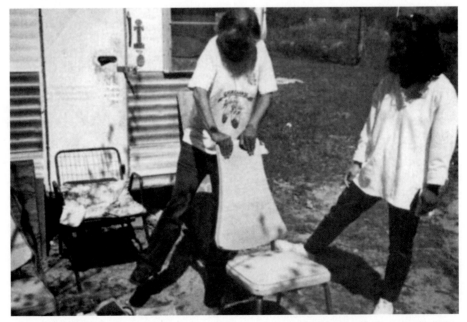

Figure 7-5 A community-based nurse teaches a Native American elder range-of-motion exercises outside his rural home. She is providing prevention and promotion strategies in her continuity of care of her client.

FORMING OUTSIDE CONNECTIONS WITH THE COMMUNITY

Developing community connections is also essential to providing effective care coordination in community-based setting. The nurse's knowledge about the community is essential to providing comprehensive, coordinated care. In addition, the nurse must know the client, the client's family and culture, and the broader community in which they live. To make appropriate referrals to ensure continuity, the nurse must know what services are available. For these outside connections to be accessed, the client and family first must know about the service and then must be willing to accept help.

> I had been making home visits to a single woman who after the birth of her twins was about to be evicted from her home. Her relationship with the father of her babies was not supportive. Every visit, she talked about the lack of progress she had made in finding a place to live. "Nobody will take someone with five kids," she would say over and over again. "I am afraid that I am going to be homeless with my kids," she exclaimed. In our community, this fear was well founded as there is virtually no low-cost housing. Together, we had explored every option available to her in our community, with no success. One day, when I went to make my weekly home visit, she didn't answer the door. I could hear the kids inside and knew she must be home. I knocked and waited. I knocked again. She finally opened the door. Both of her eyes were black and blue, and her face was bruised and swollen. She looked down at the floor and shamefully said, "He beat me up in front of the kids. I am never going to see him again, but I have no place to go. They are evicting me tomorrow." I knew about special housing available in our county for women experiencing domestic violence. I explained to her that she would have to go to a shelter for domestic abuse, but from there she could get into the special housing program. Her mother helped her pack up her kids, and she moved to the shelter the next day (Mary, a senior nursing student).

WORKING WITH OTHERS WITHIN THE COMMUNITY: COLLABORATION AND DELEGATION

Collaboration requires developing knowledge of other health care providers. This consists of becoming informed about the availability, scope of services, and referral mechanisms for various providers. Health care providers include, but are not limited to, physicians, dentists, ophthalmologists, therapists (such as occupational and physical), social workers, alternative care practitioners (such as chiropractors and acupuncturists), home health care agencies, outpatient clinics, diagnostic screening programs, and health education programs. Each health care provider has a role in ensuring continuity (Table 7-2).

When an intervention involves an interprofessional team, it is critical for the goals and plans to be structured and organized. However, it must also be flexible enough to allow for

Table 7-2 Health Care Providers Used in Discharge Referrals	
Health Care Provider	**Role**
Home health nurse	Provides assessments, direct care, client teaching and support; coordinates services; evaluates outcomes
Home health aide	Provides hygiene care, cooking, supervision, and companionship
Social worker	Assists in finding and connecting with community resources or financial resources; provides counseling and support
Physical therapist	Assists with restoring mobility, strengthens muscle groups, teaches ambulation with new devices
Occupational therapist	Helps clients adjust to limitations by teaching new vocational skills or better ways to perform activities of daily living
Nutritionist	Teaches clients about meal planning and diet restrictions
Speech therapist	Assists clients to communicate better and works with clients who have swallowing problems
Respiratory therapist	Provides home follow-up for clients with respiratory problems including assessment, oxygen administration, and home ventilator care

change as the client progresses toward health. If revisions to the plan are deemed necessary, the changes must be documented. For example, physical therapy for an older client with arthritis may be most effective in the afternoon, when the nurse is scheduled to visit. After discussing this with the client and the physical therapist, the nurse changes her visits for medication instruction to the morning to enhance the effectiveness of the physical therapy.

All members of the team are important but every team needs a leader and this team leader is often the nurse. The nurse must take the following steps of coordinating multiple disciplines to facilitate continuity of care:

- Notify all disciplines involved when there is a change in the client's health status.
- Coordinate visits with the client to avoid two professionals visiting at the same time and tiring the client.
- Integrate services to provide maximum benefit to the client; for example, have the physical therapist measure blood pressure when visiting the home to ambulate the client.
- Problem solve jointly with other team members and include the client when appropriate.

Delegation is a critical competency for the 21st century nurse and a key intervention in successful case management. Delegation requires a nurse to direct another person to perform nursing tasks and activities and is a legal concept used to empower one person to act for another (National Council of State Boards of Nursing [NCSBN], 2006). **Nursing assistive personnel** (NAP) are any unlicensed workers, regardless of title, to whom nursing tasks are, delegated (NCSBN, 2006). As more NAPs are providing care to individuals in community settings, the case manager becomes central to the issues related to delegation.

According to the NCSBN, all decisions related to delegation of nursing activities must be based on the fundamental principle of protection of the health, safety, and welfare of the patient. Licensed nurses have the ultimate accountability for the management and provision of nursing care, including all delegated decisions and tasks. This accountability is outlined in the Five Rights of Delegation, shown in Box 7-2.

Referral and follow-up is the process by which nurses in all settings assist individuals and families to identify and access community resources to prevent, promote, or maintain health (MDH, 2001). Obviously, just knowing what resources are present in the community is only the first step. For example, when caring for a client who has just had a knee replacement, the nurse learns that the client lives alone and does not have friends or family living nearby. It will be difficult for the client to cook for several weeks. Giving the client the telephone number for Meals on Wheels is one nursing intervention. In addition, the client is concerned about getting to the grocery store. There is a grocery delivery service that has a reduced rate for senior citizens. A second intervention is giving the client the name and telephone number of the referral service. Community-Based Nursing Care Guidelines 7-1 lists the steps in the referral process.

Referrals consider both the client's resources and the community's resources. A community with abundant resources has more support to offer the client and family

---

BOX 7-2	**The Five Rights of Delegation**

1. The right task
2. Under the right circumstances
3. To the right person
4. With the right directions and communication
5. Under the right supervision and evaluation

National Council of State Boards of Nursing. (2010). Joint Statement on Delegation from the American Nurses Association (ANA) and the National Council of State Boards of Nursing (NCSBN). Retrieved from https://www.ncsbn.org/Joint_statement.pdf

COMMUNITY-BASED NURSING CARE GUIDELINES 7-1

Steps in the Referral Process

1. Establish the need for referral.
2. Set objectives for the referral.
3. Explore the resources that are available.
4. Have the client make decisions concerning the referral.
5. Make the referral to the selected service.
6. Supply the agency with needed information.
7. Support the client and family in pursuing the referral.

through a recovery period or in their health promotion needs. On the other hand, the community with few resources has less to make available to citizens who require assistance with health care needs. To facilitate continuity of care when referring clients to an acute care setting, home, or community, the nurse must be aware of the assortment of individuals and organizations obtainable as community resources. Box 7-3 lists resources that can be used for the ill or older population within a community.

Resources may include a range of health-related services, from drug and alcohol treatment programs to safety education to prevent injuries. Each resource exists to provide services to meet particular needs necessitating the nurse to be knowledgeable about what these resources are and their eligibility requirements.

Community resources can be characterized as either health care providers or supportive care providers. Health care providers include all health care settings, health departments, community service agencies, and private practice physicians. Support care providers include psychological services, churches, and self-help groups with services that help people avoid problems or solve problems that interfere with their self-care and well-being. The primary service offered may not necessarily be health related and may be more difficult to recognize as compared to services directly related to health care needs. Support services are not always obvious to clients or their families, but acquiring information about them is essential to continuing care.

Ideally, the client and family participate in the referral process so they are involved in decision making and can choose the providers or organizations they prefer. But sometimes, the nurse may be in the best position to determine needs. For example, Suzie, a juvenile diabetic, is having trouble regulating her glucose levels. She asks you, "What can I eat?" Her mother says, "Sometimes I'm confused about what she can eat." Her father states, "We've been having problems with our car lately. We can't drive all the way across town to talk to someone about this." The nurse makes a referral to a dietitian located near the family's home to help determine the source of the glucose level variances and to initiate nutritional planning with Suzie and her family. Often if there are multiple referrals to make for a client, the nurse acts as a case manager for the interprofessional team.

Barriers to Successful Referrals

Because of rising health care costs, the type of referrals and resulting care plan is often driven by the client's financial resources and type of health insurance rather than by what services the client needs. Many HMOs and health insurance plans do not cover preventive care, psychiatric treatment, outpatient support services, and medications. All third-party payers limit the amount of service for which payment is made (e.g., number of home health care visits).

The nurse may need to assist clients in learning about their insurance coverage in order to create a plan of care that the payer will cover. Most health care plans employ case managers who understand health care needs and subsequently make decisions, based on diagnosis and need, about services that will be authorized for payment. Sometimes the approval or denial of payment for service conflicts with decisions made by the health care team. This interprofessional team may have to revise the plan, based not necessarily on what is felt to be best for the client but on what is optimal given the client's financial and social resources.

BOX 7-3   **Community Resources for Older and Ill Clients**

TRANSPORTATION DIFFICULTY
- Provisions for older people offered by states and city services through reduced bus fares, taxi vouchers, and van services
- Volunteer organizations: Red Cross, Salvation Army, senior citizen centers and nonprofits, church organizations for emergency or occasional transportation

PREVENTION OF HOME INJURIES
- Telephone checkup services through local hospitals, local services or friends, neighbors, or relatives
- Postal alert: register with local senior center; sticker on mailbox alerts letter carrier to check for accumulation of mail
- Private services paid for on an hourly basis
- Aide services by the Visiting Nurse Association
- Medicaid and Medicare provisions for home aides, which are limited to strict eligibility requirements
- Student help (inexpensive helpers) solicited by posting notices on bulletin boards at colleges and allied health schools
- Home sharing with another person who is willing to provide this kind of assistance in exchange for room and board

NURSING CARE OR PHYSICAL THERAPY
- Visiting nurse services provided through Medicare, Medicaid, or other health insurance (must be ordered by a physician)
- Home health services through private providers listed in the phone book; also nonprofit providers, Medicare and Medicaid reimbursement for authorized services

SHOPPING, COOKING, AND MEAL PLANNING
- Home-delivered meals delivered by Meals on Wheels or church organizations once a week, with sliding fees
- Meals served at senior centers, churches, schools, and other locations
- Cooperative arrangements with neighbors to exchange a service for meals, food shopping, and other tasks

SOCIAL ISOLATION
- Senior centers or community education programs that provide social opportunities, classes, volunteer opportunities, and outings
- Church-sponsored clubs with social activities, volunteer opportunities, and outings.
- Support groups for widows, stroke victims, and general support
- Adult day care with social interaction, classes, discussion groups, outings, and exercise

NEED FOR ASSISTANCE WITH HOME MANAGEMENT
- Homemaker services for those meeting income eligibility criteria
- Service exchanges with neighbors and friends (e.g., babysitting exchanged for housework help)
- Home helpers hired through agencies or through employment listings at senior centers, schools, etc.
- Help with housework in exchange for home sharing by renting out a room or portion of the home for reduced rent

FINANCIAL ISSUES
- Power of attorney given to a friend or relative for handling financial matters
- Joint checking account with friend or relative to facilitate paying bills
- Financial assistance available from the American Red Cross, Salvation Army, church groups, senior centers, or other organizations

LEGAL ASSISTANCE
- AARP legal services
- Legal aid or other lawyer referral services offered by the county or state bar association
- Other city/county aging services, hot lines for information, and assistance in phone book

For example, insurance companies will not pay for home health care that consists solely of a home health aide making daily visits for the client's personal care. The client must need the skilled services of an RN or physical or occupational therapist before the payer will pay for personal care needs. If the client cannot pay out of pocket for personal care, the team must reevaluate the client to determine if there are skilled nursing needs that could qualify the client for authorization of payment by the insurance carrier. Other barriers to successful use of community resources may stem from the client's prior experiences with community agencies. If a client has not had a good experience with a referral in the past, he or she may be hesitant to use this type of service again. The nurse must acknowledge the client's feelings and opinions about past experiences. If the nurse discovers that the client lacks information about the organization, then a different approach is all that is necessary. Perhaps the client's complaints about the organization are justified, in which case it may be in the client's best interest to find an alternative provider.

Another common barrier to follow-up care is accessibility. Hospitals, clinics, and other health care services are closing, especially in rural areas, and many rural communities are left with no local health care services. This loss requires clients to travel long distances to reach health care services. Conversely, a city-dwelling client who may not own a car might have difficulty getting to a suburban clinic. Many communities do not have public transportation. The nurse must get information from the client about access to transportation before making a referral. In the following situation, the nurse listens carefully to the family and client to determine their priorities and identifies a community-based service for referral. As a result of a thoughtfully developed referral, continuity is enhanced as Amy, a young teen recently diagnosed with diabetes, is able to manage self-care for her chronic condition early in the disease process.

CLIENT SITUATIONS IN PRACTICE

Supporting the Client and Family in the Referral Process

Amy is a 14-year-old Native American girl admitted to the hospital in an acute diabetic crisis from type 1 diabetes mellitus. She is afraid and does not want to face the realities of her new diagnosis. She tells the physician, "I don't want anything to do with this diet and stuff! I just want to go home, hang out with my friends, and eat what I want." The physician asks the nurse to explore this statement and Amy's general feelings about her diagnosis. Amy, her mother and father, and the nurse sit down in the conference area. As the discussion proceeds, the nurse discovers that Amy is afraid that she won't ever be able to eat out with her friends. Amy's mother says, "She loves fry bread, but she can't ever eat that again, right? What am I supposed to cook for her, anyway?"

At this point, the nurse suggests the family attend the diabetes education classes at the hospital clinic. Amy's father responds, "I don't want to go back to that clinic where there are only White people." The nurse makes several telephone calls, trying to identify a resource for a teenager with a new diagnosis of diabetes who follows a traditional Native American diet and whose family prefers a caretaker who is Indian. The nurse identifies the International Diabetes Clinic, which has a clientele and staff of many different nationalities. He also learns that there is a support group for Native American teens with diabetes at the American Indian Center near the family's home.

The nurse visits Amy's home. He gives Amy and her parents a pamphlet about managing diabetes and discusses setting an appointment with the International Diabetes Clinic. The nurse tells Amy about the support group at the neighborhood American Indian Center. Together they look up at the Web site of the clinic on the nurse's computer. He gives Amy the name of the nurse at the American Indian Center and encourages her to call and check out the support group.

ADVOCACY

Sometimes our health care system is characterized as uncaring, impersonal, and fragmented. Clients become frustrated, often feeling devalued and unable to cope with the system.

Client advocacy is defined as intervening for or acting on behalf of the client to provide the highest quality health care obtainable (MDH, 2001). A community-based nurse acts as an advocate for the client and family, providing information to the client to help ensure uninterrupted care. In many situations, the client is vulnerable, which often results in the nurse contacting a community service, other caregivers, or a physician on the client's behalf.

For example, a school nurse notices that a 13-year-old child often comes to the nurse's office on Monday mornings complaining of a stomach ache. When the girl comes in for the third week in a row, the nurse asks her, "Tell me about your weekend." The child starts crying and says, "My dad doesn't live with us anymore. My mom drinks beer and yells at me." The nurse and the child discuss the child's feelings and fears about her family situation. Then the nurse explains to the child that with her permission, she would like to talk to the school counselor about their conversation, to learn about some groups that may help her. Second, the nurse tells the child that she would like to call her mom and talk to the two of them about her stomach aches. In this situation, the nurse is acting as an advocate for the child, with the goal of facilitating self-care in the context of the student's family. The nurse is collaborating with other professionals to enhance care. Steps of Advocacy are seen in Box 7-4.

The role of the advocate involves informing clients about the nature of their health problems and the choices they have in seeking to resolve or alter their health care needs. This role is activated whenever clients are unable to take responsibility for their own health

---

BOX 7-4 **Steps of Advocacy**

UNDERSTANDING AND KNOWLEDGE OF SELF—PERSONALLY AND PROFESSIONALLY
- Knowing oneself: awareness of personal goals and how these goals may affect relationships with clients
- Realistic self-concept: awareness of one's own limitations and abilities that will affect what one can and cannot support
- Self-knowledge about values clarification: awareness of one's biases and prejudices, morals, and ethical values. This gives one a good knowledge and understanding of personal views of what is fair and acceptable and how that may affect one's approach to a relationship with the client

KNOWLEDGE OF TREATMENT AND INTERVENTION OPTIONS
- Development of knowledge base of procedures, actions, interventions, and resources.
- Awareness of rationale for specific therapies

KNOWLEDGE OF HEALTH CARE SYSTEM
- Awareness of how systems relate to each other, the client, and the community
- Awareness of the relationship of outside influences, such as politics and economics, to oneself

KNOWLEDGE OF HOW TO PUT ADVOCACY INTO ACTION
- Assessment—contextual approach:
- What does the client believe is the most important problem?
- What support or resources does the client already have in place?
- What does the client know or not know (e.g., health services, treatment options)?
- In what areas does the client feel a need for personal control to be established in his or her life?
- Planning—mobilization of resources, consultations, collaboration with other disciplines
- Implementation—education, empowerment of client (The nurse assists the client in asserting control over the variables affecting the client's life. The nurse must be a role model for assertiveness to make this important step effective.)

Adapted from Minnesota Department of Health, Section of Public Health Nursing. (2001). *Public health nursing interventions II*. Minneapolis, MN: Author.

care, lack knowledge or skill, or do not have the financial or emotional basis from which to act. The advocacy role is also one of support after clients have been informed, made choices, and need to implement these choices. Clients have an inherent right to make their own decisions and to take responsibility for those decisions. The nurse lends support and respect for clients, whether or not the nurse agrees with their decisions. To advocate for clients, the nurse must consider all aspects of the clients' lives.

Advocacy is often called for with vulnerable populations who have a weak voice within a system. Some people, because of age, cognitive abilities, lack of sophistication, or other factors, benefit from guidance in how to speak for themselves. Clarification of a do-not-resuscitate order on behalf of an elderly client who is unaware of the need to explicitly state his or her preference is one example of a nurse acting as a client advocate. The expertise and competence of nurses can also be used in supporting the needs and views of their clients and their clients' families. Nurses can be advocates for clients who feel they have been excluded from participation in health care decisions or who have little trust in the health care system or political representatives. Advocates also work to change the system by revealing gaps, opportunities, injustices, and inadequacies. Advocacy may be accomplished by engaging in some of the following activities:

- Empowering each client and family member they care for who experiences disparities in health care
- Discussing disparities in their communities with colleagues
- Writing about disparities for hospital, clinic, or professional organization newsletters
- Writing letters to, or calling and making an appointment to speak to, local or state politicians to describe evidence of health disparities that they encounter

Community-based nurses are well situated to act as an advocate for the individual and families given their knowledge of clients' needs and understanding of local services.

EVALUATION

Evaluation is the measurement of the outcomes or results of implementing the discharge plan. This involves gathering data on the client's response to interventions. Data can be collected from the client, family, physician, and referral sources. The major purpose of evaluation is to see if goals were reached. Evaluation is ongoing; reviews are made to determine if needs were met, if problems were resolved, and if the plan needs to be revised. Evaluation continues as the client moves from one setting to another.

In evaluating the effectiveness of continuity of care, it is essential to consider these points:

- Whether health planning was interprofessional and initiated when the client first obtained health care services
- Whether the client and family participated in early planning for ongoing care
- If the care being provided to the client was empathic, based on mutual trust and cultural sensitivity
- If the client and family believe they had all the information and resource they needed for self-care at home
- If there is new information that suggests the plan should be revised

Evaluation is effective only if there is a plan with goals established in collaboration with the client, family, and interprofessional team. The evaluation process is more meaningful if the expected outcomes are written in a clear, measurable way. Judgment skills are necessary when comparing real outcomes with expected outcomes. If the client's behavior matches the desired outcomes, the goal has been met. If the goals are not met, then the nurse must examine the reasons for the shortfall. Whatever the conclusion, after evaluation, the appropriate members of the interprofessional team along with the client and family must reassess and plan for the continuing needs of the client.

DOCUMENTATION

A written plan of care that incorporates elements of continuity is an essential tool to guide and document communication and coordination among team members. Although collection and evaluation of data for case management are often done in varying degrees of formality (e.g., interviews, physical examinations, questionnaires), communication is better served if the recording of such data is kept formal and organized. Use of well-constructed and consistently used planning documents across the continuum of care becomes vital to the success of coordination of disciplines and, therefore, to effective planning. At the same time, a plan must be current and dynamic to reflect the reality of the client and/or family at various points of time.

The competencies necessary for community-based care have been discussed. Competent care begins with an ability to understand what promotes and what inhibits self-care, as well as using the techniques of establishing trust, making appropriate referrals, advocating, consulting, and collaborating to facilitate self-care. People living with a chronic condition often require a great deal of assistance with health promotion to help maximize continuity and improve the quality of their lives. Because chronic diseases are the major cause of morbidity and mortality in developed countries, nurses are increasingly involved with illness prevention and health promotion. Community-based nursing occurs within the context of the client's community. The nurse is responsible for identifying resources and constraints or limitations for care that exist within the client's community. Collaboration and advocacy are important aspects of ensuring continuity of care. All combined, these elements contribute to continuity in community-based care.

Barriers to Successful Continuity of Care

The nurse must be aware of barriers that may adversely affect continuity and that stem from social factors, family matters, communication difficulties, or cultural differences. The health care system itself poses many barriers to continuity of care.

SOCIAL FACTORS

Attitude of the Health Care Worker

The health care worker's attitudes and biases can affect whether the client and family will use available resources as clients are quick to sense bias and judgment. For example, a prenatal clinic for low-income women may not have appropriate space for small children to wait while their mothers are examined implicitly discouraging children being brought to the clinic appointment. The women may sense this judgment, but most of them cannot afford child care, resulting in lack of follow-through on essential prenatal care. Thus lack of provision of child-friendly space in waiting areas in clinics may result in interrupted continuity.

Client Motivation

The client may not follow through on a suggested referral if there are more pressing matters at hand. As discussed in Chapter 4, Maslow's Hierarchy of Needs informs caregivers of the importance of prioritizing when people are ill. Often, this is seen as the client and family being only concerned with meeting basic needs. Consequently, when clients are asked to make decisions about their higher needs, their motivation may be diminished because all their energy is going toward getting their basic needs met. To address continuity issues, the nurse must be aware of the client's priorities and first assist with meeting the needs the client sees as a priority before progressing to a higher level need.

Lack of Knowledge

When clients do not understand the importance of a service, they may avoid using that service leading to poor continuity of care. This can be true in the case of prenatal care for the adolescent who is pregnant for the first time. Through conversations with the school nurse, she may know she "should" go to the clinic for checkups during pregnancy, but she may not know why. If the adolescent becomes aware of the purpose of prenatal care and the consequences of not receiving care, she is more likely to follow-up with a referral to the antenatal clinic.

FAMILY BARRIERS

When families and clients are involved in decisions about care after discharge and receive relevant self-care information, they are more likely to experience a smooth transition to the next setting. It may be helpful to realize that family involvement may either enhance or interrupt continuity. Whatever the contributing factor affecting family involvement, the nurse plays an important role in assisting the client and family in the problem-solving process to achieve quality care across the continuum.

COMMUNICATION BARRIERS

Poor communication, often attributable to language problems, health literacy, and hearing limitations, interrupts continuity of care. Communication barriers can occur when the client does not speak English. They also occur when there is a cultural difference significant enough to prohibit communication or to create misunderstandings because of factors such as the age of the client, sexual orientation, or use of nonverbal communication. A client may be offended and not listen to instructions or refuse referrals to community providers if the nurse does not practice culturally sensitive communication techniques.

TRANSCULTURAL BARRIERS

A prominent barrier may be differences in cultural orientation that exist between the provider and the client. Chapter 3 focuses on cultural care and the necessary transcultural nursing skills and competencies required of nurses in community settings. Developing transcultural skills is an ongoing process requiring a commitment to lifelong learning.

HEALTH CARE SYSTEM BARRIERS

Reimbursement

Health care services are costly in the United States, and not everyone has health insurance or has health insurance that allows service for the client's health condition. Consequently, many people do not seek health care services because they cannot afford them. This is often the case with the "working poor," who are often uninsured or underinsured, or with those who are on medical assistance but do not qualify for other needed services. Health care reform in 2010 attempted to begin to address this disparity. Gaps in care also often result from reimbursement requirements in the form of burdensome and confusing documentation regulations. In many states, the forms that have to be completed to enroll in state or federal health-related care require reading level and health literacy way beyond that of those attempting to fill out the forms. Due to these systems issues, the health care worker may be left feeling apathetic toward planning and referral with individuals and families with scare resources when services are available only when there is a source of payment. Nurses can be involved in local and state coalition building to problem solve and develop strategies to remove or modify these constraints.

Failed Systems

Sometimes systems within the health care setting create barriers to successful continuity. The primary health care team may unintentionally interrupt continuity in several different ways. First, insufficient staff may create delays. Lack of time to address continuity needs is another barrier to continuity. Third, if staff communication is poor, delays may result.

Caregivers and services outside of the primary health care team may create delays. For example, laboratory test results may not be ready on time, or transportation may not be provided during prescribed time lines. These delays are often not within the control of the primary health care team. Sometimes a lack of services may create lack of continuity when parameters for access are too stringent.

Successful Continuity of Care

Evidence illustrates that clients benefit from nursing follow-up after discharge from the hospital. For some time, the nursing literature has reported success in using telephone follow-up as a strategy for successful continuity care. Research in Community-Based Nursing Care 7-4 shows a literature review of this type of approach. Continuity between health care settings is most commonly associated with errors in communication of information related to treatment plans with frail elderly clients. LaManita et al. (2010) conducted a systematic review of research to identify and evaluate interventions to improve communication to ensure accurate and appropriate medications and advance directives for elderly clients in transition between long-term care facilities and hospitals. A standardized patient transfer form was found essential to assist with communication of an advance directive and medication list. Further, pharmacist-led review of medications is an essential component to successful transition. Researchers recommended that additional research is needed to define target populations and outcome measures to further refine successful continuity care.

Individuals with serious mental illness require complex discharge to manage their self-care, avoid rehospitalization, and remain in the community. A systematic review of eleven studies examined the effectiveness of discharge planning in mental health care (Steffen, Kösters, Becker, & Puschner, 2009). Readmission rates, adherence to out-patient treatment plans, and quality of life were the outcome measures. The researchers recommend that good clinical practice in mental health care would include at least one scheduled care conference with the interprofessional team, client, and family prior to hospital discharge with family involvement as the core element. Most discharge planning is based on a standard of care of what clients and families should get rather than a needs-based approach of what they need. Another recommendation from this research is to make every effort

RESEARCH IN COMMUNITY-BASED NURSING CARE 7-4

A Literature Review of the Potential of Telephone Follow-Up in Colorectal Cancer

The purpose of this research was to explore the efficacy of telephone follow-up with clients with colorectal cancer. Because of improved diagnosis and treatment, more individuals survive colon cancer for longer periods and need follow-up care. Via a systematic electronic search, relevant literature was identified and thematic content analysis completed. Symptom management and reassurance were the main components of the telephone follow-up care. The researcher found that telephone follow-up conducted by an experienced nurse specialist is both cost-effective and accepted by a majority of patients. Researchers concluded that telephone follow-up meets clients' satisfaction, support, and information needs and has potential to deliver care that meets high standards. This strategy was found to be at least equivalent to traditional care in meeting the needs of clients with cancer and could, for some clients, dramatically improve their care experience. Future research in the areas of nurse-led telephone follow-up as compared to nurse-led traditional follow-up is recommended. Additionally, there is a need to explore ideal structure, method, and timing of telephone follow-up as well as the skills necessary to carry out this type of care over the phone through research.

Cusack, M., & Taylor, C. (2010). A literature review of the potential of telephone follow-up in colorectal cancer. *Journal of Clinical Nursing, 19*(17/18), 2394–2405. Retrieved from CINAHL Plus with Full Text database.

to provide needs-oriented continuity of care for individuals with mental illness as well as to ensure continuity of personnel in order to avoid a fragmented therapeutic relationship.

The role of the nurse as a case manager in the care of individuals with chronic illness has evolved over the last three decades. One example is seen in the management of heart failure. Around 5.8 million people in the United States have heart failure with about 670,000 people diagnosed with it each year. In recent years, the results of heart failure costed the United States $39.2 billion, which includes the cost of health care services, medications, and lost productivity (Lloyd-Jones et al., 2010). Because the management of clients with heart failure is complex, it often requires a comprehensive, client-centered approach. Since the 1990s, numerous heart failure disease management programs have been designed and implemented to meet this need. Case management has been deemed a solution to improve outcomes for those experiencing heart failure (Annema, Luttik, & Jaarsma, 2009a, 2009b).

CLIENT SITUATIONS IN PRACTICE

Case Management

Steve, age 40, and Barb, age 37, are a couple with three children: Brook, 15; Jane, 13; and Jack, 11. Both parents are professionals. Steve works at the Veterans Administration, where he is in charge of the information systems, and Barb is a professor at a small liberal arts college. Because Steve has a family history of colon cancer (his paternal grandfather died of colon cancer at age 41 and his father and uncle had surgery for colon cancer at ages 65 and 60, respectively), he was advised to have a colonoscopy at age 40 although he was not experiencing any symptoms. One month after his 40th birthday, Steve scheduled a test. He was diagnosed with colon cancer 3 days after the test, on Christmas Eve day. Because of the size of the tumor, Steve's physician recommended that he have the surgery at a large medical center 200 miles from Steve's home. Two days after Christmas, he had a colon resection without a colostomy at Methodist Hospital. At that time, it was determined that the cancer was class C2 according to Dukes classification system (or stage 4 with the other commonly used classification). Although he was a candidate for a colostomy, he and Barb decided they wanted to try the more conservative approach, with the option of a colostomy later, if necessary.

Barb has been with Steve throughout his hospital stay while their three children have been home, 200 miles away, staying with Barb's elderly mother. It is 14 days after the operation, and he is to return home the day after tomorrow. He will begin chemotherapy at the rural hospital close to his home next week.

> *You are a staff nurse caring for Steve in the hospital. What strategies to ensure continuity of care would you use, starting from the first day?*

The first step in care management is establishing a relationship with the client and family by listening and talking. By doing this, you hope to build trust.

By now you would have established a very open relationship with Barb and Steve. You ask Barb and Steve how they anticipate the homecoming will go when they arrive home. Barb says, "We have both really missed the kids. I really want to have a normal life again—sleep in my own bed and make breakfast for everyone. Just normal stuff."

Steve says, "I can't wait to get out of here. But I am worried about the chemo. We had one conversation with the nurse at the clinic, and she said that we have to have the chemo in the morning. I have most of my meetings at work in the morning and would rather do the chemo in the afternoon."

> *How could you, as a staff nurse, respond to this comment?*

To help give some control back to the client, you might encourage him to call the clinic that day and explore whether chemotherapy could be scheduled at a time more convenient for his work schedule.

Nurse in the Outpatient Setting

You are working in a clinic as an oncology nurse, providing chemotherapy for Steve. This is the third week of his treatment, and you have established a relationship with both Barb and Steve. During Steve's visit, you ask them how things are going. Barb tells you, "Awful. Brook was picked up for shoplifting, and her grades are dropping in school." You note that Steve is unusually quiet and does not make eye contact with you. You ask, "Steve, you look down today. Are you doing okay?"

"It feels like it is all coming apart. I can't keep up at work, the kids are having trouble ...," Steve shares.

"He won't listen to me about resting. And he's throwing up all the time. That medication you gave him doesn't work," Barb reports.

    ◉ *What are some interventions you could use at this point in your care of Steve and his family?*

Possible interventions include the following:

Using the steps of the referral process to find some community resources or services to support the family with the issues the family is facing, including the daughter's shoplifting and falling grades.

Advocating for the client (with the client and family's approval) by calling the oncology nurse practitioner or physician to identify an additional antiemetic that may be helpful in controlling the nausea and vomiting.

Contacting a social worker (with the client and family's approval) to begin to collaborate and problem solve regarding the family's issues and stress.

Ten months later, Steve has completed chemotherapy and radiation therapy. Because of the intensity of the radiology treatment, he has developed interrupted bowel function. He has been to the clinic and the ED several times in the past weeks with severe cramps. You receive a call late in the afternoon from Barb. She states that the medication given at the last clinic visit is not helping; Steve has been throwing up all day, has severe abdominal cramps, and has a temperature of 103°F. You tell them to go to the local ED.

At the ED, Steve is diagnosed with a bladder and kidney infection and bowel obstruction, and he is admitted to the hospital. A complete workup is performed while he is in the hospital, and liver cancer is discovered throughout his liver, with lesions in the brain as well. He is discharged to home unable to eat, with a central line and hyperal for total parenteral nutrition.

Home Care Nurse

You are Steve's home care nurse. On the first home visit, his functional capacity for ADLs is clearly impaired. He is homebound and needs a home health care aide to help him bathe and shave. Barb is both teaching and doing consulting to try to make ends meet. The plan is for the home health aide to come every other day, with you coming once a day to start the hyperal. Two months later, at one of your visits, Steve says, "The home aide says he can do the hyperal and clean the site on the days when he is here. Then you don't have to come every day."

    ◉ *Can you delegate the administration of hyperal to the home health aide?*

According to the Five Rights of Delegation from the NCSBN (Box 7-2), this task may not be delegated for the following reasons:

The CNA is not the right person for the task. Assessment may be needed and an RN would not be immediately available for assistance or direct supervision.

Steve's condition continues to deteriorate over the next month. Steve and the family have changed the subject every time you have brought up the subject of palliative care or hospice care in the last few weeks. As you are getting ready to leave after a visit, Barb abruptly asks you, "Do you think that Steve is going to die soon?"

    ◉ *You sit down with Barb and ask her, "Are you wondering about the benefits of palliative or hospice care?" She indicates that she is feeling like she is no longer able to handle his deteriorating condition without more assistance. You conclude that Barb and Steve may be ready to talk about hospice care. How do you proceed?*

Using the steps for consultation in Box 7-1, you sit down with Steve and Barb to determine the family's desires. Through mutual problem solving, you determine if and when the family is ready to meet with the hospice nurse. As per the client and family's decision to seek hospice care, you contact her for the family and arrange for her to visit.

Conclusions

This chapter has taken a broad look at continuity of care. Discharge planning has been described as a significant process that ensures continuity of care by coordinating various aspects of a client's care beginning with admission through transition from one health care setting to another. Care management is a complex concept including a variety of roles and responsibilities. Coordination of activities involving the clients, providers, and payers is essential in providing continued care. Essential to quality health care is a mutually designed, strong, ongoing health care plan that includes appropriate use of resources and effective referrals. Identification of current and future needs leads to implementation of the referral process and continued care. Barriers to effective discharge planning include social, family, communication, health care system, and community resources issues. The care manager in community-based settings always encourages self-care with a preventive focus that is provided within the context of the client's community while following the principles of collaboration to achieve continuity.

What's on the Web

Improving Chronic Illness Care
INTERNET ADDRESS: http://www.improving chroniccare.org/change/index.html
Due to the increasing percentage of the population who develops chronic conditions, many managed care and integrated delivery systems have taken a great interest in correcting the many deficiencies in current management of diseases such as diabetes, heart disease, depression, asthma, and others. The deficiencies of lack of coordinate care and follow-up, as well as many clients being inadequately educated to manage their conditions, call for a model for managing chronic conditions. Such a model for managing chronic conditions is the subject of this Web site. There are many resources on this site sponsored by the Robert Wood Johnson Foundation.

Case Management Society of America
INTERNET ADDRESS: http://www.cmsa.org
This site offers educational opportunities, both CEU (continuing education units) and case management credential courses. It also provides extensive information on case management for consumers and nurses.

Case Management Resource Guide
INTERNET ADDRESS: http://www.cmrg.com/
This site has a comprehensive, online directory of health care organizations. It also contains an extensive case manager resource guide.

National Council of State Boards of Nursing (NCSBN) Delegation Resource Folder
INTERNET ADDRESS: http://www.ncsbn.org
The NCSBN has produced a series of excellent videos called Unlicensed Nursing Assistive Personnel Workshop Videos from a conference held in Chicago, Illinois, on June 29–30, 2010. Use the search box to find these resources.

References and Bibliography

Annema, C., Luttik, M., & Jaarsma, T. (2009a). Reasons for readmission in heart failure: perspectives of patients, caregivers, cardiologists, and heart failure nurses. *Heart & Lung, 38*(5), 427–434. Retrieved from CINAHL Plus with Full Text database.

Annema, C., Luttik, M., & Jaarsma, T. (2009b). Do patients with heart failure need a case manager? *Journal of Cardiovascular Nursing, 24*(2), 127–131. Retrieved from CINAHL Plus with Full Text database. URL: www.cinalh.com/cgi-bin/refsvc?jid=455&accno=2010220687

Agency for Healthcare Research and Quality. (2010). One in four patients experienced revolving-door hospitalizations. Retrieved from http://www.ahrq.gov/research/jul10/0710RA1.htm

Bauer, M., Fitzgerald, L., Haesler, E., & Manfrin, M. (2009). Hospital discharge planning for frail older people and their family. Are we delivering best practice? A review of the evidence. *Journal of Clinical Nursing, 18*(18), 2539–2546. Retrieved from CINAHL Plus with Full Text database.

Blaylock, A., & Cason, C. L. (1992). Discharge planning: Predicting patient's needs. *Journal of Gerontological Nursing, 18*(7), 5–10.

Cabin, W. (2010). Lifting the home care veil from depression: OASIS-C and evidence-based practice. *Home Health Care Management & Practice, 22*(3), 171–177. doi:10.1177/1084822309348693.

Carroll, Á., & Dowling, M. (2007). Discharge planning: communication, education and patient participation. *British Journal of Nursing (BJN), 16*(14), 882–886. Retrieved from CINAHL Plus with Full Text database.

Carpenito, L. J. (2010). *Handbook of nursing diagnosis* (13th ed.). Philadelphia, PA: Lippincott Williams & Wilkins.

Centers for Medicare and Medicaid Services. (2010). Your discharge planning checklist. Retrieved from http://www.medicare.gov/Publications/Pubs/pdf/11376.pdf

Commins, J. (2010, June 3). Cleveland clinic's new health center will feature 'patient navigators' to coordinate care. Retrieved from http://www.healthleadersmedia.com/content/LED-251913/Cleveland-Clinics-New-Health-Center-Will-Feature-Patient-Navigators-to-Coordinate-Care

Craven, R. F., & Hirnle, C. J. (2009). *Fundamentals of nursing: Human health and function* (6th ed.). Philadelphia, PA: Lippincott Williams & Wilkins.

Cusack, M., & Taylor, C. (2010). A literature review of the potential of telephone follow-up in colorectal cancer. *Journal of Clinical Nursing, 19*(17/18), 2394–2405. Retrieved from CINAHL Plus with Full Text database. doi: 10.1111/j.1365-2702.2010.03253.

Kempshall, N. (2010). The care of patients with complex long-term conditions. *British Journal of Community Nursing, 15*(4), 181–187. Retrieved from CINAHL Plus with Full Text database.

LaMantia, M., Scheunemann, L., Viera, A., Busby-Whitehead, J., & Hanson, L. (2010). Interventions to Improve Transitional Care Between Nursing Homes and Hospitals: A Systematic Review. *Journal of the American Geriatrics Society, 58*(4), 777–782. doi:10.1111/j.1532-5415.2010.02776.x..

Lees, L., Price, D., & Andrews, A. (2010). Developing discharge practice through education: module development, delivery and outcomes. *Nurse Education in Practice, 10*(4), 210–215. doi:10.1016/j.nepr.2009.08.008.

Liu, W., Edwards, H., & Courtney, M. (2010). Case management educational intervention with public health nurses: cluster randomized controlled trial. *Journal of Advanced Nursing, 66*(10), 2234–2244. doi:10.1111/j.1365-2648.2010.05392.x.

Lloyd-Jones D, Adams RJ, Brown TM, Carnethon M, Dai S, De Simone G, et al. (2010). Heart Disease and Stroke Statistics—2010 Update. A Report from the American Heart Association Statistics Committee and Stroke Statistics Subcommittee.˙ *Circulation.* 121:e1–e170.

Lyon, J. C. (1993). Modules of nursing care delivery and case management: Clarification of terms. *Nursing Economics, 11*(3), 163–178.

Minnesota Department of Health, Section of Public Health Nursing. (2001). *Public health nursing interventions II*. Minneapolis, MN: Author.

Mistiaen, P., Duijnhouwer, E., Prins-Hoekstra, A., Ros, W., & Blaylock, A. (1999). Predictive validity of the BRASS index in screening patients with post-discharge problems. *Journal of Advanced Nursing, 30*(5), 1050–1056.

National Council of State Boards of Nursing. (2010). Joint Statement on Delegation from the American Nurses Association (ANA) and the National Council of State Boards of Nursing (NCSBN). Retrieved from https://www.ncsbn.org/Joint_statement.pdf

Niewenhous, S. (2010). OASIS-C: new process measures promote best practices. *Home Health Care Management & Practice, 22*(3), 221–234. doi:10.1177/1084822309355903.

Rodgers, B. (2000). Coordination of care: The lived experience of the visiting nurse. *Home Healthcare Nurse, 18*(5), 301–307.

Rose, K., & Haugen, M. (2010). Discharge planning: Your last chance to make a good impression. *MEDSURG Nursing, 19*(1), 47–53. Retrieved from Academic Search Premier database.

Shear, J. (2010). Primary care medical home: Veterans Health Administration. Retrieved from www.pcpcc.net/files/PCPCC-10-09-P1-Shear.ppt

Simonet, M., Kossovsky, M., Chopard, P., Sigaud, P., Perneger, T., & Gaspoz, J. (2008). A predictive score to identify hospitalized patients' risk of discharge to a post-acute care facility. *BMC Health Services Research*, 81–9. doi:10.1186/1472-6963-8-154.

Steffen, S., Kösters, M., Becker, T., & Puschner, B. (2009). Discharge planning in mental health care: a systematic review of the recent literature. *Acta Psychiatrica Scandinavica, 120*(1), 1–9. doi:10.1111/j.1600-0447.2009.01373.x.

Tahan, H. A. (1998). Case management: A heritage more than a century old. *Nursing Case Management, 3*(2), 55–60.

Welch, G., Garb, J., Zagarins, S., Lendel, I., & Gabbay, R. (2010). Nurse diabetes case management interventions and blood glucose control: Results of a meta-analysis. *Diabetes Research & Clinical Practice, 88*(1), 1–6. doi:10.1016/j.diabres.2009.12.026.

LEARNING ACTIVITIES

JOURNALING ACTIVITY 7-1

1. In your clinical journal, describe a situation you observed or were told about in which a client or family experienced difficulty because of lack of continuity. If you have the opportunity, ask the client or family to identify what they think would have avoided these difficulties. If you were the nurse in charge, what would you have done differently to avoid these problems?

2. In your clinical journal, relate a situation in which you observed a client who received effective continuity of care in discharge planning. What made the care effective?

3. In your clinical journal, describe a situation you have observed in clinical setting where a client received effective case management. What made the care effective?

4. In your clinical journal, describe a situation where you observed or initiated two of the following intervention strategies. Discuss what happened.

   Health teaching

   Screening

   Counseling

   Referral and follow-up

   Consultation

   Collaboration

   Advocacy

5. List any barriers you have noticed that have interrupted continuity for a client you have cared for in a clinical setting. Discuss what happened and what you would do differently. Identify any system's issues that created or did not address the barriers (e.g., chart forms such as discharge forms, admission forms, unit policies).

CLIENT CARE ACTIVITY 7-2

Mr. Heaney, a 66-year-old man, is admitted for a total knee replacement. He has had constant pain in his left knee for the past 2 years secondary to osteoarthritis. Five years ago, he had coronary bypass surgery and also has a visual impairment. His wife of 45 years died just 2 months ago, and he has remained alone in their two-story home. He has visited the ED four times with cardiac symptoms in the last month related to not taking his cardiac medications regularly. Only one of their six children lives in the area. On postoperative day 1, he begins physical therapy. His left leg is in a continuous passive motion device when he is in bed. The plan is to discharge him on postoperative day 2 with outpatient physical therapy, the use of the continuous passive motion device at home, and continuation of oral analgesics for pain. He will use a walker for ambulation for at least 2 weeks and will continue to take the four cardiac drugs that he has been taking for the last 5 years. He appears to be slightly confused during the discharge planning conference when the discussion about his continuing care is discussed.

1. Describe your role as the primary nurse in Mr. Heaney's discharge planning.

2. Explain why you are in a position to coordinate continuity of care.

3. Identify the risks Mr. Heaney may have after discharge. Use the Blaylock Discharge Planning Risk Assessment Screen (Fig. 7-3) to assess for risks.

4. Propose recommendations for his living situation and home care.

5. List agencies, facilities, or individuals you would recommend for Mr. Heaney's continuing care and give your reasons.

CLIENT CARE ACTIVITY 7-3

You are a home health care nurse responsible for the care of 15 clients. It's Monday morning, and you are reviewing your phone messages as well as looking over the charts of the clients you are scheduled to visit in the next 2 days. How will you rearrange home visits for the next 2 days based on the following information?

SCHEDULED VISITS FOR MONDAY AFTERNOON AND TUESDAY

MONDAY

1:00 Mr. Carmody—routine visit to monitor symptoms of congestive heart failure.

2:30 Mrs. Gothie—routine follow-up visit after hip replacement and discharge from acute care last Wednesday, and your last visit was Friday.

4:00 Mrs. Violet—monthly blood draw for lithium levels.

TUESDAY

9:00 Mr. Perlmutter—scheduled to discharge from the hospital Monday night after open heart surgery; assessment visit and blood draw.

10:30 Mr. Toffle—follow-up visit for knee replacement surgery; discharged from the hospital last Thursday, and your last visit was Friday.

1:00 Mr. Vang—reinforcement teaching for care of a leg wound.

2:30 Mrs. O'Conner—follow-up visit for assessment after scheduled discharge from the hospital on Monday evening; administration of IV antibiotic medication.

PHONE MESSAGES ON MONDAY AT 8:00 AM

Mr. Vang called you this morning and said that he ran out of dressings on Friday. He was upset and stated that the sore on his leg looked redder, and there was some sticky green stuff dripping off of it.

Mrs. Toffle called and said her husband had severe pain in his knee over the weekend that prevented him from sleeping. She said he also has pain in the back of his calf, and she noticed it is red, and it hurts if he flexes his foot.

PRACTICAL APPLICATION ACTIVITY 7-4

Observe a nurse doing routine discharge planning with a client in the hospital, ED, or clinic. How did the nurse assess the client or the client's family? (This could be done either through questions on the discharge form or through additional questions the nurse asks.)

If you were the nurse, what would you have done differently from or in addition to the activities of the nurse you observed?

CRITICAL THINKING ACTIVITY 7-5

List at least three barriers you have observed in your clinical setting that hinder effective case management. Discuss what could be done differently to enhance case management and continuity in these situations.

CRITICAL THINKING ACTIVITY 7-6

Ask the nurse manager in the settings where you do clinical work about strategies used on his or her unit to ensure continuity of care. If the nurse manager indicates dissatisfaction with continuity of care on the unit, ask what could be done to improve it. Volunteer to do a project to assist the head nurse to explore his or her concerns. If the nurse manager asks for suggestions of projects, offer to complete a literature review of best practice continuity of care programs in the specialty area of the unit.

UNIT III

Skills for Community-Based Nursing Practice

In Chapter 2, you learned that although the U.S. health care system is the most expensive in the world, the United States lags behind other nations in key health indicators. This unit uses the recommendations from Healthy People 2020 to outline the role that the nurse must play in improving the nation's health. All three chapters in this unit address the broad goals outlined in Healthy People 2020.

Each chapter begins with a discussion of the goals of Healthy People 2020, as well as the major causes of mortality and morbidity for each age group. Nursing assessments and interventions follow. Chapter 8 discusses health promotion and disease and injury prevention for maternal/infant populations, children, and adolescents. Chapter 9 outlines health promotion and disease and injury prevention for adults, and Chapter 10 focuses on elderly adults.

The content of each chapter is organized around the leading causes of mortality for each group. Disease and injury prevention and health promotion strategies that address these causes are highlighted. Based on numerous sources, these strategies are intended for the practicing nurse to use to teach clients about health promotion and disease and injury prevention. Unit III also contains numerous Web site and organization addresses, as well as resources related to health promotion and disease prevention for clients across the life span.

Chapter 8

Health Promotion and Disease and Injury Prevention for Maternal/ Infant Populations, Children, and Adolescents

ROBERTA HUNT

Learning Objectives

1 Identify the major causes of death for maternal/infant populations, children, and adolescents.

2 Discuss the major diseases and threats to health for maternal/infant populations, children, and adolescents.

3 Summarize the major health issues for maternal/infant populations, children, and adolescents.

4 Identify nursing roles at each level of prevention for major health issues.

5 Compose a list of nursing interventions for the major health issues for maternal/ infant populations, children, and adolescents.

6 Determine health needs for maternal/infant populations, children, and adolescents for which a nurse could be an advocate.

Key Terms

Ages and Stages Questionnaire (ASQ)
fetal alcohol syndrome (FAS)
infant mortality rate
lead poisoning

low birth weight (LBW)
neural tube defects (NTDs)
sudden infant death syndrome (SIDS)

Chapter Topics

Significance of Health Promotion and Disease Prevention

Achieving Health Equity and Eliminating Disparity in Health Care

Maternal/Infant Populations

Preschool-Age Children

School-Age Children

Adolescence

Use of Complementary Therapies

Policy

Conclusions

The Nurse Speaks

For over 10 years, I worked as a school nurse at a large high school in a small Midwestern town. One day, a 15-year-old student named Jennifer came into my office. She was obviously pregnant. She told me that she was going to the doctor the next day to find out if she was pregnant. She didn't think that she was but wanted to find out for sure. I asked her if she could feel any kicking, and she said she could. I asked her if she could feel kicking when she held her hand on her stomach, and she said she could. When she left my office she said that she would let me know what the doctor said.

Several days later, she returned to see me and said that she had had an exam and was indeed pregnant and due in 1 month. I asked about the possibility of finding a prenatal class for her, but she wasn't interested. Although I saw her several times before her baby was born, she remained detached and uninterested in the baby or learning about the impending delivery. I was very concerned about Jennifer and her baby. I wondered if she would attach to the baby and thought that this family was at risk for lack of early bonding and attachment. I knew that babies born to young teen moms were at higher risk for child abuse and neglect than babies born to older women.

A month after her baby was born, I called Jennifer and asked if I could come to see her. She was living with her parents. She agreed to a home visit the next week. When I entered the home, Jennifer was holding her daughter and sitting at the kitchen table with her father. I sat down and explained that I was the school nurse and did home visits with some of the students from the high school. I kept things casual, and at first, we talked about general things. Then, Jennifer began to talk about when she would be returning to school, when she hoped to graduate, and the classes she would be taking. Jennifer's mother came in as we were talking and stated, "The baby is sleeping all night now. Jennifer is a great mom. I am working the evening shift now, so I will take care of the baby when Jennifer is in school."

All the time we were talking, I was quietly observing Jennifer with her baby daughter. She was holding her close but with a relaxed posture. She frequently looked at the baby, and when the baby woke up, Jennifer looked into her sleepy eyes and said softly, "Hi Tiffany, did you have a good nap?" Then, she fed Tiffany a bottle. As she was feeding her, Jennifer was watching Tiffany's face. As soon as the baby started to act like she wanted to stop feeding, Jennifer would take the bottle out of her mouth. She said, "Tiffany likes to just drink a little and then be burped and rest."

I left Jennifer's home confident that with the support of her parents, Tiffany would be well cared for and Jennifer would be able to finish high school. My concern about her nonchalance about being pregnant and the birth of her baby did not appear to have interfered with her attaching to her baby. I was relieved that despite the lack of prenatal care and preparation, this family had all the basics to care for this newborn.

Ashley Moore, RN, PHN
St. Paul, Minnesota

Significance of Health Promotion and Disease Prevention

Crucial issues of health are different today from what they were in the early part of the 20th century. Public health efforts have increased the life span of the average person, thanks to universal access to clean water, sanitation, and immunization and the development of effective medications, particularly antibiotics. Our focus as health care providers has changed from combating infectious diseases to addressing chronic conditions and unintentional injuries.

Health promotion is typically defined as a primary disease and injury prevention strategy. It is commonly interchanged with terms such as health education and disease prevention. Often, health promotion is discussed as the epitome of empowerment in that it is a process that enables people to use health as a resource for their lives. Health promotion is most often discussed as a strategy for an already healthy individual or population, but it applies to those with health conditions as well. Disease prevention is just as it states: preventing a disease from occurring. It also includes injury prevention, which will be foundational to the discussion in this and the following three chapters.

Recommendations from Healthy People 2020 form the foundation for all health promotion and disease prevention nursing actions. These goals include attaining higher quality, longer lives free of preventable disease, disability, injury, and premature death; achieving health equity; eliminating disparities and improving the health of all groups; creating social and physical environments that promote good health for all; and promoting quality of life, healthy development, and healthy behaviors across all life stages.

These recommendations are based on the primary causes of death, or mortality, rates and the rates of illness or injury, or morbidity, rates. The Healthy People 2020 report is based on mortality and morbidity statistics that represent the primary causes of death and illnesses and injuries experienced by the people living in the United States.

Most diseases and deaths result from preventable causes. The negative impact of many conditions can be minimized by early identification and intervention. This chapter addresses health promotion and disease prevention for pregnant women, infants, children, and adolescents.

Achieving Health Equity and Eliminating Disparity in Health Care

One of the major goals of Healthy People 2020 is to achieve health equity, eliminate health disparities, and improve health of all groups. Health disparities exist by gender, race or ethnicity, education, income, disability, rural living localities, and sexual orientation. Infant mortality (IM) is a significant indicator of such disparities. In 2008, IM was 7.0 per 1,000 live births for all infants in the United States, compared with **infant mortality rates** of 13.6 among African Americans, 8.0. for American Indians, 8.3 for Puerto Rican, and 5.8 for White, non-Hispanics. Of greater significance is the finding that, although IM rates have declined within all racial groups in the last 20 years, the proportional discrepancy between blacks and whites remains largely unchanged (MacDorman & Mathew, 2009). Comparisons between races and IM rates can be seen in Figure 8-1.

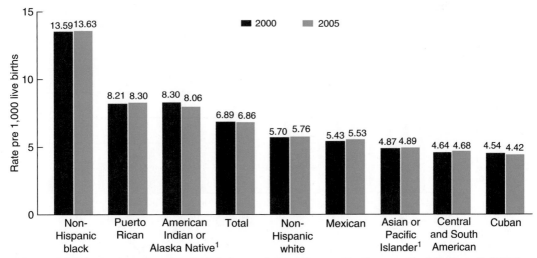

Figure 8-1 IM rates by selected racial/ethnic populations. Source: MacDorman, M., & Mathew, R. (2009). *Recent trends in infant mortality in the United States: NCHS data brief, no 9*. Hyattsville, MD: National Center for Health Statistics. Retrieved from http://www.cdc.gov/nchs/data/databriefs/db09.htm

Disparity by ethnicity is believed to result from complex interactions among genetic variations, environmental factors, and specific health behaviors. Income and education underlie many health disparities in the United States. Income and education are intrinsically related; people with the worst health status are among those with the highest poverty rates and least education. Income inequality in the United States has increased over the past three decades.

The percentage of all children living in poverty has increased, with 19% of all children ages 0 to 17 years (14.1 million) living in poverty, an increase from 18% in 2007. Nearly one in five children lived in poverty in 2008, the highest rate since 1998. In addition, 8% of children (5.9 million) lived in extreme poverty in 2008, the highest percentage since 1998 (Federal Interagency Forum on Children and Family Statistics, 2010). The U.S. child poverty rate is the highest of the top 15 richest nations (Fig. 8-2). While the poverty rate for the elderly has dropped from 35% in 1959 to 9.7% today, the rate for children has only decreased from 26% to 19% (Fig. 8-3).

Disparity in income, specifically poverty, limits children's access to equal opportunities for growing up healthy. Low-income communities are more likely to only have small convenience stores, liquor stores, and fast food where the selection and quality of fresh foods are limited. For decades, access to primary health care providers has been a problem for children living in poverty. Having a usual source of care facilitates the timely and appropriate use of pediatric services. In 2008, 6% of children had no usual source of health care; this was similar to the percentage in 2007. Children who are uninsured are nearly 10 times more likely than those with private insurance to not have a usual source of care in 2008 (30%, compared with about 3%) (Federal Interagency Forum on Children and Family Statistics, 2010).

One of the goals of Healthy People 2020 is to create social and physical environments that promote good health for all and promote quality of life for all citizens. Low-income children are more likely to live in substandard housing where they are often exposed to structural and environmental hazards. They are more likely as compared to children living in middle- or upper-income families to have lead poisoning and asthma as a result. Designing communities so that all children have access to fresh food, primary health care, safe housing, and an environment free from pollution is vital to improving all children's long-term health.

Maternal/Infant Populations

Florence Nightingale wrote in 1894 that "money would be better spent in maintaining health in infancy and childhood than in building hospitals to cure disease" (Monteiro, 1985, p. 185). The same philosophy holds true today. The health of infants and children has farther-reaching implications than that of other population groups. The health of mothers,

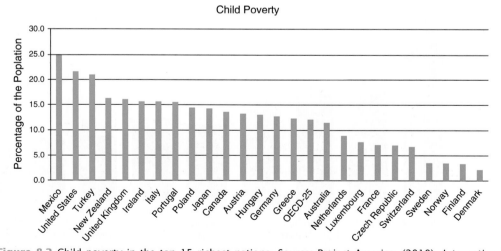

Figure 8-2 Child poverty in the top 15 richest nations. Source: Project America. (2010). *International poverty*. Retrieved from http://www.project.org/info.php?recordID=467

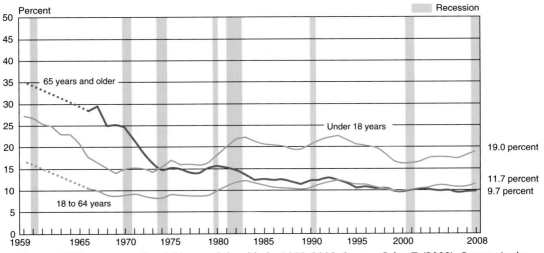

Figure 8-3 Poverty rates for children and the elderly, 1959–2008. Source: Gabe, T. (2009). *Poverty in the United States: 2008. Congressional Research Service 7-5700.* Retrieved from http://www.fas.org/sgp/crs/misc/RL33069.pdf

infants, and children is of critical importance as a predictor of the health of the next generation. Nurses are charged with creating a society where children are wanted and born with optimal health, receive quality care, and are nurtured lovingly and sensitively as they mature into healthy, productive adults. Healthy People 2020 8-1 lists the Healthy People 2020 objectives for maternal and infant health.

Healthy People 2020 8-1

OBJECTIVES FOR MATERNAL AND INFANT HEALTH

1. Reduce maternal deaths.
2. Reduce maternal illness and complications due to pregnancy (complications during hospitalized labor and delivery).
3. Increase the proportion of pregnant women who receive early and adequate prenatal care.
4. Reduce cesarean births among low-risk (full-term, singleton, vertex presentation) women.
5. Reduce low birth weight and very low birth weight.
6. Reduce preterm births.
7. Increase the percentage of healthy full-term infants who are put down to sleep on their backs.
8. Increase abstinence from alcohol, cigarettes, and illicit drugs among pregnant women.
9. Reduce the occurrence of fetal alcohol syndrome.
10. Increase the proportion of mothers who breast-feed their babies.
11. Increase the proportion of children with special health care needs who have access to a medical home.
12. Increase the proportion of children with special health care needs who receive their care in
13. Family-centered, comprehensive, coordinated systems.
14. Reduce fetal and infant deaths.
15. Increase the proportion of pregnant women who attend a series of prepared childbirth classes.
16. (Developmental) Increase the proportion of mothers who achieve a recommended weight gain during their pregnancies.
17. Reduce the proportion of children diagnosed with a metabolic disorder through newborn screening who experience developmental delay requiring special education services.

Healthy People 2020 ⚙ *8-1*

OBJECTIVES FOR MATERNAL AND INFANT HEALTH (*Continued*)

18. Decrease the proportion of children with cerebral palsy born as low-birth-weight infants (<2,500 g).

19. Reduce the occurrence of neural tube defects.

20. Increase the proportion of pregnancies begun with the recommended folic acid level.

21. Ensure appropriate newborn blood-spot screening and follow-up testing.

22. Decrease postpartum relapse of smoking among women who quit smoking during pregnancy.

23. Increase the percentage of women giving birth who attend a postpartum care visit with a health worker.

24. Among women delivering a live birth, increase the percentage that receive preconception care services and practice key recommended preconception health behaviors.

25. Increase the percentage of employers who have worksite lactation programs.

26. Decrease the percentage of breast-fed newborns who receive formula supplementation within the first 2 days of life.

27. Increase the percentage of live births that occur in facilities that provide recommended care for lactating mothers and their babies.

28. Increase the 1-year survival rates for infants with Down syndrome.

29. Reduce the proportion of persons aged 18 to 44 years who have impaired fecundity (i.e., a physical barrier preventing pregnancy or carrying a pregnancy to term).

Source: U.S. Department of Health and Human Services, National Center for Health Statistics. (2010). *Health, United States, 2010*. Washington, DC: U.S. Department of Health and Human services. Retrieved from http://healthypeople.gov/2020/default.aspx

Infant death is a critical indicator of the health of a population because it reflects the overall state of maternal health, as well as the quality of and access to primary health available to pregnant women and infants. The IM rate is the number of infants (age birth to 1 year) who die out of every 1,000 live births. Although the 1980s and 1990s saw steady declines in the IM rate in the United States, at 30th among industrialized nations, it remains among the highest in the industrialized world at 6.9 per 1,000 births (MacDorman & Mathews, 2010). Healthy People 2020 established a goal to reduce IM in the next decade.

PRENATAL CARE

The United States is the only industrialized nation that does not provide all pregnant women with prenatal care. The percentage of U.S. mothers receiving early prenatal care (in the first trimester of pregnancy) varies substantially among racial and ethnic groups, from 76% for Black and Hispanic mothers to 89% for White mothers (Kaiser Family Foundation, 2010).

Every nurse in every setting should encourage pregnant women to begin prenatal care in the first trimester. Some of the topics that are important for the nurse to assess and discuss in home visits to pregnant women are those that Healthy People 2020 has deemed the leading causes of IM: birth and congenital anomalies and **low birth weight (LBW)**.

There is a large body of research that demonstrates the importance of home visits for improving short- and long-term maternal–infant outcomes (Eckenrode et al., 2010; Olds et al., 2010). Home visiting families with infants prior to and after birth to improve birth and newborn outcomes began in the early 20th century in the United States. Today, the Nurse–Family Partnership has been replicated in 32 states that serve over 21,000 families a year. Extensive research conducted over more than 30 years has shown a high level of effectiveness and return on investment in the Nurse–Family Partnership. Three randomized controlled trials demonstrate that Nurse–Family Partnerships result in improved pregnancy outcomes, better child health and development, and increased economic self-sufficiency. These outcomes contribute to preventing child abuse, reducing juvenile crime, and increasing school readiness (Nurse–Family Partnership, 2010).

Low Birth Weight

The most important challenge facing women's and children's health in the United States is premature birth. LBW, or weight less than 2,500 g or 5.5 lb, is the leading cause of preventable neonatal death and the second cause of death of infants. This is included under disorders related to premature birth listed in Table 8-1. In the last two decades, the United States has seen a steady increase in premature births. The percentage of preterm births in the United States has risen by 36% since 1984, with one in nine infants born prematurely each year (MacDorman & Mathews, 2009). LBW is associated with long-term disabilities, such as cerebral palsy, autism, mental retardation, vision and hearing impairment, and other developmental disabilities. LBW is also the main reason premature infants require care in neonatal intensive care units. It does not take a complicated cost analysis to conclude that it is much more expensive to care for a newborn in an intensive care unit than it would have been to provide prenatal care for the infant's mother. Technological advances have been made in the care of premature infants but have resulted in enormous financial, emotional, and social costs. In 2005, preterm births cost at least $26 billion a year (Institute of Medicine, 2006).

The consequences of preterm birth over the child's lifetime can be significant and often call for a broad range of services and social support. The emotional stress to the child and family is frequently considerable. The Institute of Medicine has made several recommendations for a national policy toward preventing and managing premature births. To prepare parents for a possible premature birth, prenatal preparation including preconception risk assessment and prenatal counseling is imperative. The primary intervention to prevent LBW is early initiation of prenatal care. Care in the neonatal intensive care units should be guided by policies that support and permit development of parental involvement from the moment of birth (Institute of Medicine, 2006). In the transition from hospital to home, health care providers should encourage home health nurses to become acquainted with the families in the hospital before discharge. Discharge teaching should prepare the parents to be comfortable using any equipment that the infant will need at home. A 24-hour hotline should be available for parents to obtain advice and reassurance.

Table 8-1 Leading Causes of Death by Age Group, United States, 2007	
Age	**Cause of Death**
Younger than 1 y	Congenital anomalies Disorders related to premature birth SIDS
1–4 y	Unintentional injuries Congenital anomalies Homicide
5–9 y	Unintentional injuries Cancer Congenital anomalies
10–14 y	Unintentional injuries Cancer Homicide
15–24 y	Unintentional injuries Homicide Suicide

Source: National Center for Injury Prevention and Control, Centers for Disease Control and Prevention. (2010). *10 Leading causes of death, United States*. Retrieved from http://webappa.cdc.gov/cgi-bin/broker.exe

Neural Tube Defects

Approximately 50% of all **neural tube defects (NTDs)** may be prevented with adequate consumption of folic acid in the first trimester of pregnancy. The latest recommended daily allowance for folate recommends that all women of childbearing age consume 400 µg of folic acid daily. For women who are pregnant, 600 µg per day is recommended, while for women lactating 500 µg is advised (National Academy of Sciences, 2010). Milan and White (2010) found that Web-based instruction is an effective teaching approach for targeting college females to increase prophylactic use of folic acid for woman of childbearing age.

Smoking

Smoking during pregnancy is the single most preventable cause of illness and death among mothers and infants. A pregnant woman who smokes is more likely to have an LBW infant (Centers for Disease Control and Prevention [CDC], 2010c). Between 12% and 22% of women smoked during pregnancy with 13% continuing to smoke through the last 3 months of pregnancy (CDC, 2010c). Smoking cessation programs have been shown to be effective in reducing smoking rates. Nurses are often the best health care providers to promote smoking cessation programs, especially when the client is pregnant. Research in Community-Based Nursing Care 8-1 presents an example of research relating to a successful smoking cessation program for pregnant women. Smoking cessation programs can be found on Internet sites listed at the end of this chapter in What's on the Web. Postpartum resumption of smoking is strongly discouraged due to the detrimental impact of passive smoke on infants and children.

Alcohol and Drug Use

Moderate to heavy alcohol use by women during pregnancy has been associated with many severe adverse effects, including **fetal alcohol syndrome (FAS)** or fetal alcohol effect and other developmental delays. FAS is recognized as the leading cause of mental retardation in infants born to women who consume alcohol during pregnancy. Infants and children with FAS have characteristic facial and associated physical features attributed to excessive ingestion of alcohol by the mother during pregnancy. It is the nurse's responsibility to discuss alcohol and drug use with the client in an open and nonjudgmental manner. Currently, it is

RESEARCH IN COMMUNITY-BASED NURSING CARE 8-1

Baby BEEP: A Randomized Controlled Trial of Nurses' Individualized Social Support for Poor Rural Pregnant Smokers

For decades, pregnancy has been recognized as a time of unique opportunity for smoking cessation, with 18% to 22% of women quitting smoking once they become pregnant. Nurses are often the best health care providers to promote smoking cessation programs. This study evaluated the effect of nurses who provided individualized telephone social support on smoking prevention to low-income rural pregnant women. Half of the 695 pregnant women participants were randomly assigned to the intervention group, which provided weekly calls throughout pregnancy plus 24-7 beeper access. At monthly home visits before and after delivery, saliva cotinine samples were collected from all groups. Analysis of outcomes reflected a 4% benefit for the intervention group over the control group in producing midpregnancy and continuous abstainer. Partner smoking had no effect on late pregnancy abstinence, but postdelivery, the impact was found to be pronounced. The researchers concluded that "high abstinence rates in the controls indicate the power of biologic monitoring along with home visits to assess stress, support, depression, and intimate partner violence" (p.395).

Source: Bullock, L., Everett, K., Mullen, P., Geden, E., Longo, D., & Madsen, R. (2009). Baby BEEP: A randomized controlled trial of nurses' individualized social support for poor rural pregnant smokers. *Maternal & Child Health Journal, 13*(3), 395–406. Retrieved from CINAHL Plus with Full Text database.

recommended that women do not consume any alcohol during pregnancy. A tool kit called *Drinking and Reproductive Health*, from the American College of Obstetricians and Gynecologists (2006), which nurses can use to assist pregnant women to stop drinking, can be found at http://www.acog.org/departments/healthIssues/FASDToolKit.pdf.

NEWBORN CARE

Childs Health Guide is an excellent tool for monitoring infant and child health. It is available online at http://www.kidsource.com/kidsource/content/hg/index.html. It provides parents with explanations of child preventive care and a convenient place to keep records of health care visits, growth, and immunizations. It recommends checkups at 3 weeks; 2, 4, 6, 9, 12, 15, and 18 months; and 2, 3, 4, 5, 6, 8, 10, 12, 14, 16, and 18 years with a pediatric nurse practitioner or physician. Bright Futures Family Tip Sheets can be downloaded from http://www.brightfutures.org/TipSheets/index.html. The site contains health supervision guidelines and information, including developmental charts for children, ranging from newborn through adolescence.

Screening

All newborns should have blood tests in the hospital for phenylketonuria, thyroid disease, and sickle cell disease. The current recommendation is that all newborns should be screened for hearing impairment before they leave the hospital. In 2006, the American Optometric Association recommended that newborns have an eye examination in the first year of life (Huggins, 2006). Parents should be encouraged to ask the nurse practitioner or physician if they are unsure whether these tests were done for their infant. Healthy attachment is essential to infant mental health. Community-Based Nursing Care Guidelines 8-1 presents some helpful suggestions for promoting healthy attachment between parent and infant.

COMMUNITY-BASED NURSING CARE GUIDELINES 8-1

Nursing Interventions to Promote Attachment

The following are interventions that are directed to parents to assist them to develop an attachment with their newborn:

- Ask the parents to share the birth story and listen for words indicating that it might have been difficult so they can begin to heal.
- Explore the mother and partner's feelings of moving from pregnancy to postpartum.
- Ask the parents what they see in the newborn that were behaviors of the baby in utero.
- Remind the parents that the newborn knows their voices from hearing them when the baby was in utero.
- Tell the parents that newborns like being flexed and close to them as they were positioned before they were born.
- Emphasize the partner's role in nurturing the mother to nurture the newborn.
- Encourage the partner to get support as needed.
- Compliment both parents on their ability to read the newborn's cues, for example, the need for comfort, nourishment, and diaper change. Bring to the parent's attention the infant's response to their care.
- Comment positively regarding the newborn's progress.
- Ask both parents about the mother's well-being and what support they will have at home.

Sources: Lutz, K., Anderson, L., Riesch, S., Pridham, K., & Becker, P. (2009). Furthering the understanding of parent-child relationships: A nursing scholarship review series, part II: Grasping the early parenting experience—The insider view. *Journal for Specialists in Pediatric Nursing, 14*(4), 262–283. Retrieved from CINAHL Plus with Full Text database; O'Leary, J., & Thorwick, C. (2008). Attachment to the unborn child and parental mental representations of pregnancy following prenatal loss. *New Directions in Psychotherapy and Relational Psychoanalysis, 2*, 292–320.

All infants' growth should be monitored and plotted on a growth chart outlining the developmental status of the infant. Charts are available from the Department of Health and Human Services (DHHS) in French and Spanish at http://www.cdc.gov/growthcharts/. More information about this Web site is found at the end of this chapter. To reduce mortality and morbidity, both the parent and the nurse must be diligent in following preventive measures for normal-risk infants. In all community-based settings, the nurse can assist the parent in following basic prevention recommendations for children. Figure 8-4 outlines current recommendations for immunization schedule for infants and children.

Immunizations

Fifty years ago, many children died from what are preventable childhood diseases today. Smallpox has been eradicated, poliomyelitis has been eliminated from the Western hemisphere, and cases of measles and chickenpox in the United States are at a record low. All this progress has been made possible by the immunizations covered in Figure 8-4. The National Commission on Prevention Priorities has identified childhood immunizations as one of the most effective and cost-effective clinical preventive services. However, only if the number of vaccinated children and adults remains high will immunization programs continue to be effective. Immunizations are considered primary prevention because they prevent the occurrence of a disease. It is imperative that all children be immunized according to recommended standards. Immunizations should begin at birth and continue as recommended (Fig. 8-5).

Nutrition

Breast milk is widely acknowledged to be the most complete form of nutrition for infants (see Community-Based Teaching 8-1). The range of benefits includes health, growth, immunity, and development. Breast-fed infants have decreased rates of diarrhea, respiratory infections, and ear infections (Hale, 2007). Breast-feeding has long-term benefits in that children who are ever breast-fed are 15% to 25% less likely to become overweight and those babies breast-fed for 6 or more months are 20% to 40% less likely. Breast-feeding improves maternal health by reducing postpartum bleeding, promoting return to prepregnancy weight, and reducing the risks of breast cancer and osteoporosis long after the

Recommended Immunization Schedule for Persons Aged 0 Through 6 Years–United States • 2011
For those who fall behind or start late, see the catch-up schedule

Vaccine ▼ Age ►	Birth	1 month	2 months	4 months	6 months	12 months	15 months	18 months	19-23 months	2-3 years	4-6 years
Hepatitis B[1]	HepB	HepB				HepB					
Rotavirus[2]			RV	RV	RV[2]						
Diphtheria, Tetanus, Pertussis[3]			DTaP	DTaP	DTaP	See footnote[3]	DTaP				DTaP
Haemophilus influenzae type b[4]			Hib	Hib	Hib[4]	Hib					
Pneumococcal[5]			PCV	PCV	PCV	PCV				PPSV	
Inactiveated Poliovirus[6]			IPV	IPV		IPV					IPV
Influenza[7]						Influenza(Yearly)					
Measles, Mumps, Rubella[8]						MMR		See footnote[8]			MMR
Varicella[9]						Varicella		See footnote[8]			Varicella
Hepatitis[10]						HepA(2 doses)				HepA Series	
Meningococcal[11]											MCV4

Range of Recommended Ages for all Certain high-risk groups

Range of Recommended Ages for all Children

Figure 8-4 Recommended immunization schedule for persons aged 0 through 6 years—United States 2011. Retrieved from http://www.cdc.gov/vaccines/recs/schedules/downloads/child/0-6yrs-schedule-bw.pdf. These recommendations are subject to change. Once a year, consult Every Child by Two at http://www.ecbt.org/ or the CDC at http://www.cdc.gov/vaccines/recs/schedules/child-schedule.htm for updates.

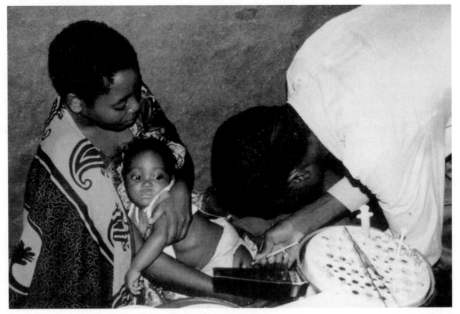

Figure 8-5 It is imperative that all children be immunized according to recommended standards.

postpartum period. The American Academy of Pediatrics (AAP) considers breast-feeding to be the ideal method of feeding and nurturing infants.

Infants and toddlers should be tested for anemia starting at 9 months of age. Hematocrit and hemoglobin screening should take place by 9 months if any of the following factors are present:

- Low socioeconomic status
- Birth weight less than 1,500 g
- Whole milk given before 6 months of age (not recommended)
- Low-iron formula given (not recommended)
- Low intake of iron-rich foods (not recommended)

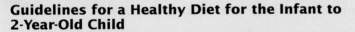

Guidelines for a Healthy Diet for the Infant to 2-Year-Old Child

- Breast milk is the single best food for infants from birth to 6 months of age. It provides good nutrition and protects against infection.
- Breast-feeding should continue for at least the first year, if possible.
- If breast-feeding is not possible or not desired, iron-enriched formula (not cow's milk) should be used during the first 12 months of life. Whole cow's milk can be used to replace formula or breast milk after 12 months of age.
- Breast-fed babies (particularly dark-skinned infants) who do not get regular exposure to sunlight may need to receive vitamin D supplements.
- Suitable solid foods should be introduced at 6 months of age. Most experts recommend iron-enriched infant rice cereal as the first food.
- Start new foods one at a time to make it easier to identify problem foods. For example, wait 1 week before adding each new cereal, vegetable, or other food.
- Use iron-rich foods, such as iron-enriched cereals, other grains, and meats.
- Do not give honey to infants during the first 12 months of life.
- Do not limit fat during the first 2 years of life.

As with any health teaching, consider the developmental stage, cognitive abilities, and culture of the client when initiating breast-feeding teaching. Teenage mothers are more interested in knowing that breast-feeding is easy, saves time, and will enhance weight loss so they can fit into their prepregnancy clothes sooner. Older mothers are typically more interested in the long-term benefits to their babies. The La Leche League is a wonderful resource for information on breast-feeding. Infant formula marketing can discourage breast-feeding, especially among low-income mothers. Infants who are breast-fed tend to gain weight more slowing compared to formula-fed infants, and formula has been associated with the increase in obese infants over the last decade. Encouraging new mothers to breast-feed is a simple intervention that can have a strong and lasting effect on the health of the mother and baby, second only to early prenatal care.

Safety

Because more children die of unintentional injuries than any other cause, it is important to counsel parents on home safety (see Community-Based Teaching 8-2). The primary issue related to safety of the infant is sleep positioning. Parents should put newborns to sleep on their backs. This position dramatically reduces deaths from **sudden infant death syndrome (SIDS)**, a leading cause of death in infants.

Parents should never smoke in the home if they have an infant or small child. Nor should a child or infant be in any environment where there is secondhand smoke. Secondhand smoke is known to be a risk factor for SIDS in infants and asthma and other respiratory conditions and otitis media in infants and children. More information for parents on reducing the risk of SIDS is available from the National Institute of Child Health and Human Development at http://www.nichd.nih.gov/sids/.

Preschool-Age Children

The leading cause of death in children ages 4 to 20 years is motor vehicle traffic crashes. Among children ages 1 to 4 years, the leading injury-related causes of death are motor vehicle crashes, drowning, and fires and burns. These deaths are, for the most part, preventable. Healthy People 2020 objectives for child health are listed in Healthy People 2020 8-2. Nurses working in community-based settings with children can use these objectives as a basis for assessing and intervening health promotion activities.

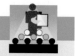

COMMUNITY-BASED TEACHING 8-2

Safety Guidelines for Infants and Young Children

- Use a car safety seat at all times until your child weighs at least 40 lb.
- Car seats must be properly secured in the back seat, preferably in the middle.
- Keep medication, cleaning solutions, and other dangerous substances in childproof containers, locked up, and out of reach of children.
- Use safety gates across stairways (top and bottom) and guards on windows above the first floor.
- Keep hot-water heater temperatures below 120°F.
- Keep unused electrical outlets covered with plastic guards.
- Use safety latches and locks, doorknob covers, and door locks.
- Keep objects and foods that cause choking away from your child, such as coins, balloons, small toy parts, hot dogs (unmashed), peanuts, and hard candies.
- Use fences that go all the way around pools, and keep gates to pools locked.
- Use window guards and safety netting to prevent falls from windows.

Source: U.S. Consumer Product Safety Commission. (2010). *Childproofing your home.* Retrieved from http://www.cpsc.gov/CPSCPUB/PUBS/SHOWER/206.pdf

SCREENING

In all community-based settings, the nurse can assist the parent in following basic prevention recommendations for children to reduce mortality and morbidity. All young children's growth should be monitored and plotted on a growth chart.

Periodic screening benefits all children. Most screening programs are developed and run by nurses in community-based settings. Preschool screening, which typically includes vision, hearing, height and weight, immunization status, and developmental screening, is an important preventive intervention. The cost of preschool screening is minimal when compared with the cost of undetected deficits that result in hardship and monetary costs to the child, parents, and society. The earlier a condition is identified, the greater the chances of lessening or eliminating the long-term effects.

Ages and Stages Questionnaires (ASQ) are used to screen infants and children from 4 to 60 months of age, covering the topics of communication, gross motor, fine motor, problem solving, and personal–social development. This easy-to-administer screening tool has the potential to identify developmental issues early for prompt intervention. The AAP recognized over a decade ago that screening and early identification leads to more effective therapy for children with developmental disabilities (AAP, 1995). The ASQ is an excellent example of secondary prevention.

Lead Screening

Lead has been present in our environment since industrialization. Children are particularly sensitive to the toxic effects of lead. Most often, **lead poisoning** is silent, with the individual having no symptoms until systemic damage has occurred. Decreased stature or growth, decreased intelligence, impaired neurobehavioral development, and adverse effects on the central nervous system, kidneys, and hematopoietic system are some of the common symptoms. Three percent of all black children compared to 1.3% of all white children had lead blood levels above safe levels in 2005. More than half of occupied, privately owned housing built before 1980 contains lead-based paint. In general, screening and assessment for lead poisoning should focus on children younger than 24 months and should begin at 12 months because children at these ages are the most vulnerable (CDC, 2010b). Assessment of high-dose lead exposure should take place at birth.

Healthy People 2020 ✳ *8-2*

OBJECTIVES FOR EARLY AND MIDDLE CHILDHOOD

- (Developmental) Increase the proportion of children who are ready for school in all five domains of healthy development: physical development, socioemotional development, approaches to learning, language, and cognitive development.
- Increase the proportion of parents who use positive parenting and communicate with their doctors or other health care professionals about positive parenting.
- (Developmental) Decrease the proportion of children who have poor sleep quality.
- Increase the proportion of elementary, middle, and senior high schools that require health education.
- Reduce the rate of child deaths.
- Increase the proportion of children with special health care needs who have access to a medical home.
- Increase the proportion of children with special health care needs who receive their care in family-centered, comprehensive, coordinated systems.
- Increase the percentage of young children with an autism spectrum disorder and other developmental delays who are screened, evaluated, and enrolled in early intervention services in a timely manner.

Source: U.S. Department of Health and Human Services, National Center for Health Statistics. (2010). *2020 topics and objectives: United States, 2020.* Washington, DC: U.S. Department of Health and Human services. Retrieved from http://www.healthypeople.gov/2020/default.aspx

Vision and Hearing Screening

Vision and hearing screening should be performed at 3 or 4 years of age and repeated once a year. Screening should be done earlier or more frequently than recommended if any of the following warning signs of visual or hearing impairment is present:

- Inward- or outward-turning eyes
- Squinting
- Headaches
- Decline in quality of schoolwork
- Blurred or double vision
- Hold objects close to eyes to see
- Poor response to noise or voice
- Hear some sounds but not others
- Slow language and speech development
- Abnormal sounding speech

IMMUNIZATIONS

Immunizations are important preventive health measures for the preschool child. The current recommended immunization schedule is found in Figure 8-4.

NUTRITION AND ACTIVITY

Nutritional status should be assessed. Key concepts related to children include independence and formation of habits that influence the futures. As children become more independent in food choices they are often more heavily influenced by media and peer pressure. Along with food choices, physical activity during these years is often critical to development of lifelong exercise along with creating a home and community environment that readily allows a child to be physically active. A combination of healthy eating habits and physical activity is essential for maintenance of normal weight throughout a lifetime.

SAFETY

Injury is the leading cause of death in young children. Many of the dangers for young children are in the home (see Community-Based Teaching 8-3). In most states, the law requires that infants and children be restrained in a safety seat when riding in a car and parents who are not compliant may be fined. Table 8-2 provides information on general child seat use for infants to 12-year-olds. These change yearly so check the Highway Traffic Safety Administration recommendations for children for updates.

COMMUNITY-BASED TEACHING 8-3

Safety Guidelines for Parents of Children of All Ages

- Use smoke detectors in your home. Change the batteries every year, and check once a month to see that they work.
- If you have a gun in your home, make sure that the gun and ammunition are locked up separately and kept out of children's reach.
- Never drive after drinking alcohol.
- Use car safety belts at all times.
- Teach your child traffic safety. Children under 9 years of age need supervision when crossing streets.
- Teach your children how and when to call 911.
- Learn basic lifesaving skills (cardiopulmonary resuscitation).
- Post the telephone number of the poison control center near your telephone.

Table 8-2 Child Passenger Safety: A Parent's Primer			
	Age/Weight	**Seat Type/Seat Position**	**Usage Tips**
Infants	Birth to at least 1 y and at least 20 lb	Infant-only seat/rear-facing	• Never use in a front seat where an air bag is present. • Tightly install child seat in rear seat, facing the rear. • Child seat should recline at approximately a 45-degree angle. • Harness straps/slots at or below shoulder level. • Harness straps snug on child; harness clip at armpit level.
Toddler/preschoolers	1–4 y/at least 20 lb to approximately 40 lb	Keep child in rear-facing seat as long as possible. Forward-facing only or high back booster/harness	• Tightly install child seat in rear seat, facing forward. • Harness straps/slots at or above child's shoulders (usually top set of slots for convertible child safety seats).
Young children	4 to at least 8 y/unless they are 4 ft 9 in (57 in) tall	Belt-positioning booster (no back, only) or high back belt-positioning booster	• Booster used with adult lap and shoulder belt in rear seat. • Shoulder belt should rest snugly across chest, rest on shoulder, and should NEVER be placed under the arm or behind the back. • Lap-belt should rest low, across the lap/upper thigh area—not across the stomach.
Child	Over 8 y or over 4 ft 9 in	Keep child in a booster seat until big enough to fit in a seat belt properly.	Belt lies across the upper thighs, and the shoulder belt fits across the chest.

Source: Highway Traffic Safety Administration. (2010). Car seat recommendations for children. Retrieved from http://www.nhtsa.gov/Safety/CPS. These change yearly so check the Highway Traffic Safety Administration recommendations for children for updates.

OTHER PREVENTIVE HEALTH MEASURES

Child abuse is a serious concern in the United States, where more than 772,000 children are victims of abuse and neglect each year. Of these, approximately 1,740 fatalities resulted from child abuse or neglect (CDC, National Center for Injury Prevention and Control [NCIPC], 2010b). Even when an adult's account of how a child is injured seems plausible, it is imperative that the nurse reassess the situation for possible child abuse. See Community-Based Teaching 8-4 for ways to prevent child abuse. Infants and children of all ages should be protected from the harmful effects of the sun.

As the most common type of cancer in the United States, skin cancer is a significant public health issue. Anyone can get skin cancer, but individuals with certain risk factors are particularly vulnerable. Some risks for skin cancer are the following (CDC, National Center for Chronic Disease Prevention and Health Promotion [NCCDPHP], 2010b):

- Lighter natural skin color
- Skin that burns, freckles, gets red easily, or becomes painful in the sun
- Blue or green eyes
- Blond or red hair
- Certain types of and a large number of moles
- Family history of skin cancer
- Personal history of skin cancer

COMMUNITY-BASED TEACHING 8-4

Child Maltreatment Prevention Strategies Focusing on Positive Parenting

For Parents

One key way to prevent child maltreatment is for nurses to assist parents to develop positive parenting skills. Through health teaching, modeling, and counseling, the nurse can encourage nurturing parental behaviors such as the following:

- Engaging in empathetic communication with their children
- Giving physical signs of affection such as hugs
  - Developing self-esteem in their children
  - Recognizing and understanding their children's feelings
  - Responding to their children's physical and emotional needs
  - Learning alternative methods to shaking, hitting, or spanking
- Provide parents with social support
- Notify the parent that if they are afraid they might harm their child, to get help by calling someone and asking for help. Suggest talking with a friend or relative, other parents, clergy, or health care providers. Encourage parents to take time for themselves. The 24-hour National Child Abuse Hotline number is 1-800-4-A-CHILD or 1-800-252-2873, 1-800-25ABUSE

For Communities

To help prevent child maltreatment, community resources and services to support families should be available and accessible. Programs can take many forms. They may occur in homes, schools, medical or mental health clinics, or other community settings. They may be one-on-one meetings or group sessions. This can be accomplished by the nurse by

- Encouraging volunteer efforts at organizations that provide family support services
- Collaborating with or sponsoring organizations such as sports teams and local businesses to communicate prevention messages
- Community organizing by working with prevention organizations and local media to develop community strategies that support parents and prevent abuse
- Providing health education to teach children, parents, and educators preventions strategies that can help keep children safe
- Participating in policy development by engaging local legislators in increasing child maltreatment prevention efforts

Centers for Disease Control and Prevention, National Center for Injury Prevention and Control. (2010a). *Understanding child maltreatment: Fact sheet.* Retrieved from http://www.cdc.gov/ViolencePrevention/pdf/CM-FactSheet-a.pdf

- Exposure to the sun through work and play
- A history of sunburns early in life

Epidemiologic studies suggest that skin cancers can be prevented if children, adolescents, and adults are protected from ultraviolet radiation. At the end of the chapter in What's on the Web, there is a Web site where you can read more about community prevention strategies. CDC recommends five options for individuals and families to protect them from sun exposure:

- Seek shade especially during midday
- Cover up with clothing to protect exposed skin
- Get a hat with a wide brim
- Grab shades
- Put on sunscreen

Poor nutrition and dental hygiene contribute to dental caries. Dental caries represent the single most common chronic disease of childhood, occurring five times as frequently as asthma, the second most common chronic condition among children. Unless identified and addressed early, caries are irreversible. More than 19% of all children have untreated caries. Poor children have nearly 12 times more restricted activity days because of dental-related illness than children from higher-income families. Pain and suffering due to untreated tooth decay can lead to difficulties eating, speaking, and attending to learning (CDC, 2010d).

Asthma is the second most common chronic condition in children. Over 10 million U.S. children aged 17 and under (14%) have ever been diagnosed with asthma; 7.1 million children still have asthma (10%). In the last 20 years, the prevalence of asthma in children has increased by over 75%. Disparity is seen in the incidence of asthma with non-Hispanic Black children being more likely to have ever been diagnosed with asthma (22%) or to still have asthma (17%) than Hispanic children (13% and 8%) or non-Hispanic White children (12% and 8%). Poverty also predicts which children will have asthma; children in poor families were more likely to have ever been diagnosed with asthma (18%) or to still have asthma (14%) than children in families that were not poor (13% and 8%) (U.S. Department of Health and Human Services, 2010).

Both the immediate environment and the quality of the air in the home contribute to children developing asthma. In many sections of the United States, poor air quality and air pollution endanger the respiratory health of children and exacerbate symptoms in children who have asthma. Because respiratory diseases send more American children to the hospital than any other illness, there is ample opportunity for disease prevention and health promotion. Nurses play a vital role in assisting children and parents in managing the symptoms of asthma.

One way to prevent flare-ups of asthma is by avoiding colds and upper respiratory infections. Handwashing is a simple and effective disease-prevention measure (Fig. 8-6). It is important to teach children handwashing skills. To explore different curriculum for teaching children about how, when, and why to wash hands, see Web sites listed in What's on the Web at the end of the chapter.

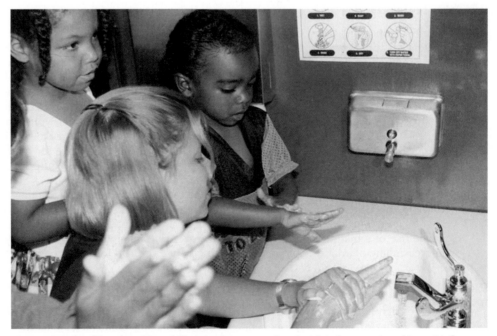

Figure 8-6 Good handwashing skills have been associated with a decrease in colds and influenza.

As with all assessments, the effectiveness lies in the strength of the questions asked. There are many resources that include general interview and developmental surveillance questions for children of all ages and their parents at http://www.brightfutures.org/.

School-Age Children

The leading cause of death for all children between ages 5 and 14 years is motor vehicle accidents. Factors that contribute to these fatalities include drunk drivers and unrestrained children. Pedestrian deaths account for 25% of all motor vehicle–related deaths sustained by children (CDC, NCCDPHP, 2010a). Healthy People 2020 objectives for school-age children are listed in Healthy People 2020 8-2.

SCREENING

Children's readiness for school depends on their experiences in the first 5 years of life. Nurses should assess the achievement of the child and provide guidance to the family on anticipated tasks. See the Bright Futures Web site for information on developmental tasks.

At age 5, screening should include vision and hearing, blood pressure, risk for lead exposure (with blood draw if deemed necessary), blood cholesterol, and developmental screening. Weight and height should also be assessed. The growth rate of children slows somewhat in the middle childhood years.

IMMUNIZATIONS

The current recommended immunization schedule for children and adolescents is shown in Figure 8-4. In 2006, the U.S. Food and Drug Administration licensed the first vaccine developed to prevent human papillomavirus and cervical cancer. The Advisory Committee on Immunization Practices recommends the use of this vaccine in females ages 9 to 26 years, with the ideal age of administration between 11 and 12 years of age and administered before onset of sexual activity. There is also information on the CDC Web site about who should not be vaccinated (CDC, 2010a).

PREVENTION OF INJURY

The most important topic to cover with all families with children is safety, and the one intervention that prevents the most loss of life and injury is using appropriate restraints when riding in an automobile. Child safety seats reduce the risk of death in passenger cars by 71% for infants and 54% for preschool children. Seatbelt laws vary from state to state. In some states, children are required to be in a booster seat until they are over 70 lb, while other states require them to ride in a booster seat until they are 80 lb. Contact your jurisdiction's department of motor vehicles for the seatbelt law in your state. At this time, air bags are not safe for children younger than 13 years and can cause fatalities. Until passenger vehicles are equipped with air bags that are safe and effective for children, those younger than 13 years should not ride in a front passenger seat that is equipped with an air bag (CDC, NCCDPHP, 2010c).

Another important safety intervention is the use of a bike helmet. Bicycling is a popular activity in the United States. About half a million people are injured in bike mishaps each year. Of these injuries, head injury is the most common cause of death and serious disability. The use of a bike helmet is effective in preventing head injury. Community programs to increase bike helmet use can reduce the incidence of head injury among bicycle riders.

PREVENTION OF CHRONIC CONDITIONS

There are significant data that many children in the United States are not adopting healthy lifestyle behavior, as obesity rates have doubled among children and teens since 1980. Among children and adolescents, annual hospital costs related to obesity were four times as much in the early 2000s as in the early 1980s. Because there is a strong relationship between obesity in childhood and the development of chronic illness in adulthood, there are numerous initiatives to prevent obesity in childhood. These initiatives for children focus on increasing physical activity, increasing daily intake of fruits and vegetables, reducing fat intake, and ensuring that children get adequate sleep every night. As the child enters middle childhood, even more emphasis should be placed on secondary prevention, which allows early intervention for health conditions that may develop into chronic conditions in adulthood. The primary contributors to chronic conditions that can be addressed are weight, nutrition, and physical activity level.

Nutrition and Weight

Overweight and obesity are increasing among children and adolescents in the United States. The rate of those overweight among preschool children aged 2 to 5 years has doubled from 5% to 10%; for school-age children aged 6 to 11 years, the rate has tripled from 2% to 6%; and for adolescents aged 12 to 19 years, the rate has more than tripled from 5% to 18% in the last 35 years, with most of the increase since the late 1970s (Ogden & Carroll, 2010). There are significant racial and ethnic disparities in obesity prevalence among U.S. children and adolescents (Figs. 8-7 and 8-8).

Obesity puts individuals at risk for elevated blood cholesterol and high blood pressure, which, in turn, are associated with heart disease and stroke, two leading causes of death in adulthood. Children who are overweight are more likely to develop type 2 diabetes, asthma, sleep apnea, and social discrimination. Being overweight in childhood and adolescence has been associated with increased adult morbidity. Disease prevention and health promotion activities that decrease the incidence of obesity are directed at improving nutrition and increasing physical activity levels. Inadequate sleep is also associated with being overweight. The suggested number of hours of sleep for various age groups is given in Table 8-3.

Reviewing basic information about the recommended intake by food groups with parent and child is an important intervention in helping families improve their nutrition and avoid overweight and obesity. Because children cannot change their exercise and eating habits by themselves, they need the help and support of their families. Parents can encourage healthy eating habits by following some simple tips:

- Provide plenty of vegetables, fruits, whole-grain products, and low-fat dairy products.
- Choose lean meats, poultry, fish, lentils, and beans for protein.

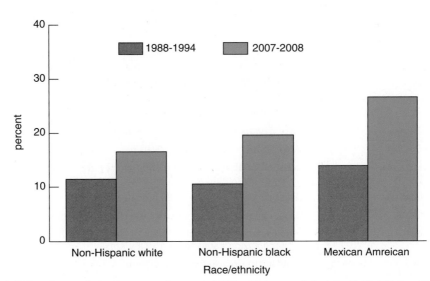

Figure 8-7 Prevalence of obesity among boys aged 12 to 19, by race/ethnicity, United States, 1988–1994 and 2007–2008.

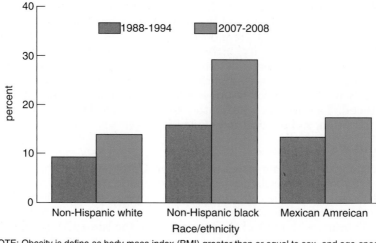

NOTE: Obesity is define as body mass index (BMI) greater than or equal to sex- and age-specific 95th percentile from the 2000CDC Growth Charts.
Souces: CDC/NCHS, National Health and Nutrition Examination Survey (NHANES) III 1988-1944 and NHANES 2007-2008.

Figure 8-8 Prevalence of obesity among girls aged 12 to 19, by race/ethnicity, United States, 1988–1994 and 2007–2008.

- Serve reasonably sized portions.
- Encourage drinking water as a beverage.
- Have no or a limited supply of sugar-sweetened beverages and high sugar or fat snacks.

Another part of balancing calories is to engage in an appropriate amount of physical activity and to avoid too much sedentary time. Playing outside, going for walks, playing tag, jumping rope, playing soccer, swimming, and dancing are all examples of free or inexpensive ways for children to be more active.

Physical Activity

In an era when increasing obesity and rising health care costs are threatening the health of the nation, programs that could reverse this trend are being cut. Schools can play a critical role in increasing physical activity through daily physical education and other opportunities

Table 8-3 All About Sleep	
Age	**Suggested Number of Hours per Night**
Newborn	Generally sleep or drowse for 16–20 h a day, divided about equally between night and day. Longest sleep is generally about 4–5 h.
6–12 mo	May nap about 3 h during the day and sleep about 11 h at night
1–3 y	Most toddlers sleep about 10–13 h.
Preschoolers	Most sleep about 10–12 h a night. If they are not napping during the day they may benefit from quiet time.
School-age	Most children 6–9 y need 10 h of sleep a night.
Children	Most children 10–12 y need a little over 9 h a night.
Teens	Adolescents need about 8–9.5 h of sleep per night (Note: they need more sleep as compared to 10- to 12-y-olds).

Adapted from KidsHealth. (2010). *All about sleep*. Retrieved from http://kidshealth.org/parent/general/sleep/sleep.html

to recreate. Unfortunately, many states have eliminated physical education programs and after-school sports programs. Physical education programs are determined by state, and the American Heart Association is working at the state level and the federal level to require that quality physical education be offered in all grades (American Heart Association, 2010). In addition, physically active children are more likely to thrive academically and socially.

Discussing the need for daily physical activity with parents is an important strategy for nurses in community-based settings. Children should participate in 60 minutes or more of age-appropriate moderate or vigorous physical activity each day (CDC, NCIPC, 2010a). Activities that provide an aerobic component include riding bikes every day (wearing a helmet, of course), walking instead of riding in a car from place to place, and playing outside everyday. Swimming, playing organized or unorganized sports, or doing physical activities together as a family is another way to increase a child's activity level.

Nurses can guide parents to help their children be active through setting an example by leading an active lifestyle themselves. This is accomplished by making physical activity part of the family's daily routine by taking family walks or playing active games together (Fig. 8-9). Children should be provided with simple equipment that encourages physical activity and then be taken to places where they can be active, such as public parks or community centers.

Pointing out the benefits of exercise may also help parents encourage children to be more physically active. Helping parents understand the relationship between activity and normal weight, future health, and the threat of developing chronic disease are a few of the strategies the nurse can use to help parents understand the importance of structuring family life and the child's life to include physical activity (visit http://www.brightfutures-forfamilies.org/materials.html).

There is an excellent Web site (listed at the end of the chapter) related to physical activity called Fitness for Kids: Getting Your Children Off the Couch. It can be found at http://www.mayoclinic.com/health/fitness/fl00030.

Adolescence

Adolescence is one of the most dynamic stages of human development. It is accompanied by dramatic physical, cognitive, social, and emotional changes that present both opportunities and challenges for the adolescent, the family, and the broader community. Nurses must be sensitive to the dynamic nature of this stage and the increasing need for independence balanced with dependence. Further, as adolescents progress through the teen years, they become increasingly able to make their own health care decisions, and they want to make these choices.

Almost half of all deaths among adolescents aged 16 to 20 years are from unintentional injuries. The majority of the total mortality in this age group can be attributed to preventable causes. Teens are far less likely to use seatbelts than any other age group (National Highway Traffic Safety Administration, 2010a). Alcohol is involved in about 31% of adolescent motor vehicle fatalities. Suicide is the third leading cause of death among those aged 10 to 24 years. As with the 15- to 19-year-old group, most of the deaths in this age group can be attributed to preventable causes (NCIPC, CDC, 2010b). At this time, most of the new human immunodeficiency virus (HIV) infections occur each year among those between ages 13 and 29 years (National Center for HIV/AIDS, 2010).

The latest National Youth Risk Behavior Survey reported that high school students responded that 85% rode bicycles without a helmet, 18% carried a weapon, and 6% had attempted suicide in the 12 months preceding the survey. Twenty percent smoked cigarettes, 41% had at least one drink of alcohol, and 25% had five or more drinks of alcohol on at least one occasion during the 30 days preceding the survey (Eaton et al., 2010).

The survey reported that of the 46% of teens who had had sexual intercourse during their lifetime, 61% used a condom during the last intercourse. As far as dietary behaviors were concerned, 12% were overweight, 22% ate five or more servings of fruits and vegetables during each of the 7 days preceding the survey, and 4% took laxatives or vomited to lose weight during the 30 days preceding the survey. As far as physical activity was concerned, 18% did vigorous physical activity for at least 60 minutes on 7 days preceding the survey, and 56% were enrolled in physical education class with 33% attending physical education class daily.

When results from 1991 are compared with results from the 2009 survey, it is noted that the percentage of students who use seatbelts has increased; those who *never* buckle up decreased from 25% to 9.7%. The percentage of students who report using alcohol has declined dramatically from 51% in 1991 to 41% in 2009. Reported binge drinking in 1991 at 31% decreased in 2009 to 24%. In 1991, 54% of youth responded never having intercourse, compared to 46% in 2010. In addition, 61% of sexually active students used a condom during last sexual intercourse compared to 46% in 1991. These changes are encouraging as they show that persistent efforts to get young people to adopt healthier behaviors can achieve positive results.

When different ethnic groups are compared, Black students, when compared to White and Hispanic high school students, are least likely to use tobacco, alcohol, or binge drink but most likely to report sexual risk behaviors and sedentary behaviors. White students are the least likely to report physical fighting, sexual risk behaviors, and being overweight but more likely to smoke cigarettes and binge drink. Hispanic students are more likely than other students to report attempted suicide, to ride in a car with a driver who had been drinking, or to use drugs such as cocaine, heroin, and methamphetamines (Eaton et al., 2010).

Healthy People 2020 objectives for adolescent health are listed in Healthy People 2020 8-3. Nurses working in community-based settings with adolescents can use these objectives as a basis for assessing and intervening health promotion activities.

Healthy People 2020 🔆 8-3

OBJECTIVES FOR ADOLESCENT HEALTH

- Increase the proportion of adolescents who have had a wellness checkup in the past 12 months.
- Increase the proportion of adolescents who participate in extracurricular and out-of-school activities.
- Increase the proportion of adolescents who are connected to a parent or other positive adult caregiver.
- (Developmental) Increase the proportion of adolescents and young adults who transition to self-sufficiency from foster care.
- Increase educational achievement of adolescents and young adults.
- Increase the proportion of schools with a school breakfast program.
- Reduce the proportion of adolescents who have been offered, sold, or given an illegal drug on school property.
- Increase the proportion of adolescents whose parents consider them to be safe at school.
- (Developmental) Increase the proportion of middle and high schools that prohibit harassment based on a student's sexual orientation or gender identity.
- Decrease the proportion of public schools with a serious violent incident.
- Reduce adolescent and young adult perpetration of, as well as victimization by, crimes.

Source: U.S. Department of Health and Human Services, National Center for Health Statistics. (2020). *2020 topics and objectives: United States, 2020*. Washington, DC: U.S. Department of Health and Human services. Retrieved from http://www.healthypeople.gov/2020/default.aspx

SCREENING

Recommendations for screening in early and later adolescence are found in the Bright Futures guidelines. Some other areas for screening adolescent clients include questions concerning smoking, alcohol and drug use, sexual activity, and injury prevention behaviors. Teens' behaviors often place them at risk for serious injury, sexually transmitted diseases (STDs), and chronic diseases. Bright Futures provides excellent developmental surveillance questions that address these issues. It is also important to keep developmental tasks in mind when assessing health issues and planning health promotion and disease prevention activities.

Because such a large proportion of deaths in this age group are preventable, safety should be the number one priority for health promotion and injury prevention. However, because of the nature of the adolescent client, this is a formidable challenge.

PREVENTION OF CHRONIC CONDITIONS

Smoking Cessation

Several excellent resources on the Internet address smoking cessation. Some are very colorful, specifically designed by teens for teens. One site is http://kidshealth.org/teen/drug_alcohol/tobacco/quit_smoking.html. Others are found at the end of the chapter. See Community-Based Teaching 8-5 for community-based teaching strategies for adolescents who want to know more about the dangers of tobacco.

Nutrition

Teaching teens about nutrition is challenging (Fig. 8-10). Bright Futures in Practice: Nutrition is an excellent resource for nutrition information for infancy through adolescence. This resource called Family Pocket Guide: Raising Healthy Infants, Children and Adolescents is available through http://www.brightfuturesforfamilies.org/materials.html.

COMMUNITY-BASED TEACHING 8-5

What You(th) Should Know About Tobacco

Tobacco and Athletic Performance

- Don't get trapped. Nicotine in cigarettes, cigars, and spit tobacco is addictive.
- Nicotine narrows your blood vessels and puts added strain on your heart.
- Smoking can wreck lungs and reduce oxygen available for muscles used during sports.
- Smokers suffer shortness of breath almost three times more often than do nonsmokers.
- Smokers run slower and can't run as far, affecting overall athletic performance.
- Cigars and spit tobacco are NOT safe alternatives.

Tobacco and Personal Appearance

- Yuck! Tobacco smoke can make hair and clothes stink.
- Tobacco stains teeth and causes bad breath.
- Short-term use of spit tobacco can cause cracked lips, white spots, sores, and bleeding in the mouth.
- Surgery to remove oral cancers caused by tobacco use can lead to serious changes in the face. Sean Marcee, a high school star athlete who used spit tobacco, died of oral cancer when he was 19 years old.

Source: Centers for Disease Control and Prevention. (2009). *Information sheet: Youth and tobacco.* Retrieved from http://www.cdc.gov/tobacco/youth/information_sheet/

Figure 8-9 Family life can be intentionally structured to include more physical activity such as taking walks with young children.

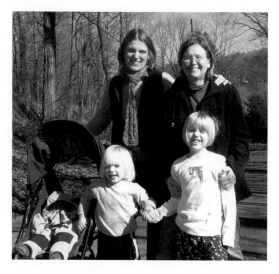

Physical Activity

Nearly half of American youth ages 12 to 21 years are not vigorously active on a regular basis. Adolescents and young adults benefit from physical activity, particularly considering that 18% of all adolescents are overweight. Adolescents should participate in 60 minutes

Figure 8-10 Suggestions for teaching adolescents about nutrition include instilling a sense of pride in identifying and choosing healthy meals and snacks.

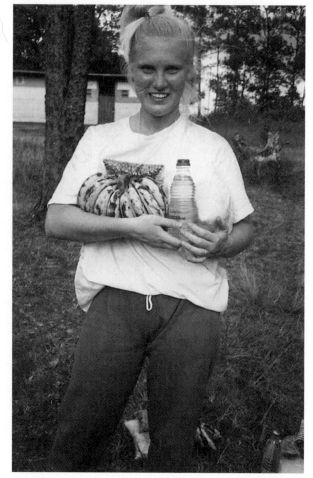

or more of age-appropriate moderate or vigorous physical activity each day (CDC, NCIPC, 2010a). Regular participation in physical education classes helps reduce obesity among low-income teenagers (Madsen, Gosliner, Woodward-Lopez, & Crawford, 2009). In addition, physically active children are more likely to thrive academically and socially.

Activities that provide an aerobic component including riding bikes every day (wearing a helmet, of course), walking instead of riding in a car from place to place, swimming, playing organized or unorganized sports, or doing physical activities as a family are other ways to increase a teen's activity level.

Nurses can guide parents to help their children be active through setting an example by leading an active lifestyle themselves. This is accomplished by making physical activity part of the family's daily routine by taking family walks or playing active games together. Physical activity helps build and maintain healthy bones, muscles, and joints; controls weight; builds lean muscle; and reduces fat. Most importantly, physical activity prevents or delays the development of high blood pressure, helps reduce blood pressure in some adolescents with hypertension, and prevents the development of type 2 diabetes.

HEALTH PROMOTION

Sexual Health Promotion

The incidence of STDs has skyrocketed, and most new HIV infections occur in people between 13 and 21 years of age (National Center for HIV/AIDS, 2010). Teens exhibit high behavioral risks for acquiring most STDs. Teenagers and young adults are more likely than other age groups to have multiple sex partners, to engage in unprotected sex, and (for young women) to choose sexual partners older than themselves. As part of holistic care, nurses in community-based settings should always assess sexuality. When discussing the topic of sexuality, take an open, frank, direct, and nonjudgmental approach. Talking openly and frankly with young teens about the benefits and risks of being sexually active may allow teens, especially girls, to understand that being sexually active is a choice. Early age of first coitus is a well-established risk factor for STDs because there is greater opportunity for exposure to pathogens. Early coitus is also associated with later high-risk cognitive, affective, and behavioral choices. Opportunities to interact with caring adults outside of their families, self-esteem building, and empowerment activities contribute to delay of first intercourse.

Other primary prevention strategies to promote sexual health include comprehensive sex education beginning in primary school. Abstinence is a highly positive choice for both sexes until they are ready to deal with the responsibility of being sexually active. However, it is not realistic as a sole strategy. The emphasis must be that sexual health promotion is a lifestyle choice and that contraception is useless if not practiced consistently. Use of condoms should be encouraged for every sexual encounter.

Some sexuality health promotion programs use a dramatic approach, with speakers who are HIV-positive or have acquired immunodeficiency syndrome (AIDS). These speakers tell their stories to teen groups, often with great success. Nurses can develop audiovisual aids (e.g., diagrams, pictures, computer-assisted instruction, PowerPoint presentations, and videos) to make sex education unforgettable. Nurses can explore with teens the differences between the facts of physiology and untrue but fervently held myths and beliefs about sex. Helping teens understand the relationship between substance abuse and STDs is another important issue to address. Peer education is a program model that is highly successful and inexpensive to implement.

Nurses can play a critical role in supporting sexual health through counseling with a direct and frank approach in all interactions with individual teens, parents, groups, and peers. Nurses in community-based settings can have an enormous impact on sexual health promotion by acting as a positive role model for sexual health and being involved in issues related to sexual health.

Suicide and Violence Prevention

Suicide, the third leading cause of death among 15- to 24-year-olds, is a complex problem that can, in some cases, be prevented by early recognition and treatment of mental disorders. Most people who kill themselves have mental or substance abuse disorders. Thus, early identification and treatment of these disorders is paramount in the prevention of suicide.

Violence is a critical public health issue in the United States. In 2007, homicide was the third leading cause of death for children aged 10 to 14 years, and the second leading cause of death for youth aged 15 to 24 years. Violence among adolescents is a critical public health issue in the United States. Youth violence refers to harmful behaviors that begin in childhood and continue into young adulthood. Behaviors such as bullying, slapping, punching, and weapon use are some common examples. One way nurses can be involved in violence prevention in the community is through school-based violence prevention programs. These programs, delivered to all students in a school or particular grade, focus on topics such as emotional self-awareness, emotional control, self-esteem, positive social skills, social problem solving, conflict resolution, and teamwork. The intent of these programs is to help children to develop social skills by providing opportunities for them to observe and interact with others. Approaches incorporate teaching, modeling, and role playing to enhance social interaction; teaching nonviolent methods for resolving conflict; and strengthening nonviolent beliefs among young people (CDC, Division of Adolescent and School Health, 2010).

Health Promotion and Disease Prevention Activities With Teens

When teaching teens about health, it is particularly important to base the teaching on what the teen already knows about the subject. It is also helpful to determine what the teen wants to learn about and begin with these topics. Cognitively, many teens are not able to conceptualize or hypothesize. This, coupled with the fact that teens tend to be egocentric, complicates determining the best teaching modalities to reach the teen population. Successful disease prevention and health promotion activities for teens incorporate these considerations. Thus, it is most effective when teaching teens about physical activity or nutrition to talk about the immediate, particular, personal impacts in areas of importance to them.

For instance, a teenage girl who is overweight may respond to information on nutrition with the incentive of losing weight so she can wear the latest clothing styles. A boy may respond to the suggestion to increase physical activity in his daily life if the nurse talks about the benefits of belonging to a team or being a sports hero. When taught about smoking cessation, teens respond to the idea that if they smoke, they are less desirable to kiss, or that their hands, clothes, and hair will smell, but not to the notion that smoking increases the chances of developing lung cancer when they are older adults. Nor do teens respond to the idea that if they are not physically fit and well nourished there is an increased chance that they will develop heart disease, diabetes, stroke, and cancer. Most teens are developmentally unable to value such notions.

Use of Complementary Therapies

The benefits of complementary and alternative modes of therapy are increasingly reported in empirical research. Complementary therapies may be advantageous as primary, secondary, or tertiary prevention strategies. Research in Community-Based Nursing Care 8-1 describes one example.

Policy

Public policy may appear, at first glance, to evolve primarily from the government, but policy makers consider many sources when developing public policy related to the health of women and children. For example, being vocal and involved in public policy issues such as gun control, allocation of health care dollars for health promotion and disease prevention programs for children, requiring daily physical education in the schools, or creating walking and bike paths are all ways that nurses can improve the health of children in our country. Supporting political candidates who value public health is another way that nurses can make a difference at the community level.

RESEARCH IN COMMUNITY-BASED NURSING CARE 8-1

School-Based Meditation Practices for Adolescents: A Resource for Strengthening Self-Regulation, Emotional Coping, and Self-Esteem

Many adolescents have unique academic, social, emotional, and behavioral needs stemming from serious personal and family challenges. School-based interventions have been established as efficacious for health promotion activities for children and adolescents. An innovative health promotion practice that is currently being introduced into school settings is meditation. This includes various types of meditation such as mindfulness meditation, the relaxation response, and transcendental meditation. These practices are readily available to school nurses and social workers as cognitive–behavioral interventions to help students enhance academic and psychosocial strengths. Further, they have been found to improve self-regulation capacities and coping abilities. This article reviews the literature on the topic, defines meditation and meditative practices, and describes the benefits and challenges of offering meditation to adolescents in a school-based setting. The researchers conclude that meditation as a cognitive–behavioral intervention improves the functioning of students. This is particularly true for students experiencing high levels of stressful life circumstances such as chronic illness, learning problems, or low self-esteem. Meditation as a regular practice has the potential to help students to manage behavior, thinking, and emotions. Meditation can be learned fairly quickly and is efficacious even for relatively brief periods of time (4–8 weeks.) Investigation of the effectiveness of meditation used in school-based programs for adolescents is a developing area of research that is expected to show much growth in the future.

Source: Wisner, B., Jones, B., & Gwin, D. (2010). School-based meditation practices for adolescents: A resource for strengthening self-regulation, emotional coping, and self-esteem. *Children & Schools*, *32*(3), 150–159. Retrieved from CINAHL Plus with Full Text database.

Nurses are considered valued professionals whose opinions and input are often sought by those who participate in the policy-making process. Participation may involve a variety of approaches from calling or sending a letter to a city, state, or federal lawmaker to testifying at a public hearing to informing a client about proposed changes in the law related to health care. Often, through public education and social marketing, the nurse may influence public opinion and, in turn, public policy. It is a professional responsibility of the graduate nurse to stay current on health care issues, particularly in their own area of professional expertise and to share that information with other members of the community. Numerous issues offer nurses the opportunity to act as advocates for maternal and child health. Through advocacy, social marketing, and education, the nurse may influence public opinion and health care public policy.

Conclusions

The primary issues involved in health promotion and disease prevention, based on Healthy People 2020, have been discussed from infancy through adolescence. Providing early prenatal care would eliminate many health conditions for newborn babies, save precious health care dollars, and improve the quality of life for countless infants. During infancy and childhood, periodic screening allows for early identification and intervention of common and preventable conditions. Helping young children and teens value and adopt healthy lifestyle choices by improving nutrition, increasing physical activity, and following basic safety recommendations is an important contribution that nurses in community-based settings can make. Advocating and participating in activities related to these issues in their own communities is another way nurses can contribute to the health of children. Lastly, being vocal and involved in public policy issues such as gun control and allocation of health care dollars for public health, as well as supporting political candidates who value public health, are all ways that nurses can improve the health of the nation's children.

What's on the Web

Administration for Children and Families Resources
INTERNET ADDRESS: http://www.acf.hhs.gov/acf_services.html
This site provides an exhaustive list of resources for families through the U.S. DHHS.

American Social Health Association (ASHA)
INTERNET ADDRESS: http://www.iwannaknow.org
This site is a part of ASHA. It is designed for teens and provides answers to questions about teen sexual health and STDs. The site provides information about relationships, sexual health, reducing risk for sexually transmitted infections and unplanned pregnancy, and more. Many resources are available on this site.

Body Mass Index: About BMI for Children and Teens
INTERNET ADDRESS: http://www.cdc.gov/nccdphp/dnpa/bmi/childrens_BMI/about_childrens_BMI.htm
This site (from the CDC) describes the concept of body mass index (BMI) and how it can be used with children and teens. It is a very helpful resource for nurses when intervening with overweight and obese children and teens.

Bright Futures
INTERNET ADDRESS: http://www.brightfutures.org
This Web site provides information about preventive and health promotion needs of infants, children, adolescents, families, and communities. The Toolkit of Resources for Families is a great resource (found at http://www.brightfutures.org/wellchildcare/toolkit/family.html). A number of publications, including handouts in Spanish, can be downloaded or ordered through the site. The Family Tip Sheets are an excellent resource when working with families with children and adolescents (found at http://www.brightfutures.org/TipSheets/index.html). These materials are written in family-friendly language and may be used by families and children as well as professionals in a range of disciplines including health, education, and child care. The companion Referral Tool and Locating Community-Based Services for Children and Families are tailored to help providers and families connect with the service they need.

CDC Growth Charts
INTERNET ADDRESS: http://www.cdc.gov/growthcharts/
This site includes growth charts as well as educational materials to prepare professionals to use and interpret the growth charts. The World Health Organization child growth standards are also on this site.

CDC Tobacco Information and Prevention Source Resources for Children and Teens
INTERNET ADDRESS: http://www.cdc.gov/tobacco/resources_for_you/children/index.htm
A list of resources to help anyone interested in teaching children, adolescents, and teens about the negative health effects associated with tobacco.

Childhood Obesity: Make Weight Loss a Family Affair
INTERNET ADDRESS: http://www.mayoclinic.com/print/childhood-obesity/FL00058
Childhood obesity is caused by eating too much and exercising too little. The solution is eating healthier foods and increasing physical activity, but it'll be tough for your child to do it alone. The most effective way to treat—and prevent—childhood obesity is to adopt healthier habits for the entire family.

Handwashing Curriculum
INTERNET ADDRESS: http://www.health.state.mn.us/handhygiene/curricula/curriculum.html
This site is very well organized and has handwashing curriculum for children aged 3 years to teens.
INTERNET ADDRESS: http://www.hummingbirded.com/freebies/Handwashing-Curriculum.pdf
This document includes numerous handouts and songs to use when teaching children about handwashing.

Health and Human Services for Kids
INTERNET ADDRESS: **http://www.hhs.gov/kids/**
This is the first site to check out when looking for health teaching materials or Web sites to use with any age child. There are numerous materials for health care professionals and educators to use on an exhaustive list of health topics.

Community Preventive Services: The Community Guide
INTERNET ADDRESS: **http://www.thecommunityguide.org/index.html**
The Guide to Community Preventive Services is a free resource to help choose programs and policies to improve health and prevent disease in your community. Systematic reviews are used to answer these questions:

• Which program and policy interventions have been proven effective?
• Are there effective interventions that are right for my community?
• What might effective interventions cost; what is the likely return on investment?

There is also a section for public health care professionals.

Healthfinder
INTERNET ADDRESS: **http://www.healthfinder.gov**
Healthfinder is a search engine for consumer health education material, maintained by the U.S. DHHS. Resources for many of the topics covered in the chapter can be found on this site.

Healthy People 2020
INTERNET ADDRESS: **http://www.healthypeople.gov/2020/default.aspx,**
http://www.healthypeople.gov/2020/topicsobjectives2020/default.aspx
This site introduces Healthy People 2020. There are resources for early and middle childhood and adolescent health under the appropriate topic headings.

Healthy People 2020 Maternal, Infant, and Child Health Interventions and Resources
INTERNET ADDRESS: **http://www.healthypeople.gov/2020/topicsobjectives2020/ebr. aspx?topicid=26**
This site provides suggested interventions, resources, and clinical recommendations to address the maternal, infant, and child health objectives of Healthy People 2010.

Kids and Asthma
INTERNET ADDRESS: **http://www.cdc.gov/asthma/children.htm**
This site is intended as a health education site for children and parents related to asthma. Here are some games and learning activities that are fun and easy to do at home or in the classroom, whether you are a child, childcare provider, parent, or teacher.

Fitness for Kids: Getting Your Children Off the Couch
INTERNET ADDRESS: **http://www.mayoclinic.com/health/fitness/fl00030**
For many children, biking to the playground and playing kickball in the backyard have given way to watching television, playing video games, and spending hours online. But it's never too late to get kids off the couch. Use these simple tips to help children develop a lifelong appreciation for activities that strengthen their bodies.

La Leche League
INTERNET ADDRESS: **http://www.llli.org**
This Web site provides information on breast-feeding, online discussion groups, and listings of local resources and groups.

Media Smart Youth
INTERNET ADDRESS: **http://www.nichd.nih.gov/msy/**
This is an interactive after-school program for children aged 11 to 13 years. It is designed to teach them about the relationship between the media and health, especially in the areas of nutrition and physical activity.

National Asthma Control Program
INTERNET ADDRESS: **http://www.cdc.gov/asthma/interventions.htm**
Client education is imperative for effective management of asthma. This is one of many Web sites offering health education about asthma. If you find that there is a need for an asthma education program in your community, this is the Web site for you. Also check out http://www.cdc.gov/asthma/faqs.htm for podcasts, videos, and other materials to use with parents.

CDC Vaccination and Immunization Home Page
INTERNET ADDRESS: http://www.cdc.gov/vaccines/
Parents often have questions about vaccinations. Unfortunately, information is sometimes published that is inaccurate or can be misleading when taken out of context. This site helps provide accurate information about immunizations.

National Institute of Child Health and Human Development
INTERNET ADDRESS: http://www.nichd.nih.gov
This site is an excellent resource for health education information for nurses to use with parents and families. It includes research about the health status of children.

The Foundation for a Smoke Free America
INTERNET ADDRESS: http://www.anti-smoking.org/info.htm
This site offers numerous resources for nurses to use to motivate youth to remain tobacco free and empower smokers to quit.

Tips for Parents About Obesity
INTERNET ADDRESS: http://www.cdc.gov/healthyweight/children/index.html
This site suggests steps parents can take to help prevent obesity in children. This page provides answers to some of the questions parents may have and provides resources to help keep families healthy.

Tips4Youth Web Page Smoking Cessation
INTERNET ADDRESS: http://www.cdc.gov/tobacco/tips4youth.htm, http://www.womenshealth.gov/quit-smoking/teens/
These two Web sites compile sites listing smoking cessation programs geared toward children, teens, and pregnant women.

The Women, Infants, and Children (WIC) Program
INTERNET ADDRESS: http://www.fns.usda.gov/wic/
WIC provides Federal grants to States for supplemental foods, health care referrals, and nutrition education for low-income pregnant, breast-feeding, and non-breast-feeding postpartum women and to infants and children up to age 5 years who are found to be at nutritional risk. The WIC program saves lives and improves the health of nutritional at-risk women, infants, and children. Numerous studies prove that the WIC program is one of the nation's most successful and cost-effective nutrition intervention programs. Since its beginning in 1974, the WIC program has earned the reputation of being one of the most successful federally funded nutrition programs in the United States. All nurses working in community-based settings benefit from knowing about the WIC program and sharing that information with the clients they serve.

References and Bibliography

American Academy of Pediatrics, Committee on Practice and Ambulatory Medicine. (1995). Recommendations for pediatric health care. *Pediatrics, 96*(2, Pt. 1), 373–374.

American College of Obstetricians and Gynecologists. (2006). *Drinking and reproductive health: A fetal alcohol spectrum disorders prevention tool kit.* Retrieved from http://www.acog.org/departments/healthIssues/FASDToolKit.pdf

American Heart Association. (2010). *Physical education in the schools.* Retrieved from http://www.americanheart.org/presenter.jhtml?identifier=3010854

Bullock, L., Everett, K., Mullen, P., Geden, E., Longo, D., & Madsen, R. (2009). Baby BEEP: A randomized controlled trial of nurses' individualized social support for poor rural pregnant smokers. *Maternal & Child Health Journal, 13*(3), 395–406. Retrieved from CINAHL Plus with Full Text database.

Centers for Disease Control and Prevention. (2009). *Information sheet: Youth and tobacco.* Retrieved from http://www.cdc.gov/tobacco/youth/information_sheet/

Centers for Disease Control and Prevention. (2010a). *HPV vaccination.* Retrieved from http://www.cdc.gov/vaccines/vpd-vac/hpv/default.html# recs

Centers for Disease Control and Prevention. (2010b). *Lead.* Retrieved from http://www.cdc.gov/nceh/lead

Centers for Disease Control and Prevention. (2010c). *Tobacco use and pregnancy.* Retrieved from http://www.cdc.gov/reproductivehealth/tobaccoUsePregnancy/index.htm

Centers for Disease Control and Prevention. (2010d). *Untreated dental caries (cavities) in children ages 2-19, United States.* Retrieved from http://www.cdc.gov/Features/dsUntreatedCavitiesKids/

Centers for Disease Control and Prevention. (2011). *Recommendations and guidelines: 2011 child & adolescentImmunization schedules*. Retrieved from http://www.cdc.gov/vaccines/recs/schedules/child-schedule.htm

Centers for Disease Control and Prevention, Division of Adolescent and School Health. (2010). *Understanding school violence: Fact sheet*. Retrieved from http://www.cdc.gov/violenceprevention/pdf/SchoolViolence_FactSheet-a.pdf

Centers for Disease Control and Prevention, National Center for Chronic Disease Prevention and Health Promotion. (2010a). *Pedestrian safety: Fact sheet*. Retrieved from http://www.cdc.gov/motorvehiclesafety/Pedestrian_Safety/factsheet.html

Centers for Disease Control and Prevention, National Center for Chronic Disease Prevention and Health Promotion. (2010b). *Skin cancer prevention*. Retrieved from http://www.cdc.gov/cancer/skin/basic_info/prevention.htm

Centers for Disease Control and Prevention, National Center for Chronic Disease Prevention and Health Promotion. (2010c). *Child passenger safety: Fact sheet*. Retrieved from http://www.cdc.gov/MotorVehicleSafety/Child_Passenger_Safety/CPS-Factsheet.html

Centers for Disease Control and Prevention, National Center for Injury Prevention and Control. (2010a). *Making physical activity a part of a child's life*. Retrieved from http://www.cdc.gov/physicalactivity/everyone/getactive/children.html

Centers for Disease Control and Prevention, National Center for Injury Prevention and Control. (2010b). *Understanding child maltreatment: Fact sheet*. Retrieved from http://www.cdc.gov/ViolencePrevention/pdf/CM-FactSheet-a.pdf

Clancy, C. (2008). Quitting smoking: Helping patients kick the habit. *Nursing for Women's Health, 12*(4), 282–285. Retrieved from CINAHL Plus with Full Text database.

Eaton, D. K., Kann, L., Kinchen, S., Shanklin, S., Ross, J., Hawkins, J., et al. (2010). Youth risk behavior surveillance, United States, 2009. *MMWR Surveillance Summaries, 59*(5), 1–142. Retrieved from http://www.cdc.gov/mmwr/pdf/ss/ss5905.pdf

Eckenrode, J., Campa, M., Luckey, D., Henderson, C., Cole, R., Kitzman, H., et al. (2010). Long-term effects of prenatal and infancy nurse home visitation on the life course of youths: 19-year follow-up of a randomized trial. *Archives of Pediatrics & Adolescent Medicine, 164*(1), 9–15. Retrieved from CINAHL Plus with Full Text database.

Federal Interagency Forum on Children and Family Statistics. (2010). *American's children: Key national indicators of well-being, 2010*. Washington, DC: U.S. Government Printing Office. Retrieved from http://www.childstats.gov

Ferguson, C., Langwith, C., Muldoon, A., & Leonard, J. (2010). *Improving obesity management in adult primary care: Executive summary. Strategies to Overcome and Prevent (STOP) Obesity Alliance. George Washington University School of Public Health and Health Services, Department of Health Policy*. Retrieved from http://www.stopobesityalliance.org/wp-content/assets/2010/03/STOP-Obesity-Alliance-PC-Paper-Executive-Summary-FINAL.pdf

Gabe, T. (2009). *Poverty in the United States: 2008. Congressional Research Service 7-5700*. Retrieved from http://www.fas.org/sgp/crs/misc/RL33069.pdf

Guthrie, K., Gaziano, C., & Gaziano, E. (2009). Toward better beginnings: Enhancing healthy child development and parent-child relationships in a high-risk population. *Home Health Care Management & Practice, 21*(2), 99–108. Retrieved from CINAHL Plus with Full Text database.

Hale, R. (2007). Infant nutrition and the benefits of breastfeeding. *British Journal of Midwifery, 15*(6), 368–371.

Huggins, C. (2006). *Early screening spots vision problems in infants*. Retrieved from http://www.hlm.nih.gov/medlineplus/news/fullstory_35187.html

Institute of Medicine. (2006). *Preterm birth: Causes, consequences, and prevention. Report brief*. Retrieved from http://www.iom.edu/Reports/2006/Preterm-Birth-Causes-Consequences-and-Prevention.aspx

Kaiser Family Foundation. (2010). *Percentage of mothers beginning prenatal care in the first trimester*. Retrieved from http://www.statehealthfacts.org/comparebar.jsp?ind=45&cat=2

KidsHealth. (2010). *All about sleep*. Retrieved from http://kidshealth.org/parent/general/sleep/sleep.html#

Lutz, K., Anderson, L., Riesch, S., Pridham, K., & Becker, P. (2009). Furthering the understanding of parent-child relationships: A nursing scholarship review series, part II: Grasping the early parenting experience—The insider view. *Journal for Specialists in Pediatric Nursing, 14*(4), 262–283. Retrieved from CINAHL Plus with Full Text database.

MacDorman, M., & Mathew, R. (2009). *Recent trends in infant mortality in the United States: NCHS data brief, no. 9.* Hyattsville, MD: National Center for Health Statistics. Retrieved from http://www.cdc.gov/nchs/data/databriefs/db09.htm

MacDorman, M., & Mathew, R. (2010). *Behind international rankings of infant mortality: How the United States compares with Europe. International health rankings: A look behind the numbers. National Conference on Health Statistics. August 16–18, 2010.* Retrieved from www.cdc.gov/nchs/ppt/nchs2010/44_MacDorman.pdf

Madsen, K., Gosliner, W., Woodward-Lopez, G., & Crawford, P. (2009). Physical activity opportunities associated with fitness and weight status among adolescents in low-income communities. *Archives of Pediatrics & Adolescent Medicine, 163*(11), 1014–1021. Retrieved from CINAHL Plus with Full Text database.

Milan, J., & White, A. (2010). Impact of a stage-tailored, web-based intervention on folic acid-containing multivitamin use by college women. *American Journal of Health Promotion, 24*(6), 388–395. Retrieved from CINAHL Plus with Full Text database.

Monteiro, L. A. (1985). Florence Nightingale on public health nursing. *American Journal of Public Health, 75*(2), 181–186.

National Academy of Sciences. (2010). *Dietary reference intakes (DRIs): Recommended intakes for individuals, vitamins.* Retrieved from http://iom.edu/Activities/Nutrition/SummaryDRIs/~/media/Files/Activity%20Files/Nutrition/DRIs/DRISummaryListing3.ashx

National Center for HIV/AIDS. (2010). *HIV in the U.S.* Retrieved from http://www.cdc.gov/hiv/resources/factsheets/PDF/us.pdf

National Center for Injury Prevention and Control, Centers for Disease Control and Prevention. (2010a). *10 Leading causes of death, United States.* Retrieved from http://webappa.cdc.gov/cgi-bin/broker.exe

National Center for Injury Prevention and Control, Centers for Disease Control and Prevention. (2010b). *Youth suicide.* Retrieved from http://www.cdc.gov/ncipc/dvp/Suicide/youthsuicide.htm

National Highway Traffic Safety Administration. (2010a). *Teen drivers: Seat belt use.* Retrieved from http://www.nhtsa.gov/Driving+Safety/Driver+Education/Teen+Drivers/Teen+Drivers+-+Seat+Belt+Use

National Highway Traffic Safety Administration. (2010b). *Traffic safety facts: Teen drivers.* Retrieved from http://www-nrd.nhtsa.dot.gov/Pubs/811169.PDF

Nurse–Family Partnership. (2010). *Fact sheets.* Retrieved from http://www.nursefamilypartnership.org/about/fact-sheets

Ogden, C., & Carroll, M. (2010). *Prevalence of obesity among children and adolescents: United States: Trends 1963–1965 through 2007–2008. National Center for Health Statistics.* Retrieved from http://www.cdc.gov/nchs/data/hestat/obesity_child_07_08/obesity_child_07_08.pdf

Olds, D., Kitzman, H., Cole, R., Hanks, C., Arcoleo, K., Anson, E., et al. (2010). Enduring effects of prenatal and infancy home visiting by nurses on maternal life course and government spending: Follow-up of a randomized trial among children at age 12 years. *Archives of Pediatrics & Adolescent Medicine, 164*(5), 419–424. Retrieved from CINAHL Plus with Full Text database.

Project America. (2010). *International poverty.* Retrieved from http://www.project.org/info.php?recordID=467

Rauzon, S., Wang, M., Studer, N., & Crawford, P. (2010). An evaluation of a school lunch initiative. Retrieved from http://cwh.berkeley.edu/

U.S. Consumer Product Safety Commission. (2010). *Childproofing your home.* Retrieved from www.cps.gov

U.S. Department of Health and Human Services, National Center for Health Statistics. (2010). *Health, United States, 2010.* Washington, DC: U.S. Department of Health and Human services. Retrieved from http://healthypeople.gov/Default.htm

U.S. Department of Health and Human Services, National Center for Health Statistics. (2020). *2020 topics and objectives: United States, 2020.* Washington, DC: U.S. Department of Health and Human Services. Retrieved from http://www.healthypeople.gov/2020/default.aspx

U.S. Department of Health and Human Services, Centers for Disease Control and Prevention, National Center for Health Statistics. (2010). *Summary health statistics for U.S. children: National Health Interview Survey, 2009.* Retrieved from http://www.cdc.gov/nchs/data/series/sr_10/sr10_247.pdf

Wisner, B., Jones, B., & Gwin, D. (2010). School-based meditation practices for adolescents: A resource for strengthening self-regulation, emotional coping, and self-esteem. *Children & Schools, 32*(3), 150–159. Retrieved from CINAHL Plus with Full Text database.

LEARNING ACTIVITIES

JOURNALING ACTIVITY 8-1

1. In your clinical journal, describe a situation you have encountered when doing health screening or health promotion activities.
   - What did you learn from this experience?
   - How will you practice differently based on this experience?
2. In your clinical journal, describe a situation in which you have observed infants or children not receiving the disease prevention or health promotion services that they needed.
   - How could or would you like to advocate for this issue when you begin to practice as an RN?
   - What could you do now?

CLIENT CARE ACTIVITY 8-2

You are working as a community-based nurse making home visits to pregnant teens through the clinic where you are employed. A school nurse from a school in your community calls the clinic and requests that a home visit be made to Shantrell, who has shared with the school nurse that she is pregnant. She has not had any prenatal care. All you know is that Shantrell is 16 years old, pregnant, and no longer going to school. When you drive to the client's home, you notice that the house is very old, with old cars and debris in the yard.

- What else do you assess as you drive through the neighborhood?

You knock on the door. You notice that the paint is peeling on the outside of the house, and it looks like it hasn't been painted in a long time. Your client, Shantrell, comes to the door. You greet her, tell her your name, the name of the clinic you work for, and why you are visiting. During the first part of the visit, you spend some time getting to know Shantrell.

- What could you use for a guide for interview questions?

You learn that Shantrell found out that she was pregnant 1 month ago, and she is now 3 months pregnant. She has not come into the clinic because she thought that she only needed to see the doctor the month before the baby was born.

- What would you want to screen for?
- What topics would you want to address during the rest of the visit?
- What other questions would you ask?
- What will be your number-one priority?
- What do you hope to screen for and teach about in the next visit?

CLIENT CARE ACTIVITY 8-3

Shantrell gave birth to a baby girl weighing 7 lb 6 oz last week. She named the baby Precious. Both mom and baby did well during and after delivery. The baby is crying when you arrive for the visit. Shantrell picks up the baby, holds her close, and quietly talks to her.

- What does this tell you about Shantrell's ability to comfort the newborn?
- What do you do at this point?

Shantrell says she is breast-feeding Precious because "Remember we talked about it and I thought I didn't want to do it. You told me that if I breast-feed my baby, I will lose my big tummy and look slimmer faster." You ask how the feeding is going, and she states, "Good. When I am at school, my mom gives her a bottle of milk."

- What screening would you do at every visit?
- What special risks may this infant have?
- What would your priority be at this visit?

PRACTICAL APPLICATION ACTIVITY 8-4

Contact the director of a day care center in a community where there is a high rate of low-income families or that serves low-income families. These families are likely to have limited access to well child care and health care. Talk to the day care director about the health teaching that he or she sees as important to the kids and parents they serve. Develop a class or classes according to the director's request. One idea is to use the handwashing curricula listed in What's on the Web. (Some of these curricula are in Spanish and Hmong as well as English.) Another approach is to develop a teaching sheet according to the topics that the day care staff members identify as important for them. Check the Bright Futures Web site for teaching materials once you decide on a topic.

CLIENT CARE ACTIVITY 8-5

Make a home visit to a family with a newborn baby. Use Community-Based Nursing Care Guidelines 8-1 to assess and intervene with issues related to attachment. Identify family strengths or assets and needs and formulate one or more short- and long-term nursing diagnoses. Use at least one of the nursing interventions listed in the guidelines and evaluate how well it worked, why it did or didn't work, and what other things you would do on the next visit. Document your care.

Chapter 9

Health Promotion and Disease and Injury Prevention for Adults

ROBERTA HUNT

Learning Objectives

1 Identify the leading causes of death for adults.

2 Discuss the major diseases and threats to health for adults.

3 Summarize the primary health issues for adults.

4 Identify nursing roles for each level of prevention for primary health issues for adults.

5 Compose a list of nursing interventions for the primary health issues for adults.

6 Determine health needs for adults for which a nurse could be an advocate.

Key Terms

health indicator
moderate physical activity
obese
overweight

Chapter Topics

Health Status of Adults

Eliminating Disparity in Health Care

Health Screening for Adults

Interventions for Leading Health Indicators

Use of Complementary Therapies

Policy

Conclusions

The Nurse Speaks

My first job working as a staff nurse was on the oncology unit for a large teaching hospital in New York. Many of our patients did not have insurance. One day I floated to a general medical–surgical unit, where I took care of a 50-year-old woman named Linda who was admitted for cholecystitis. It was a quiet day on the unit, so as I was doing my morning assessment, I took some time to talk to her. She told me that her husband was disabled and that they had four children. Although she worked full time as a nurse's aide, to get family insurance, she had to pay $800 a month, and they could not afford to pay such a large premium. Consequently, no one in her family was insured except her husband. Her younger sister passed away the year before from breast cancer. She told me, "It was my third sister who has died of breast cancer. Two of my mother's sisters and my grandma died of breast cancer." We talked about the importance of yearly mammography for women over 50, particularly if they have a family history of breast cancer. She said she was aware of the need for the screening but had never had mammography because she could not afford to pay $900 for the test. I told her about the National Breast and Cervical Cancer Early Detection Program (NBCCEDP) and gave her the number to call. She told me she would contact them and make an appointment.

Three months later I saw Linda on the oncology unit. She had contacted the NBCCEDP and had mammography. She was in the hospital for surgery for early-stage breast cancer. I never appreciated the importance of early screening and detection so much as I did that day.

Susan Larson, RN
Oncology Nurse, St. Paul, Minnesota

Health Status of Adults

The major causes of death in the United States (Table 9-1) often result from behaviors and lifestyle choices that contribute to injury, violence, and illness. Environmental factors, such as lack of access to quality health services, also contribute to the major causes of death. For the nurse, this underscores the importance of understanding and monitoring health behaviors, environmental factors, and community health systems. This chapter will assist the nurse to understand and learn to monitor health behaviors that affect health and contribute to the major causes of death and disability. Ultimately, nursing interventions in community-based care are intended to encourage healthy behaviors.

Because the average person is living longer, more attention is now focused on preserving quality of life rather than simply extending length of life. Chief among the factors involving preserving quality of life is the prevention and treatment of musculoskeletal conditions. Demographic trends also indicate that people will need to continue to work to an older age. Nurses will increasingly be involved in efforts to decrease the adverse social and economic consequence of high rates of activity limitation and disability of older persons.

As discussed in Chapter 2, health is determined by the interrelationships among the determinants of health. These determinants fall into the broad categories of policy making, social factors, health services, individual behavior, and biology and genetics. This chapter focuses on the individual behavioral determinants of health. Common examples of individual behavioral determinants of health are diet, physical activity, hand washing, alcohol, cigarette, and other drug use. Individual behavior is the determinant of health most frequently addressed by nurses working in the community. An example being if the nurse assists an individual to quit smoking, his or her risk of developing heart disease is greatly reduced.

Table 9-1 Leading Causes of Death According to Age, United States, 2007	
Age	**Cause of Death**
25–34 years	Unintentional injuries
	Suicide
	Homicide
35–44 years	Unintentional injuries
	Malignant neoplasm
	Heart disease
45–54 years	Malignant neoplasm
	Heart disease
	Unintentional injuries
55–64 years	Heart diseases
	Malignant neoplasm
	Chronic low respiratory disease
65 years and over	Malignant neoplasm
	Cerebrovascular diseases

Source: Office of Statistics and Programming, (2011). National Center for Injury Prevention and Control, Centers for Disease Control and Prevention Data Source: National Center for Health Statistics (NCHS), National Vital Statistics System. Leading causes of death. Retrieved from http://webappa.cdc.gov/cgi-bin/broker.exe

Eliminating Disparity in Health Care

Recommendations from Healthy People 2010 offer a foundation for all health promotion and disease prevention nursing actions. This chapter focuses on three of the goals from Healthy People 2020 as they relate to adult health. These are attaining higher quality, longer lives free of preventable disease, disability, injury, and premature death; achieving health equity, eliminating disparities, and improving the health of all groups; and promoting quality of life, healthy development, and healthy behaviors across all life stages.

The first goal of Healthy People 2020 is to attain higher quality, longer lives free from preventable disease, disability, injury, and premature death. For adult health, a combination of unhealthy behaviors that include smoking, lack of exercise, poor diet, and substantial alcohol consumption greatly increase the risk of premature death (Kvaavik, Batty, Ursin, Huxley, & Gale, 2010). Differences in health and access to health care services by gender, age, race or ethnicity, education or income, disability, geographic location, or sexual orientation also must be considered in order to improve the health of all individuals. For example, men have a life expectancy that is 5 years less than that for women. Likewise, information about the biologic and genetic characteristics of African Americans, Hispanics, Native Americans, Alaska Natives, Asians, Native Hawaiians, and Pacific Islanders do not explain the health disparities experienced by these groups compared with the White, non-Hispanic population in the United States.

Disparity in health in the United States is well documented with numerous federal initiatives undertaken in an attempt to reduce these disparities. Despite the fact that one of the goals in Healthy People 2000 and in 2010 was to reduce health disparities, analysis of disparities between non-Hispanic Black and non-Hispanic White populations nationwide shows it widened for 6 of the 15 health status indicators from 1990 to 2005. Leading **health indicators** for Healthy People 2020 are given in Healthy People 2020 9-1.

Income and education underlie many health disparities in the United States. The two are intrinsically related; people with the worst health status are among those with the highest poverty rates and least education. Poverty disproportionately affects women. Income inequality in the United States has increased over the past three decades. Minorities are more likely to be uninsured and less likely to have a regular source of, or access to, specialty

Healthy People 2020 ❋ *9-1*

LEADING HEALTH INDICATORS

1. Physical activity	6. Mental health
2. Overweight and obesity	7. Injury violence
3. Tobacco use	8. Environmental quality
4. Substance abuse	9. Immunization
5. Responsible sexual behavior	10. Access to health care

care. Uninsured people are less likely to be recommended care for disease prevention and management. There are differences between individuals with private insurance and no insurance for measures related to preventive services, including cancer screening, dental care, counseling about diet and exercise, and flu vaccination as well as diabetes management (Agency for Healthcare Research and Quality [AHRQ], 2009a).

People with disabilities are identified as people who have activity limitations, people who need assistive devices, or people who perceive themselves as having a disability. Roughly, 16% of the adult population reports some level of limitation in physical functioning. Many people with disabilities lack access to health services and medical care (Centers for Disease Control and Prevention, National Center for Disease Statistics, 2010a).

Twenty-five percent of Americans live in rural localities. In rural and remote areas, many people with mental illnesses have less adequate access to care, more limited availability of skilled care providers, lower family incomes, and greater societal stigma for seeking mental health treatment as compared to their urban counterparts. Those living in rural areas are less likely to use preventive screening services, exercise regularly, or wear seat belts, and are more likely to be uninsured. Compared to urban counterparts, residents in rural communities have a higher chance of chronic conditions such as diabetes but are less likely to receive recommended services to manage their condition and die more frequently from heart disease (AHRQ, 2009a).

In addition, rural Americans are less likely to have private health insurance benefits for mental health care. Even those individuals living in rural communities who have insurance policies are more likely to have limited or no mental health coverage.

Gay men and lesbians have health problems unique to their populations. Gay men are more likely than heterosexual men to have acquired human immunodeficiency virus (HIV) and other sexually transmitted diseases (STDs), and they are at an increased risk for substance abuse, depression, and suicide. Gay and bisexual individuals account for more than half (53%) of all new HIV infections in the United States each year, as well as nearly half (48%) of people living with HIV (National Center for HIV/AIDS, 2010). In some parts of the United States, lesbians, gay men, bisexual individuals, and transgender people are reluctant to reveal their sexual orientation or gender identity to health care providers and will avoid health care settings because of lack of trust.

Health Screening for Adults

As with clients at other ages, health screening for adults may be intended for primary, secondary, or tertiary prevention. Primary prevention to prevent the initial occurrence of a disease with an adult client could be immunization screening and recommendation of an annual flu shot. Secondary prevention could be screening for hypertension at a health fair or yearly mammography for women over 40 years of age. Tertiary prevention could be initiating an exercise program for an **obese** client who has type 2 diabetes.

Table 9-2 Ranking of Preventative Services for Cost-Effectiveness
Discuss daily aspirin use—men 40+, women 50+
Childhood immunizations
Smoking cessation advice and help to quit—adults
Alcohol screening and brief counseling—adults
Colorectal cancer screening—adults 50+
Hypertension screening and treatment—adults 18+
Influenza immunization—adults 50+
Vision screening—adults 65+
Cervical cancer screening—women
Cholesterol screening and treatment—men 35+, women 45+
Pneumococcal immunizations—adults 65+
Breast cancer screening—women 40+
Chlamydia screening – sexually active women under 25 years of age
Discuss calcium supplementation—women
Vision screening—preschool children
Discuss folic acid use—women of childbearing age
Obesity screening—adults
Depression screening—adults
Hearing screening—adults 65+
Injury prevention counseling—parents of children ages 0–4
Osteoporosis screening—women 65+
Cholesterol screening—men <35, women <45 at high risk
Diabetes screening—adults at risk
Diet counseling—adults at risk
Tetanus-diphtheria booster—adults

Source: Rankings of preventive services for the US population. Partnership for Prevention. Retrieved from http://www.prevent.org/National-Commission-on-Prevention-Priorities/Rankings-of-Preventive-Services-for-the-US-Population.aspx

The nurse should encourage all clients to actively practice prevention. One strategy is to use the Women/Men: Stay Healthy at Any Age screening guide available at no cost from http://www.ahrq.gov/ppip/adguide/. There are two versions: one for men and one for women. This resource is a simple tool for the nurse to guide clients in identifying and planning health promotion and disease prevention activities. The guide contains information on screening as well as topics related to the leading health indicators. There are questions throughout the guide to empower the client to take charge of his or her own health care.

The American College of Preventive Medicine has identified the most cost-effective clinical preventive services (Table 9-2). Nurses working in the community setting can use this list as a guide for setting priorities for disease prevention interventions.

GENERAL SCREENING

Major areas of adult health screening covered in the Women/Men: Stay Healthy at Any Age screening guide include blood pressure, cholesterol, weight, and immunizations. Maintaining a normal blood pressure protects people from heart disease, stroke, and kidney problems. It is recommended that all adults have their blood pressure checked regularly.

Recommended Immunizations for Adults

- Tetanus–diphtheria: every 10 years.
- Measles–mumps–rubella: For women considering pregnancy, if born after 1956.
- Pneumococcal (pneumonia): At about age 65 or before for those with a chronic condition.
  - Depending on health problems, a pneumonia shot at a younger age or shots to prevent diseases such as whooping cough or shingles may require additional immunizations.
- Influenza: Most people 50 or older need a flu shot every year. If under 50 years of age, a flu shot is recommended for those who work with high-risk populations or live with someone who works with high-risk populations and pregnant women after the first trimester. Those who have a chronic condition, such as lung, heart, or kidney disease; diabetes; HIV; or cancer may need both influenza and pneumococcal immunizations.
- Hepatitis B: For people who have contact with human blood or body fluids, have unprotected sex, or share needles during intravenous drug use. Health professionals should also consider hepatitis B immunization. Those who travel to areas where hepatitis B is common.
  - Additional vaccinations may be necessary as determined by the individual's health care team.
  - To guide individuals to find what specific immunizations they might need, go to www2.cdc.gov/nip/

Source: Agency for Healthcare Research and Quality. (2010). *Adult resources.* Retrieved from http://www.ahrq.gov/ppip/adguide/

Those with high blood pressure should work with their health care provider to lower it by changing their diet, losing weight, exercising, and, if prescribed, taking medication.

Cholesterol should be checked in men over 35 years of age and women from ages 45 years. If it is within a normal range, it should be checked every 5 years. If it is not, there are many strategies to lowering it by changing diet, losing excess weight, and getting exercise. Weighing too much or too little can lead to health problems. Healthy diet and regular exercise are factors that contribute to weight loss. Assessment should include the evaluation of body mass index (BMI), waist circumference, and overall medical risk.

Immunization is cited as one of the greatest achievements of public health in the 20th century. It is important to continue to increase the proportion of children who receive all vaccines, as well as the proportion of adults who update all vaccines as well as are vaccinated annually against the flu (Box 9-1).

Oral health care is also important for overall general health. Not only will proper oral care preserve teeth for a lifetime, but flossing every day contributes to a longer life (Community-Based Teaching 9-1). Poor oral hygiene and gum disease is associated with heart disease (Andriankaja, 2009), as well as diabetes, blood infection, and even low birth weight infants.

COMMUNITY-BASED TEACHING 9-1

Basic Principles of Oral Health

- Visit your dentist regularly for checkups.
- Brush after meals.
- Use dental floss daily.
- Limit the intake of sweets, especially between meals.
- Do not smoke or chew tobacco products.

CANCER SCREENING

Colorectal cancer is the second leading cause of death from cancer. If colorectal cancer is caught early, it can be treated. The risk of developing colorectal cancer increases with advancing age. Risk factors include inflammatory bowel disease and a family or personal history of colorectal cancer or polyps. Lack of regular physical activity, low fruit and vegetable intake, a low-fiber diet, obesity, and alcohol consumption are other contributing factors. Reducing the number of deaths from colorectal cancer chiefly depends on detecting and removing precancerous colorectal polyps, as well as detecting and treating the cancer in its early stages. People 50 to 75 years of age should be screened regularly using a combination of the three recommended screening tests: high sensitivity fecal occult blood test, sigmoidoscopy, or colonoscopy (Centers for Disease Control and Prevention [CDC], 2009b).

There are three main strategies used to screen the breasts for cancer. Risk factors such as dense breast tissue and family history are all variables to be considered when determining the best screening protocol. Regular mammography is one method to detect breast cancer early, when it is easier to treat but before it is big enough to feel or cause symptoms. Having regular mammograms can lower the risk of dying from breast cancer. The U.S. Preventive Services Task Force (2010) recommends that women age 50 to 74 years have a mammogram every 2 years. Women age 40 to 49 years should consult their physician about the recommended frequency depending on their risk factors. Some women may require beginning mammograms at an earlier age and more frequently, depending on individual health history and density of breast tissue.

All women should have an annual Pap smear starting at age 18 or when they become sexually active. Those who have three or more normal annual tests may be tested less frequently, at the discretion of the nurse practitioner or the physician. National Breast and Cervical Cancer Early Detection Program (NBCCEDP) offers free or low-cost mammograms and education about breast cancer. Consult the Web site at http://apps.nccd.cdc.gov/cancercontacts/nbccedp/contacts.asp for more information or to find out where your clients can get free or low-cost clinical breast examinations, mammograms, pap tests, pelvic examinations, diagnostic testing if results are abnormal, or referrals to treatment in your area.

Prostate cancer is the most commonly diagnosed form of cancer, second to skin cancer, and is second to lung cancer as a cause of cancer-related death among men. The two most common tests used by physicians to detect prostate cancer are the digital rectal exam and the prostate-specific antigen (PSA). Medical experts do not universally support the PSA screening for prostate cancer for all men because the test can be abnormal for reasons other than prostate cancer. This means while a potential benefit of PSA is finding cancer early, when treatment may be more effective, one of the potential risks include false-positive test results. False-positive results can lead to initiating treatment for prostate cancer that may never impact health or longevity (Wolf et al., 2010). Therefore, men should talk to their physician or nurse practitioner about screening if they are from 50 to 75 years old, have a father or brother with prostate cancer, or are African American (CDC, 2010a).

Skin cancer is the most common form of cancer in the United States with more than one million new cases of skin cancer diagnosed each year. Exposure to the sun's ultraviolet rays appears to be the most important environmental factor in the development of skin cancer. Skin cancer can be prevented by following consistent sun-protective practices. Risk factors include the following:

- Light skin color, red or blond hair color, and blue or green eye color
- Family history of skin cancer
- Personal history of skin cancer
- Chronic exposure to the sun through work or play
- History of sunburns early in life
- Certain types and a large number of moles
- Skin that burns, freckles, reddens easily, or becomes painful in the sun, which indicate sun sensitivity and sun damage (CDC, 2010b)

SCREENING FOR HIGH-RISK VULNERABLE GROUPS

In the last decade, disparity in some areas of health screening has widened or gotten worse. The percentage of Black, Asian, American Indian, and Hispanics adults age 50 and over who received a colonoscopy, sigmoidoscopy, proctoscopy, or fecal occult blood test decreased, while at the same time, Blacks and Hispanics both had worsening disparities in colorectal cancer mortality. Disparities in pneumococcal vaccination have been worsening for Asians and Hispanics at a rate of 4.7% per year and 2.4% per year, respectively. Further, mammography rates remain significantly lower for Hispanic women compared to non-Hispanic White women (58.9% compared with 68.2%), while mammography rate for poor women is about two thirds that for high-income women (48.5% compared with 75.3%). The only groups to achieve the Healthy People 2010 target of 70% of women age 40 and over receiving a mammogram within the past 2 years were women with high income (75.3%), women with at least some college education (72.5%), and women with private insurance (74.2%) (AHRQ, 2010). These data provide compelling evidence that more effort should be directed to screening programs and initiatives for high-risk vulnerable groups.

Interventions for Leading Health Indicators

Evidence reflects that some of the leading causes of death and disability in the United States—such as heart disease, cancer, stroke, some respiratory diseases, unintentional injuries, HIV, and AIDS—can often be prevented by making lifestyle changes. About two thirds of all mortalities and a great amount of morbidity, suffering, and rising health care costs among adults result from three causes. Heart disease and cancer are the leading causes of death in adults. Three behaviors are the primary contributors to these causes of death: tobacco use, dietary patterns, and physical inactivity. Staying physically active, eating right, and not smoking (or quitting if you do smoke) are the three most important strategies to better health (Fig. 9-1). Hypertension, smoking,

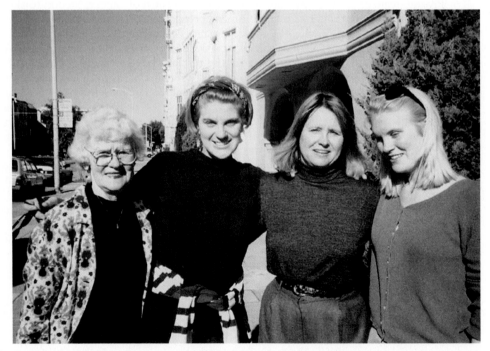

Figure 9-1 A healthy lifestyle incorporating physical activity, good nutrition, social support, and avoidance of activities that are detrimental to health can improve the quality of life for adults of all ages.

abdominal obesity, diet, and physical inactivity are responsible for a full 80% of all stroke risk, with stroke being the third most common cause of death (O'Donnell, 2010).

PHYSICAL ACTIVITY

Engaging in regular physical activity on most days of the week reduces the risk of developing or dying from some of the leading causes of illness and death. Box 9-2 presents an overview of the relationship between physical activity and morbidity and mortality.

More than 65% of adults in the United States do not engage in recommended amounts of physical activity. Physical inactivity is more common among women than men, African American and Hispanic adults than White adults, older adults than younger adults, and less affluent people than more affluent people.

"How much activity?" and "How do I start?" are two common questions clients ask about physical activity. Clients who have been sedentary or are obese may want to start by reducing sedentary time and gradually building physical activity into each day. A client may begin by gradually increasing daily activities such as taking the stairs or walking or swimming at a slow pace.

The need to avoid injury during physical activity is a high priority. Before beginning an exercise program, all adults over 40 years of age should speak to their physician or nurse practitioner. Walking is an ideal activity to increase physical activity because it is safe and accessible to most people. For those who have been physically inactive, a starting point can be walking 10 minutes, 3 days a week, building to 30 to 45 minutes of more intense walking and gradually increasing to a total of 250 minutes a week. Table 9-3 shows the current recommendations for physical activity for adults. **Moderate physical**

BOX 9-2   **The Effects of Physical Activity on Health**

Regular physical activity reduces the risk of the following:
- Dying prematurely
- Dying prematurely from heart disease
- Developing diabetes
- Developing high blood pressure
- Developing colon cancer

Regular physical activity helps in the following ways:
- Reduces blood pressure in those with hypertension
- Reduces feelings of depression and anxiety
- Controls weight
- Builds and maintains healthy bones, muscles, and joints
- Promotes psychological well-being

These health burdens could be reduced through regular physical activity:
- 95,000 people are newly diagnosed with colon cancer each year
- 250,000 people suffer from a hip fracture each year
- 50 million people have high blood pressure
- 13.5 million people have coronary heart disease
- 1.5 million individuals have a myocardial infarction each year
- 8 million people have type 2 diabetes (adult onset)
- More than 60 million individuals (one third of the population) are overweight

Source: Centers for Disease Control and Prevention. (2010c). *The link between physical activity and morbidity and mortality. Physical activity and health: A report of the Surgeon General.* Retrieved from: http://www.cdc.gov/nccdphp/sgr/pdf/mm.pdf

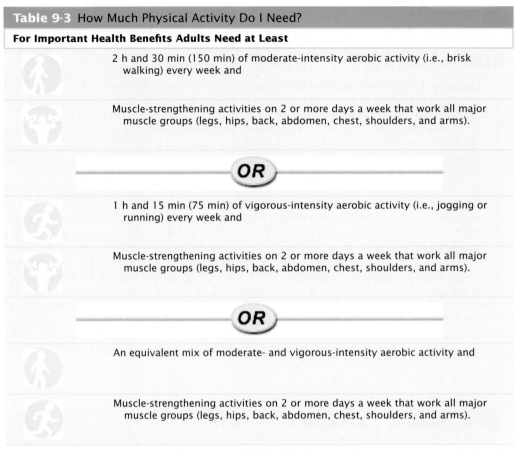

Table 9-3 How Much Physical Activity Do I Need?

For Important Health Benefits Adults Need at Least

2 h and 30 min (150 min) of moderate-intensity aerobic activity (i.e., brisk walking) every week and

Muscle-strengthening activities on 2 or more days a week that work all major muscle groups (legs, hips, back, abdomen, chest, shoulders, and arms).

OR

1 h and 15 min (75 min) of vigorous-intensity aerobic activity (i.e., jogging or running) every week and

Muscle-strengthening activities on 2 or more days a week that work all major muscle groups (legs, hips, back, abdomen, chest, shoulders, and arms).

OR

An equivalent mix of moderate- and vigorous-intensity aerobic activity and

Muscle-strengthening activities on 2 or more days a week that work all major muscle groups (legs, hips, back, abdomen, chest, shoulders, and arms).

Source: Center for Disease Control and Prevention. (2010d). Physical activity for everyone: How much physical activity do adults need. Retrieved from http://www.cdc.gov/physicalactivity/everyone/guidelines/adults.html

activity for 30 to 45 minutes, 3 to 5 days per week, is a reasonable initial goal. Most adults should be encouraged to set a long-term goal of 30 minutes or more of moderate-intensity physical activity on most, preferably all, days of the week. Table 9-4 shows examples of moderate amounts of physical activity achieved from both common chores and sporting activities.

With time, weight loss, and increased functional capacity, a client may want to engage in more strenuous activities. These include fitness walking, cycling, rowing, cross-country skiing, aerobic dancing, and jumping rope. If jogging is desired, the client's ability to jog must be assessed first. Competitive sports such as tennis, soccer, and volleyball provide enjoyable physical activity for some individuals, but again, care must be taken to avoid injury. There is no such thing as one "magic" exercise. Rather, to get the greatest health and fitness benefits a mix of moderate and vigorous exercise as well as strength training is required. Individuals who are not physically active cite many reasons for their inactivity. Box 9-3 provides some suggestions that nurses can follow to assist clients to overcome obstacles to regular activity.

Social support from family and friends has been consistently and positively related to regular exercise. Walking with a friend is often the best way to begin a simple and doable exercise program. Nurses who work closely with individuals in community-based settings have ample opportunity to encourage moderate physical activity for 30 minutes a day for all adults.

Table 9-4 Examples of Moderate Amounts of Physical Activity[a]

Common Chores	Sporting Activities	
Washing and waxing a car for 45–60 min	Playing volleyball for 45–60 min	Less vigorous, more time
Washing windows or floors for 45–60 min	Playing touch football for 45 min	
Gardening for 30–45 min	Walking 1¼ miles in 35 min (20 min/mile)	
Wheeling self in wheelchair for 30–40 min	Basketball (shooting baskets) for 30 min	
Pushing a stroller 1½ miles in 30 min	Bicycling 5 miles in 30 min	
Raking leaves for 30 min	Dancing fast (social) for 30 min	
Walking 2 miles in 30 min (15 min/mile)	Water aerobics for 30 min	
Shoveling snow for 15 min	Swimming laps for 20 min	
Stair walking for 15 min	Basketball (playing a game) for 15–20 min	More vigorous, less time
	Jumping rope for 15 min	
	Running 1½ miles in 15 min	
	(10 min/mile)	

NOTE: Some activities can be performed at various intensities; the suggested durations correspond to expected intensity of effort.
[a]A moderate amount of physical activity is roughly equivalent to physical activity that uses approximately 150 calories of energy per day, or 1,000 calories per week.
Source: National Institutes of Health. (2000). *The practical guide: Identification, evaluation, and treatment of overweight and obesity in adults* (NIH Publication Number 00-4084). National Heart, Lung and Blood Institute Obesity Education Initiative.

BOX 9-3 **Counseling Strategies to Encourage More Physical Activity**

EXCUSE	SUGGESTED RESPONSE
I don't have time to exercise.	Exercise does take time but think of all the time you spend watching TV. Many forms of exercise can be done while watching TV (riding a stationary bike, using hand weights).
I don't have the energy to be more active.	Once you are more active, you will have more energy.
It's hard to remember to exercise.	Leave your sneakers near the door to remind you to walk, bring a change of clothes to work and head straight for exercise on the way home. Put a note on your calendar to remind you.
I can't go because of my kids.	Walking is free and can be done even with small children by putting them in a stroller or wagon. Children over 4 years old benefit from walking as much as adults. They will become accustomed to taking walks with a parent as it becomes a part of the family routine. In states with colder or rainy climates, malls are a great place to walk or many public schools have open gym when the weather does not allow walking outside.

size and weight status	NHANES I 1971-1974	NHANES II 1976-1980	NHANES III 1988-1994	NHANES 1999-2000	NHANES 2001-2002	NHANES 2003-2004	NHANES 2005-2006	NHANES 2007-2008
Sample (n)	12,911	11,765	14,468	3,603	3,916	3,756	3,835	4,881
Overweight (25 ≤ BMI < 30)	32.3	32.1	32.7	33.6	34.4	33.4	32.2	33.6
Obese (BMI ≥ 30)	14.5	15.0	23.2	30.9	31.3	32.9	35.1	34.3
Extremely obese (BMI ≥ 40)	1.3	1.4	3.0	5.0	5.4	5.1	6.2	6.0

Figure 9-2 Age-adjusted prevalence of overweight and obesity among U.S. adults, ages 20 to 74. NHANES, National Health and Nutrition Examination Survey. Source: Ogden, C., & Carroll, M. (2010). *Prevalence of overweight, obesity, and extreme obesity among adults: United States, Trends 1976–1980 through 2007–2008*. Retrieved from http://www.cdc.gov/NCHS/data/hestat/obesity_adult_07_08/obesity_adult_07_08.pdf

OVERWEIGHT AND OBESITY

Estimates of the percentage of obese American adults in the U.S. population have been steadily increasing, from 19.4% in 1997, 24.5% in 2004 to 26.7% in 2009 (Fig. 9-2). Over 75% of all Americans are **overweight** or obese. Over 27% of all Americans report a weight that puts them in the obese category. Rates of obesity vary from state to state with a low of 15% to 19% in Colorado to a rate of over 30% in most of the states in the southern part of the United States (Mortality and Mobidity Weekly Report, 2010).

The rates of obesity and overweight continue to increase, but this trend varies by race, gender, income, and age. Women from lower income households are more likely to be overweight. Obesity is more common among African American and Hispanic women than among White women and more common among women than among men.

Obesity is a major contributor to many preventable causes of death, with a general rule that higher body weight is associated with higher death rates. Obesity is a risk factor for a variety of chronic conditions including diabetes, hypertension, high cholesterol, stroke, heart disease, certain cancers, and arthritis. Being morbidly obese is associated with excess mortality, primarily from cardiovascular disease, diabetes, and certain cancers (Malnick & Knobler, 2006).

Health care provider–based exercise and diet counseling is an important component of effective weight loss interventions shown to produce increased levels of physical activity among sedentary patients. Not every obese person needs counseling about exercise and diet, but many would likely benefit from improvements in these activities. Nearly one in four overweight women of reproductive age inaccurately perceives her body weight as normal, thus affecting her weight-related behavior (Rahman & Berenson, 2010). This misperception of normal versus weight that is above the normal range has implications for nurses doing health counseling and teaching in community settings. When counseling about weight loss, a logical place to begin is to plot the clients' weight on a BMI chart to assist them to have a realistic understanding of how their weight compares to standard healthy, overweight, obese, and very obese weight. A person with a BMI between 25.0 and 29.9 is considered *overweight*. A person with a BMI of 30.0 or greater is considered *obese*. Box 9-4 shows how to calculate BMI and waist circumference. Table 9-5 provides a BMI estimation table.

Weight loss therapy is not appropriate for some individuals, including most pregnant or lactating women, people with uncontrolled psychiatric illness, and those with serious

---

BOX 9-4 **Calculating BMI and Waist Circumference**

BMI measures your weight in relation to height, and it is closely associated with measures of body fat. You can calculate your BMI using this formula:

$$BMI = \frac{weight\,(pounds) \times 703}{height\,squared\left(inches^2\right)}$$

For example, for someone who is 5 feet, 7 inches tall and weighs 220 lb, the calculation would look like this:

$$BMI = \frac{220\,lb \times 703}{67\,inches \times 67\,inches} = \frac{154,660}{4,489} = 34.45$$

A BMI of 18.5–24.9 is considered to be in the healthy range. A person with a BMI of 25–29.9 is considered overweight, and a person with a BMI of 30 or more is considered obese.

Another way to calculate BMI is plot weight and height using Table 9-5. The chart applies to all adults. The higher weights in the healthy range apply to people with more muscle and bone, such as men. Even within the healthy range, weight gain could increase your risk for health problems. Because BMI does not show the difference between fat and muscle, it does not always accurately predict when weight could lead to health problems. For example, someone with a lot of muscle (such as a body builder) may have a BMI in the overweight or obese range, but still be healthy and have little risk of developing diabetes or having a heart attack.

Waist Circumference Measurement
Excess weight as measured by BMI is not the only risk to health. Where excess fat is located on the body may be another risk. If weight is mainly carried around your waist, there is a greater likelihood to develop health problems than if when fat is mainly in the hips and thighs. This is true even if the BMI falls within the normal range. Women with a waist measurement of more than 35 inches or men with a waist measurement of more than 40 inches may have a higher disease risk than people with smaller waist measurements because of where their fat lies.

To measure waist circumference, place a tape measure around the bare abdomen just above the hip bone. Be sure that the tape is snug (but does not compress the skin) and that it is parallel to the floor. Tell the person to relax, exhale, and measure the waist.

High-Risk Waist Circumference
Men: >40" (>102 cm)
Women: > 36" (>88cm)

Source: U.S. Department of Health and Human Services. (2008). *National Institute of Health weight and waist measurement tools for adults.* Retrieved from http://win.niddk.nih.gov/publications/tools. htm#bodymassindex or http://win.niddk.nih.gov/publications/PDFs/Weightandwaist.pdf

---

illnesses that might be exacerbated by caloric restriction. Clients with active substance abuse or a history of anorexia nervosa or bulimia nervosa should receive care by a specialist.

Regular exercise and a healthy diet aid in maintaining normal blood cholesterol levels, weight loss, and blood pressure control efforts, reducing the risk of heart disease, stroke, diabetes, and other comorbidities of obesity (AHRQ, 2010). Dietary therapy, physical activity, and behavioral therapy are the usual interventions for those who are overweight or obese. There are numerous resources found in What's on the Web at the end of the chapter for counseling and health teaching. For the morbidly obese, pharmacotherapy and weight loss surgery may be considered. A combination of diet modification, increased physical activity, and behavior therapy can be effective for most obese individuals.

There are some simple behavior changes that promote weight loss. Eating a high-fiber diet improves health by lowing cholesterol and enhancing weight loss. There is a relationship between obesity and sleep, with those individuals who get at least 7 hours of sleep less

Table 9-5 Body Mass Estimation

BMI	Normal						Overweight					Obese										Extreme Obesity		
	19	20	21	22	23	24	25	26	27	28	29	30	31	32	33	34	35	36	37	38	39	40	41	42
Height (feet-inches)	Weight (lb)																							
4'10"	91	96	100	105	110	115	119	124	129	134	138	143	148	153	158	162	167	172	177	181	186	191	196	201
4'11"	94	99	104	109	114	119	124	128	133	138	143	148	153	158	163	168	173	178	183	188	193	198	203	208
5'00"	97	102	107	112	118	123	128	133	138	143	148	153	158	163	168	174	179	184	189	194	199	204	209	215
5'01"	100	106	111	116	122	127	132	137	143	148	153	158	164	169	174	180	185	190	195	201	206	211	217	222
5'02"	104	109	115	120	126	131	136	142	147	153	158	164	169	175	180	186	191	196	202	207	213	218	224	229
5'03"	107	112	118	124	130	135	141	146	152	158	163	169	174	180	186	191	197	203	208	214	220	225	231	237
5'04"	110	116	122	128	134	140	145	151	157	163	169	175	180	186	191	197	204	209	215	221	227	232	238	244
5'05"	114	120	126	132	138	144	150	156	162	168	174	180	186	192	198	204	210	216	222	228	234	240	246	252
5'06"	118	124	130	136	142	148	155	161	167	173	179	186	192	198	204	210	216	223	229	235	241	247	253	260
5'07"	121	127	134	140	146	153	159	166	172	178	185	191	198	204	211	217	223	230	236	242	249	255	261	268
5'08"	125	131	138	144	151	158	164	171	177	184	190	197	203	210	216	223	230	236	243	249	256	262	269	276
5'09"	128	135	142	149	155	162	169	176	182	189	196	203	209	216	223	230	236	243	250	257	263	270	277	284
5'10"	132	139	146	153	160	167	174	181	188	195	202	209	216	222	229	236	243	250	257	264	271	278	285	292
5'11"	136	143	150	157	165	172	179	186	193	200	208	215	222	229	236	243	250	257	265	272	279	286	293	301
6'00"	140	147	154	162	169	177	184	191	199	206	213	221	228	235	242	250	258	265	272	279	287	294	302	309
6'01"	144	151	159	166	174	182	189	197	204	212	219	227	235	242	250	257	265	272	280	288	295	302	310	318
6'02"	148	155	163	171	179	186	194	202	210	218	225	233	241	249	256	264	272	280	287	295	303	311	319	326
6'03"	152	160	168	176	184	192	200	208	216	224	232	240	248	256	264	272	279	287	295	303	311	319	327	335
6'04"	156	164	172	180	189	197	205	213	221	230	238	246	254	263	271	279	287	295	304	312	320	328	336	344

Adapted from Bray G. (1998). Pennington Biomedical Research Center. Clinical guidelines on the identification, evaluation, and treatment of overweight and obesity in adults: The evidence report. Bethesda, MD: National Institutes of Health, National Heart, Lung, and Blood Institute. U.S. Department of Health and Human Services. National Institute of Health. Weight-control Information Network. Getting on track. Retrieved from http://win.niddk.nih.gov/publications/gettingontrack.htm#healthyweight.

BOX 9-5

Tips for Talking With Clients About Weight Control

1. **Address the clients' concerns or complaints first, independent of weight.** No one wants health care professionals to place blame or attribute all of their health problems to weight.

2. **Open the discussion.** Open the conversation by finding out if the client is willing to talk about weight, or by expressing your concerns about how his or her weight affects health. Next, you might ask the client to describe his or her weight. Here are some sample discussion openers:

   "Mr. Lopez, could we talk about your weight? What are your thoughts about your weight right now?"

   "Mrs. Brown, I'm concerned about your weight because I think it is causing health problems for you. What do you think about your weight?"

   Be sensitive to cultural differences that your patients may bring to the discussion regarding weight, food preferences, social norms and practices, and related issues. Patients may be more open when they feel respected.

3. **Decide if your patient is ready to control weight.** Ask more questions to assess a patient's readiness to control weight. Some sample questions are as follows:

   "What are your goals concerning your weight?"

   "What changes are you willing to make to your eating and physical activity habits right now?"

   "What kind of help would you like from me regarding your weight?"

   A person who is not yet ready to attempt weight control may still benefit from a discussion about healthy eating and regular physical activity, even if he or she is not ready to make behavioral changes. A talk focusing on the ways weight may affect health may also be appropriate because it may help bring weight loss to the forefront of his or her mind. A person who is ready to control weight will benefit from setting a weight loss goal, receiving advice about healthy eating and regular physical activity, and follow-up.

4. **Set a weight goal.** A 5–10% reduction in body weight over 6 months is a sensible weight loss goal. One half to 2 lb per week is a safe rate of weight loss. A goal of maintaining current weight and preventing weight gain may be appropriate for some people.

   It may be beneficial to focus on improving other diet- and exercise-related risk factors too. Some patients may lose weight very slowly, which can be discouraging. Improving risk factors such as cholesterol levels may motivate clients, especially if changes are achieved in the face of slow weight loss.

5. **Prescribe healthy eating and physical activity behaviors.** Give concrete actions to take to meet his or her weight goal over the next 6 months. Write specific suggestions for healthier eating and increased physical activity. You can also bring the WIN's online resources about weight, healthy eating, and physical activity to the person's attention.

   Another option is to refer to a weight loss program, a registered dietitian who specializes in weight control, or a certified fitness professional. The American Dietetic Association (*www.eatright.org*) offers referrals to registered dietitians throughout the United States, and the American College of Sports Medicine (*www.acsm.org*) offers a search engine for certified fitness professionals. In addition, the online WIN document *Choosing a Safe and Successful Weight loss Program* can help during this process. This publication offers a list of questions clients may ask their health care providers before deciding on a weight loss plan, as well as various tips on what to look for in such programs.

6. **Follow up.** When you see the client again, note progress made on behavior changes, such as walking at least 5 days a week. For any progress noted, offer praise to boost self-esteem and keep him or her motivated. Likewise, discuss setbacks to help the individual overcome challenges and be more successful. Set a new weight goal with your client. This may be for weight loss or prevention of weight gain. Discuss eating and physical activity habits to change or maintain to meet the new weight goal.

Source: U.S. Department of Health and Human Services. (2007). *National Institute of Health tips for talking about weight control.* Retrieved from http://win.niddk.nih.gov/publications/talking.htm#staff

likely to be overweight or obese. Therefore, by addressing a variety of health habits the nurse can assist individuals to reach a normal weight. Of course, it is important to address one issue at a time in small incremental steps. For example, encourage a client to go to bed 15 minutes earlier for a month. The next month, move the bedtime another 15 minutes earlier. Or encourage clients to add one piece of fruit per day to their diet for a month. After a month, advance to having two pieces of fruit a day.

Studies show that short 3-to-5-minute conversations during routine contact can contribute to patient behavior change. In one study, patients who were obese and were advised by their health care professionals to lose weight were three times more likely to try to lose weight than patients not advised. Research has also shown that patients who were counseled in a primary care setting about the benefits of healthy eating and physical activity lost weight, consumed less fat, and exercised more than patients who did not receive counseling. Unfortunately, the majority of primary care professionals do not talk with their patients about weight (U.S. Department of Health and Human Services, 2007). Box 9-5 has some suggestions for health care professionals about how to talk to clients about weight control.

Approach the subject of weight loss if the individual has

- A BMI of 30 or above
- A BMI between 25 and 30 and two or more weight-related health problems, such as a family history of coronary heart disease or diabetes
- A waist measurement over 35 inches (women) or 40 inches (men)—even if BMI is less than 25—and two or more weight-related health problems, such as a family history of coronary heart disease or diabetes

TOBACCO USE

Cigarette smoking, responsible for more than 440,000 deaths annually, continues to be the main preventable cause of disease and death in the United States (American Heart Association, 2010). Smoking is a major risk factor for developing heart disease, stroke, lung cancer, and chronic lung disease. Most smokers begin as teenagers and become addicted to tobacco. Half of all adolescent smokers who continue to smoke in adulthood will die from smoking-related illness. Primary prevention is a critical strategy in reducing the number of teens who ever begin smoking, which, in turn, reduces the mortality and morbidity associated with cigarette smoking. Although high-school smoking declined 40% from 1997 to 2003, that decline has dramatically slowed to 11% from 2003 to 2009. Much of this trend is attributed to the elimination of state and federal funding for smoking cessation programs.

Coupled with this enormous health toll is the significant economic burden of tobacco use. More than $96 billion per year in medical expenditures and another $97 billion per year resulting from lost productivity. About 14% of all Medicaid expenditures are for smoking-related illnesses. It is estimated that approximately 18.2 billion packs of cigarettes were sold in the United States in 2007. Each pack cost the nation an estimated $10.60 in medical care costs and lost productivity.

Tobacco cessation is the most cost-effective method of preventing disease among adults. Each smoker who successfully quits reduces the anticipated medical costs associated with heart attack and stroke by an estimated $47 in the first year and $853 during the following 7 years. When compared with nonsmokers, men who smoke have nearly $16,000 more in lifetime medical expenses; women who smoke incur more than $17,000 (CDC, 2008).

For several decades, nurses have been providing health education about how to quit smoking to clients in community settings. An integrative literature review of 29 studies was conducted to determine the effectiveness of nursing-delivered smoking cessation interventions. It was found that smokers who were offered advice by nursing professionals had an increased likelihood of quitting compared to smokers without such nursing interventions. This result reflected a significantly positive effect for smoking cessation interventions by nurses, especially in the hospital setting. The challenge to nurses is to incorporate smoking

---

COMMUNITY-BASED NURSING CARE GUIDELINES 9-1

Quick Reference Guide for Clinicians Treating Tobacco Use and Dependence

Ask	Systematically identify all tobacco users at every visit.
Advise	Strongly urge all tobacco users to quit.
Assess	Determine willingness to make a quit attempt.
Assist	Aid the client in quitting.
Follow up	Ask clients if they still smoke. Give ex-smokers a pat on the back. Send cards or call clients soon after their visit and just before their original quit day.

Source: Centers for Disease Control and Prevention. (2006). *A practical guide to working with health-care systems on tobacco-use treatment.* Atlanta, GA: U.S. Department of Health and Human Services, Centers for Disease Control and Prevention, National Center for Chronic Disease Prevention and Health Promotion, Office on Smoking and Health. Retrieved from http://www.cdc.gov/tobacco/quit_smoking/cessation/practical_guide/pdfs/practical_guide.pdf

---

cessation interventions as part of standard practice so that the nurse discusses tobacco use with all clients, gives advice to quit, and uses behavioral counseling. Nurses interface with clients in numerous settings, allowing them to play an important role in reducing cigarette smoking by adults (Rice & Stead, 2008).

The community-based nurse should screen for tobacco use and encourage cessation with every client. The literature continues to document the leadership role that nurses working in the community play in developing and implementing smoking cessation programs. One approach to smoking cessation comes from recommendations from the CDC. These guidelines feature five "As" (ask, assess, advise, assist, and arrange) and five "Rs" (relevance, risk, rewards, roadblocks, and repetition), which provide a logical framework for supporting smoking cessation efforts and improving success (Malucky, 2010). These guidelines for clinicians assisting clients with smoking cessation are shown in Community-Based Nursing Care Guidelines 9-1.

ALCOHOL AND SUBSTANCE USE AND ABUSE

There were 9.1 cirrhosis deaths per 100,000 populations reported in 2007. Healthy People 2020 set a goal of improving this mortality rate by 10% to 8.2 per 100,000 (U.S. Department of Health and Human Services, 2010). Only 16.0% of persons aged 12 years and older who needed illicit drug treatment reported that they received specialty treatment for abuse or dependence in 2008. Healthy People 2020 set a target goal of improving this percentage by 10% in the next decade.

For individuals over 18 years of age, over 40% of men and 20% of women report drinking five or more alcoholic drinks on at least 1 day (binge drinking) in the past year. Whites and Hispanics are more likely than African Americans to use alcohol. Whites are more likely than African Americans and Hispanics to use illicit drugs (National Institute of Alcohol Abuse and Alcoholism, 2008).

There is a great deal of confusion about the benefits and detriments of alcohol consumption. In the last decade, some research suggested that moderate alcohol use might provide some protection from coronary artery disease. However, research has established that it is the pattern of drinking, or having a drink every day, that may provide health benefit. Drinking large quantities of alcohol at one sitting has a negative impact on health, and is what determines the effects of alcohol on one's health. These findings are consistent with what we have known for some time—binge drinking creates health problems.

COMMUNITY-BASED TEACHING 9-2

Tips to Reduce Substance Abuse Behaviors

- Don't use illegal (street) drugs of any kind, at any time.
- Use prescription drugs only as directed by a health care provider.
- Use nonprescription drugs only as instructed on the label.
- Tell your health care provider all of the medications you are currently taking.
- If you drink alcohol, have no more than two drinks per day if you are a man and one drink a day if you are a woman. A standard drink is one 12-oz bottle of beer or wine cooler, one 5-oz glass of wine, or 1.5-oz of 80-proof distilled spirits.
- Do not drink alcohol before or while driving a motor vehicle.
- If you have concerns about your alcohol or drug use, talk to your health care provider.

Agency for Healthcare Research and Quality. (2010). *Prevention and care management: Resources and tools. Women/Men: Stay healthy at any age screening guide.* Retrieved from http://www.ahrq.gov/clinic/ppipix.htm

Many serious problems are associated with alcohol and illicit drug abuse. In the last year that data were available, the financial costs of substance abuse were estimated at $276 billion per year (Harwood, 2000). Substance abuse is associated with child and spousal abuse, STDs, motor vehicle accidents, escalation of health care costs, low worker productivity, and homelessness. Alcohol abuse alone is associated with motor vehicle accidents, homicides, suicides, and drowning. For several decades, the positive association between chronic alcoholism and heart disease, cancer, liver disease, and pancreatitis has been found in large population studies.

Assessment and intervention with substance-related health issues is an important role for the nurse in community-based settings. The more direct, honest, and open the nurse is when addressing this issue, the more likely clients will be to view their own patterns of alcohol use as an important aspect of health promotion. *Rethinking Drinking* is an assessment tool for exploring alcohol use and abuse with clients. This tool is available at www.RethinkingDrinking.niaaa.nih.gov and http://pubs.niaaa.nih.gov/publications/Rethinking-Drinking/Rethinking_Drinking.pdf. Teaching the client about avoiding substance abuse is the next step after assessment (see Community-Based Teaching 9-2).

Interventions targeted at groups and communities have demonstrated some efficacy in reducing substance abuse. School-based prevention programs directed toward altering perceived peer-group norms about alcohol use and helping develop skills in resisting peer pressure to drink are successful in reducing alcohol use among participants. Raising the minimum legal drinking age has reduced alcohol consumption, traffic accidents, and related fatalities among persons younger than 21 years of age. Laws that prohibit sale of alcohol to minors that are consistently enforced are another effective method to reduce alcohol abuse. Higher cost and additional taxes on alcohol are also associated with lower alcohol consumption and lowered adverse outcomes. In college settings, one-to-one motivational counseling has been effective in reducing alcohol-related problems. It is important that the nurse direct efforts to reduce the proportion of adults using illicit drugs and engaging in binge drinking of alcoholic beverages.

RESPONSIBLE SEXUAL BEHAVIOR

STDs remain a major public health challenge in the United States, with more than 19 million new infections each year, almost half among young adults aged 15 to 24 (CDC, 2009a). Unprotected sex can result in unintended pregnancies and STDs, including HIV. About half of all new HIV infections in the United States are among individuals over 25 years of age, with the majority being infected through sexual behavior. Women bear the greatest burden of STDs, suffering more frequent and more serious complications than men. The highest rates are found among Blacks (51%), Whites (29%). and Hispanics (18%). Condoms, used correctly and consistently, can prevent STDs, including HIV. However, it is estimated that one in five persons in the United States who are HIV-positive do not know they are infected. Since 2006, the CDC has recommended screening all individuals aged 13 to 64 and yearly screening for people at high risk for HIV (CDC, 2006).

Nurses should never hesitate to assess sexual health. Here are some simple questions:

- Are you concerned you might have a sexually transmitted disease?
- Do you have questions about tests or treatment?
- Do you need to find a doctor or clinic where you can get private, personal, and confidential care? You can call the CDC:

  1-800-CDC-INFO

  (1-800-232-4636)

  TTY: 1-888-232-6348

  In English and Spanish (*en Español*)

Health teaching is the most important disease prevention activity the nurse can use to address health issues related to sexual behavior. Again, sexuality must always be assessed, with teaching and interventions based on the client's knowledge base, concerns, and cultural sensitivities. As discussed in Chapter 8, young teens should be encouraged to delay the age of first intercourse. Teaching about the effectiveness of various contraceptive methods and providing condoms to be used with every sexual encounter are interventions that have been shown again and again to be essential to sexual health promotion and a strategy that saves lives.

MENTAL HEALTH

Twenty-six percent of the population is affected by mental illness during a given year, with depression as the most common disorder (Kessler et al., 2005). Over a 12-month period, 60% of those with a mental disorder receive no treatment at all. Improvements are needed to speed initiation of treatment as well as enhance the quality and duration of treatment (Wang et al., 2005).

Adults and older adults have the highest rates of depression, with about 1 in 20 American adults experiencing major depression in a given year. Major depression affects twice as many women as men. Research suggests that for women menopausal transition is linked to new onset of depressive symptoms (Cohen et al., 2006). There is a high rate of depression among those with chronic conditions. One in three people who have survived a heart attack develop depression. Major depression is the leading cause of all disabilities and the cause of more than two thirds of suicides each year. Financial costs from lost work time are high. Unfortunately, there is still widespread misunderstanding about mental illness and associated stigmatization, which often prevents individuals with depression from getting professional help.

Depression affects daily functioning and, in some cases, incapacitates the individual. Depression is a common condition that is often not recognized by health care providers in the community. Home care nurses use the OASIS-C (discussed in Chapter 12) method of assessment that requires ongoing screening for depression. The nurse asks the client, "Over the past 2 weeks, how often have you been bothered by little interest or pleasure in doing things or feeling down, depressed, or hopeless?" A frequent positive response requires a referral for further evaluation.

Depression is a treatable condition—medications and psychological treatment are effective for most people suffering from depression. But to receive treatment, people with depression have to be identified and encouraged to seek help. An important role of the nurse in community-based care is to identify those experiencing depression and convince them to seek assistance early.

There is an urgent need for improving detection and treatment of depression and other mental illness as a means of reducing suicide. At least 90% of people who commit suicide have had or are experiencing mental illness, a substance abuse disorder, or a combination; therefore, it is essential that health care professionals be diligent about screening and intervention when mental illness is suspected. Again, nurses should not be afraid to ask questions regarding mental health concerns and to refer clients accordingly. It is important that the proportion of adults with recognized depression who receive treatment continues to rise.

INJURIES AND VIOLENCE

Injury and violence are a serious threat to the health of American adults. Motor vehicle accidents are the most common cause of serious injury among adults. Nearly 40% of all traffic fatalities were related to alcohol use, with drivers between 21 and 24 years of age having the highest intoxication rate. About 3 in 10 Americans will be involved in an alcohol-related crash in their lifetimes. Every day, 32 people in the United States die in motor vehicle crashes that involve an alcohol-impaired driver. This amounts to one death every 45 minutes. The annual cost of alcohol-related crashes totals more than $51 billion. But there are effective measures that can help prevent injuries and deaths from alcohol-impaired driving (National Center for Injury Prevention and Control [NCIPC], CDC, 2010).

Certain types of injuries appear to affect some groups more frequently. Native Americans and Alaskan Natives have disproportionately high death rates from motor vehicle accidents, residential fires, and drowning. There are higher rates of death from unintentional injury among African Americans. In every age group, drowning rates are almost two to four times greater for males than females. Homicide is especially high among African American and Hispanic youths. Nurses must be involved in efforts to reduce death caused by motor vehicle accidents and homicide. Community-Based Teaching 9-3 provides general recommendations for preventing injuries.

Injuries are among the leading causes of death for women in the United States. Many injuries to women result from violent acts; others are caused by unintentional events such as falls, motor vehicle accidents, burns, drowning, and poisonings. Some injuries affect women more frequently than men, with hip fractures and partner violence being the most common.

Violence is a significant problem in the United States. From infants to the elderly, it affects people in all stages of life. Homicide and suicide are leading causes of death for those aged 15 to 34. The number of violent deaths tells only part of the story. Many more survive violence and are left with permanent physical and emotional scars. Violence also erodes communities by reducing productivity, decreasing property values, and disrupting social services.

COMMUNITY-BASED TEACHING 9-3

Recommendations for Preventing Injuries

- Always wear a seatbelt while in the car.
- Never drive after drinking alcohol.
- Always wear a safety helmet while riding a motorcycle or bicycle.
- Use smoke detectors in your home; check to make sure they work every month, and change the batteries every year.
- Keep the temperature of hot water less than 120°F, particularly if there are children or older adults living in your home.
- If you choose to keep a gun in your home, make sure that the gun and the ammunition are locked up separately and are out of the reach of children.
- Prevent falls by older adults by repairing slippery or uneven walking surfaces, improving poor lighting, and installing secure railings on all stairways.

BOX
9-6

Abuse Assessment Screen

1. WITHIN THE LAST YEAR, have you been hit, slapped, kicked, or otherwise physically hurt by someone?   YES   NO

   If YES, by whom? _____
   Total number of times _____

2. SINCE YOU'VE BEEN PREGNANT, have you been hit, slapped, kicked, or otherwise physically hurt by someone?   YES   NO

   If YES, by whom? _____
   Total number of times _____

MARK THE AREA OF INJURY ON THE BODY MAP. SCORE EACH INCIDENT ACCORDING TO THE FOLLOWING SCALE:

SCORE

1. = Threats of abuse including use of a weapon   _____
2. = Slapping, pushing; no injuries and/or lasting pain   _____
3. = Punching, kicking, bruises, cuts and/or continuing pain   _____
4. = Beating up, severe contusions, burns, broken bones   _____
5. = Head injury, internal injury, permanent injury   _____
6. = Use of weapon; wound from weapon   _____

If any of the descriptions for the higher number apply, use the higher number.

3. **WITHIN THE LAST YEAR,** has anyone forced you to have sexual activities?   YES   NO

   If YES, by whom? _____
   Total number of times _____

Source: Nursing Network Violence Against Women. (2010). *Abuse assessment screen.* Retrieved from http://www.nnvawi.org/page.cfm/assessment-tools. Developed by the Nursing Research Consortium on Violence and Abuse. With permission.

Intentional injury, or physical assault, is a leading cause of injury to women, with more women than men experiencing intimate partner violence (IPV). IPV is a major public health issue. Each year, women experience about 4.8 million intimate partner–related physical assaults and rapes. Men are the victims of about 2.9 million intimate partner–related physical assaults. Yearly mortality rates for IPV are a leading cause of death, with 78% of victims being women and 22% men (CDC, NCIPC, 2009).

The first and foremost responsibility of the nurse is to use refined assessment skills in cases where intimate partner abuse is suspected. Nurses should never be afraid to ask the question, "are you afraid (or concerned) that someone at home or someone you love has (or may have) tried to hurt you?" In order to be comfortable with this type of assessment, the nurse should acquire basic information about IPV as well as develop basic clinical skills for identifying and assessing this type of situation. Next, the nurse must be familiar with resources within his or her own community for referral phone numbers and contact persons. A simple quick assessment tool that has been found to be highly effective is found in Box 9-6.

ENVIRONMENTAL QUALITY

An estimated 25% of preventable illnesses worldwide can be attributed to poor environmental quality. Poor air quality, including both ozone (outside air) and tobacco smoke (inside air), is one of the prime contributors. In the United States, epidemiological studies suggest that more than 500,000 Americans die each year from cardiopulmonary disease linked to breathing fine particle air pollution. Incidence of asthma has been on the rise for the past few decades among adults and children.

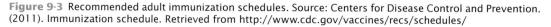

VACCINE▼ AGE GROUP▶	19-26 Year	27-49 Year	50-59 Year	60-64 Year	≥65 Year
Influenza[1,*]	1 dose annualy				
Tetanus, diphtheria, pertussis (Td/Tdap)[2,*]	Substitutb 1-time dose of Tdap for Td booster; then boost with Td every 10 years				Td booster every 10 year
Varicella[3,*]	2 doses				
Human papillomavirus (HPV)[4,*]	3 doses (Females)				
Zoster[5]				1 dose	
Measles, mumps, rubella (MMR)[6,*]	1 or 2 doses		1 dose		
Pneumococcal (polysaccharied)[7,8]	1 or 2 doses				1 dose
Meningococca[9,*]	1 or more doses				
Hepatitis A[10,*]	2 doses				
Hepatitis B[11,*]	2 doses				

*Coverd by the Vaccine Injury Compensation Program

For all persons in this category who meet the age requirements and who lack evidence of immunity (e.g, lack document of Vaccination or have no evidence of previous infection)

Recommended if some other risk factor is present (e.g., based on medical, occupational, lifestyle, or other indications)

NO recommendation

Figure 9-3 Recommended adult immunization schedules. Source: Centers for Disease Control and Prevention. (2011). Immunization schedule. Retrieved from http://www.cdc.gov/vaccines/recs/schedules/

It is important that the proportion of individuals exposed to poor air quality be reduced, as well as the proportion of nonsmokers exposed to secondhand smoke. One intervention involves teaching clients about the importance of maintaining smoke-free indoor air and the hazards of secondhand smoke. Second, the nurse can teach clients the threat that poor outdoor air quality poses for health and the importance of supporting political candidates and legislation that protect air quality. This topic is discussed in more detail in Chapter 15.

IMMUNIZATIONS

Immunization is cited as one of the greatest achievements of public health in the 20th century. It is important to continue to increase the proportion of children who receive all vaccines, as well as the proportion of adults who are vaccinated annually against the flu. Figure 9-3 summarizes recommended screening, immunization, and health promotion activities.

ACCESS TO HEALTH CARE

According to Healthy People 2020, access to quality care is important to eliminate health disparities and increase the quality and years of healthy lives for all Americans. One way to improve access is to improve the continuum of care. Until the 1980s, the proportion of people without health insurance gradually declined. Since the late 1980s, this proportion has increased to 28% of the population uninsured at some point during the previous year. Half of all young adults aged 18 to 29 do not have health insurance (Roberts & Rhoades, 2010). The variation in access to health care by race and ethnicity is shown in Figure 9-4.

Use of Complementary Therapies

Increasingly, the benefits of complementary and alternative modes of therapy are reported in empirical research. Complementary therapies are advantageous as primary, secondary, or tertiary prevention strategies. For instance, a single session of Swedish massage impacts neuroendocrine and immune function by increasing oxytocin levels, which, in turn, decrease hypothalamic–pituitary–adrenal (HPA) activity and enhances immune function (Rapaport, Schettler, & Bresee, 2010). Research examining the effects of a workplace Tai Chi (TC) intervention on musculoskeletal fitness and psychological well-being among

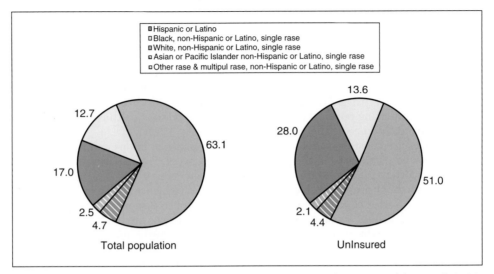

Figure 9-4 Percentage distribution in the total population and in the uninsured by race/ethnicity of people under age 65, in 2009. Source: Roberts, J., & Rhoades, J. A. (2010). *The uninsured in America, first half of 2009: Estimates for the U.S. civilian noninstitutionalized population under age 65.* Agency for Healthcare Research and Quality. Retrieved from http://www.meps.ahrq.gov/mepsweb/data_files/publications/st291/stat291.pdf

female university employees who were computer users found significant improvements in physiological and psychological measures after 12 weeks. The researchers concluded that TC has considerable potential as an economic, effective, and convenient workplace intervention for workers spending long periods of time each day working at the computer (Tamim et al., 2009). Research in Community-Based Nursing 9-1 illustrates another example of a complementary therapy that can be used in any setting.

RESEARCH IN COMMUNITY-BASED NURSING 9-1

Chair Massage for Treating Anxiety in Patients Withdrawing From Psychoactive Drugs

Therapeutic massage has been reported to be an effective, nonpharmacologic alternative for managing anxiety in a variety of clinical situations. This study investigated the effectiveness of chair massage for reducing anxiety in persons participating in an inpatient withdrawal management program for psychoactive drugs. Using a randomized, controlled clinical trial 82 adult patients received inpatient treatment for psychoactive drug withdrawal (alcohol, cocaine, and opiates). Random assignment to either receive chair massage (*n* = 40) or a relaxation control condition (*n* = 42) was used. Participants received massage 3 consecutive days with standard treatments also offered concurrently to patients in both groups. Anxiety was assessed using Analysis of the Spielberger State–Trait Anxiety Inventory. Findings indicated that anxiety was significantly reduced and sustained for 24 hours in the chair massage group. This study indicates that chair massage may be more effective in reducing anxiety when compared to standard treatment. The authors recommend additional research exploring chair massage as a potential nonpharmacologic adjunct in the management of withdrawal related anxiety.

Source: Black, S., Jacques, K., Webber, A., Spurr, K., Carey, E., Hebb, A., et al. (2010). Chair massage for treating anxiety in patients withdrawing from psychoactive drugs. *Journal of Alternative & Complementary Medicine, 16*(9), 979–987. Retrieved from EBSCO*host*.

Policy

Public policy may appear, at first glance, to evolve primarily from the government, but policy makers consider many sources when developing public policy related to adult health. For example, being vocal and involved in public policy issues such as gun control, allocation of health care dollars for health promotion, and disease prevention programs and creating walking and bike paths are all ways that nurses can improve the health of adults in our country. Supporting political candidates who value public health is another way that nurses can make a difference at the community level.

Nurses are considered valued professionals whose opinions and input are often sought by those who participate in the policy-making process. Participation may involve calling or sending a letter to a city, state, or federal lawmaker; testifying at a public hearing; informing a client about proposed changes in laws related to health. For example, laws to increase taxes on cigarettes to discourage smoking or alcohol to discourage drinking impacts smoking rates and alcohol abuse rates, which, in turn, improve the health of populations. Often, through public education and social marketing, the nurse may influence public opinion and, in turn, public policy. So, nurses can bring to public attention how enforcing laws prohibiting driving with a certain blood alcohol level reduces motor vehicle accidents. It is a professional responsibility of the graduate nurse to stay current on health care issues, particularly in their own area of professional expertise and to share that information with other members of the community. Through advocacy, social marketing, and education, the nurse may influence public opinion and health care public policy.

Conclusions

Current critical issues of health and health care have changed dramatically in the past 100 years. Today, most diseases and deaths result from preventable causes. The nurse plays an essential role in early identification of and intervention in these conditions. Nurses can be successful in this charge through screening, particularly in high-risk groups. By identifying conditions early in their course, nurses can provide interventions that will substantially minimize the effects of these conditions. Once a chronic illness or injury has already occurred, tertiary prevention has the potential to avoid additional exacerbations and maximize quality of life. By employing health promotion and disease prevention strategies for all the health indicators identified by Healthy People 2020, nurses can facilitate longer and healthier lives for more adults in the United States.

What's on the Web

American Association of Dermatology
INTERNET ADDRESS: http://www.aad.org/media/background/factsheets/fact_skincancer.html
This Web site has a fact sheet on skin cancer that is a good source of updated information about skin cancer.

American Social Health Association (ASHA)
INTERNET ADDRESS: http://www.ashastd.org
The ASHA has been providing health information to the American public since 1914. They are recognized by the public, clients, providers, and policy makers for developing and delivering accurate, medically reliable information about STDs. Public and college health clinics across the United States order ASHA's educational pamphlets and books to give to clients and students. Community-based organizations depend on ASHA, too, to help communicate about risk, transmission, prevention, testing, and treatment.

Men/Women Stay Healthy at Any Age
INTERNET ADDRESS: http://www.ahrq.gov/ppip/adguide/
This online consumer guide from the AHRQ explains preventive care for adults. The guide is also available in Spanish.

Cookbooks

Heart-Healthy Home Cooking African American Style
INTERNET ADDRESS: http://www.nhlbi.nih.gov/health/public/heart/other/chdblack/cooking.htm
Download for free or order print copies for a small fee.

Delicious Heart-Healthy Latino Recipes (bilingual cookbook)
INTERNET ADDRESS: http://www.nhlbi.nih.gov/health/public/heart/other/sp_recip.htm
Download for free or order print copies for a small fee.

Obesity Education Initiative
INTERNET ADDRESS: http://www.nhlbi.nih.gov/about/oei/index.htm
This excellent Web site offers abundant information for providers, clients, and public educators related to obesity, produced by the National Heart, Lung, and Blood Institute.

Resources for Alcoholism

Al-Anon Family Group Headquarters, Inc.
INTERNET ADDRESS: http://www.al-anon.alateen.org/
This Web site makes referrals to local Al-Anon groups, which are support groups for sponsors and other significant adults in an alcoholic person's life.

Alcoholics Anonymous (AA) World Services, Inc.
INTERNET ADDRESS: http://www.aa.org
This Web site provides numerous resources for Alcoholics Anonymous: what it is; group membership; how to find a group.

National Council on Alcoholism and Drug Dependence (NCADD)
INTERNET ADDRESS: http://www.ncadd.org
This Web site provides links and contact information of local NCADD affiliates that can provide information on local treatment resources and educational materials on alcoholism.

National Institute on Alcohol Abuse and Alcoholism (NIAAA)
INTERNET ADDRESS: http://www.niaaa.nih.gov
This site offers free publications on all aspects of alcohol abuse and alcoholism, with some in Spanish.

Resources for Cancer Screening

American Cancer Society
INTERNET ADDRESS: http://www.cancer.org
The American Cancer Society Web site provides information various types of cancer, treatment and research as well as volunteer opportunities.

National Cancer Institute
INTERNET ADDRESS: http://www.nci.nih.gov
National Cancer Institute provides information for health care providers as well as other interested individuals about most types of cancer. There are many resources on this site.

National Breast and Cervical Cancer Early Detection Program
INTERNET ADDRESS: http://www.cdc.gov/cancer/nbccedp/
CDC's National Breast and Cervical Cancer Early Detection Program (NBCCEDP) provides access to breast and cervical cancer screening services to underserved women in all 50 states, the District of Columbia, 5 U.S. territories, and 12 tribes.

National Cancer Institute Cervical Cancer Information
IINTERNET ADDRESS: http://www.cancer.gov/cancertopics/types/cervical
This is the National Cancer Institute site for cervical cancer offering in-depth information and resources.

National Cervical Cancer Coalition
INTERNET ADDRESS: http://www.nccc-online.org
This Web site provides information and resources through the NCCC, a grassroots nonprofit organization dedicated to serving women with, or at risk for, cervical cancer and HPV disease.

Resources for Chronic Disease Prevention
INTERNET ADDRESS: http://www.cdc.gov/chronicdisease/index.htm
This Web site contains information about chronic disease through statistics, state profiles,and tools and research.

Resources for Intimate Partner Violence
National Domestic Violence Hotline
Hotline number: 1-800-799–SAFE (7233)
1-800-787-3224 (TTY)
INTERNET ADDRESS: http://www.thehotline.org/
The Web site and hotline number provide information for individuals experiencing domestic abuse. The hotline is available 24 hours a day and 365 days a year. There is a database of 4,000

shelters and services across the United States, Puerto Rico, Alaska, Hawaii, and the U.S. Virgin Islands. With just one contact, those experiencing domestic violence can find out about the options available in their own community. Bilingual services are available.

The Nursing Network on Violence against Women (NNVAW)
INTERNET ADDRESS: http://www.nnvawi.org/

The Nursing Network on Violence against Women (NNVAW) was formed to encourage the development of nursing practice that focuses on health issues relating to the effects of violence on women's lives. The abuse and exploitation of women is a social problem of epidemic proportions that adversely affects the health of millions of women each year. The Network's ethic fosters the ideal of nursing practice designed to provide assistance and support to women in the process of achieving their own personal empowerment. The ultimate goal of NNVAWI is to provide a nursing presence in the struggle to end violence in women's lives.

Resources for Obesity Management and Prevention

Weight-Control Information Network
INTERNET ADDRESS: http://win.niddk.nih.gov/publications/index.htm#public

On this Web site, there are hundreds of publications for the general public and health care professionals on nutrition, physical activity, and weight control. There are also numerous promotional flyers. These are excellent teaching tools and available in English and Spanish.

Weight Loss for Life
INTERNET ADDRESS: http://win.niddk.nih.gov/publications/PDFs/WeightLossforLife_04.pdf or http://win.niddk.nih.gov/publications/for_life.htm

This is a simple but comprehensive booklet that can be used as a health teaching tool for weight control. Topics covered include activity, nutrition, assessment of healthy weight, and how to evaluate weight loss programs and strategies. It can be downloaded and shared with clients in any setting. For nurses having classes on weight control, free copies can be ordered.

Talking to Patients about Weight Control
INTERNET ADDRESS: http://win.niddk.nih.gov/publications/PDFs/TalkingWPAWL.pdf

This site is for professionals to guide them in how to assess whether the client is ready to talk about weight control and how to successfully discuss the topic.

Seasonal Flu
INTERNET ADDRESS: http://www.cdc.gov/flu/

This site provides information on a variety of topics, including weekly and seasonal surveillance information about cases of the flu in the United States and globally. There are also numerous resources for health professionals and for health teaching purposes.

Resources for Smoking Cessation

American Lung Association: Primary, secondary and tertiary strategies
INTERNET ADDRESS: http://www.stateoftobaccocontrol.org/

How does your state rate as compared to other states in tobacco control? Find out by looking at this Web site. Mounting scientific evidence shows that effective tobacco control policies lead to fewer kids starting to smoke and more smokers quitting. However, elected officials continue to fail to enact these proven measures. The American Lung Association's State of Tobacco Control report tracks progress on key tobacco control policies at the state and federal levels and gives grades to tobacco control laws and regulations.

American Lung Association
INTERNET ADDRESS: http://www.lungusa.org/stop-smoking/how-to-quit/

Numerous resources are found on this Web site related to smoking cessation and how to talk to children and adolescents about smoking and many others.

National Heart Blood Lung Institute.
INTERNET ADDRESS: http://www.nhlbi.nih.gov/health/dci/index.html

This Web-based health index gives you a quick and easy way to get complete and dependable information about heart, lung, and blood diseases and sleep disorders. There are a variety of resources including podcasts, videos, quizzes, and widgets.

Tobacco Free Nurses/Tobacco Control Resources for Nurses
INTERNET ADDRESS: http://www.tobaccofreenurses.org/resources/

This Web site was designed to provide nurses with smoking cessation information, smoking research, international links, and information about trying to quit. There are informative and useful tools for nurses to use as a reference and resource for tobacco intervention.

Nursing Center for Tobacco Intervention
INTERNET ADDRESS: **http://www.projectmainstream.net/index.asp**
This site is an authoritative source for teaching and learning about alcohol, tobacco, and other drug problems. There are thousands of resources for identification, prevention, and treatment of substance use disorders developed and reviewed by experts. An interactive forum for health professions educators and others who want to learn and teach about substance abuse is also available on this site. Further, there is a vehicle for peer review and e-publication of original educational materials.

Quick Reference Guide for Clinicians: Treating Tobacco Use and Dependence
INTERNET ADDRESS: **http://www.ahrq.gov/clinic/tobacco/tobaqrg.pdf**
A guide that summarizes strategies for providing appropriate treatments for every client who could benefit from a smoking cessation program can be downloaded from this site.
Calculating the Cost of Smoking

University of Maryland Medical System
INTERNET ADDRESS: **http://www.healthcalculators.org/calculators/cigarette.asp**
This is an outstanding site to use when counseling and health teaching about the expense associated with smoking. The site has a calculator that can be used to calculate the cost of smoking depending on how much the person smokes a day.

Additional Web sites for Clients Interested in Information about Smoking Cessation
INTERNET ADDRESS: **http://www.cancer.org/docroot/subsite/greatamericans/smokeout.asp**
INTERNET ADDRESS: **http://www.smokefree.gov/**
INTERNET ADDRESS: **http://www.surgeongeneral.gov/tobacco/**
INTERNET ADDRESS: **http://www.cdc.gov/tobacco/quit_smoking/cessation/index.htm/**
INTERNET ADDRESS: **http://www.cdc.gov/tobacco/**
INTERNET ADDRESS: **http://apps.nccd.cdc.gov/osh_pub_catalog/PublicationList.aspx**
INTERNET ADDRESS: **http://www.healthfinder.gov/scripts/SearchContext.asp?topic=860**
INTERNET ADDRESS: **http://www.4woman.gov/QuitSmoking/index.cfm**

References and Bibliography

Agency for Healthcare Research and Quality. (2009a). *National health care disparity report*. Retrieved from http://www.ahrq.gov/qual/nhdr09/nhdr09.pdf

Agency for Healthcare Research and Quality. (2009b). *Key themes and highlights. National health care quality report*. Retrieved from http://www.ahrq.gov/qual/nhqr09/Key.htm

Agency for Healthcare Research and Quality. (2010). *Prevention and care management: Resources and tools. Women/Men: Stay healthy at any age screening guide*. Retrieved from http://www.ahrq.gov/clinic/ppipix.htm

American Heart Association. (2010). *Cigarette smoking and cardio-vascular disease*. Retrieved from http://www.americanheart.org/presenter.jhtml?identifier=4545

Andriankaja, O. (2009). The more oral bacteria, the higher the risk of heart attack, study shows. *ScienceDaily*. Retrieved from http://www.sciencedaily.com/releases/2009/04/090401101848.htm

Centers for Disease Control and Prevention. (2006). *CDC releases revised HIV testing recommendations in healthcare settings*. Retrieved from http://www.cdc.gov/hiv/topics/testing/resources/factsheets/pdf/healthcare.pdf

Centers for Disease Control and Prevention. (2008). *Preventing chronic disease: Investing in health. Preventing tobacco use*. Retrieved from http://www.cdc.gov/nccdphp/publications/factsheets/Prevention/pdf/tobacco.pdf

Centers for Disease Control and Prevention. (2009a). *Trends in sexually transmitted diseases in the United States. 2009*. Retrieved from http://www.cdc.gov/std/stats09/trends.htm

Centers for Disease Control and Prevention. (2009b). *Basic fact sheet: Colorectal cancer screening*. Retrieved from http://www.cdc.gov/cancer/colorectal/pdf/Basic_FS_Eng_Color.pdf

Centers for Disease Control and Prevention. (2010a). *Prostate cancer: Should I get screened?* Retrieved from http://www.cdc.gov/cancer/prostate/pdf/prostate_fs_final.pdf

Centers for Disease Control and Prevention. (2010b). *Skin cancer: Risk factors*. Retrieved from http://www.cdc.gov/cancer/skin/basic_info/risk_factors.htm

Centers for Disease Control and Prevention. (2010c). *The link between physical activity and morbidity and mortality. Physical activity and health: A report of the Surgeon General*. Retrieved from http://www.cdc.gov/nccdphp/sgr/pdf/mm.pdf

Centers for Disease Control and Prevention. (2010d). *Physical activity for everyone: How much physical activity do adults need*. Retrieved from http://www.cdc.gov/physicalactivity/everyone/guidelines/adults.html

Centers for Disease Control and Prevention, National Center for Injury Prevention and Control. (2009). *Understanding intimate partner violence fact sheet.* Retrieved from http://www.cdc.gov/violenceprevention/pdf/IPV_factsheet-a.pdf

Centers for Disease Control and Prevention, National Center for Disease Statistics. (2010). *Faststats: Adults with disabilities.* Retrieved from http://www.cdc.gov/nchs/fastats/disable.htm

Cohen, L. S., Soares, C. N., Vitonis, A. F., et al. (2006). Risk for new onset of depression during the menopausal transition: The Harvard Study of moods and cycles. *Archives of General Psychiatry, 63,* 385–390.

Ferguson, C., Langwith, C., Muldoon, A., & Leonard, J. (2010). *Improving obesity management in adult primary care: Executive summary. Strategies to Overcome and Prevent (STOP) Obesity Alliance.* George Washington University School of Public Health and Health Services, Department of Health Policy. Retrieved from http://www.stopobesityalliance.org/wp-content/assets/2010/03/STOP-Obesity-Alliance-PC-Paper-Executive-Summary-FINAL.pdf

Gaffney, K., Baghi, H., & Sheehan, S. (2009). Two decades of nurse-led research on smoking during pregnancy and postpartum: Concept development to intervention trials. *Annual Review of Nursing Research, 27,* 195–219. doi:10.1891/0739–6686.27.195.

Harwood, H. (2000). *Updating estimates of the economic costs of alcohol abuse in the United States: Estimates, update methods, and data.* Report prepared by The Lewin Group for the National Institute on Alcohol Abuse and Alcoholism. Retrieved from http://pubs.niaaa.nih.gov/publications/economic-2000/printing.htm

Kessler, R. C., Berglund, P., Demler, O., et al. (2005). Lifetime prevalence and age-of-onset distributions of DSM-IV disorders in the National Comorbidity Survey Replication. *Archives of General Psychiatry, 62*(6), 593–602.

Kvaavik, E., Batty, G. Ursin, G., Huxley, R., & Gale, CR. (2010). *Influence of individual and combined health behaviors on total and cause-specific mortality in men and women:* The United Kingdom health and lifestyle survey. *Archives of Internal Medicine 170,*(8). 711-718.

Malnick, S., & Knobler, H. (2006). The medical complications of obesity. *Quarterly Journal of Medicine., 99*(9), 565–579.

Malucky, A. (2010). Brief evidence-based interventions for nurse practitioners to aid patients in smoking cessation. *Journal for Nurse Practitioners, 6*(2), 126–131. doi:10.1016/j.nurpa.2009.05.017.

Mortality and Mobidity Weekly Report. (2010). *Vital signs: State-specific obesity prevalence among adults, United States, 2009.* Retrieved from http://www.cdc.gov/mmwr/pdf/wk/mm59e0803.pdf

National Center for HIV/AIDS. (2010). *HIV in the US.* Retrieved from http://www.cdc.gov/hiv/resources/factsheets/PDF/us.pdf

National Center for Injury Prevention and Control, Centers for Disease Control and Prevention. (2010). *10 leading causes of death, United States.* Retrieved from http://webappa.cdc.gov/cgi-bin/broker.exe

National Center for Injury Prevention and Control. (2010). *Injury prevention and control: Motor vehicle injuries.* Retrieved from http://www.cdc.gov/MotorVehicleSafety/Impaired_Driving/impaired-drv_factsheet.html

National Institute of Alcohol Abuse and Alcoholism. (2008). *Percent reporting heavy alcohol use in the past month by age group and demographic characteristics: NSDUH (NHSDA), 1994–2008.* Retrieved from http://www.niaaa.nih.gov/Resources/DatabaseResources/QuickFacts/AlcoholConsumption/Pages/default.aspx

National Institutes of Health, National Heart, Lung, and Blood Institute, Obesity Education Initiative. (1998). *The practical guide: Identification, evaluation, and treatment of overweight and obesity in adults.* Bethesda, MD: U.S. Department of Health and Human Services.

National Institutes of Health. (2000). *The practical guide: Identification, evaluation, and treatment of overweight and obesity in adults. National Heart, Lung, and Blood Institute Obesity Education Initiative* (NIH Publication Number 00-4084). Retrieved from http://www.nhlbi.nih.gov/guidelines/obesity/prctgd_c.pdf

Nidich, S., Fields, J., Rainforth, M., Pomerantz, R., Cella, D., Kristeller, J., et al. (2009). A randomized controlled trial of the effects of transcendental meditation on quality of life in older breast cancer patients. *Integrative Cancer Therapies, 8*(3), 228–234. Retrieved from CINAHL Plus with Full Text database. doi:10.1177/1534735409343000

Ogden, C., & Carroll, M. (2010). *Prevalence of overweight, obesity, and extreme obesity among adults: United States, Trends 1976–1980 through 2007–2008.* Retrieved from http://www.cdc.gov/NCHS/data/hestat/obesity_adult_07_08/obesity_adult_07_08.pdf

O'Donnell, M., Xavier, D., Lisheng, L., Zhang, H., Chin, S., & Yusuf, S. (2010). Risk factors for ischaemic and intracerebral haemorrhagic stroke in 22 countries (the INTERSTROKE study): A case-control study. *The Lancet, 376*(9735), 112–123. Online publication. doi:10.1016/S0140-6736(10)60834-3.

Rahman, M., & Berenson, A. (2010). Self-perception of weight and its association with weight-related behaviors in young, reproductive-aged women. *Obstetrics & Gynecology, 116*(6), 1274–1280. doi:10.1097/AOG.0b013e3181fdfc47.

Rapaport, M., Schettler, P., & Bresee, C. (2010). A preliminary study of the effects of a single session of Swedish massage on hypothalamic-pituitary-adrenal and immune function in normal individuals. *Journal of Alternative & Complementary Medicine, 16*(10), 1079–1088. doi:10.1089/acm.2009.0634.

Rice, V., & Stead, L. (2008). Nursing interventions for smoking cessation. Cochrane Database of Systematic Reviews, (1), Retrieved from EBSCOhost.

Roberts, J., & Rhoades, J. A. (2010). *The uninsured in America, first half of 2009: Estimates for the US civilian noninstitutionalized population under age 65.* Retrieved from http://www.meps.ahrq.gov/mepsweb/data_files/publications/st291/stat291.pdf

Tamim, H., Castel, E., Jamnik, V., Keir, P., Grace, S., Gledhill, N., et al. (2009). Tai Chi workplace program for improving musculoskeletal fitness among female computer users. *Work, 34*(3), 331–338. doi:10.3233/WOR-2009-0931.

U.S. Department of Health and Human Services. (2007). *National Institute of Health tips for talking about weight control.* Retrieved from http://win.niddk.nih.gov/publications/talking.htm#staff

U.S. Department of Health and Human Services. (2010). *Healthy People 2020.* Washington, DC: U.S. Government Printing Office. Retreived from http://www.healthypeople.gov/2020/default.aspx

U.S. Preventive Services Task Force. (2010). Screening for breast cancer, topic page. Retrieved from http://www.uspreventiveservicestaskforce.org/uspstf/uspsbrca.htm

Wang, P. S., Berglund, P., Olfson, M., et al. (2005). Failure and delay in initial treatment contact after first onset of mental disorders in National Comorbidity Survey Replication. *Archives of General Psychiatry 62*(6), 603–613.

Wolf, A., Wender, R., Etzioni, Thompson, I., D'Amico, S., Volk, R., Durado, B., Chiranjeev, S., Guessous, I., Andrews, K.,DeSantis, C., & Smith R. (2010). American Cancer Society Guideline for the early detection of prostate cancer: Update 2010. CA: A Cancer Journal for Clinicians, 60(2). 70-98. DOI: 10.3322/caac.20066

LEARNING ACTIVITIES

JOURNALING ACTIVITY 9-1

In your clinical journal, describe a situation where you have observed an adult client who was not receiving the health promotion or disease prevention care that he or she needed.

- What screening or intervention would the client have benefited from receiving?
- How would you advocate for these issues when you begin to practice as an RN?
- What could you do now?
- Do you see evidence that the current health care system values and provides prevention and health promotion care? Why do you think that this type of care is or is not valued or provided? What arguments would you make that health care should provide such an emphasis in care?

JOURNALING ACTIVITY 9-2

In your clinical journal, describe a situation you have encountered when screening and doing health promotion and disease prevention teaching and planning with an adult client.

- What did you learn from this experience?
- How will you practice differently based on this experience?

CLIENT CARE ACTIVITY 9-3

You are working as a home care nurse, caring for Richard, a 45-year-old client who has advanced chronic obstructive pulmonary disease and is on oxygen constantly. Richard, a former smoker, has had several upper respiratory infections this winter, with one resulting in hospitalization for a week. Richard lives with his 25-year-old daughter and her husband, who are both teachers and heavy smokers.

- Which health indicators contribute to Richard's health status?
- What could you as the nurse for this family do to promote Richard's health?
- What community health interventions would you use?
- What steps will you take to address this issue?

PRACTICAL APPLICATION ACTIVITY 9-4

A local community agency has contacted your instructor to ask that a team of students survey some of the clients at their facility to determine health promotion and disease prevention needs as well as the best way to provide health promotion and disease prevention teaching and care.

- What would you like to know about this group before planning this project?
- When forming a group to work on this task, whom would you invite to participate?
- How would you involve the various community partners in the planning?
- How would you go about determining what to include and how to develop the survey?
- What resources could you consult to develop teaching and standard of care materials based on the findings of the survey?

CLINICAL REASONING ACTIVITY 9-5

You are visiting with a family friend who asks you about your studies in your nursing classes. You explain that you are studying about disease prevention and health promotion. The friend, who is 45 years old, says, "I am not sick. What would someone my age need to do to prevent disease?"

- What would be your response to his question?
- What could you tell him about the leading health indicators?
- What simple assessment could you make?
- What suggestions could you make based on what you learned about his present health indicators?

Chapter 10

Health Promotion and Disease and Injury Prevention for Older Adults

ROBERTA HUNT

Learning Objectives

1. Identify the major causes of death for the older adults.
2. Discuss the major diseases and threats to the health of older adults.
3. Summarize the major health issues for older adults.
4. Identify nursing roles for each level of prevention for major health issues affecting older adults.
5. Compose a list of nursing interventions for the major health issues of older adults.
6. Determine health needs of older adults for which a nurse could be an advocate.

Key Terms

life expectancy at ages 65 and 85
life expectancy at birth
medication safety
polypharmacy

Chapter Topics

Health Status of Older Adults

Eliminating Disparity in Health Care

Health Screening in Older Adults

Interventions for Leading Health Indicators

Policy

Conclusions

The Nurse Speaks

Bea was unforgettable. She was a woman who had lived a hard life, which was reflected in her face and physical condition. She was short, thin, missing several teeth, and appeared older than her 73 years. Most remarkable was Bea's short vibrant red–orange hair, which spiked out in all directions. There were never any cards or flowers or visitors in Bea's room, but it was reported that her husband visited in the evening. Bea was not the kind of patient to inspire extra staff support, but Bea's continued presence on the unit and her weekly assignment to one of the students resulted in visits by almost all of the students each week. The students found her mysterious past, red hair, and one-of-a-kind smile hard to resist.

Spring break and on-campus activities had resulted in several weeks away from the unit. On our return, I was surprised to find Bea still on the unit. She had undergone additional major surgery and once again spent time in intensive care on mechanical ventilation. The staff noted that she was supposed to be up and walking, but when brought to a standing position, she would throw herself back on the bed, dead weight and hard to move despite her less than 100-lb weight. The nursing staff felt I might be able to find a more interesting patient than Bea, so I assigned Bea to a student who had not yet cared for her. The next morning, I went in to check on the student and Bea. Bea still had that amazing red hair (which seemed a little more gray at the base), she was thinner (if that could be possible), she looked tired, and there was no smile. She was alone in a dark double room in the bed farthest from the door, a central line was infusing a variety of fluids, and she wore a nasal cannula for oxygen.

Two students were talking to Bea about their plans for the summer, beginning with a much-anticipated massage. I joined the conversation and agreed there was nothing more relaxing than a day at the spa. I asked Bea if she would like to have a spa day and suggested that if she did, she and the student plan it for the next day. Bea was noncommittal. In postconference, Bea's spa day was discussed. The next morning, each of the students asked me if Bea's student was going ahead with the spa day.

About 9 o'clock, I finally made it to Bea's room. I had brought my lavender essential oil and planned to demonstrate how to use the oil to provide a hand massage. The student noted that Bea was presently resting, having received a complete bath and a long massage. Prior to the bath, the student had suggested that Bea get up for a short walk. According to the student, and to the amazement of the staff, Bea popped out of bed and circled the unit, leaving the student struggling to keep up. No wonder Bea was resting. Around 10 o'clock, we got Bea up in a chair, wrapped her in a warm bath blanket obtained from preop, and washed her hair using the hair-wash-in-a-hat. Bea's hair looked great—soft, shiny, clean, and, of course, very red. A foot soak was prepared using a few drops of lavender essential oil. The aroma of lavender began to fill the room. The student asked Bea if she would like a hand massage, and Bea agreed after some convincing. As the student began the steps of the hand massage, using Jane Buckle's "M" Technique and a 5% lavender essential oil solution, Bea closed her eyes and snuggled into her blanket. When it came to massaging the second hand, Bea was ready. The aroma of lavender now filled the room and wafted into the hall. The students started stopping by. They reminded Bea who they were and asked her how her spa day was going. The students told Bea how relaxed and comfortable she looked and expressed some envy.

Eventually, Bea was returned to a fresh bed with the curtains pulled back. Staff walking by the door started stopping in, wondering what was going on. They told Bea she smelled great and so did her room. The student told the staff about Bea's spa day as she reported off. Each of the nursing staff commented that this was what they had gone into nursing for and never had the time to do.

Staff members also observed that they had never seen Bea look so great. During postconference, Bea's student shared how excited the staff was about Bea's spa day. The staff noted she looked much better and were definitely impressed by her walk around the unit, the first in a long time. The social worker decided she wanted to see for herself what this was all about, so she went in to see Bea and asked her how her morning had gone. Bea stated, "This is the first time I have felt like a real person in a long time."

Now whether this change in Bea was due to the massage, the hair wash, the warm blanket, the essential oil, an increase in positive social interaction, or Bea's own self-determination, it is hard to know. I like to think that it was a holistic intervention plan focused on Bea, helping her and those about her find Bea, a woman with strength, a great smile, a mysterious past, and amazing hair.

Mary Kathryn Moberg, MS, RN
Associate Professor
St. Catherine University

Health Status of Older Adults

Life expectancy at birth, as well as **life expectancy at ages 65 and 85**, has increased over time as death rates for many causes of death have declined. Life expectancy at birth is the number of years that a person born in that year can expect to live. Life expectancy at 65 or 85 is the number of years that a person who is 65 or 85 years old can expect to live. The leading causes of death for older adults are listed in Table 10-1.

The elderly population in the United States is growing. Life expectancies at ages 65 and 85 have increased over the past 50 years. People who live to age 65 can expect to live, on average, nearly 18 more years. Since 1900, the percentage of people 65 years and older has tripled with the aging of the baby boomers born between 1946 and 1964 accelerating this growth. In 1994, about one in eight Americans were elderly but about 1 in 5 will be elderly by the year 2030. There is an increase in the proportion of men 85 years and older who are veterans. In addition, the elderly population will continue to be more and more diverse. This growing segment of the population has health care needs that are different from those of other segments of the population. Of people older than 70 years, 80% have one or more chronic conditions (Administration on Aging, 2010; Centers for Disease Control and Prevention [CDC], 2010b; Interagency Forum on Aging Related Statistics, 2011, p. 54).

Living arrangements of persons over 65 years of age show that as people age, they are more likely to live alone. Further, they are more likely to have difficulty performing one or more physical activities, activities of daily living (ADL), or instrumental ADL. Figure 10-1 shows selected chronic conditions limiting activity for people older than 65 years. All of these factors have implications for the ability of older adults to perform self-care and live independently while managing a chronic illness and the amount of nursing care this population may need as they age.

Table 10-1 Leading Causes of Death in Adults 65 Years and Older, United States, 2007
Cause of Death Age 65 and above
Heart disease
Malignant neoplasms
Cerebrovascular

Source: Office of Statistics and Programming, (2011). National Center for Injury Prevention and Control, Centers for Disease Control and Prevention.
Data Source: National Center for Health Statistics (NCHS), National Vital Statistics System. Leading causes of death. Retrieved from http://webappa.cdc.gov/cgi-bin/broker.exe

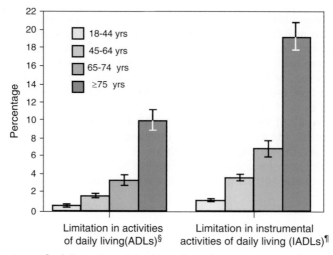

Figure 10-1 Percentage of adults with activity limitations, by age group and type of limitation. From Percentage of adults with activity limitations, by age group and type of limitation. National Health Interview Survey, United States, 2008. *Mortality and Morbidity Weekly Report, 58*(48), 1357. Retrieved from http://www.cdc.gov/mmwr/preview/mmwrhtml/mm5848a6.htm

Eliminating Disparity in Health Care

Recommendations from Healthy People 2020 offer a foundation for all health promotion and disease prevention nursing actions. This chapter focuses on the goals from Healthy People 2020 as they relate to older adult health. These include attaining higher quality, longer lives free of preventable disease, disability, injury, and premature death; achieving health equity; eliminating disparities and improving the health of all groups; and promoting quality of life (QOL), healthy development, and healthy behaviors across all life stages.

Health Screening in Older Adults

As with clients at other ages, health screening for the older adults is intended for primary, secondary, or tertiary prevention. Primary prevention (to prevent the initial occurrence of a disease) with an elderly client could be immunization screening, recommendation of an annual flu shot, or a safety assessment of the home to identify areas where a fall could occur. Examples of secondary prevention are screening for hypertension and teaching breast self-examination to a group or an individual. Tertiary prevention could be initiating an exercise program for an older client who has heart disease or a home safety check to eliminate hazards that may result in falls. Screening is always performed so that people at risk for certain conditions can be identified, with interventions provided as appropriate.

One way to encourage the older client to put prevention into practice is to use *Men Stay Healthy at 50+* or *Women Stay Healthy at 50+* available online at http://www.ahrq.gov/ppip/men50.htm or http://www.ahrq.gov/ppip/women50.htm. It is also available in Spanish. It includes recommendations about lifestyle choices that prevent certain chronic diseases, primary prevention screening, and immunizations. It is an excellent tool for guiding health promotion and disease prevention activities.

GENERAL SCREENING

All screening discussed for adults in Chapter 9 also applies to older adults. This section discusses screening that is particularly important for older adults. The American College of

Preventive Medicine has identified the most effective and cost-effective clinical preventive services. Among the services that apply to the elderly are aspirin to prevent heart disease; screening and counseling for tobacco use and problem drinking; screening for colorectal cancer, cervical cancer, vision impairment, blood pressure, and cholesterol; and pneumococcal and influenza immunizations.

High blood pressure is more common in people over age 55, especially African Americans. Therefore, older adults should have their blood pressure checked periodically, with the frequency determined by their nurse practitioner or physician. Cholesterol levels start to increase in middle-aged men, in women just before menopause, and in anyone who has just gained weight; cholesterol should be measured in people meeting these descriptions.

Heart disease is the leading cause of death for people over 65 years of age. Heart disease is the number 1 killer of women, yet only 8% of women realize that it is a greater threat than cancer. More than 200,000 women die each year from heart attacks, which is five times as many as women who die of breast cancer. More than 42 million women are currently living with some form of cardiovascular disease, with 35.3% of deaths in American women over the age of 20 caused by cardiovascular disease each year.

Disparity by gender exists in terms of mortality and morbidity rates for heart disease. Women are more likely than men to die of heart disease each year. Twenty-three percent of women and 18% of men die within 1 year of the first recognized heart attack, while 22% to 32% of female and 15% to 27% of male heart attack survivors die within 5 years. Women are less likely than men to receive appropriate treatment after a heart attack, and women are almost twice as likely as men to die after bypass surgery. Despite this documented disparity in mortality and morbidity for heart disease, women comprise only 27% of participants in all heart-related research studies (National Coalition of Women with Heart Disease, 2010).

As with other chronic conditions, the risk factors for developing heart disease should be identified and addressed in childhood (e.g., poor diet, lack of exercise, smoking, and weight gain). It is essential that every adult be aware of his or her own risk factors for heart disease.

Type 2 diabetes is more common in people over age 45, with one in five individuals over age 65 developing diabetes. Screening for diabetes is recommended for people who have a family member with diabetes, those who are overweight, and those who have had diabetes during pregnancy. Type 2 diabetes is a risk factor for developing heart disease.

Hearing impairment is common in older adults: More than 35% of people over age 65 and 50% of people over age 75 have some degree of hearing loss. Hearing loss can lead to miscommunication, social withdrawal, confusion, depression, and reduction in functional status. Likewise, older adults have more vision problems such as glaucoma, cataracts, or macular degeneration. Older people are more likely than younger adults to suffer accidental injuries because of vision problems, making regular eye exams important.

Older individuals should also be screened for risk of osteoporosis, depression, alcohol abuse, and violence as discussed in Chapter 9.

The adult immunization schedule applies to older adults as well. However, the current recommendation is that everyone older than 50 years receives an annual flu shot, and, if over age 65, he or she receives a pneumonia shot besides being vaccinated against whooping cough and shingles. However, each individual should consult a primary care provider about the vaccines they might need. Older people should be screened for tuberculosis (TB) if they have been in close contact with someone who has TB; have recently moved to the United States from Asia, Africa, Central or South America, or the Pacific Islands; have kidney failure, diabetes, or alcoholism; are positive for human immunodeficiency virus (HIV); or have injected or now inject illegal drugs. Making vaccinations more convenient is known to increase immunization rates among elderly and at-risk people. Nurses working in community-based settings are often the professionals who initiate, implement, and evaluate this type of service.

CANCER SCREENING

Most breast cancer occurs in women older than 50 years, so mammography is recommended every 2 years after a woman reaches 50 years of age unless family history suggests otherwise. Women who have ever been sexually active should have a Pap test every 3 years except in the presence of genital warts, multiple sex partners, or an abnormal Pap test, in which case, testing should be done annually. Women over age 65 with a history of normal Pap smears or with a hysterectomy may stop having Pap tests after consulting with a nurse practitioner or physician. For women without health insurance, the National Breast and Cervical Cancer Early Detection Program (NBCCEDP) offers free or low-cost mammograms and education about breast cancer. Consult the Web site at http://apps.nccd.cdc.gov/cancercontacts/nbccedp/contacts.asp for more information or to find out where your clients can get a free or low-cost clinical breast examinations, mammograms, Pap tests, pelvic examinations, diagnostic testing if results are abnormal, or referrals to treatment in your area.

Colon cancer is more common in older than in younger adults. Starting at age 50, fecal occult blood testing should be done every year in combination with other screening tests as recommended by the health care provider.

Prostate cancer is most common in men over age 50, African Americans, and men with a family history of prostate cancer. Screening includes digital rectal examination and prostate-specific antigen blood testing. Other information on this topic is found in Chapter 9.

ADDITIONAL SCREENING

Environmental screening with a home safety check is an essential component of health promotion and disease prevention for the older client. As discussed in Chapter 5, other screening that is important for older clients is hearing and vision screening, functional assessment, and cognition status. With all clients, it is important to screen for all leading health indicators. Refer to Healthy People 2020 9-1 in Chapter 9 for a list of the leading health indicators from Healthy People 2020. Interventions to address these indicators are covered in the next section.

Interventions for Leading Health Indicators

Once screening has been done, conditions that put the client at risk are addressed. Many factors have contributed to the decline in mortality from heart disease and stroke. Some of these include changes in health behaviors such as not smoking, improvements in nutrition, being physically active, drinking alcohol in moderation, and maintaining a healthy weight.

Because the average person is living longer, more attention is now focused on preserving QOL than on extending length of life. Most older people have one or more chronic conditions, and as a result of increased longevity, they will be living longer with these conditions (Fig. 10-2). Nurses will continue to be involved in efforts to decrease the adverse social and economic consequences of a high rate of activity limitation and disability of older persons. Thus, health promotion and disease prevention interventions for this segment of the population are important.

Using disease prevention and health promotion interventions requires questioning assumptions commonly held about older adults, including seeing them as sick and sedentary, sexless, and senile. Nurses can facilitate healthy aging by considering the older client holistically and maximize functioning by addressing physical and psychological well-being, as well as competence in adaptation (Fig. 10-3).

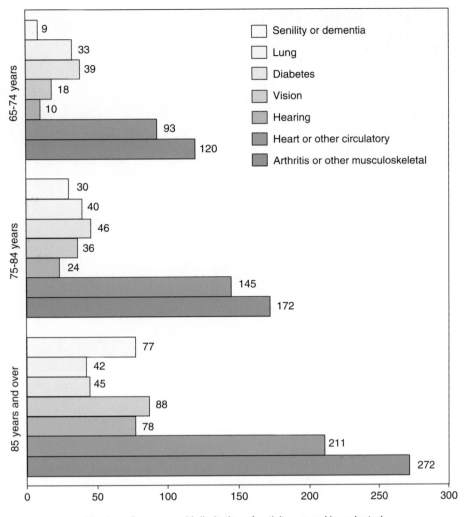

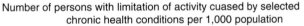

Number of persons with limitation of activity cuased by selected
chronic health conditions per 1,000 population

Figure 10-2 Limitation of activity caused by selected chronic health conditions among older adults, by age: United States. From National Center for Health Statistics. (2009). *Health, United States, 2009 with chartbook on trends in the health of Americans.* Retrieved from http://www.ncbi.nlm.nih.gov/books/NBK19623/

PHYSICAL ACTIVITY

Older adults, both men and women, obtain significant health benefits from a moderate amount of daily physical activity. Additional health benefits are gained through even greater amounts of physical activity. Care should always be taken to avoid injury.

Previously sedentary older adults who begin physical activity programs should first consult with their health care provider. Then they should begin with start with short intervals of moderate physical activity, from 5 to 10 minutes, and gradually build up to the desired amount. Benefits of physical activity include cardiorespiratory endurance and muscle strengthening. Stronger muscles reduce the risk of falling and improve the ability to perform routine tasks of daily life. Other benefits of physical activity include the following:

- Helps maintain the ability to live independently and reduces the risk of falling and fracturing bones

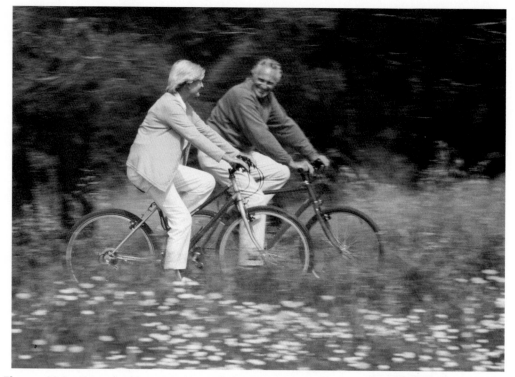

Figure 10-3 Using health promotion and disease prevention strategies can create a longer and healthier life. Used with permission from U.S. Administration on Aging, Department of Health and Human Services (from the photo archive at the Administration on Aging: http:aoa.gov)

- Reduces the risk of dying from coronary heart disease and of developing high blood pressure, colon cancer, and diabetes
- Helps reduce blood pressure in some people with hypertension
- Helps people with chronic, disabling conditions improve their stamina and muscle strength
- Reduces symptoms of anxiety and depression and fosters improvements in mood and feelings of well-being
- Helps maintain healthy bones, muscles, and joints
- Helps control joint swelling and pain associated with arthritis

For several decades, recommendations regarding ways that communities can promote physical activity for older adults have been commonly known (Box 10-1). Nurses have an important role to play in ensuring that these simple suggestions are implemented in their own communities.

OVERWEIGHT AND OBESITY

Because no consensus exists regarding optimal weight for older persons, it is difficult to make recommendations regarding weight loss in the older adult. In the past, it was believed that lean body weight throughout life is optimal, but stability in weight after age 50 is also important. Obesity has been tied to dozens of health problems: hypertension, diabetes, knee replacement surgery, heart failure, cholecystitis, pulmonary embolism, chronic fatigue, and insomnia (CDC, 2009). For more than a decade, the literature has documented an urgent

---

BOX 10-1   ## What Communities Can Do to Promote Physical Activity in Older Adults

- Provide community-based physical activity programs that offer aerobic, strengthening, and flexibility components specifically designed for older adults.
- Encourage mall and other indoor or protected locations to provide safe places for walking in any weather.
- Ensure that facilities for physical activity accommodate and encourage participation by older adults.
- Provide transportation for older adults to parks or facilities that provide physical activity programs.
- Encourage health care providers to talk routinely to their older adult clients about incorporating physical activity into their lives.
- Plan community activities that include opportunities for older adults to be physically active.

From Centers for Disease Control and Prevention. (1999). *Physical activity and health: A report of the Surgeon General.* Retrieved from http://www.cdc.gov/nccdphp/sgr/olderad.htm

---

need for effective and practical public health approaches to preventing weight gain and treating obesity across the life span.

TOBACCO USE

Smoking among adults has declined, but older smokers continue to suffer a large proportion of the health consequences from smoking. Because smoking remains the health indicator that is known to most negatively affect health, it is important to address the question of smoking with older clients and encourage them to quit. Research has shown that older smokers, particularly those hospitalized with cardiovascular disease, can quit at high rates when provided an intervention (Doolan & Froelicher, 2008). Nurses are well positioned to facilitate smoking cessation. Community-Based Teaching 10-1 can be used for teaching older clients about the advantages of quitting at any age.

SUBSTANCE ABUSE

Older adults tend to drink less than other age groups. However, current research suggests that alcohol use among this group is on the rise, thus problems in older adults are anticipated to become a national health issue. Not everyone who drinks regularly has a drinking problem. However, older adults are more vulnerable to harm from consuming alcohol compared to individuals at other points along the life span.

As age increases, alcohol is metabolized more slowly; as a result, alcohol remains in the body longer. Older adults are more likely to have health conditions that can be exacerbated by alcohol, including stroke, hypertension, neurodegeneration, memory loss, mood disorders, and cognitive or emotional problems. Compared to younger people, older adults take more medications, putting them at risk for interactions that can be dangerous or even life threatening. Alcohol also may decrease the effectiveness of some medications (United States Department of Health and Human Services [USDHHS], 2008).

A comprehensive nursing assessment includes exploring alcohol use with the client. Older individuals respond well to cognitive behavioral therapy and group treatment with other older adults. Social isolation is associated with alcohol abuse. It is helpful to involve the family in the treatment process because family support might have been lacking or even exacerbating the patient's alcohol use (USDHHS, 2008).

COMMUNITY-BASED TEACHING 10-1

Check Your Smoking IQ

If you or someone you know is an older smoker, you may think that there is no point in quitting now. Think again. By quitting smoking now, you will feel more in control and have fewer coughs and colds. On the other hand, with every cigarette you smoke, you increase your chances of having a heart attack, a stroke, or cancer. Need to think about this more? Take this older smokers' IQ quiz. Just answer "true" or "false" to each statement below.

True or False

1. ○ True ○ False   If you have smoked for most of your life, it's not worth stopping now.
2. ○ True ○ False   Older smokers who try to quit are more likely to stay off cigarettes.
3. ○ True ○ False   Smokers get tired and short of breath more easily than nonsmokers of the same age.
4. ○ True ○ False   Smoking is a major risk factor for heart attack and stroke among adults 60 years of age and older.
5. ○ True ○ False   Quitting smoking can help those who have already had a heart attack.
6. ○ True ○ False   Most older smokers don't want to stop smoking.
7. ○ True ○ False   An older smoker is more likely to smoke more cigarettes than a younger smoker.
8. ○ True ○ False   Someone who has smoked for 30 to 40 years probably won't be able to quit smoking.
9. ○ True ○ False   Very few older adults smoke cigarettes.
10. ○ True ○ False   Lifelong smokers are more likely to die of diseases such as emphysema and bronchitis than nonsmokers.

Answers

1. False.   Nonsense! You have every reason to quit now and quit for good—even if you've been smoking for years. Stopping smoking will help you live longer and feel better. You will reduce your risk of heart attack, stroke, and cancer; improve blood flow and lung function; and help stop diseases such as emphysema and bronchitis from getting worse.
2. True.   Once they quit, older smokers are far more likely than younger smokers to stay away from cigarettes. Older smokers know more about both the short- and long-term health benefits of quitting.
3. True.   Smokers, especially those over 50 years old, are much more likely to get tired, feel short of breath, and cough more often. These symptoms can signal the start of bronchitis or emphysema, both of which are suffered more often by older smokers. Stopping smoking will help reduce these symptoms.
4. True.   Smoking is a major risk factor for four of the five leading causes of death including heart disease, stroke, cancer, and lung diseases such as emphysema and bronchitis. For adults 60 years and older, smoking is a major risk factor for 6 of the top 14 causes of death. Older male smokers are nearly twice as likely to die from stroke as older men who do not smoke. The odds are nearly as high for older female smokers. Cigarette smokers of any age have a 70% greater heart disease death rate than do nonsmokers.
5. True.   The good news is that stopping smoking does help people who have suffered a heart attack. In fact, their chances of having another attack are smaller. In some cases, ex-smokers can cut their risk of another heart attack by half or more.

Continued on following page

COMMUNITY-BASED TEACHING 10-1

Check Your Smoking IQ (Continued)

6. False.   Most smokers would prefer to quit. In fact, in a recent study, 65% of older smokers said that they would like to stop. What keeps them from quitting? They are afraid of being irritable, nervous, and tense. Others are concerned about cravings for cigarettes. Most don't want to gain weight. Many think it's too late to quit—that quitting after so many years of smoking will not help. But this is not true.

7. True.   Older smokers usually smoke more cigarettes than younger people. Plus, older smokers are more likely to smoke high-nicotine brands.

8. False.   You may be surprised to learn that older smokers are actually more likely to succeed at quitting smoking. This is truer if they're already experiencing long-term smoking-related symptoms such as shortness of breath, coughing, or chest pain. Older smokers who stop want to avoid further health problems, take control of their life, get rid of the smell of cigarettes, and save money.

9. False.   One of five adults 50 years or older smokes cigarettes.

10. True.   Smoking greatly increases the risk of dying from diseases such as emphysema and bronchitis. In fact, over 80% of all deaths from these two diseases are directly due to smoking. The risk of dying from lung cancer is also a lot higher for smokers than nonsmokers: 22 times higher for males, 12 times higher for females.

From National Heart, Lung, and Blood Institute. *Campaign resources.* Retrieved from http://www.nhlbi.nih.gov/health/public/lung/copd/campaign-materials/index.htm

Older problem drinkers have a good chance for recovery because once they decide to seek help, they usually stay with treatment programs. Alcohol dependence is often not appreciated as relevant to the care of older adults. There is emerging evidence that reduction in alcohol use among older adults abusing alcohol can enhance health-related QOL. Because of the comorbidity of alcohol abuse and depression, it is important to screen for alcohol abuse in all cases where depression is suspected. For additional information on substance abuse, see Chapter 9.

RESPONSIBLE SEXUAL BEHAVIOR

Understanding normal changes in sexual response is the first step to sexual health promotion. With aging, women may notice changes in the shape and flexibility of the vagina and a decrease in vaginal lubrication. This can be addressed by using a vaginal lubricant. Men may find that it takes longer to get an erection or that the erection may not be as firm or large as in earlier years. As men get older, impotence increases, with some chronic conditions contributing to this change (e.g., heart disease, hypertension, and diabetes). For many men, impotence can be managed and reversed. Many pharmaceutical and mechanical options are available to enhance sexual enjoyment. Nurses and nurse practitioners are often the trusted member of the health team to whom a client may first direct his or her question about sexuality.

Having safe sex is imperative for people at all ages. In some areas of the country, the incidence of HIV among the elderly is on the rise. It is always essential that the nurse discuss the importance of safe sex, particularly regarding having sex with a new partner or multiple partners. Before having sex with a new partner, the client should be encouraged to be tested for sexually transmitted diseases and talk to the new partner about doing the same.

MENTAL HEALTH

Many issues related to mental health emerge as individuals age. The losses associated with aging, including loss of health, friends, and spouse, all contribute to the development of depression among the elderly. The risk of depression in the older adult increases when chronic illness impairs functional abilities. Estimates of major depression in older people living in the community range from less than 1% to about 5%, but rises to 13.5% in those who require home health care and to 11.5% in older hospital patients (National Institute of Mental Health [NIMH], 2010). Depression can and should be treated, and there are many effective therapies available. Unfortunately, depression is commonly underdiagnosed and undertreated in the older adult population. Interrupting depression in the elderly significantly extends life.

Depression is one of the most common conditions associated with suicide in older adults. Older Americans are disproportionately likely to die by suicide; they make up only 12% of the U.S. population but account for 16% of suicide deaths (NIMH, 2010). The highest rate of suicide in the Unites States is found in White men 85 years and older, which is five times the national rate (NIMH, 2010).

Home care nurses use the OASIS-C (discussed in Chapter 5 and 12) method of assessment, which requires ongoing screening for depression. The nurse asks the client, "in the past 2 weeks, how often have you experienced little interest or pleasure in doing things or feeling down, depressed, or hopeless?" A frequent positive response requires a referral for further evaluation. This same simple assessment and referral can be used by nurses in any setting.

Once depression is identified, it can be treated successfully. Support groups, other talk therapy, antidepressant drugs, and electroconvulsive therapy are some forms of treatment that may be used for clients with depression.

Preparing for major changes in life, keeping and maintaining friendships, developing interests or hobbies, and keeping the mind and body active may help prevent depression. Exploring and cultivating opportunities for social interaction and social support maintains mental health (Fig. 10-4). Being physically fit, eating a balanced diet, and following the nurse practitioner or physician's recommendations regarding medication can also minimize depression. Other suggestions for the client facing depression include the following:

- Accept the fact that help is needed.
- Consult a health care provider who has special training in mental health issues of the older adult.
- Do not be afraid of getting help because of the cost.

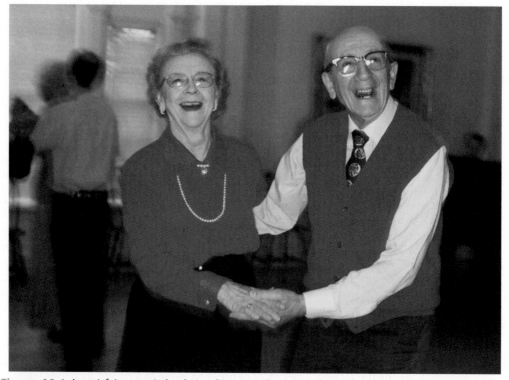

Figure 10-4 A satisfying marital relationship contributes to longevity. Used with permission from U.S. Administration on Aging, Department of Health and Human Services (from the photo archive at the Administration on Aging: http:aoa.gov).

If the depressed older person will not seek help, friends or relatives may facilitate self-care by explaining to the person how treatment may help them feel better. Sometimes, the family can arrange for the health care provider to call the family member or make a home visit to start the process. Community mental health centers offer treatment and often have resources for depression.

SAFETY AND INJURY PREVENTION

Injuries are a leading cause of morbidity and mortality among older adults. The primary causes of injury among this age group are motor vehicle accidents, falls, and mishaps. Risk factors related to injuries include polypharmacology, depression, vision and hearing impairments, and reduced reaction time.

Motor vehicle–related death rates for older adults are the highest of any age group. The risk of being killed in a motor vehicle accident increases with age. Per miles driven, adults older than 75 years have higher rates of vehicle-related death than all other age groups except teenagers. Measures that could benefit older people as well as other age groups are increased use of public transportation and restricted driving privileges when circumstances warrant. For example, in some states, the length of the license term for older drivers has been reduced from 4 years to 2 years. In some states, physicians are required to report to the state's licensing agency cases of certain medical conditions that could affect a person's ability to drive.

Falls are recognized as a leading cause of injury and death among older adults. In the United States, one of every three people 65 years and older falls each year. Half of those older than 75 years who fracture a hip as a result of a fall die within 1 year of the incident (CDC, 2010a). By 2020, the cost of fall injuries is expected to reach $32 billion. The general risk factors for falling include fall history, gait and balance impairment, the use of sedative and hypnotic medications, incontinence, difficulties in performing ADL, inactivity, visual impairment, home hazards, and reduced lower limb strength. The elderly are at increased risk for injury from falls because of the high incidence of osteoporosis in this age group. Prevention of fractures is related to increasing bone density and preventing falls. See Community-Based Teaching 10-2 for tips to prevent fractures in older adults.

Polypharmacy, or the prescription of more than one medication, resulting in a complex medication regimen, is becoming more common. Older clients typically take more

---

COMMUNITY-BASED TEACHING 10-2

Tips for Prevention of Fractures in Older Clients

Osteoporosis can be prevented by
- Doing weight-bearing exercises, such as walking, stair climbing, jogging, yoga, and lifting weights
- Getting 1,000 to 1,300 mg of calcium per day
- Not smoking

In adults 65 years or older, 60% of all falls happen at home, 30% in public places, and 10% in health care institutions.
The risk of falling can be reduced by

- Maintaining a regular exercise program
- Taking steps to make living areas safer:
  - Remove tripping hazards
  - Use nonskid mats in the bathtub
  - Have handrails on both sides of all stairs
  - Reviewing all medications with the nurse practitioner or physician to reduce side effects and interactions
  - Having a vision check every year

Adapted from Centers for Disease Control and Prevention. (2010a). *Falls among adults: An overview.* Retrieved from http://www.cdc.gov/HomeandRecreationalSafety/Falls/adultfalls.html

medications than other age groups. Medication errors are increasingly recognized as a potential for injury. Taking medication the wrong way or with other medications that cause harmful interactions can make the client worse rather than better. **Medication safety** should be practiced by all those taking a number of medications. *Your Medication: Play It Safe Patient Guide,* is an excellent guide designed to help avoid medication errors and get the most from the medication (AHRQ, 2004). See What's on the Web for information on how to obtain a copy.

ENVIRONMENTAL QUALITY

Because older clients are more vulnerable to alterations in environmental conditions, poor air quality has a greater impact on this age group. As people age, their bodies are less able to compensate for the effects of all environmental hazards. The proportion of older individuals exposed to poor air quality, both secondhand smoke and other air pollution, must be reduced. Further, older adults benefit from reducing their own exposure to poor air quality. This can be accomplished by avoiding tobacco smoke, smoke from wood-burning stoves, mold, dust mites, and cockroaches and keeping pets out of sleeping areas. Indoor air quality in the home must be maintained. This is accomplished by checking and cleaning furnace and heating units and fixing water leaks promptly. Last of all, monitoring outdoor air quality through the Air Quality Index (http://www.epa.gov/airnow) and avoiding outdoor activity on poor air quality days is an important strategy. With the older population increasing, maintaining air quality is even more essential to maintaining and improving the health of the nation.

IMMUNIZATIONS

The most important intervention to improve the health of the elderly related to immunizations is to increase the number of older people vaccinated against influenza every year. Nurses play an important role in organizing, staffing, and evaluating immunization clinics. The recommended immunization schedule for adults is found in Chapter 9, Figure 9-3. It is recommended that older adults receive a flu shot every year.

ACCESS TO HEALTH CARE

Access to care increases the quality and years of healthy life for all Americans. Disparity in access to care remains a significant issue for older Americans. For example, the percentages of individuals who report being vaccinated for influenza and pneumococcal disease by rate are given in Figure 10-5. Non-Hispanic Whites were more likely to have a pneumonia vaccination (64%) compared with non-Hispanic Blacks (45%) or Hispanics (36%).

Older individuals may perceive that they do not have access because they have unfounded concerns about cost for services. They also may have limited mobility as a result of either a chronic condition or lack of transportation. Perhaps the older person has a limited ability to speak English or is distrustful of health care providers. These are all issues of access that may affect the client's health. The nurse must always assess the client's perception of access and intervene accordingly.

Use of Complementary Therapies

The benefits of complementary and alternative modalities are increasingly reported in empirical research. These modalities are advantageous as primary, secondary, or tertiary prevention strategies.

For instance, research suggests that Tai Chi Chuan has a positive effect on cardiorespiratory function (Taylor-Piliae, 2008), muscle strength and balance and motor control (Wong & Lan, 2008), improved immune function (Yeh et al., 2009), and fall prevention (Gillespie et al., 2009). In addition to the physical benefits, Tai Chi Chuan's impact on mental health is evident in a reported positive effect on QOL (Deschamps, Onifade,

Percentage of population age 65 and over vaccinated against influenza and pneumococcal disease, by race and Hispanic origin, selected years 1989–2008

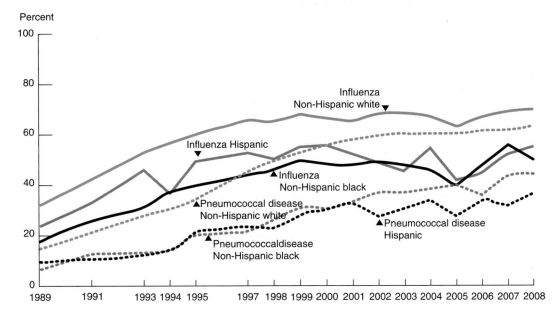

NOTE: For influenza, the percentage vaccinated consists of people who reported having a flu shot during the past 12 months and does not include receipt of nasal spray flu vaccinatiors. For pneumococcal disease, the percentage refers to people who reported ever having a pneumonia vaccination.
See Appendix B for the definiion of race and Haspanic origin in the National Health Interview Survey.
Reference population: These data refers to the civilian noninstitutionalized population.
SOURCE: Centers for Disease Control and Prevention, National Center for Health Statistics,
National Health Interview Survey.

Figure 10-5 Percentage of people age 65 and older who reported having been vaccinated against influenza and pneumococcal disease, by race and Hispanic origin. From Federal Interagency Forum on Aging Related Statistics. (2011). *Older Americans update 2010: Key indicators of well-being* (p. 54). Retrieved from http://www.agingstats.gov/agingstatsdotnet/Main_Site/Data/2010_Documents/Docs/OA_2010.pdf

Decamps, & Bourdel-Marchasson, 2009) and reduction in anxiety-related stress (Rogers, Larkey, & Keller, 2009).

An illustration of primary prevention is found in research that suggests that martial arts training may be a safe way to teach osteoporosis patients how to reduce the risk of injury when they fall. It is postulated that because martial arts techniques reduce hip impact forces and can be learned by older persons, martial arts training may prevent hip fractures among persons with osteoporosis (Groen, Smulders, de Kam, Duysens, & Weerdesteyn, 2010).

Other commonly used complementary therapies that have been shown to enhance health with older adults are massage, yoga, and transcendental meditation. Massage is simple to use in any setting. Research establishes massage as efficacious for a variety of purposes including pain relief, enhancing well-being, and relaxation (Nelson & Coyle, 2010; Robertshawe, 2007; Weaver, 2009). Yoga is physiologically equivalent to very light- to moderate-intensity exercise. Yoga used in longer duration in standing postures has the potential to improve cardiovascular fitness for older adults. During warm-up, the relaxation component of yoga may improve psychological well-being (Buranruk et al., 2010). One case control study found that use of transcendental meditation with older women with breast cancer improved physical function, spiritual well-being, and mental health when used over an 18-month period of time (Nidich et al., 2009). See Research in Community-Based Nursing Care 10-1 for more details.

RESEARCH IN COMMUNITY-BASED NURSING CARE 10-1

A Randomized Controlled Trial of the Effects of Transcendental Meditation on Quality of Life in Older Breast Cancer Patients

This randomized controlled trial examined the impact of transcendental meditation on the quality of life (QOL) of women 55 years and older with stage II to IV breast cancer. One hundred and thirty women were randomly assigned to either the intervention group or the control group. Transcendental meditation was taught to the intervention group to be done at home twice a day for 20 minutes. Every six months Functional Assessment of Cancer Therapy-Breast (FACT-B), Functional Assessment of Chronic Illness Therapy-Spiritual Well-Being (FACIT-SP), and 36-Item Short Form Health Survey (SF-36) mental health and vitality scales were administered. The researchers found significant improvements in the group that received transcendental meditation compared with controls in overall QOL, emotional well-being, social well-being, and mental health. The researchers recommended that this easy to implement stress reduction program is appropriate for many types of community settings.

From Nidich, S., Fields, J., Rainforth, M., Pomerantz, R., Cella, D., Kristeller, J., et al. (2009). A randomized controlled trial of the effects of transcendental meditation on quality of life in older breast cancer patients. *Integrative Cancer Therapies, 8*(3), 228–234. Retrieved from CINAHL Plus with Full Text database.

Policy

Policy makers consider many sources when developing public policy related to the health of older adults. Since the late 1950s, older Americans have been represented in the policy arena by the powerful advocacy of the American Association of Retired Persons. This vocal group is one of the largest membership organizations in the United States involved in public policy issues.

Nurses are considered valued professionals whose opinions and input are often sought by those who participate in the policy-making process. Participation may involve calling or sending letters to a city, state, or federal lawmaker; testifying at a public hearing; or informing a client about proposed changes in laws related to health. Related to older adult health, an example might be proposed legislation related to Medicare coverage for health promotion or disease prevention services. Often, through public education and social marketing, nurses may influence public opinion and, in turn, public policy. It is a professional responsibility of the graduate nurse to stay current on health care issues, particularly in their own area of professional expertise and to share that information with other members of the community. Through advocacy, social marketing, and education, nurses influence public opinion and health care public policy.

Conclusions

Life expectancy at birth, as well as at 65 and 85 years of age, has increased over the past decades. The population of older adults is growing in number and has special health needs. Because older people are living longer with more chronic conditions, attention is now focused on preserving their QOL. Nurses can use the leading health indicators to illuminate individual behaviors and physical, social, and environmental factors that require intervention to prevent disease and promote health in the older segment of the population.

What's on the Web

AgePage: Depression: Don't Let the Blues Hang Around
INTERNET ADDRESS: http://www.nia.nih.gov/HealthInformation/Publications/depression.htm
This document from the National Institute on Aging addresses depression as it relates to older people and provides a list of resources.

Alzheimer's Association
INTERNET ADDRESS: http://www.alz.org
This site provides consumer and professional information, including a section dedicated to family caregivers and friends of people with Alzheimer disease. It contains links to local chapters and other support groups and resources and also includes information in Spanish.

Diabetes Education: Centers for Disease Control and Prevention
INTERNET ADDRESS: http://www.cdc.gov/diabetes
Information about diabetes statistics and state programs can be found at this CDC site.

Centers for Disease Control, National Center for Injury Prevention and Control
INTERNET ADDRESS: http://www.cdc.gov/ncipc/
The mission of the National Center for Injury Prevention and Control is to prevent injuries and violence and reduce their consequences. There are various sites related to the health of older adults.

National Council on Aging
INTERNET ADDRESS: http://www.ncoa.org/index.cfm
This site provides information geared toward improving health, enhancing economic security, and promoting independence and dignity of older adult as well as strengthening community organization advocating for older Americans.

National Institute of Diabetes and Digestive and Kidney Diseases
INTERNET ADDRESS: http://www2.niddk.nih.gov/HealthEducation/InteractiveTools/
This National Institutes of Health (NIH) site provides educational resources and tools related to a variety of chronic conditions.

National Diabetes Education Program
INTERNET ADDRESS: http://www.ndep.nih.gov/
Consumer information and health education material for individuals, families, and health professionals related to diabetes are all available on this Web site supported by the NIH, USDHHS, and the CDC.

Older Americans 2010: Key Indicators of Well-Being
INTERNET ADDRESS: http://www.agingstats.gov/agingstatsdotnet/Main_Site/Default.aspx
This report of the Federal Interagency Forum on Aging-Related Statistics provides information on indicators that address the lives of the older population, including access to health care, home care, vaccinations, social activity, and dietary quality. It is updated yearly, so find the most recent version. There are slides, statistics, and other resources related to older adult health on this site.

Women Stay Healthy at 50+/Men Stay Healthy at 50+
INTERNET ADDRESS: http://www.ahrq.gov/ppip/men50.htm or http://www.ahrq.gov/ppip/women50.htm.
This guide is available online. It is also available in Spanish. It includes recommendations about lifestyle choices that prevent certain chronic diseases, primary prevention screening, and immunizations. It is an excellent tool for guiding health promotion and disease prevention activities.

Health and Aging Organization Online Directory
INTERNET ADDRESS: http://www.nia.nih.gov/HealthInformation/ResourceDirectory.htm
This online, searchable database lists more than 300 national organizations that provide help to older people.

Your Medicine: Play It Safe Patient Guide
INTERNET ADDRESS: http://www.ahrq.gov/consumer/safemeds/safemeds.htm
This site is intended as a client or caregiver education site. This consumer guide from the National Council on Patient Information and Education and the Agency for Healthcare Research and Quality can be used as a teaching tool to facilitate medication safety.

Potential Partners for Health Promotion Activities for Older Adults

American Association of Retired Persons
INTERNET ADDRESS: http://www.aarp.org

American Council on Science and Health
INTERNET ADDRESS: http://www.acsh.org

American Society on Aging
INTERNET ADDRESS: http://www.asaging.org

National Association for Home Care and Hospice
INTERNET ADDRESS: http://www.nahc.org

National Health Policy Forum
INTERNET ADDRESS: http://www.nhpf.org

National Wellness Institute
INTERNET ADDRESS: http://www.nationalwellness.org

References and Bibliography

Administration on Aging. (2010). *Aging statistics.* Retrieved from http://www.aoa.gov/AoARoot/Aging_Statistics/index.aspx

Agency for Healthcare Research and Quality. (2010). *Consumers and patients.* Retrieved from http://www.ahrq.gov/consumer/

Agency for Healthcare Research and Quality. (2004). *Your medicine: Play it safe.* Retrieved from http://archive.ahrq.gov/consumer/safemeds/safemeds.htm

Buranruk, O., Grow, S., Ladawan, S., Makarawate, P., Suwanich, T., & Leelayuwat, N. (2010). Thai yoga as an appropriate alternative physical activity for older adults. *Journal of Complementary & Integrative Medicine, 7*(1), article 6. doi:10.2202/1553-3840.1290.

Centers for Disease Control and Prevention. (1999). *Physical activity and health: A report of the Surgeon General.* Retrieved from http://www.cdc.gov/nccdphp/sgr/olderad.htm

Centers for Disease Control and Prevention. (2007). *Health information for older adults.* Retrieved from http://www.cdc.gov/aging/info.htm#3

Centers for Disease Control and Prevention. (2009). *Overweight and obesity: Health consequences.* Retrieved from http://www.cdc.gov/obesity/causes/health.html

Centers for Disease Control and Prevention. (2010a). *Falls among older adults: An overview.* Retrieved from http://www.cdc.gov/HomeandRecreationalSafety/Falls/adultfalls.html

Centers for Disease Control and Prevention. (2010b). *The state of aging and health in America.* Retrieved from http://www.cdc.gov/aging/data/stateofaging.htm

Deschamps, A., Onifade, C., Decamps, A., & Bourdel-Marchasson, I. (2009). Health-related quality of life in frail institutionalized elderly: Effects of a cognition-action intervention and Tai Chi. *Journal of Aging and Physical Activity, 17*(2), 236–248.

Doolan, D., & Froelicher, E. (2008). Smoking cessation interventions and older adults. *Progress in Cardiovascular Nursing, 23*(3), 119–127. Retrieved from EBSCOhost.

Gillespie, L. D., Robertson, M. C., Gillespie, W. J., Lamb, S. E., Cumming, R. G., & Rowe, B. H. (2009). Interventions for preventing falls in older people living in the community. *Cochrane Database of Systematic Reviews, 15*(2), CD007146.

Groen, B., Smulders, E., de Kam, D., Duysens, J., & Weerdesteyn, V. (2010). Martial arts fall training to prevent hip fractures in the elderly. *Osteoporosis International, 21*(2), 215–221. Retrieved from EBSCOhost.

Interagency Forum on Aging Related Statistics. (2011). *Older Americans update 2010: Key indicators of well-being.* Retrieved from http://www.agingstats.gov/agingstatsdotnet/Main_Site/Data/2010_Documents/Docs/OA_2010.pdf

National Center for Health Statistics. (2009). *Health, United States, 2009 with chartbook on trends in the health of Americans.* Retrieved from http://www.ncbi.nlm.nih.gov/books/NBK19623/

National Center for Injury Prevention and Control, Centers for Disease Control and Prevention. (2010). *10 leading causes of death, United States.* Retrieved from http://webappa.cdc.gov/cgi-bin/broker.exe

National Coalition for Women with Heart Disease. (2010). *Women and heart disease fact sheet.* Retrieved from http://womenheart.org/resources/cvdfactsheet.cfm

National Heart, Lung, and Blood Institute. (2010). *Campaign resources.* Retrieved from http://www.nhlbi.nih.gov/health/public/lung/copd/campaign-materials/index.htm

National Institute of Mental Health. (2010). *Older adults: Depression and suicide facts.* Retrieved from http://www.nimh.nih.gov/health/publications/older-adults-depression-and-suicide-facts-fact-sheet/index.shtml

Nelson, R., & Coyle, C. (2010). Using massage to reduce use of sedative-hypnotic drugs with older adults: A brief report from a pilot study. *Journal of Applied Gerontology, 29*(1), 129–139. Retrieved from EBSCOhost.

Nidich, S., Fields, J., Rainforth, M., Pomerantz, R., Cella, D., Kristeller, J., et al. (2009). A randomized controlled trial of the effects of transcendental meditation on quality of life in older breast cancer patients. *Integrative Cancer Therapies, 8*(3), 228–234. Retrieved from CINAHL Plus with Full Text database.

Percentage of adults with activity limitations, by age group and type of limitation. National Health Interview Survey, United States, 2008. (2010). *Mortality and Morbidity Weekly Report, 58*(48), 1357. Retrieved from http://www.cdc.gov/mmwr/preview/mmwrhtml/mm5848a6.htm

Robertshawe, P. (2007). Massage vs guided relaxation on wellbeing and stress of older adults. *Journal of the Australian Traditional-Medicine Society, 13*(4), 215. Retrieved from EBSCOhost.

Rogers, C. E., Larkey, L. K., & Keller, C. (2009). A review of clinical trials of Tai Chi and Qigong in older adults. *Western Journal of Nursing Research, 31*(2), 245–279.

Taylor-Piliae, R. E. (2008). The effectiveness of Tai Chi exercise in improving aerobic capacity: An updated meta-analysis. *Medicine and Sport Science, 52,* 40–53.

United States Department of Health and Human Services. (2008). *Alcohol research: A lifespan perspective.* Retrieved from http://pubs.niaaa.nih.gov/publications/AA74/AA74.pdf

Weaver, D. (2009). Minimizing pain and promoting comfort for older adults in care. *Nursing & Residential Care, 11*(7), 329–332. Retrieved from EBSCOhost.

Wong, A. M., & Lan, C. (2008). Tai Chi and balance control. *Medicine and Sport Science, 52,* 115–123.

Yeh, S. H., Chuang, H., Lin, L. W., Hsiao, C. Y., Wang, P. W., Liu, R. T., et al. (2009). Regular Tai Chi Chuan exercise improves T cell helper function of patients with type 2 diabetes mellitus with an increase in T-bet transcription factor and IL-12 production. *British Journal of Sports Medicine, 43*(11), 845–850.

LEARNING ACTIVITIES

JOURNALING ACTIVITY 10-1

In your clinical journal, describe a situation where you have observed an older client who was not receiving the health promotion or disease prevention care that he or she needed.

- What assessment and screening do you believe should have been completed?
- What interventions do you think should have been pursued?
- How would or could you advocate for these issues when you begin to practice as an RN?

JOURNALING ACTIVITY 10-2

1. In your clinical journal, describe a situation you have encountered when screening and doing health promotion and disease prevention teaching and planning with an older adult.
   - What did you learn from this experience?
   - How will you practice differently based on this experience?

CLIENT CARE ACTIVITY 10-3

Roberta is a 62-year-old Black woman employed as a housekeeper in a hotel. She does not have health insurance. As you are reviewing *Women Stay Healthy at 50+* with her, you learn that she has not had a pelvic or breast examination in 10 years.

- What do you do?
- What do you recommend?

Roberta says, "I used to be more active. I used to play basketball when I was a teenager, and now I can hardly walk up a flight of stairs. I would like to be more active and lose some weight. Would that help my high blood pressure?"

- What do you say and do?
- What do you recommend?
- What resources do you use?

She tells you that she has smoked since she was 16 years old and has decided that she wants to quit.

- What do you say and do?
- What do you recommend?
- What resources do you use?

PRACTICAL APPLICATION ACTIVITY 10-4

You are working at a city clinic that serves many older adults. Last year, you noted that in November through March, most of the clinic visits were for colds, influenza, sore throats, bronchitis, and pneumonia, in order of frequency. As you are reviewing the clinic records, you learn that 80% of the clinic visits resulting in hospitalization resulted from bronchitis, pneumonia, and influenza.

1. How would you go about assessing and planning for the coming influenza season? (Consult Chapter 5 for some ideas.)
2. What clinic activities related to health promotion and disease prevention would you plan for the next year in the late fall?
3. Develop a plan for the activities with a list of who would be involved in planning, formulating the goals and objectives of the plan, a timeline, and a method for evaluating the results.

PRACTICAL APPLICATION ACTIVITY 10-5

A local senior citizens center has contacted your instructor and asks that a team of students provide a health fair for the center's fall festival held in late October or early November.

- What would you like to know about this group before planning this project?
- When forming a group to work on this task, whom would you invite to participate?
- How would you involve the various community partners in the planning?
- How would you go about determining which screening activities to include in the health fair?
- What other activities would be important to offer based on the time of the year and the typical health needs of older adults?

UNIT IV

Settings for Practice

The settings and roles of the nurse have changed over time. In the late 1800s, a nurse was a woman in a black dress and a long black cape, carrying a black satchel, visiting homes to care for the sick. As health care shifted toward care of the ill in the hospital, the nurse was a woman dressed in a severely starched white uniform, white stockings, and a starched white cap, bending over the bed of a sick person.

Today, male and female nurses work in a wide variety of settings, taking on many roles. These are discussed in Chapter 11. The nurse working in the community is no longer recognizable by sex, uniform, or setting. Nurses practice in all levels of health care delivery including corporations, neighborhood schools, day surgery centers, churches, long-term care facilities, and a variety of ambulatory clinics. Their clients may be well children or they may be older people, victims of partner abuse, families experiencing homelessness, incarcerated individuals, or drug addicts.

Increasingly, the home is again becoming a common setting for nursing practice. Descriptions of types of agencies providing home care, the significance of home care, and the transfer of acute care nursing to home care nursing skills are discussed in Chapter 12. Purposes and goals of home care as well as the advantages and disadvantages of this type of service are explored. Barriers to successful home care and skills and competencies are also addressed. The first visit is described, along with safety issues and lay caretaker involvement. Chapter 13 provides an overview of specialized home health care nursing, where hospice care, pain management, wound care, disease management, infusion therapy, telehealth, maternal/child care, and case management in the home setting.

In Chapter 14, the role of the mental health nurse in community-based settings is outlined. This includes a discussion of the historical perspective, significance of community mental health, nursing competencies and skills, agencies and service available in community-based settings, mental health care with vulnerable populations, and challenges to successful implementation of nursing care in these settings.

The global community as a setting for practice in community care will be the focus of Chapter 15. This chapter will address the millennium development goals, the global nature of health and disparity, and emergency preparedness. All nurses benefit from understanding the global nature of health, particularly related to advocacy, when working with immigrants, refugees, and new Americans.

Chapter 11 ◌ **Practice Settings and Specialties**

Chapter 12 ◌ **Home Health Care Nursing**

Chapter 13 ◌ **Specialized Home Health Care Nursing**

Chapter 14 ◌ **Mental Health Nursing in Community-Based Settings**

Chapter 15 ◌ **Global Health and Community-Based Care**

Chapter 11

Practice Settings and Specialties

ROBERTA HUNT

Learning Objectives

1 Describe different settings in which nursing care is provided.

2 Identify three settings in which children receive nursing care and the services that these settings offer.

3 Identify three settings in which elderly clients receive nursing care and the services that these settings offer.

4 Compare the roles of the advanced practice nurse and the registered nurse.

5 Contrast the roles of the nurse in a school setting with the roles in the work setting.

6 Discuss the trends in settings for practice.

Key Terms

adult day care
adult foster care homes
advanced practice nurses
ambulatory care centers
assisted living facilities
boarding care homes
case manager
certified nurse midwife
clinical nurse specialists
day surgery centers
detoxification facilities
employee assistance programs
employee wellness programs
extended care facilities
home health care
homeless shelters

nurse practitioners
nursing centers
nursing-managed health centers
occupational health nurse
outpatient services
parish nursing
rehabilitation center
residential center
retirement communities
school nurse
skilled nursing facilities
specialized care centers
subacute rehabilitation centers
transitional housing
wellness promotion
work-site health promotion

Chapter Topics

Practice Settings and Practice Opportunities

Nursing Specialties

Conclusions

The Nurse Speaks

We offered an ongoing "Faithfully Fit" exercise class at the church as part of the Parish Nurse program. It is an exercise class mostly for older, retired people. Afterward, we meet at the church and have devotions. One of the regular participants brought her neighbors, Warren and Colette, who eventually became a big part of the class. They both grew up in a faith different from ours but had not been to church for over 40 years. Warren had had three or four bouts of different kinds of cancer before this, and about a year after joining the exercise class, he came up with esophageal cancer. I brought a card the first day after we heard about this, and we all signed the card in class. From there, the class took over and we sent cards almost every day either to Warren or to Colette for support. They had three daughters who lived in Chicago, Madison, and California and no family in the area. When he came home from the hospital, he had a feeding tube. We started bringing supper for her every night. Some nights whoever brought it stayed with them and ate, while some nights they just left the meal. He got well enough to come back to the class and, of course, this was really fun even though he was pretty weak. So we watched him get better and better. Then they moved into a condominium next to our church. They hadn't been there 2 weeks, and she was diagnosed with lung cancer. This was almost a year after his diagnosis. Someone in the class coordinated rides and the food, and we all participated and, of course, prayed for them. When they were too ill to come to the class, they looked out from their condo onto our exercise class that was held in the church. They would wave at us. Then we did things such as take Colette to coffee and Warren to the library, to spend time with them. It was not just the parish nurse or the exercise group that was involved in this process by then but the whole neighborhood. The realtor who sold the house, her hairdresser, and two of his work colleagues all began to help, so it became a community thing. For me, that is what parish nursing is all about. It should start inside the church and move to outside the church into the community.

Anyway, they died in the spring within a few weeks of each other. Warren had hooked up with the priest from his own faith near the end of his life and had last rites. Colette would have none of that and she huffed around that apartment. Colette had a great deal of spirit and did not hesitate to express her opinions. Prior to All Saints Day, St. Cecelia sent us an invitation to their All Saints mass. It was a beautiful celebration and they listed all the people, either members or people with whom they had contact with for the prior year who had died. Warren and Colette were listed in the program. In the church, there were beautiful wrought iron candle holders with little candles in them, each labeled with the name of the person remembered in the service. Of course, we could not see the names during the service. During the service, one candle kept sputtering and was so noisy and finally went out. After the service, they encouraged us to find the name of our loved one and see the candle. When we discovered that it was Colette's candle that was making all the ruckus, those of us there from our neighborhood laughed. She was speaking even after her death.

Lynda Morlock, RN, PHN
Former Parish Nurse,
St. Anthony Lutheran Church,
St. Anthony, Minnesota

The settings for health care delivery have undergone rapid and dramatic changes in the past decade primarily designed to contain escalating health care costs. The self-care movement is also attributed to this shift. Reduced infant mortality, control of communicable diseases, and medical technology and pharmaceutical advancements have increased the percentage of the population in the United States living to older age. Life span has increased for those with specific chronic diseases, such as cystic fibrosis, sickle cell anemia, diabetes, heart disease, and acquired immunodeficiency syndrome (AIDS), and for those who have been paralyzed by stroke or trauma.

These changes make it possible for nurses to work in an ever-expanding number of specialized areas of care and settings for practice. The U.S. Department of Labor, Bureau of Labor Statistics (2010) anticipates that the need for nurses will increase by 22% by 2018, with many new jobs being created. Although there will always be a need for traditional hospital nurses, a large number of new graduates will be employed in home care, long-term care, primary care, and ambulatory care. The fastest growing category of jobs for nurses will be in physician offices (48% growth rate), home health (33% growth rate), and long-term care facilities (25% growth rate) (U.S. Department of Labor, Bureau of Labor Statistics, 2010a). Further, given the changes in health care delivery, it is expected that more nurses will work in nursing-based clinic practice, health maintenance organizations (HMOs), federal agencies, health planning agencies, prisons and jails, insurance companies, and pharmaceutical and durable medical equipment companies. Technological advances in client care, which allows a greater number of health problems to be treated, will drive this growth. Further, as discussed in Chapter 10, the number of older people, who typically have more health care needs than other segments of the population, is increasing.

This chapter discusses the different settings for practice that a nurse may encounter. Although schools of nursing are expanding placement for clinical training of their students well beyond what was typical one or two decades ago, no one school can cover all these settings within its curriculum. People entering nursing today must seek out ways of venturing into new and different nursing roles by reading about, observing, and volunteering in their own community.

Practice Settings and Practice Opportunities

With the increased emphasis on self-care, disease prevention, and health promotion, health care is provided in settings other than traditional hospitals as an effort has been made to extend to underserved areas (e.g., to people who live in remote rural areas of the country) and populations. As the need for local health care facilities that provide comprehensive services intensifies, the way the services are made available to consumers will evolve. The growing number of nontraditional health care facilities reflects this trend as a glance at our social systems shows that almost every established institution provides some type of health service. Industrial plants, businesses, schools, prisons, churches, and civic groups provide varying degrees of care, usually with a focus on prevention. Although state laws govern the tasks nurses may perform, it is usually the work setting or the agency that determines day-to-day activities.

It will be impossible to offer a complete description of every practice setting for community-based nursing, so an overview will be provided. Further, it is difficult to place health care settings in precise categories, any of them overlap. For instance, a clinic may be located in a hospital, or some long-term care facilities may be specialized facilities. The categories in this section are arbitrary and were chosen for ease in identifying some of the settings and types of care that community-based nurses may provide (see Community-Based Nursing Guidelines 11-1).

HOSPITAL CARE

Hospitals remain the major site in which nurses practice. A little more then half of all nurses are employed in hospitals. The role of the nurses in hospitals continues to be to provide bedside care through performing delegated medical functions prescribed by physicians, identifying collaborative problems, and utilizing independent nursing diagnosis. In addition, nurses also supervise licensed practical nurses and other nursing assistive personnel. Typically, nurses in larger facilities are assigned to one specialty area, while in smaller community hospitals, nurses provide care across the age span and specialty area.

COMMUNITY-BASED NURSING CARE GUIDELINES 11-1

Sampling of Variety of Nursing Functions in Health Care Settings

Hospital: Acute Care
Serves as administrator or manager
Assesses and monitors client's health status
Provides direct care
Coordinates care by others
Teaches client and family
Provides support for family members
Makes referrals

Home Care
Assesses client, family, and culture
Assesses home and community environment
Develops relationship based on mutual trust
Contacts physician regarding client's condition
Plans, implements, and evaluates plan of care
Provides direct care
Coordinates care given by others
Teaches client and family
Provides support for family members
Makes referrals

Clinic (Ambulatory) Care
Makes health assessments
Assists primary care provider (may be primary care provider)
Provides direct care
Coordinates care given by others
Teaches client and family
Plans, implements, and evaluates the plan of care
Provides health promotion and disease prevention
Serves as a client advocate

Extended Care Facility
Serves as administrator
Coordinates care of others
Assesses client's condition
Develops treatment plans
Provides direct care
Maintains contact with the client's physician

Residential Centers
Provides direct care
Provides health assessments
Provides health promotion and prevention
Provides counseling and support
Makes referrals
Collaborates with other health care team members
Coordinates services

COMMUNITY-BASED NURSING CARE GUIDELINES 11-1

Sampling of Variety of Nursing Functions in Health Care Settings *(Continued)*

Schools and Industry
Conducts health screening
Completes health assessments
Provides first aid or initial emergency care
Provides health education
Provides health promotion and disease prevention
Provides counseling and support
Makes referrals

Pharmaceutical and Durable Medical Devices
Conducts research
Provides education about new medication and devices
Outreach
Provides consultation
Insurance Companies
Case management
Outreach
Provides counseling and consultation

Technically, acute care nursing is community-based nursing because acute care nurses do take care of individuals and families in a specific community. They also perform the initial assessment to prepare the client for discharge from the hospital. Further, as discussed in Chapters 6 and 7, it is the hospital nurse who does most of the preliminary teaching of clients and caregivers for procedures to be done in the home. Hospital nurses often provide information about resources in the community allowing clients and families to become proficient in self-care with a disease prevention focus and within the context of their culture and community.

CARE IN THE HOME: THE HOME VISITING NURSE

Since the middle of the 19th century, home visiting nurses have worked in community-based care both as occupational health nurses and as maternal and child care nurses. Currently, home visiting has numerous applications in the community, but the major one is seen in maternal/child care and home health care.

Foundational goals and purposes of maternal and child visiting run parallel to those of community-based care in that through collaborative action self-care is promoted with an emphasis on prevention and continuity within the context of the community. In many industrialized nations, the home visiting nurse plays a vital role in promoting health and preventing disease in the maternal/child population. In fact, in the past few decades, various studies have demonstrated how home visits improve outcomes for high-risk pregnancies and at-risk infants. As discussed in Chapter 8, one of the goals of Healthy People 2020 is to reduce the rate of low-birth-weight infants. Pregnant teenagers receiving home visits from nurses are less likely to deliver low-birth-weight babies compared to teenagers who are not visited by a nurse. Women who smoked before pregnancy who receive home visits are less likely to smoke during pregnancy than women without home visits, which decreases the risk of having a low-birth-weight infant. Numerous studies over the last 20 years have shown that postpartum home visits are associated with a decrease in recorded physical child abuse and neglect in the first 2 years of life, especially in unmarried teen mothers of low socioeconomic status (Olds, Henderson, & Kitzman, 1994; Olds, Henderson, Tatelbaum, & Chamberlin, 1986, 1988). Research demonstrates enduring effects of nurse home visiting over a 19-year period in improved maternal life course and reduced government spending for mothers and lower rates of arrests and convictions and fewer children born to the female children of the mothers (Eckenrode et al., 2010; Kitzman et al., 2010).

Unfortunately, in the last decade, the role of the home visiting nurse in maternal/child care in the United States has been eroded by a lack of funding resulting in a dramatic reduction in services provided to low-income women. This is particularly tragic considering the increase in the rate of low-birth-weight infants. Home visiting is proven to be an effective means to enhance health outcomes, yet it is used relatively infrequently in the United States compared with many other countries. The Affordability Care Act of 2010 allocated a dramatic increase in funding for home visiting services that is anticipated to address this disparity.

The European Union [EU], through the World Health Organization, promotes the role of the maternal/child home visiting nurse and coined the term "family nurse." As a result, countries in the EU widely using home visiting for maternal/child care have lower infant mortality rates, low rates of low-birth-weight infants, and more extensive use of family planning compared to the United States. At the same time, the percentage of the national expenditure on health care in these nations is less compared to the United States. In addition to home health care and maternal/child care, there are other populations and roles for home visitors. Home visiting allows the nurse to establish a trusting relationship with the family and the child so that additional interventions may follow. Home visits with any individual or family across the lifespan facilitates case finding as well as provide more intense assessment and intervention for individuals with chronic conditions. It enhances continuity of care for all populations with all conditions.

HOME CARE NURSING

Home health care has been a growing area for the last three decades, with service provided mainly through home visits. Agencies contract directly with clients, or with Medicare or private insurance plans, to provide a selected number of visits to a particular client. Chapters 12 and 13 discuss home health care nursing in more depth. Currently, this type of home visiting is most commonly seen with those recently hospitalized or those with chronic illnesses, primarily the elderly receiving home health care services.

Most seniors prefer to stay in their own homes and communities rather then enter long-term care or **assisted living facilities**. There are other nonnursing community-based programs designed to lengthen the period of time that seniors are able to remain in their homes.

Living at Home Network/Block Nurse Program

This program is a community-based service that depends on professional and volunteer services of neighborhood residents to provide information, social and support services, skilled nursing care, and other assistance to the elderly in order to promote self-sufficiency and avoid nursing home placement. This can range from arranging for a neighborhood Boy Scout to do yard work, to contacting Meals on Wheels to deliver meals, to providing grocery shopping assistance, to making a referral for transportation to medical appointments.

It is important to note that this program was developed by a group of nurses in 1982 who wanted to provide better care for the elderly living in their neighborhood. The concept depends on grassroots community interest and active commitment of service groups, churches, businesses, schools, colleges, and universities. Evaluation of data from over two decades ago demonstrated that $3 is saved for every $1 spent keeping the elderly at home and out of long-term care facilities, which are primarily funded by Medicare. In the 37 sites in Minnesota evaluated, $30 million was saved by preventing premature nursing home placement. This model has been duplicated throughout the United States with great success. The Block Nurse program provides skilled nursing, case management, and supervision of home health aides and homemakers, often with nursing students as the care providers (Elderberry Institute, 2010).

Adult Day Care Centers/Adult Foster Care

Adult day care centers offer social, recreational, and therapeutic activities to seniors who are in need of supervision during the day. Nurses are frequently part of the professional staff and are responsible for health assessments and design and management of therapeutic regimens and medications. Often, physical care (e.g., bathing) takes place at the day care center. These vital organizations offer more personal attention and have a quieter atmosphere than most senior centers. In addition, they provide care for the dependent individual who cannot manage alone but is not in need of nursing home placement. Medicare does not always cover day care costs but can pay all the costs in a licensed day care center with a medical model or an Alzheimer's environment if the senior qualifies financially. In some facilities, need-based scholarships are available, while others may use a sliding fee scale based on income. Private medical insurance policies sometimes cover a portion of day care costs when registered, licensed medical personnel are involved in the care. In addition, long-term care insurance may also pay for adult day services, depending upon the policy. Dependent care tax credits may be available to the caregiver as well. (National Respite Network, 2010). **Adult foster care homes** (AFCHs)—also known as board and care homes or family care homes—are safe, small (usually fewer than six clients per home) residential sites that provide housing and protective oversight. Many AFCHs provide care to frail elderly adults and those with dementia. Nationwide, these facilities may be referred to by many names, including residential, adult, foster, family, boarding, or assisted living. Adult foster care homes are optional elements of state Medicaid programs. Therefore, states determine what services are covered, who may be eligible, and what services they receive.

The Older American Act from Administration on Aging (AoA) provides funding for both adult day care and adult foster care homes (U.S. Department of Health and Human Services, 2010). Locating adult foster care or day care centers can be facilitated by contacting the local Area Agency on Aging. In a few States, the State Unit or Office on Aging serves as the Area Agency on Aging. Appropriate Area Agency on Aging or local service providers can be found through Eldercare Locator, the AoA-supported nationwide, toll-free information and assistance directory. Table 11-1 provides specific suggestions for identifying these resources within the community.

Table 11-1 Resources for Community-Based Care		
Resource	**Description**	**Contact Information**
Eldercare Locator	A federal government service for identifying resources for respite care	The Eldercare Locator phone number is 1-800-677-1116, Monday through Friday, 9:00 AM to 8:00 PM, Eastern time. For 24-hour access to the locator, visit http://www.eldercare.gov
The Family Caregiver Alliance	A San Francisco nonprofit that tracks respite programs	http://www.caregiver.org (under tab for Public Policy & Research, click on National Center for Caregiving) across the states or call 1-800-445-8106 or 415-434-3388
Disease-specific groups: National Association of Chronic Diseases	For many chronic illnesses, there may be advocacy groups. For example, Alzheimer disease	http://www.chronicdisease.org/i4a/pages/index.cfm?pageid=3849
Professional care managers	For example, the National Association of Professional Geriatric Care Managers	http://www.caremanager.org (under the button Find a Care Manager)
State or local agencies on aging	Senior service, elder services, or public or private agencies	Check online phone book blue pages or yellow pages

Parish Nursing

Parish nursing is "a health promotion and disease prevention role based on the care of the whole person which encompasses seven functions" (Solari-Twadell, 1999, p. 3). These functions require integrating faith and health in the roles of health educator, health counselor, referral agent, trainer of volunteers, and health advocate. Parish nursing finds its historical roots in the late 1800s, when nurses sent by religious organizations practiced in many rural mountainous areas of the Southeast.

Many churches have nurses on their staffs, while others use volunteer nurses. Almost 70% of parish nurses are over 55 years of age. Parish nurses offer the interventions of screening, health education, resource and referral services, counseling, consultation, outreach, collaboration, and case management to parishioners (McGinnis & Zoske, 2008).

Parish nurses reach out to vulnerable populations: older adults, single parents and their children, and grieving individuals. Because parish nurses are a source of client empowerment, they have an important role in promoting self-care and self-advocacy. Parish nurses are playing an increasingly vital role in addressing health care inequities in the community by working with underserved populations, as shown in Research in Community-Based Nursing Care 11-1. With appropriate support, this model of nursing could be expanded into other settings within the community and has the potential to draw on the skills of experienced registered nurses (RNs) to provide communities with services that address unmet health care needs (Mayernik, Resick, Skomo, & Mandock, 2010).

RESIDENTIAL CARE FOR THE ELDERLY

Some older adults, particularly those with chronic conditions, may be very isolated living at home. Living arrangements for these individuals in a **residential center** may be a better option. Successful placement, however, requires research, client and family involvement, planning, and a focus on the client's maintaining control of his or her own life. There are multiple levels of residential living from which to choose.

Extended care facility residents were queried in a study about factors that influence the quality of care they receive. They responded that the most important aspect was their ability to retain control of their lives. To provide effective care, the nurse must be familiar with the resident's health problems and needs. Aging is a normal, irreversible process. Many of the problems of aging can be prevented by considering that the older adult's physical, emotional, social, and spiritual needs are complex and interrelated. These factors are important to any older adult living in any kind of residential setting.

Residential facilities provide a unique setting for community-based nursing because the nurse has a captive audience. Here the nurse can take advantage of the close proximity of the residents to do health teaching, health promotion, and disease prevention. By building trust through good relationships with the residents, nurses expand their roles to become counselors and advocates, providing direct support.

Retirement Communities

Designed for the functionally and socially independent, **retirement communities** provide a community living style for individuals who choose to live with other seniors. Accommodations include homes or apartments with supportive services provided by the retirement community.

Assisted Living Facilities

Geared toward the individual who has need for some assistance in daily activities (e.g., medications, meals, dressing, bathing), but who is able to function fairly independently, assisted living facilities generally house residents in bedrooms located in a homelike environment.

Extended Care Facilities and Skilled Nursing Facilities

More institutional in their design, with ongoing medical and nursing services and supervision, **extended care facilities** (also known as nursing homes) provide care for individuals who need ongoing daily care, generally for the rest of their lives. **Skilled nursing facilities**

RESEARCH IN COMMUNITY-BASED NURSING CARE 11-1

Parish Nurse–Initiated Interdisciplinary Mobile Health Care Delivery Project

The role and scope of parish nursing has evolved to extend service from the immediate church community to the community at large. Expanding care for vulnerable populations includes inner-city neighborhoods and declining small towns that are home to many of society's marginalized individuals. A creative initiative to reach the individuals most at risk in these communities is outlined. This article describes a collaboration between parish nurses and a university school of pharmacy faculty with a mobile health project to bring screening and preventive services to low-income neighborhoods. Funding for the project was shared among the parish nurse collaboration and the school of pharmacy. Monthly visits began with interprofessional teams to food pantries in churches with the target population of low-income women. Churches are typically a trusted location in most communities by members. Over 1,600 client visits were recorded from September 2005 to December 2008. Various free health screenings followed by consultation services were offered. Of these visits, a group of 502 women received 1,915 screenings. Those with moderately abnormal results received counseling to modify diet, increase exercise, and come back to the van for a recheck the next month. Individuals with very high abnormal results were advised to see their doctor. The parish nurse assisted the uninsured with information regarding resources in their community. Pharmacists provided medication consultation, as well as a brief depression screening when needed. Follow-up by phone to monitor health status and assess progress was offered for those with abnormal results. I Incidence and prevalence rates for hypertension, hyperlipidemia, diabetes, and obesity observed in the population of women screened in the mobile project were comparable to the general population. Despite the fact that many of these women were being treated for hypertension, their blood pressure was not in the appropriate range. Health education and counseling on medication adherence and life style changes were common interventions by both the nurses and the pharmacist. Delivering screening services to low-income neighborhoods via mobile van was successful for several reasons. First, using the church, a location that is familiar and comfortable for community members, facilitates establishing the trust between client and health care provider enhances motivation necessary to make needed lifestyle changes. Second, an accessible health promotion program allows ease in participation and follow-up. Many individuals who have limited income also experience challenges in securing transportation to health promotion services. The authors concluded that delivering screening and follow-up services in trusted community settings is enhanced markedly by interprofessional collaboration.

Source: Mayernik, D., Resick, L., Skomo, M., & Mandock, K. (2010). Parish nurse-initiated interdisciplinary mobile health care delivery project. *JOGNN: Journal of Obstetric, Gynecologic & Neonatal Nursing, 39*(2), 227–234. doi:10.1111/j.1552–6909.2010.01112.x.

provide nursing, medical, and therapy services for elderly people requiring ongoing medical or rehabilitative services but not hospitalization. Most individuals stay for a few weeks in a skilled facility and are then discharged home or transferred into an extended care facility because they can no longer manage at home after an acute illness or injury or due to a chronic condition. For guidelines for consumers choosing a nursing home, see Community-Based Nursing Care Guidelines 11-2.

For more than two decades, nursing research has demonstrated a link between lower nurse staffing levels in hospitals and adverse client outcomes. In 2005, researchers published evidence that increased direct care by RNs improves outcomes for nursing home residents (Horn, 2005). More RN direct care was associated with fewer pressure ulcers, fewer

COMMUNITY-BASED NURSING CARE GUIDELINES 11-2

A Consumer Guide to Choosing a Nursing Home

1. Determine the alternatives (sources include www.eldercare.gov or www.eldercare.gov or www.nursinghomeaction.org).
2. Consult long-term care ombudsman (a person who investigates and resolves complaints) and citizen advocacy groups in your community.
3. Compare staffing information and quality measures from nursing home. Compare at www.medicare.gov/NHCompare/home.asp
4. Consult state nursing home inspection reports.

From National Citizens' Coalition for Nursing Home Reform. (2009). *A consumer guide to choosing a nursing home: Consumer information sheet.* Retrieved from www.nursinghomeaction.org. or http://www.theconsumervoice.org/sites/default/files/advocate/A-Consumer-Guide-To-Choosing-A-Nursing-Home.pdf

hospitalizations, and fewer urinary tract infections; decreased weight loss, catheterization, and deterioration in the ability to perform activities of daily living; and increased use of nutritional supplements. Better care translates to lower cost. There is an urgent need for additional research to confirm these findings. Further evidence suggests that quality of care can be improved by enhancing nurses' working conditions and that organizational initiatives should be aimed at reducing time pressures and promoting fair managerial procedures that engage all nursing staff in the decision making in long-term care settings (Pekkarinen, Sinervo, Elovainio, Noro, & Finne-Soveri, 2008). If future studies find similar relationships, it is likely that the same concern that has required high nurse–patient ratios in the hospital setting will be recommended for long-term care facilities. Further, this research highlights the importance of families inquiring about the resident/RN ratio when assessing the quality care of a long-term care facility.

Subacute Rehabilitation Centers

Focused on the rehabilitation of individuals who have suffered an illness or accident, **subacute rehabilitation centers** provide longer term rehabilitative services, such as nursing and medical care, as well as physical, occupational, and speech therapy. Generally, the length of stay in this type of facility is limited. Individuals are discharged when they have reached established rehabilitation goals or when they are no longer making progress. The following situation describes this setting.

CLIENT SITUATIONS IN PRACTICE

Several years ago, I fractured my hip and had to have it nailed back together. Because of my age (77 years), the doctor and the physical therapist wanted to put me in a nursing home. I told one of the nurses that I did not want to go to a nursing home. He made some suggestions for an alternate plan encouraging me to insist on a referral to a rehabilitation center. The social service department helped me find the best one in my own community. Today, I can walk again, not as well as I used to, but I am walking and living at home. If that nurse had not taken the time to help me problem solve and encouraged me to ask for the plan I thought was best for me, I'd be immobile in a nursing home today.

Boarding Care Homes

This type of facility provides personal custodial care for residents who are not able to live independently. **Boarding care homes** do not have nursing or medical supervision or care. Residents generally stay indefinitely.

RESIDENTIAL CARE ACROSS THE LIFE SPAN

Residential programs provide health care services across the life span in the areas of chemical dependency treatment facilities, group homes for the mentally ill or developmentally delayed, halfway houses for recovery from addiction, detoxification units for safe withdrawal from alcohol or drugs, shelters for battered women, and hospices for the terminally ill. Nursing functions and roles vary with the type of residential program or facility. Personnel may include direct caregiver (who may provide delegated medical functions), **case manager**, health educator, discharge planner, counselor, collaborator, consultant, or advocate.

Shelters for Partner Violence

Domestic violence crosses all social, economic, racial, and ethnic boundaries. Although most individuals experiencing partner violence are women, men also may be the target of abuse. Shelters have been built around the country to house individuals experiencing partner violence and their children. They provide a safe place where families will have an advocate and easy access to counseling. The nurse functions primarily as advocate, case manager, health educator, and collaborator for the women or men and their children. Individual and group meetings with residents are part of the nurse's regular routine. This role requires good communication skills and familiarity with community resources available to meet the needs of these families. Box 11-1 describes one nurse's personal experience with partner violence.

Homeless Shelters and Transitional Housing

The percentage of people in the United States who are homeless has been growing since 1970. Increases in the number of families experiencing homelessness have been reported in many cities with the current recession, high unemployment, and rising home foreclosures

---

BOX 11-1 A Nurse's Personal Experience With Violence

I was 9 years old when I walked into the bathroom and saw him beating her over the bathtub. I began screaming, leave her alone. He looked at me and kept on hitting her. At that moment I knew that I hated him. I promised myself that I would never allow a man to put his hands on me. Thirteen years later, I married a man who was just like my stepfather. Even though he did not physically abuse me, the words that came from his mouth were very poisonous. Each day, he broke down my self-worth by telling me that I was a terrible mother, that I did not love my children, and that I would be nothing without him.

I stayed with him for 12 years, isolated from my family and friends. I believed his lies even though I was an educated nurse. Finally, I gathered up enough strength to leave him. I packed my bags and left with my two children. We moved into a small apartment, and I was so afraid because I did not know how I was going to make it on my own. Gradually I regained my self-esteem and self-confidence. I was able to return to school and obtained my MSN degree. It wasn't easy, but with the support of my family and friends, I made it. In retrospect, I asked my 13-year-old son the other day, "If you could do one thing differently in your life what would it be?" He thought about it for a few moments and then he looked at me and said, "I wish you would have listened when I tried to tell you about daddy." Imagine that, my son observed the verbal abuse and chaos in the family, he tried to tell me about his father looking at other women, and printing pornography from the Internet, and I didn't listen. Imagine if I had listened.

It took a lot out of me to share this story because I had to confront the demons of my past. It is so important for us as nurses to be alert to the signs of domestic violence. When the opportunity presents itself, we must be brave enough to ask the question: Do you feel safe at home? Not only must we be prepared to ask the question, but we must also be able to provide the resources for obtaining help. So, my message to women of all ages, ethnicity, and socioeconomic background is that it is not OK for someone to abuse you. It is not OK for someone to demoralize you. You did not do anything wrong. You are just a victim. Seek help. Take care of yourself. Most importantly, be safe.

likely to continue to impact these increasing trends (U.S. Conference of Mayors, 2009; U.S. Department of Housing and Urban Development, 2009). Most are single-parent, female-headed families with up to three children who are primarily preschoolers. There is an urgent need for **transitional housing** to facilitate the move from crisis housing in **homeless shelters** to permanent stable housing. Over the last 20 years, correlations between poor health and homelessness have been reported in research studies with homeless populations experiencing three to six times higher rates of physical illness compared to housed populations (National Health Care for the Homeless Council [NCHC], 2008). A national sample of homeless adults reported substantial unmet health care needs including inability to obtain needed medical or surgical care (32%), prescription medications (36%), mental health care (21%), eyeglasses (41%), and dental care (41%) (Baggett, O'Connell, Singer, & Rigotti, 2010). In addition, the health of homeless individuals is complicated by barriers to effective health treatment plans and access to health care. Further, individuals without homes are exposed to nature's elements and to society's violence, placing them at increased risk for illness or injury. They also may be addicted to drugs and alcohol, have poor nutrition and hygiene, and live in overcrowded facilities. Children in homeless shelters have critical and chronic health needs while at the same time limited access to health care services (NCHC, 2008).

There is an urgent need for preventive approaches to alleviate homelessness and the health consequences that follow. In treating illnesses and injuries in the homeless population, the nurse may offer a variety of services, such as screening or health teaching. Assessing and completing immunization status of children who are homeless is an important primary prevention intervention. Screenings for skin conditions and evidence of early signs of chronic conditions such as diabetes and hypertension are secondary prevention interventions. Another example is screening for normal development in children by using the developmental screening tools such as the Ages and Stages Questionnaire to identify developmental delays. When the community-based nurse assists clients to follow up with existing health issues and access to care, such as obtaining medication for mental health conditions including depression, it is tertiary prevention. The social determinants of health, in this case safe housing, impacts health. It follows that nurses have a role in promoting safe and affordable housing in their own communities. Nurses play an important role as advocates in the care of individuals and families who are homeless.

Camps

Camp programs for children and adults employ nurses in private, church, YWCA, YMCA, and Girl Scout and Boy Scout programs to mention a few examples. Nurses may be employed in camps for children with chronic illnesses, such as asthma, seizure disorders, AIDS, or numerous other chronic conditions. Camp nursing offers a unique setting to apply a variety of interventions, including health teaching, collaborating, counseling, case management, and delegated medication functions.

Camps for children with chronic conditions are now more common, serving children often previously precluded from having a camp experience. These camps hire staff familiar with the issues facing these children. Oversight and assistance for whatever needs the children or teens may have are combined with typical camp pastimes. For instance, at a camp for children with asthma, the nurse may assist the children with a nebulizer treatment or help them to decide when to use an inhaler before a particular camp activity. Significant improvements in children's symptoms control and life experiences as well as increased knowledge are documented outcomes from attending an educational asthma camp (Holsey & Cummings, 2008). Additionally, camp experiences provide assistance with social, emotional, and self-care challenges facing children related to their particular conditions.

Rehabilitation Centers

A freestanding or hospital-associated **rehabilitation center** for drug dependency treatment or for physical or emotional rehabilitation is another setting for care. The goal of this type of facility is to help clients reach optimal health so they can become part of the productive community again. Rehabilitation centers often have a philosophy of improving quality of life and facilitating independent self-care to the client's full ability. An interdisciplinary health care team collaborates to plan and implement care. The role of the nurse frequently calls for interventions of direct care, teaching, and counseling.

Detoxification Facilities

Clients are admitted to **detoxification facilities** for the express purpose of detoxifying their bodies from chemicals. Medication administration and ongoing monitoring of the client's physical well-being from the day of admission are critical delegated medical functions to ensure the client's safety. Nurses are responsible for health assessment, identification of immediate physical needs, and referral to community organizations at the time of discharge.

Treatment Facilities for Addictions

Clients in treatment facilities for addictions usually do not require close monitoring for physiologic changes after the first 48 to 72 hours of the detoxification period. The goal of treatment is for clients to begin their own recovery process to allow them to return to the community as better functioning and productive members of society. Recovery from substance abuse is a lifelong commitment that clients must make to address their addiction. The nurse is responsible for health assessment, planning, and management of identified problems. Direct care is provided through medication administration and management of acute problems. In some programs, the nurse acts as a case manager or counselor. A multidisciplinary approach is typically used, and the focus for discharge planning is the successful reentry of the client into society.

✳ CLIENT SITUATIONS IN PRACTICE

Role of the Nurse in a Residential Treatment Center for Teenagers

Jason is a nurse at a residential chemical dependency treatment program for male and female adolescents. Criteria for admission require that clients be between 11 and 17 years old and diagnosed as chemically dependent or chronic substance abuse with legal consequences.

Jason has a small office close to the dormitory-style rooms where the clients stay. His responsibilities include the delegated medical functions of medication supervision and oversight of self-administration of medications and obtaining health histories and assessments on each new admission. Other common interventions he is involved in are health education, disease prevention, health promotion, and collaboration with the other services in the facility during the treatment phase and for discharge planning. Another important role is that of formal and informal counselor. He enjoys working with adolescents who have varied emotional and physical problems.

It is important that the teens trust Jason and develop a therapeutic relationship with him. Establishing trust is always a challenge, but it is particularly so with teens who have addiction problems. Another challenge in this particular facility is that the population is coed. Sex education is imperative, as is problem solving about the many "attachments" the clients develop among each other. Jason states with a smile, "I just did not learn how to handle problems like this at nursing school. Some days, I really need to use every ounce of imagination I can muster." Jason reports both independence and challenge in his practice.

AMBULATORY CARE OR OUTPATIENT SERVICES

Clinics

Clients who do not require inpatient care in an acute setting can receive treatment, care, and education on an outpatient basis. **Outpatient services**, also called **ambulatory care centers**, are rapidly expanding and are now provided by private and public hospitals, HMOs, physicians' offices, community agencies, and public health departments (city, state, and federal). Services cover a broad range and include medical care, surgery, diagnostic tests, administration of medications (including intravenous therapy), physical therapy, kidney

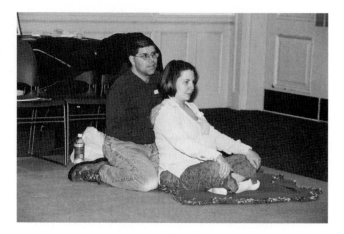

Figure 11-1 Expectant parents learn techniques to promote relaxation and comfort during birth. Classes in breastfeeding, infant care, and child care are also provided by many maternity centers. From Ricci, S. (2007). *Essentials of maternity, newborn, and women's health nursing.* Philadelphia, PA: Lippincott Williams & Wilkins.

dialysis, counseling, outpatient substance abuse treatment, various health education classes such as birthing classes (Fig. 11-1), aerobics classes, well-child care, and health education for management of chronic illness.

Ambulatory care centers are located around the community for ease of access. They may be found in hospitals, low-income neighborhoods, and shopping malls. They may be provided in conjunction with a physician's practice and a managed care facility. Some settings, such as urgent care centers, offer walk-in emergency care during extended hours when physicians' offices may be closed.

Some ambulatory clinics offer services to select groups or specific populations, for instance, community-based nurses practice in migrant camps (Fig. 11-2). Native American reservations, correctional facilities, and remote rural settings such as coal mining towns are other examples. Nurses can provide the impetus for improved health and quality of life for a wide range of client populations. In some clinics, nurses have the primary role in conducting assessments and caring for clients who need health maintenance or health promotion.

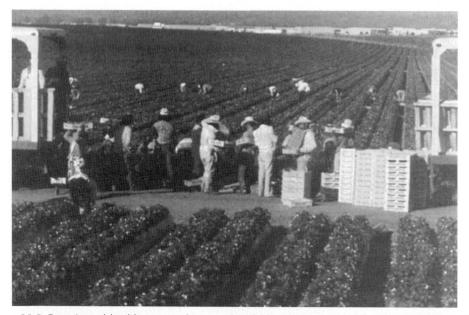

Figure 11-2 Experienced health care workers need to find ways to reach underserved people, such as these migrant workers. Migrant workers are defined by their common occupation and lifestyle, but they may cross various ethnic or racial lines.

In some locations, **nurse practitioners** have established their own independent ambulatory services while others may work in a large HMO or physician practice. Clinic nurses take on a variety of roles, depending on the medical specialty of the physician in charge and the type of clients served. For example, a nurse working in an HMO wound care clinic may care only for clients with private insurance. Community clinics may have a more heterogeneous population, with some clients insured and some uninsured. Client ability for self-care may vary between the two populations, depending on the individual client, family and social support, and other resources. Further, continuity of care may differ depending on what the insurance coverage will pay for as well as the family and community support that is available for the client.

Physicians' Offices

Physicians in individual and group practices, in primary care or specialties, also employ nurses. These nurses prepare clients, perform some assessments and routine laboratory work, assist with examinations, administer injections and medications, change wound dressings, assist with minor surgery, and maintain records. In some cases, they use telephone triage to direct clients to a clinic or emergency department immediately or recommend a simple intervention and call back the next day. Occasionally, physician offices will employ RNs to work as case managers.

Day Surgery Centers

Advanced technologies have influenced both the care of the client and the environment where care is provided. Minimally invasive procedures (e.g., laparoscopy, use of flexible endoscopes and lasers, and microwave therapies) now allow surgical procedures to be done in an ambulatory setting rather than in the hospital. Nurses working in **day surgery centers** have a range of duties: case management and delegated functions such as admission and assessment, preoperative and postoperative monitoring, and discharge planning and teaching. All these responsibilities are compressed into a very short time frame, requiring a high level of skill.

Community Health Centers

For more than three decades, a network of federally subsidized community health centers have served as a major safety net provider for low-income Americans. Community health centers are private, nonprofit, community-based organizations. Most health center patients have low incomes, are uninsured or publicly insured, and are members of racial/ethnic minority groups. Health care reform in 2010 substantially increased funding for community health centers (Fig 11-3). By 2015, health centers will double their current capacity to 40 million patients (National Association of Community Health Centers, 2010).

Working in community health centers provides rich transcultural opportunities with a diverse population, while at the same time offering challenges for the most experienced health care professionals. Innovative approaches to develop appropriate services for uninsured Americans include working with community partners to identify community needs and secure grants and funding sources to address these needs. There are numerous opportunities to affiliate with community health centers in addition to employment. Nurses volunteer to staff free clinics; participate in outreach, such as launch campaigns on health education; and speak to neighborhood gatherings, community forums, and church groups.

Specialized care centers provide health care for specific population or condition. Some of these are walk-in clinics; others provide residential care. For instance, a walk-in clinic may serve only teens or homeless teens.

Specialized clinics for individuals with cancer, human immunodeficiency virus (HIV) and AIDS, or orthopedics issues such as sports medicine or back conditions, are some examples of specialized care centers available in most cities. For another example, oncology clinics offer diagnosis, treatment, and care, including chemotherapy and are generally associated with a hospital or an HMO. Nurses provide direct client care, treatment, monitoring, and assistance with planning of interventions; they also attempt to minimize discomfort, manage pain, and maximize quality of life. The members of the multidisciplinary

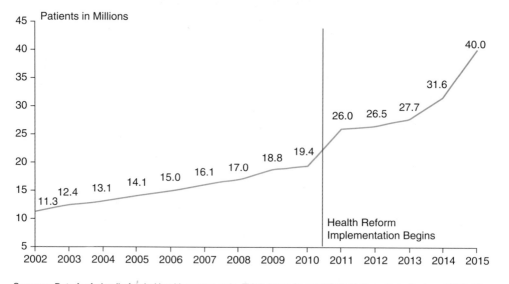

Estimated Number of Total Health Center Patients under Health Reform

Figure 11-3 Estimated number of total health center patients under health reform.

Sources: Data for federally-funded health centers only. FY00-08are from HRSA's Uniform Data System. FY09 -15 are NACHC projected estimates based on new federal funding. NACHC estimates future health center patients as a function of new federal funding.

Note: Other factors are difficult to predict and include payer mix, growth in non-federal grant sources, and the costs of care, which may be related to new patients having unmet health needs.

team collaborate closely. Nurses focus their time on care and support for the clients and families. Thus, the interventions of health teaching, counseling, collaborating, delegated medical functions, screening, and sometimes outreach are typical of this role regardless of the type of clinic.

Day Care Centers

Day centers for older adults were discussed at the beginning of this chapter. More commonly, day care centers provide services for infants, children, or disabled adults. Care may be provided for children while their parents work or after school before parents return from work. Some specialized day care centers provide care for children with minor illnesses when the parents must work. Other centers provide day care for children with chronic illnesses who cannot attend public school or for adults who because of physical, mental, or developmental disabilities cannot find employment. Nurses usually serve on the staff, as the center manager or develop a business providing specialized day care.

Mental Health Services

Mental health centers may be connected to a hospital or may be independent agencies. They may be part of a network of other coordinated social and health care services. Treatment provided may be short-term or long-term care or crisis intervention. The nurse is commonly involved in assessment, health teaching, counseling, and delegated functions such as administration of medications. Knowledge of the community for referral is necessary. In some cases, nurses function as case managers. Nurses may be involved in 24-hour hotline services. Generally mental health care is interdisciplinary, thus calling for the nurse to use collaboration skills. Clients may vary from mentally healthy people in a situational crisis to those with acute or chronic schizophrenia or Alzheimer disease. Often the nurse acts as an advocate in various capacities. Chapter 14 discusses community-based mental health nursing in more detail.

Maternal and Well-Child Services

Maternal and well-child health care programs may be conducted at a specialized center. Prenatal and postnatal care may be provided in which assessment and education are the focus. Postnatal follow-ups are sometimes made by telephone or with home visits. The nurse may advise clients on exercise, nutrition, and family planning. These services are discussed in more detail in Chapter 8.

Nutrition Services

Nutrition services address both issues of food insecurity and various health conditions that require specialized nutritional information across the life span. Food insecurity is addressed through government-sponsored Women, Infants, and Children (WIC) Programs that help fortify the dietary intake of infants, children, and pregnant women. For decades, research has demonstrated that for every $1 spent on WIC, $3 is saved in the improved health status of the women and children receiving the food vouchers. Meals on Wheels and food pantries may be part of the program for older adults, homebound individuals, or clients and families living in poverty. Food pantry use fluctuates with economic conditions rising in times of high unemployment. Nutrition centers may provide health teaching and counseling for mothers and children, older adults, and homeless or addicted clients. Programs for adolescents with eating disorders, nutrition counseling for people with diabetes, and programs for the overweight client illustrates the variety of nutrition programs that can be offered in specialized clinics. Many diseases, celiac disease, congestive heart disease, kidney disease, hypertension being a few examples, require specific diets.

Senior Citizens Centers

Senior citizen health clinics, designed to provide health care for seniors, are found in senior high-rise buildings, neighborhood senior centers, and other locations where high concentrations of elderly citizens live. These clinics provide blood pressure screening, medication review, hospital discharge follow-up, chronic disease management, basic nursing screening and assessment, and disease prevention and health promotion interventions. Some clinics offer home visits by nurses.

In this setting, the clinic nurse may identify older adults who are socially isolated and in need of companionship or friendship. In some community-based senior citizen clinics, volunteers provide friendship on a one-to-one basis. These types of programs have demonstrated success by reducing depression and the number of clinic visits by older adults.

Nursing Centers

Among the newer forms of community-based care are **nursing centers** or **nursing-managed health centers**. With the health care reform act of 2010, health insurance coverage was expanded to 31 million Americans. At the same time, a shortage of primary care physicians is projected to reach 35,000 to 44,000 by 2025. Given that the present percentage of Americans with chronic health conditions is 45% and is expected to continue to increase in the coming decades, the need to fill this lack of primary care providers is acute (Hansen-Turton, Bailey, Torres, & Ritter 2010). Nurse-managed health centers are increasingly offering communities another option for access to high-quality primary care to those individual with limited access.

A **nursing center** is not only a setting. It is also a philosophy of care. A nursing center is managed by nurses in partnership with the community; they serve by shaping broader services offered to the community. Nursing centers are the perfect design to meet this charge (Fig. 11-4).

Most academic nursing centers focus on outreach, disease prevention, management of chronic conditions, and **wellness promotion**, and many operate out of schools of nursing, with faculty and students providing the services. As mentioned, they often provide services to the underserved, uninsured, and disadvantaged populations, including women and children, the homeless, and minorities. However, there are nursing centers that serve insured populations as well. See Box 11-2 for a description of the development and success of a community nursing center.

Figure 11-4 Nurses counsel men and women, children, and elderly clients in community health centers across the nation.

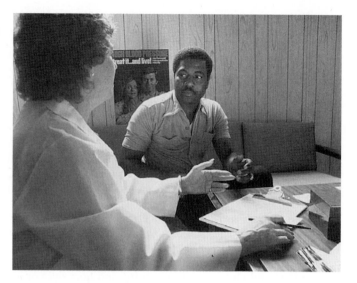

BOX 11-2 — A Community Nursing Center for the Health Promotion of Senior Citizens

Community nursing centers provide contact between members of vulnerable populations and health care. This cost-effective model offers direct access to nurses who offer holistic, client-centered health services. A community nursing center was developed in Chester, Pennsylvania, in 1997 as a partnership between the faculty at Neumann College Division of Nursing and Health Sciences and Widener University School of Nursing, and the Health Advisor Committee of Chester. The intent of the collaboration was to determine health care needs of underserved senior citizens in this community and develop a system to meet these needs. The needs assessment identified "health needs in the county as early cancer detection; expansion of support at the home for the frail elderly; expansion of support for chronic psychiatric, drug, and alcoholic clients; prevention of sexually transmitted diseases; provision of better health promotion for the public; and the reduction of premature cardiovascular deaths" (p. 221). From these needs, the goals for the nursing center became as follows:

- Identify the unmet health promotion needs of elderly men and women.
- Establish a nurse-managed center to provide health promotion activities and research and placement of nursing students to focus on the health of elderly men and women.
- Provide culturally competent health promotion activities to elderly residents.
- Promote relationships with existing health maintenance organizations to meet the health promotion needs of elderly men and women (p. 222).

Students and faculty worked from the inception of the partnership to develop the program. Forms were developed to track the progress of the client, including an intake form, admission record, and nursing visit report. The faculty and undergraduate and graduate nursing students from both universities worked in the center to meet the identified needs and serve as an effective referral system to services within the community. From 1997 to 2001 over 400 clients were seen at the center. The authors reported that the center had a positive impact on the health of the clients at the primary, secondary, and tertiary levels of prevention.

Source: Newman, D. M. (2005). A community nursing center for the health promotion of senior citizens based on the Neuman systems model. *Nursing Education Perspectives, 26*(4), 221–223.

SCHOOLS

In 1902, Lillian Wald placed a nurse, Lina Rogers, in a school setting in New York City as an experiment. The experiment, to determine if placing nurses in schools could reduce the spread of contagious diseases, proved to be successful. This was the beginning of the school nursing movement that has provided the backbone of nursing-related health promotion activity in the school setting. Today, schools of all kinds comprise a major sector of practice for community-based nursing: day care centers, preschools, elementary schools, secondary schools, colleges, and universities. Children seen by school nurses reflect the changing society of the nation, with different racial and ethnic backgrounds, varying socioeconomic backgrounds, and complex disabilities. Often school nurses are the most important source of health assessment, health education, and emergency care for the nation's children.

The **school nurse** focuses on the healthy, growing individual, or in some cases specializes in educational settings for the mentally or physically disabled. State laws determine if the school can provide emergency treatment for injuries, maintenance of health records, immunizations, referral for health and social services, physical assessments, and teaching (Fig. 11-5).

One school nurse describes her position as follows:

> I am responsible for about 1,200 high school students. Our office is open daily, and we serve 50 to 60 students each day with such complaints as headaches, sore throats, and fever. The biggest change over the past few years has been the decrease in the number of high school-age single mothers we serve. A decade ago I developed a program for these young women that includes safe sex, birth control options, child care, and child health. The decrease in the pregnancy rate is related to this program. The best evaluation data from the program shows that only one of the young women who have completed the classes has had another unintended pregnancy. I would say I am nurse, mother, confidante, baby-sitter, first-aid giver, record keeper, and friend as a school nurse.

Many school nurses become "drop-in" counselors as public school funding for school counselors has dramatically decreased in the last decade. Consequently the school nurse is often the one to whom a child or adolescent goes with personal questions and problems. These nurses use an established network of referrals for students' personal needs. A school nurse may refer to speech and hearing services, individual and family counseling, gay and lesbian support and youth

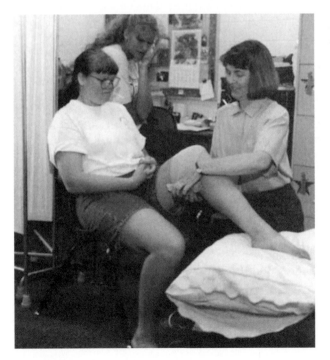

Figure 11-5 A school nurse assesses and treats an injured child. This is essential to a comprehensive school health program.

groups, the department of social services, crisis drop-in centers, drug and alcohol programs, foster care, drop-in health clinics, mental health services, and parents-in-training groups.

A school health program may include identification of communicable, chronic, and disabling diseases, immunizations, safety, and health education. School nursing requires competence in health teaching, delegated medical functions, collaboration, counseling, case finding, consultation, referral and follow-up, advocacy, and case management. Required educational preparation varies from that of an RN to an nurse practitioner with a graduate degree. From state to state, school nurse coverage ranges from comprehensive to inadequate with some jurisdictions providing direct access to RNs to all students to others where there is never a nurse on site at the school. There is a trend toward increasing the number of school-based health centers (SBHCs) in the United States. SBHCs provide a nurse-managed clinic in a school that offers primary care with a disease prevention/health promotion model. Some employ an nurse practitioner or physician's assistant (Hansen-Turton et al., 2010; Robert Wood Johnson Foundation, 2010). Most families are already associated with and trust the schools in their community. Expansion of school-based clinics into comprehensive neighborhood health and social service centers offers easy access to nursing care for families in their own community.

OCCUPATIONAL HEALTH NURSE

Occupational health nursing began in 1895 when Ida M. Steward was hired by the Vermont Marble Company to visit mothers and infants, care for the ill at home, and curb communicable diseases. During the same time period, Margaret Sanger, PHN, was instrumental in advocating for women factory workers in the lower East Side of Manhattan. This role was soon expanded to include disease and injury prevention and first aid in the work place.

Currently, the toll of workplace injuries and illness remains significant. Every year, almost 5,000 people die from work-related diseases (U.S. Department of Labor, Bureau of Labor Statistics, 2010b). Employers acknowledge that the health and well-being of employees are vital to morale and enhance the productivity of the company. Consequently, most companies provide health insurance, and many have developed programs to enhance health through the promotion of healthy lifestyles. This has spawned new language and a new focus for health care with programs such as **work-site health promotion**, **employee wellness programs**, and **employee assistance programs**, all of which focus on the health of employees. Healthy snacks and meals, exercise programs and facilities, and educational classes are all used by companies to promote health.

A survey of almost 6,000 occupational health nurses throughout the United States and Canada provides an interesting picture of occupational health nursing (Strasser, Maher, Knuth, & Fabrey, 2006). First, it shows that the educational level varies, with 36% having a diploma, 31% an associate degree, 29% a bachelor's degree, and 3% a master's degree. Second, as to time spent in various roles and activities: 27% was spent in direct care, 43% as a case manager, 14% as a health educator or counselor, and 9% as a consultant.

The focus of the **occupational health nurse** is on keeping employees healthy, preventing illness and accidents, providing assistance to the employee who is returning to work after an illness or injury, and ensuring a safe business or industrial environment. Given the expanding opportunities in this type of service, nurses can market their expertise to employers. They can provide programs aimed at job-related safety, weight reduction, and addiction-free lifestyles as well as promote nutrition, exercise, smoking cessation, and family planning.

DISASTER NURSING

Traditionally disaster nursing has been provided through the American Red Cross. Nurses have been central to the provision of services through the American Red Cross throughout the history of disaster nursing. Beginning with the 1880 Johnstown flood and the 1888 yellow fever epidemic, nurses have provided assistance during times of crisis. More than 30,000 nurses are involved in the American Red Cross in paid and volunteer positions. These activities consist of providing direct assistance in times of crisis, developing and teaching courses, and acting in management and supervisory roles. There are opportunities for both RNs and nursing students (American Red Cross, 2010).

There is renewed interest and appreciation for this type of nursing care following the attacks on the World Trade Center on September 11, 2001; Hurricane Katrina in 2005; and the earthquake in Haiti in 2010. Although we know more today about disaster nursing, terrorism, and bioterrorism preparedness than we did in September of 2001, some believe there is a need for additional education, training, and other preparation for all health care workers in anticipation of another terrorist event.

To be prepared, nurses benefit from first developing their own individual family and home disaster plan. They must understand medical management of those exposed to biological agents as well as how to protect themselves when treating victims. Protection varies according to the agent and provides education for the appropriate precautions depending on the agent on its Web site: http://www.bt.cdc.gov/ (Centers for Disease Control and Prevention, 2010). Additional discussion of disaster nursing is found in Chapter 15.

Nursing Specialties

Although all nurses working in community-based settings benefit from developing skills in assessment, program planning, communication, cultural competency, dimensions of communities, public health science, management, and leadership, nurses may choose to develop an area of expertise. A nurse's title may reflect the practice setting, such as school nurse, home care nurse, or occupational health nurse. Other times the expertise of the role in a setting, such as health educator, case manager, discharge planner, or continuity of care nurse reflects a nursing specialty. A nursing specialty may also be defined by level of education or completion of additional certification.

SPECIALTIES REQUIRING REGISTERED NURSE LICENSE

Advanced practice nurses include nurse practitioners and **clinical nurse specialists**. The number of nurse practitioners and certified nurse midwives increased dramatically in the last two decades. In 2000, there were an estimated 95,000 nurse practitioners and 8,000 certified nurse midwives practicing in the United States, an increase of about 160% from the early 1990s. By 2008, there were more than 158,000 advanced practice nurses in the United States. Over this duration, these two professions have become more widely accepted by physicians, clients, and the general public as key members of the health care delivery team (U.S. Department of Health and Human Services, 2010). There are several underlying forces that have contributed to this dramatic change. First, the concerns about the rising cost of health care along with the growing recognition that advanced practice nurses provide cost-effective, high-quality care created a dramatic increase in job opportunities. Second, consumers are better educated about health care diagnosis and treatment as more health information has become widely available to the general public. Third, consumers began to play a more active role in the purchase of health services, the utilizations of services, and the choice of care providers. Fourth, the dramatic increases in the number of advanced practice nurses occurred as consumers are more open to practitioners, interventions, and approaches beyond the traditional ones. A fifth factor stems from the growing number of uninsured and underinsured people in need of health care and the increased demand for advanced practice nurses to work with underserved populations. Sixth, nurse practitioners are more commonly used instead of medical residents in primary care (Health Resources and Services Administration, Bureau of Health Professions, 2006).

An **nurse practitioner** is an RN who has graduated from a nurse practitioner program and successfully completed the advanced practice licensing examination. Nurse practitioners first began to appear in the United States and Canada in the late 1960s. Nurse practitioners may be generalists or may specialize in the care of particular types of clients (Table 11-2).

Not only do nurse practitioners provide quality health care, but they do so at a fraction of the cost of physician care. Nurse Practioners have consistently been found to be the solution to wellness and preventive health care with 45 years of evidence supporting NPs as

Table 11-2 Primary Clinical Specialties of Employed Nurse Practitioners With Job Title of Nurse Practitioner	
Clinical Specialty*	**Percentage (%)**
Critical care	5.8
Cardiac care	8.6
Chronic care	6.9
Emergency/trauma care	3.5
Gastrointestinal	3.4
General medical surgical	12.1
Gynecology (women's health)	12.1
Infectious/communicable disease	3.7
Neurological	3.2
Obstetrics/labor and delivery	8.6
Oncology	4.4
Primary care	36.1
Psychiatric/mental health	6.3
Other specialties**	16.7

From U.S. Department of Health and Human Services, Health Resources and Services Administration. (2010). *The registered nurse population: Findings from the 2008 national sample survey of registered nurses.* Retrieved from http://bhpr.hrsa.gov/healthworkforce/rnsurveys/rnsurveyfinal.pdf; (**includes dermatology, endocrinology, hospice, occupational health, ophthalmology, orthopedic, otolanryngoglogy, plastic surgery, radiology, pulmonary/respiratory, renal/idalysis, urology, no specific area).

cost-effective providers of high-quality health care (American Academy of Nurse Practitioners, 2010). For example, the potential for NPs to control costs associated with the health care of older adults has been recognized by United Health Group (2009), which recommends that by providing NPs to manage nursing home patients, $166 billion savings in health care would result. This suggests greater opportunities for geriatric nurse practitioners in the future.

Certified nurse midwifes have provided care for women during normal pregnancy, labor, and delivery since the inception of the certification and accreditation process in the early 1970s. The certified nurse midwife practices in connection with a health care agency in which medical services are available if the client develops complications. In the United States, a nurse midwife is required by law to have a baccalaureate degree in nursing and a graduate degree from an accredited nurse midwife program, and he or she must pass the certification examination from the American College of Nurse Midwives. The number of certified nurse midwives more than tripled, from 3,000 in 1995 to over 10,000 in 2008 (U.S. Department of Health and Human Services, 2010).

A clinical nurse specialist can practice in an acute care or a community setting. First formally recognized as a nursing specialty in 1965, such positions today generally focus on a particular expertise (e.g., diabetes or oncology). In contrast to nurse practitioners, in the last 20 years, there has been a decrease in the number of clinical nurse specialists (U.S. Department of Health and Human Services, 2010). The CNS or Clinical Nurse Specialist education and role focuses on improving clinical care, primarily in hospitals and extended care facilities by having an expert nurse. The CNS coordinates care for individuals, educates nursing personnel who provided direct care, and helps identify and improve aspects of the health system patients and nursing staff. CNSs have expertise in one or more clinical areas such as oncology, pediatrics, geriatrics, psychiatric/mental health, adult health, obstetrics, acute/critical care, and community health. The specialist may develop and oversee a specialty program, act as a resource and consultant for other staff, and establish educational programs for the general public. Nurses have different degrees of autonomy and responsibility, depending on the setting. Educational and professional role requirements differ as well. Most states require the nurse to have a master's degree to be a clinical nurse specialist. National certification by professional associations may be available. The role of the clinical nurse specialist is evolving as the health care delivery system continues to be transformed.

Conclusions

Rapid and dramatic changes have occurred in health care delivery in the community. Today, opportunities exist for men and women to assume many roles in different settings with a variety of clients. Because of the increasing elderly population, many nurses are entering the field of geriatric nursing, but many other opportunities exist for the practicing nurse. The nurse may specialize in primary care, as a case manager, clinical nurse specialist, or nurse practitioner. The dramatic expansion in the use of advanced practice nurses in the last two decades suggests that the importance of the role of the nurse in community-based settings will continue to expand in the coming years. The principles of community-based care apply to all nursing roles in all settings. All of this points to the expanding opportunities our profession presents for each of us to develop an exciting and evolving career in nursing.

What's on the Web

All Nurses
INTERNET ADDRESS: **http://allnurses.com/**
To find an exhaustive array of information on different specialty roles in nursing, consult allnurses.com and click on the Nursing Specialties category. This site provides access to resources for more than 50 nursing specialties, including but not limited to many community-based nursing roles, such as school, ambulatory care, parish, and correctional health nursing; telephone triage; intravenous therapy; and advanced practice nursing or nurse practitioner duties.

Community Preventative Services for Worksite Health Promotion
INTERNET ADDRESS: **http://www.thecommunityguide.org/worksite/index.html**
This site provides resources for worksite policies and programs to help employees reduce health risks and improve their quality of life. These worksite interventions can be delivered:

- *At the worksite (e.g., signs to encourage stair use, health education classes)*
- *At other locations (e.g., gym membership discounts, weight management counseling)*
- *Through the employee health benefits plan (e.g., flu shots, cancer screenings)*

American Academy of Ambulatory Care Nursing
INTERNET ADDRESS: **http://aaacn.inurse.com/**
This organization advances and influences the art and science of ambulatory care nursing practice and health care delivery systems to improve the health of individuals and communities.

American Academy of Nurse Practitioners (AANP)
INTERNET ADDRESS: **http://www.aanp.org/**
This organization promotes high standards of health care as delivered by NPs and acts as a forum to enhance the identity and continuity of NPs.

American Association of Occupational Health Nurses (AAOHN)
INTERNET ADDRESS: **http://www.aaohn.org/**
This site provides information about occupational health nursing and the professional organization. AAOHN's mission is to advance the profession of occupational and environmental health nursing as the authority on health, safety, productivity, and disability management for worker populations. Online (CEUs) modules are available.

American Holistic Nurses Association (AHNA)
INTERNET ADDRESS: **http://www.ahna.org/**
The mission of AHNA is to unite nurses in healing. AHNA serves as a bridge between the traditional medical paradigm and universal complementary and alternative health practices. AHNA supports the concepts of holism: a state of harmony between body, mind and emotions, and spirit within an ever-changing environment.

American School Health Association (ASHA)
INTERNET ADDRESS:**http://www.ashaweb.org/**
ASHA unites many school professionals who are committed to safeguarding the health of school-age children. The goals of the organization are to advocate for children and youth, represent all school health care professionals, and promote professional education, public education, research, and service to children and youth. The Web site offers information about publications and conferences related to school health.

Visiting Nurse Associations of America (VNAA)
INTERNET ADDRESS: **http://vnaa.org/vnaa/siteshelltemplates/homepage_navigate.htm**
   This Web site has information about visiting nurse agencies, conferences, and professional information, as well as caregiver information and home care resources.

References and Bibliography

American Academy of Nurse Practitioners. (2010). *Cost effectiveness of nurse practitioners*. Retrieved from http://www.aanp.org/NR/rdonlyres/197C9C42-4BC1-42A5-911E-85FA759B0308/0/CostEffectiveness4pages.pdf

American Red Cross. (2010). *Nursing.* Retrieved from http://www.redcrosstc.org/detalle_noticias.asp?id=5919&SN=10910&OP=10911&IDCapitulo=073V3P7593

Baggett, T., O'Connell, J., Singer, D., & Rigotti, N. (2010). The unmet health care needs of homeless adults: A national study. *American Journal of Public Health, 100*(7), 1326–1333. Retrieved from MEDLINE database.

Centers for Disease Control and Prevention. (2010). *Emergency preparedness and response.* Retrieved from http://www.bt.cdc.gov/

Cooper, J., Loeb, S., & Smith, C. (2010). The primary care nurse practitioner and cancer survivorship care. *Journal of the American Academy of Nurse Practitioners, 22*(8), 394–402. doi:10.1111/j.1745-7599.2010.00528.x.

Eckenrode, J., Campa, M., Luckey, D., Henderson, C., Cole, R., Kitzman, H., et al. (2010). Long-term effects of prenatal and infancy nurse home visitation on the life course of youths: 19-year follow-up of a randomized trial. *Archives of Pediatrics & Adolescent Medicine, 164*(1), 9–15. Retrieved from CINAHL Plus with Full Text database.

Elderberry Institute. (2010). *Living at home network reorganizes to better promote neighborhood-based care for elders.* Retrieved from http://www.elderberry.org/breakingNews.asp

Hansen-Turton, T., Bailey, D., Torres, N., & Ritter, A. (2010). Policy & politics: Nurse-managed health centers. *American Journal of Nursing, 110*(9), 23–26. Retrieved from CINAHL Plus with Full Text database.

Health Resources and Services Administration, Bureau of Health Professions. (2006). *A comparison of changes in the professional practice of nurse practitioners, physician assistants, and certified nurse midwives: 1992 and 2000.* Retrieved from http://www.bhpr.hrsa.gov/healthworkforce/reports/scope/scope1-2.htm

Holsey, C., & Cummings, L. (2008). Evaluating a residential asthma camp program and ways to increase physical activity. *Pediatric Nursing, 34*(6), 459. Retrieved from CINAHL Plus with Full Text database.

Horn, S. D. (2005). RN staffing time and outcomes of long-stay nursing home residents: Pressure ulcers and other adverse outcomes are less likely as RNs spend more time on direct patients care. *The American Journal of Nursing, 105*(11), 58–71.

Kitzman, H., Olds, D., Cole, R., Hanks, C., Anson, E., Arcoleo, K., et al. (2010). Enduring effects of prenatal and infancy home visiting by nurses on children: Follow-up of a randomized trial among children at age 12 years. *Archives of Pediatrics & Adolescent Medicine, 164*(5), 412–418. Retrieved from CINAHL Plus with Full Text database.

Kitzman, H., Olds, D. L., Sidora, K., et al. (2000). Enduring effects of nurse home visitation on maternal life course. *JAMA, 283*(15), 1983–1989.

Mayernik, D., Resick, L., Skomo, M., & Mandock, K. (2010). Parish nurse-initiated interdisciplinary mobile health care delivery project. *JOGNN: Journal of Obstetric, Gynecologic & Neonatal Nursing, 39*(2), 227–234. doi:10.1111/j.1552-6909.2010.01112.x.

McGinnis, S., & Zoske, F. (2008). The emerging role of faith community nurses in prevention and management of chronic disease. *Policy, Politics & Nursing Practice, 9*(3), 173–180. Retrieved from CINAHL Plus with Full Text database.

National Association of Community Health Centers. (2010). *Expanding health centers under health care reform: Doubling patient capacity and bringing down costs.* Retrieved from http://www.nachc.org/client/HCR_New_Patients_Final.pdf

National Citizens' Coalition for Nursing Home Reform. (2009). *A consumer guide to choosing a nursing home: Consumer information sheet.* Retrieved from www.nursinghomeaction.org; http://www.theconsumervoice.org/sites/default/files/advocate/A-Consumer-Guide-To-Choosing-A-Nursing-Home.pdf

National Health Care for the Homeless Council. (2008). *Health care for the homeless: Comprehensive services to meet complex needs.* Retrieved from http://www.nhchc.org/Publications/HCHbrochure2008.pdf

National Respite Network. (2010). *Adult day care: One form of respite for older adults.* Retrieved from http://www.archrespite.org/images/docs/Factsheets/fs_54-adult_day_care.pdf

Newman, D. M. (2005). A community nursing center for the health promotion of senior citizens based on the Neuman systems model. *Nursing Education Perspectives, 26*(4), 221–223.

Olds, D. L., Henderson, C. R., Jr., & Kitzman, H. (1994). Does prenatal and infancy home visitation have enduring effects on qualities of parental care giving and health at 25 to 50 months of life? *Pediatrics, 93,* 89–98.

Olds, D. L., Henderson, C. R., Jr., Tatelbaum, R., & Chamberlin, R. (1986). Improving the delivery of prenatal care and outcomes of pregnancy: A randomized trial of home visitations. *Pediatrics, 77,* 16–28.

Olds, D. L., Henderson, C. R., Jr., Tatelbaum, R., & Chamberlin, R. (1988). Improving the life course development of socially disadvantaged mothers: A randomized trial of home visitations. *American Journal of Public Health, 78*(11), 1436–1445.

Pekkarinen, L., Sinervo, T., Elovainio, M., Noro, A., & Finne-Soveri, H. (2008). Drug use and pressure ulcers in long-term care units: Does nurse time pressure and unfair management increase the prevalence? *Journal of Clinical Nursing, 17*(22), 3067–3073. Retrieved from CINAHL Plus with Full Text database.

Ricci, S. (2007.) Essentials of maternity, newborn, and women's health nursing. Philadelphia, PA: Lippincott Williams & Wilkins.

Robert Wood Johnson Foundation. (2010). *School nurses: Keeping children healthy and ready to learn.* Retrieved from http://www.rwjf.org/pr/product.jsp?id=67388

Solari-Twadell, P. (1999). The emerging practice of parish nursing. In P. Solari-Twadell & M. A. McDermott (Eds.), *Parish nursing: Promoting whole person health within faith communities* (pp. 3–24). Thousand Oaks, CA: Sage.

Strasser, P. B., Maher, H. K., Knuth, G., & Fabrey, L. J. (2006). Occupational health nursing 2004 practice analysis report. *American Association of Occupational Health Nurses, 54*(1), 14–23.

United Health Group. (2009). *Federal health care cost containment: How in practice can it be done? Options with a real world track record of success.* Retrieved from http://www.unitedhealthgroup.com/hrm/unh_workingpaper1.pdf

U.S. Conference of Mayors. (2009). *Hunger and homelessness survey.* Retrieved from http://usmayors.org/pressreleases/uploads/USCMHungercompleteWEB2009.pdf

U.S. Department of Health and Human Services. (2010). *Administration on aging fact sheet on agency for older Americans.* Retrieved from http://www.aoa.gov/aoaroot/Press_Room/Products_Materials/fact/pdf/AoA.pdf

U.S. Department of Health and Human Services, Health Resources and Services Administration. (2010). *The registered nurse population: Findings from the 2008 National Sample Survey of Registered Nurses.* Retrieved from http://bhpr.hrsa.gov/healthworkforce/rnsurvey/2008/nssrn2008.pdf

U.S. Department of Housing and Urban Development. (2009). *The 2008 annual homeless assessment report to Congress.* Retrieved from http://www.hudhre.info/documents/4thHomelessAssessment Report.pdf

U.S. Department of Labor, Bureau of Labor Statistics. (2010a) *National census of fatal occupation injuries in 2009: Preliminary results.* Retrieved from http://www.bls.gov/news.release/pdf/cfoi.pdf

U.S. Department of Labor, Bureau of Labor Statistics. (2010b). *Occupational outlook handbook, 2010–2011 edition: Registered nurses.* Retrieved from http://www.bls.gov/oco/ocos083.htm#projections_data

LEARNING ACTIVITIES

JOURNALING ACTIVITY 11-1

Contact a nurse in a specialty area of interest to you. Set up an appointment to interview him or her, and spend some time observing the nurse in his or her clinical role.

- Explore http://allnurses.com/ to learn more about the role in preparation for your interview.

- Develop questions prior to the interview (at least four to eight questions about aspects of the role that interest you). Take notes during the interview, or with permission from the nurse, audiotape the interview and transcribe it into written form. Complete a summary of the interview.

- As soon as you are home from observation of the nurse, answer the following questions in your clinical journal.
  - What did you see, hear, and feel today?
  - How does it compare to what you expected?
  - What roles that you observed would you enjoy doing?
  - Is this the type of practice that you would enjoy? Why or why not?
  - If you are interested in this role, what is the next step that you will take to further explore this area of nursing?

JOURNALING ACTIVITY 11-2

1. In your clinical journal, identify a practice setting that you would like to know more about. Identify three ways you can learn more about this setting and the roles that nurses have in it. Implement this plan.
2. Discuss the strategies you used to explore this setting and the roles of the nurse.
3. What did you learn from this experience?
4. How will you use this information?

PRACTICAL APPLICATION ACTIVITY 11-3

Interview a nurse in one of the settings described in this chapter. Use one or more of the following questions as a part of the interview.

1. How do you assist your clients to improve their self-care? Can you tell me a story about when you assisted or did not assist one of your clients to improve his or her self-care?
2. How do you alter care according to the context of the client's family, culture, and community? Can you tell me about a situation when you or someone else you work with did or did not alter care according to the context of the client's family, culture, or community?
3. How do you incorporate the concept of disease prevention and health promotion in the care you provide to your clients and families? Can you give me some examples?
4. How do you enhance continuity for your clients? Can you tell me about a time when you were or you weren't successful creating continuity?

Chapter 12

Home Health Care Nursing

ROBERTA HUNT

Learning Objectives

1. Identify the purpose and goals of home care nursing.

2. Discuss types of home care agencies.

3. Outline the advantages and disadvantages of home care.

4. Discuss barriers to successful home care nursing.

5. Define the nursing skills and competencies needed in home care.

6. Describe the home visit and its main components.

7. Summarize methods the community-based nurse can use in meeting needs of the lay caregiver.

Key Terms

financial assessment
home care agencies
home care equipment vendors
hospital-based home care agencies
lay caregiving
official home care agencies
respite care

Chapter Topics

Historical Perspective

Significance of Home Health Care

Agencies That Provide Home Care

Acute Care Nursing Versus Home Care Nursing

Nursing Skills and Competencies in Home Health Care

Support of the Lay Caregiver

The Future of Home Care

Conclusions

THE NURSE SPEAKS

"Please go out and see him. He's refusing hospitalizations and hospice, so there's not much more I can do." This was a fairly common request from acquired immunodeficiency syndrome (AIDS)-specialized physicians in the early to mid-1990s, so I was not surprised to find a very cachectic, disoriented patient when I arrived. Tom was lying in soiled sheets in an upstairs bedroom. He was too weak to be walked to the bathroom by his partner, and he had fallen twice in the past 3 days. He could answer some questions but frequently drifted off to sleep midsentence. Physical inspection revealed a severely wasted male in his middle years with a stage IV decubitus ulcer on his coccyx and 4+ pitting edema bilaterally to midthigh. When he was able to talk, he conveyed a strong will to live and gratitude for a supportive partner who was willing to assist in all of his care. Tom had tried the AIDS medications, but he had stopped them because he felt too weak to keep up with the regimen.

I immediately realized Tom still had a curative versus comfort focus. I also recognized it would take the effort of many people working together if we were to pull him back from the edge of death. Complex cases require thoughtful and effective case management, and Tom's case was no exception. I pulled in as many home health aide hours as his insurance would cover. I called and got orders for a dietitian consult, which led to nasogastric tube feedings. From there, I involved a wound care specialist, who prescribed the best products to heal the decubitus ulcer. Tom was moved to the first floor of his home, providing more space for a hospital bed, commode, and wheelchair. This also allowed his partner to get more sleep, so the family did not face the frequent problem of burnout. When the insurance company balked at the cost of all these services, I reminded them of the expense that would be incurred if Tom were staying in a hospital or long-term care facility for weeks on end.

Slowly, Tom's level of strength began to return and with it his ability to take his antiretroviral medications. Three months later, I was called to the front office by our receptionist. There stood Tom with a big smile on his face and a bouquet of flowers in his hand. He gave me a warm hug and asked me to wish him luck as he returned for his first day back at his job. The combined efforts of home care professionals guided by nursing case management had indeed helped Tom follow his desire to continue to focus on living.

Teddie M. Potter, RN, MS,
Home Care Nurse,
Instructor, Minneapolis Community and Technical College

Home health care is the provision of health services to individuals and families in their places of residence for the purpose of promoting, maintaining, and restoring health. It is one of the most rapidly growing service industries in the United States. Home care nurses must be competent communicators, teachers, managers, and physical caregivers. This chapter begins with a brief introduction to the history of home health care. **Home care agencies**, the goals, advantages and disadvantages of home care, as well as the barriers to successful home care are discussed. A large section of the chapter deals with nursing skills and competencies, together with a summary of the first visit. Safety issues and lay caretaker involvement conclude the chapter.

Historical Perspective

Home care nursing as it is practiced today is a relatively new phenomenon. However, providing health care in the home is a very old concept. Florence Nightingale is credited with developing the concept of nursing care provided in the home in the 1860s. In the

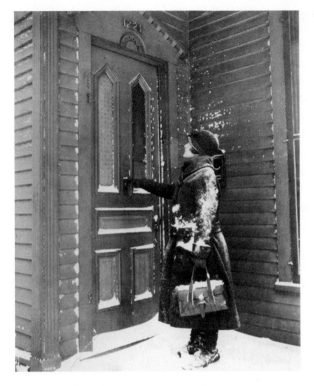

Figure 12-1 A Minnesota home health nurse paying a visit to a client at the beginning of the 20th century. Copyright the Minnesota Historical Society. Used with permission.

United States, Lillian Wald and Mary Brewster established nurse home visiting in the late 1800s that later evolved into the New York City Visiting Nurse Association. Almost 100 years later, changes in federal reimbursement for health care brought about vast growth in home health care. Figure 12-1 is a charming reminder of the long and rich history of the home care nursing profession.

Modern home care evolved from the Visiting Nurse Association (VNA), which originated at the beginning of the 20th century in New York City. The mission of home care has changed from that of the VNA in the early part of the 20th century, when nurses were caring for mostly women and their infants before and after birth. In addition, the VNA cared for indigent tuberculosis clients in the tenements. Physicians were involved in home care before World War II. The war produced a shortage of physicians, however, so the use of nurses for home care services expanded. In the 1940s, **hospital-based home care agencies** were established. A pivotal change in home care came from the 1965 Medicare and Medicaid legislation that allowed payment for some home care services for qualified recipients. With this legislation, home care became more narrowly defined as a medical model alternative to extended hospital care. The impact of this legislation was the first factor to contribute to the growth in the home care industry. In 1963, there were 1,100 home health agencies; today, there are more than 10,500 (Table 12-1).

The second factor that contributed to the growth in the home care industry was the implementation of diagnosis-related groups (DRGs) for Medicare during the late 1970s and early 1980s. This legislation was intended as a cost containment measure. As most hospitals and health maintenance organizations (HMOs) were required to follow Medicare's DRG reimbursement guidelines, home care began to be viewed as a vital aspect of the health care system. Again, home care became a more central aspect of health care as a cost-containment strategy. Gradually, throughout the United States, insurance companies and HMOs adopted home care as part of their standard health insurance package because of the cost efficiency of care at home versus institutional care. With the trend toward shorter hospital stays, continuing care needs, and available reimbursement for home health care, the home care boom was born. Further, the increasing number of noninstitutionalized

Table 12-1 Number of Medicare-Certified Home Care Agencies

| Year | Freestanding Agencies | | | Facility Based | |
	VNA	Public	Proprietary	Hospital	Total
1967	549	939	0	133	1,753
1975	525	1,228	0	273	2,242
1985	514	1,205	832	1,277	5,983
1995	575	1,182	3,951	2,470	9,120
2000	436	909	2,863	2,151	7,152
2003	439	888	3,402	1,776	7,265
2007	459	1,132	4,919	1,547	8,838

Adapted from National Association for Home Care & Hospice. (2010). *Basic statistics about home care.* Washington, DC: Author. Retrieved from http://www.nahc.org/facts/10HC_Stats.pdf

individuals over age 65, living longer and with multiple chronic conditions, has intensified the need for more home health care services. The acceleration in development of sophisticated technology that allows people to be kept alive and relatively comfortable in their own homes has also added to the need for nursing care in the home, as has consumer demand for improved end-of-life care at home.

Significance of Home Health Care

The goal of home health care nursing is to provide services to individuals and families and to promote, maintain, and restore health. In most cases, this is achieved through short-term, intermittent, direct nursing care made in home visits. Home care nurses provide direct services or supervise direct services to assist with activities of daily living (ADL); teach clients, families, and caregivers how to provide self-care; and use communication skills to enhance continuity of care.

Governmental, private, and hospital-based programs employ home health care nurses. Home health care nurses come from all levels of educational preparation, with 40% bachelor's, 24% diploma, 23% associate, and 5% with a master's degree. Only 6% of all home care nurses are under 30 years of age (Anthony & Milone-Nuzzo, 2005). Home health care includes not only skilled nursing care but also the services of physical, occupational, and speech therapists; social workers; and home health aides.

More than 69% of clients served in home care are older than 65 years, and 17% are over 85 years of age. Hospitalized clients make up a large proportion of home care clients within 30 days of discharge. Diseases of the circulatory system account for almost 26% of those receiving home care services with Medicare reimbursement (National Association for Home Care & Hospice, 2010). There are also an increasing number of clients requiring high-technology medical interventions (e.g., intravenous therapy, mechanical ventilation, and parenteral nutrition).

Agencies That Provide Home Care

Home health care has evolved into a major industry, with three key components: home care agencies, **home care equipment vendors**, and home infusion therapy companies. Home infusion therapy is discussed in Chapter 13. A change in the types of agencies that provide home care resulted from the federal legislation enacted in 1965 and 1983. Agency types today include official, hospital-based, and proprietary.

Official home care agencies are often housed in city and county departments and only provide service certified by federal government mandates. Hospital-based agencies have no mandate and can offer services of their own choosing, or Medicare and Medicaid service if they are certified by the federal government. They receive no direct tax support and operate as a unit or department of a hospital. Proprietary agencies are freestanding and for-profit home care agencies that provide services based on third-party reimbursement or self-pay.

All three types of agencies may be certified by the federal government to provide services for clients with Medicare and Medicaid insurance. The services have to be skilled and provide home visits by nurses; physical, occupational, and speech therapists; medical social workers; and home health aides. Most insurance companies pay for home health care services, but few will pay for 24-hour nursing care. Few, if any, insurance carriers will pay for paraprofessional care without skilled care services. The growing managed care movement follows the Medicare guidelines for the development of home health care services, although the number of visits may be fewer and may vary among insurance companies or managed care organizations. Medicare will not cover 24-hour-a day care at home or meals delivered to the home. Neither will it cover homemaker services such as shopping, cleaning, and laundry or personal care if these are the only services needed (Centers for Medicare & Medicaid Services, 2010).

Private duty agencies that primarily provide shift relief at health care institutions and for private clients are generally described as home care agencies. Private sources or private insurance pays for most of the care; time is scheduled in hourly blocks, and services are largely provided by paraprofessionals (aides and homemakers) and nurses. Home care is also a generic term used for the entire industry and can include all types of agencies. In this text, the term home care is used to include all at-home nursing services.

Medicare is the largest single payer of home care services (Table 12-2).

Clients who are homebound and under the care of a physician are eligible for home care services under Medicare (Box 12-1).

Some states have lifted the homebound restriction, so it is important for the nurse to know the requirements where he or she is practicing. Many insurance companies follow the Medicare criteria. For the most part, home care has become medical care in the home; clients are given care and treatment under the specific orders of a physician. Thus, over time, the focus in home care has changed from a broad public health nursing model characterized in the role of the VNA to medical care in the home that addresses specific needs of the individual that have to be accomplished in a limited amount of time.

Acute Care Nursing Versus Home Care Nursing

There are major differences between nursing practice in the hospital and in the home. The nature of providing care in the home is described in Research Box 12-1. One obvious difference between the two settings is the environment or the location of care. In the home setting, the nurse is a guest in the client's home, unlike the hospital or clinic setting, where the nurse is in control of the environment. The need to be flexible and adaptable is essential in the home setting, as the nurse visits many different clients living in a variety of home situations. While hospitals recruit new graduates, home care agencies normally hire only experienced nurses because of the need for the practitioner in the home to be a self-reliant

Table 12-2 Sources of Payment for Home Care	
Source of Payment	**Percentage**
Medicare	41.0
Medicaid	24.0
State and local government	15.0
Private insurance	8.0
Out-of-pocket	10.0
Other	2.0

From National Association for Home Care & Hospice. (2010). *Basic statistics about home care.* Washington, DC: Author. Retrieved from http://www.nahc.org/facts/10HC_Stats.pdf

---

BOX 12-1

Medicare Home Care Coverage Criteria

To be eligible for Medicare reimbursement for home health care services, clients must meet the following criteria:

1. Under the care of a physician, and getting services under a plan of care established and reviewed regularly by a doctor
2. Certification from a physician that one of the following is needed:
   a. Intermittent skilled nursing care
   b. Physical therapy
   c. Speech–language pathology services
   d. Continued occupational therapy
3. Home health agency must be Medicare-certified
4. Physician certification of homebound status

From Centers for Medicare & Medicaid Services. (2010). *Medicare and home health care*. Retrieved from http://www.cms.hhs.gov/center/hha.asp

---

and autonomous decision maker. When emergencies arise, unlike in the hospital where there is a large cadre of professionals to confer with, there is no backup for consultation in the home. When teaching clients in their homes, the nurse must be competent in developing the client and family's efficacy regarding self-care. Even charting is different in home care where reimbursement often drives all documentation.

RESEARCH BOX 12-1

Defining Roles, Relationships, Boundaries, and Participation Between Elderly People and Nurses Within the Home: An Ethnographic Study

Although the literature suggests that interactions between nurses and elderly individuals are often disempowering for the individuals in many settings for care, there has been comparatively scant evidence published regarding elderly clients experiences with nursing care in the home. Over 1 year, 16 community nurses and 13 elderly adults receiving home care services were interviewed using a semi structured format. Three themes were identified from data analysis. First, were the advantages of providing and receiving care in the home. Nurses reported that being in the home allowed them to emphasize personal and professional values while the elderly clients appreciated that sense of self and personal identify is preserved when receiving care in the home. The second theme focused on the nature of the relationship in the home setting. For the nurses, this meant caring for clients who had a "nursing need," while having the opportunity to develop a deeper relationship with the client and family. The nature of the relationship was described by the clients as a reciprocal, "kin like" connection. Finding meaning in being ill was the third theme with the nurses describing this as the client accepting illness or impaired condition as a daily part of life. Elderly clients described finding meaning as becoming less passive in managing their own health by having the opportunity to participate in a mutual process of problem solving and identifying alternatives that had an impact on their daily life. The researchers concluded that as more care is provided in the home, the implicit qualities valued within the nurse–client relationship that occur within the context of home care must be identified and made more explicit at the agency and policy level.

From McGarry, J. (2009). Defining roles, relationships, boundaries and participation between elderly people and nurses within the home: An ethnographic study. *Health & Social Care in the Community, 17*(1), 83–91. Retrieved from CINAHL Plus with Full Text database.

Even the nurse–client relationship is not the same in acute care settings as in home care because in home care the client and family may be cared for over a long period of time. This allows for the development of a therapeutic relationship built on trust and caring that is much closer than in other settings. The type and amount of family involvement is not the same in the hospital when compared to care in the home. In the acute care setting, the staff makes decisions regarding the client's care; in the home, the client and family must by necessity participate in the decision-making process regarding care. Goals in home care aim for long-term rather than short-term outcomes with decision making and priority setting mutual endeavors.

CLIENT SITUATIONS IN PRACTICE

Significance of Home Care

Rafael is a home care nurse who visits 91-year-old Norma Wilkinson three times a week. Ms. Wilkinson has several medical problems, the major ones being hypertension, severe congestive heart failure, and arthritis. Rafael takes Ms. Wilkinson's blood pressure, weighs her, sometimes draws blood, and checks on Ms. Wilkinson's general well-being. Ms. Wilkinson never married and has no relatives nearby, but Ruth, a woman from her church, looks in on her now and then and takes her shopping. Ruth has a key to the apartment. Ms. Wilkinson does not always take her medications as prescribed because some of her friends tell her she is taking too many pills.

As usual, Rafael telephones Ms. Wilkinson before the scheduled Friday morning visit. There is no answer, but he decides to make the visit anyway. When he knocks on the door, there is no response and the door is locked. Should he leave? He knows Ms. Wilkinson has had some dizzy spells lately and has fallen several times in the apartment. Rafael decides to call Ruth to bring the key and check the apartment with him. They search the apartment, but Ms. Wilkinson is not there, and she has not slept in her bed. They notice when looking at her medication dispenser that Ms. Wilkinson did not take her pills for the previous 2 days. They begin a search of the building and discover Ms. Wilkinson in a remote part of the basement. She had fallen and is confused. If the home health nurse had not made his regular visit, had not established a close relationship, and had not known her history so well, Ms. Wilkinson could have died before anyone discovered she was missing.

ADVANTAGES OF HOME HEALTH CARE

There are a number of advantages to providing care in the home as opposed to the acute care setting. The primary advantage is the lower cost. Table 12-3 shows the cost of inpatient care compared with home care for selected conditions. For clients, one advantage is the less-threatening, familiar comfort of home, which enhances care and the quality of life.

Table 12-3 Cost of Inpatient Care Compared With Home Care, Selected Conditions

Condition	Hospital Costs per Patient, per Month ($)	Home Care Costs per Patient, per Month ($)	Savings per Patient, per Month ($)
Low birth weight	26,190	330	25,860
Ventilator-dependent adults	21,570	7,050	14,520
Oxygen-dependent children	12,090	5,250	6,840
Chemotherapy for children with cancer	68,870	55,950	13,920
Congestive heart failure among the elderly	1,758	1,605	153
Intravenous antibiotic therapy for cellulitis, osteomyelitis, others	12,510	4,650	7,860

From National Association for Home Care & Hospice. (2010). *Basic statistics about home care*. Washington, DC: Author. Retrieved from http://www.nahc.org/facts/10HC_Stats.pdf

Home care allows for easier access to loved ones and their support, and clients are taught self-care and encouraged to be independent, which maximizes their quality of life. Being at home also removes the family burden of traveling to and from the hospital and allows for maintenance of normal daily routine. Additionally, it contributes to the restoration of family control for the care being provided and allows for ease in personalizing education to fit with the family's circumstances. These advantages are supported by the philosophy of community-based care, which focuses on enhancing self-care in the context of the family and the community. Furthermore, families experience lower levels of stress when a family member is cared for at home compared to being cared for in acute care in hospital (Leff et al., 2008; Leff et al, 2009).

Working in home care creates benefits for nurses. One benefit is seen in higher job satisfaction. This is attributed to the independent nature of this type of practice as well as the opportunity to provide one-on-one care in a flexible work environment. Home care nurses are most satisfied with their relationships with clients and peers, professional pride, and the autonomy and independence of the role (Ellenbecker, Porell, Samia, Byleckie, & Milburn, 2008).

CHALLENGES TO SUCCESSFUL HOME HEALTH CARE

Providing care in the home has a downside for families and nurses. For several decades, research has demonstrated that stress caused by multiple unfamiliar professionals coming into the home can also affect members of the family. The presence of the nurse or other professional is an intrusion on the family's privacy. This may affect family decision making and interaction among members. For instance, family members express concerns about privacy, interruption of the family routine, loss of control, personality conflicts with the home care staff, and concerns about the competency of the nurses. Families express their difficulties with statements such as, "It changed our lives totally" as loss of privacy interrupts the family structure, function, and communication patterns. In some instances, conflict may result if the nurse or other professional is not sensitive to the family's wishes and boundaries. Further, caring for a child at home may also have a negative impact on siblings and may result in aggressive behavior.

These challenges are not insurmountable as the nurse uses a family-centered approach in providing care in the home. All members of the family are impacted by the presence of nurses in the home. Families may understand the importance of regularity in the client's routine. Nurses can respect this concern by arriving on time for appointments and performing procedures consistent with the family's desire as long as they are within the parameters of safe care. Families tend to resent nurses who are too pushy or who try to control everything. They want the nurse to listen to them and respect the knowledge they have accumulated from being involved in care on a 24-hour-a-day, 7-day-a-week basis. However, as mentioned, families experience lower levels of stress when a family member is cared for at home compared to being cared for in acute care in hospital (Leff et al., 2007).

Out-of-pocket expenses may accumulate as the result of home care not reimbursed by the third-party payer. These expenses may cause stress for the family. Financial pressure is often a precursor to the family assuming total responsibility for their loved one's care. Nurses working in the home setting have a responsibility to be aware of resources in the community to assist families with financial concerns and refer to these services as needed.

Another challenge that nurses cite is that the amount of paperwork or documentation required in home care is excessive. Further, dealing with inclement weather and wear and tear on one's automobile are also mentioned as negative aspects of working as a home care nurse. Further, nurses who leave home care do so because of job stress and workload as well as lack of satisfaction with salary and benefits (Leff et al., 2008).

The advantages of home care far outweigh the disadvantages. Disadvantages of nursing care in the home are more of an issue if the family member is ill for a long period of time. In home care although the client and family experience a loss of privacy and interruption of the normal family decision-making process, they still can enjoy a life together that is not possible if the client is hospitalized.

Nursing Skills and Competencies in Home Health Care

The basic concepts of professionalism apply to nursing care in the home as they do in every setting. Promptness is imperative to good work habits. Nursing competency is critical. Families want procedures done carefully and in a manner similar to what was performed or taught in the hospital or clinic. Needs of the home care client and family are most often psychosocial and learning needs: information about community resources, techniques of physical care, and management of care. Thus, as in other settings, familiarity with community resources for making appropriate referrals, counseling, health teaching, care management, and delegated medical functions are important interventions. Figure 12-2 shows "Don'ts for Young Nurses," an excerpt taken from a historic 1919 text for home care nurses. It is interesting that the tips provided are just as true today as they were so many years ago.

COMMUNICATION

A comfortable relationship between the nurse and the client is essential to successful home care. First and foremost, the successful nurse communicates effectively with the client and family to build a trusting relationship. A myriad of psychosocial issues characteristic of the home care client requires that the nurse wear many hats when providing care in the

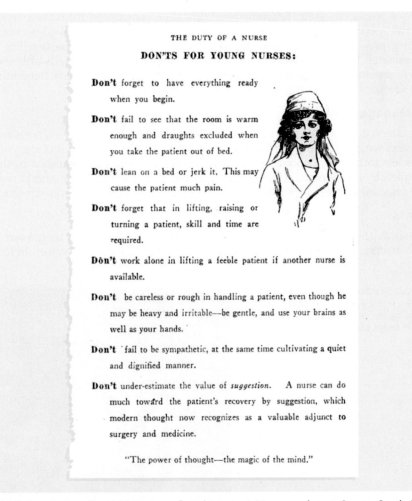

THE DUTY OF A NURSE

DON'TS FOR YOUNG NURSES:

Don't forget to have everything ready when you begin.

Don't fail to see that the room is warm enough and draughts excluded when you take the patient out of bed.

Don't lean on a bed or jerk it. This may cause the patient much pain.

Don't forget that in lifting, raising or turning a patient, skill and time are required.

Don't work alone in lifting a feeble patient if another nurse is available.

Don't be careless or rough in handling a patient, even though he may be heavy and irritable—be gentle, and use your brains as well as your hands.

Don't fail to be sympathetic, at the same time cultivating a quiet and dignified manner.

Don't under-estimate the value of *suggestion*. A nurse can do much toward the patient's recovery by suggestion, which modern thought now recognizes as a valuable adjunct to surgery and medicine.

"The power of thought—the magic of the mind."

Figure 12-2 Suggestions for visiting nurses from historic visiting nurse's text. Source: South, L. H. (1919). *Nurses in the home* (11th ed.). Buffalo, NY.

home, including but not limited to: social worker, friend, spiritual comforter, psychologist, financial counselor, and translator of medical information. One home care nurse says this:

> I was not prepared for the numerous psychosocial demands of the job. I thought I was pretty good at dealing holistically with the clients I cared for in the hospital, but it was nothing like caring for someone in the home with the family present.

The psychosocial needs of the home care client primarily revolve around the client's adjustment to the illness or injury, the anxiety it produces, and the possible social isolation that results. Counseling is the primary public health nursing intervention that addresses psychosocial needs of the client and family and assists the nurse in building trusting, therapeutic relationships. It is also helpful to elicit the client and family's thoughts and feelings about the situation they are facing, which has taken control away from them.

HEALTH TEACHING

Health teaching is an important intervention for the home care nurse (Fig. 12-3). Chapter 6 addresses teaching in detail. Teaching includes explaining and demonstrating care and treatment at a comprehensible level. The nurse remains open minded by listening and showing respect for the client and family's knowledge.

When determining learning needs, remember that the learner may be the client, family member, or other caregiver. The learner's readiness to learn, need to learn, and past experiences are assessed. Learning needs are then considered from the perspective of the affective, psychomotor, or cognitive domain. Finally, the learning need is validated, and the teaching plan is developed with the learner. After instruction, the teaching and learning are evaluated for their effectiveness. Common areas of learning needs of home care clients revolve around disease process, treatments, and medication but vary depending on the client's specific condition and the complexity of the diagnosis.

Disease Management

Most clients and families need assistance understanding the client's diagnosis and any related disease processes. The client who requires only two or three home visits after routine surgery needs less information about managing his or her condition as compared to the client with multiple chronic diseases. Disease management is a relatively new reimbursable aspect of skilled nursing home care provided in the home and is discussed in more depth in Chapter 13.

Treatments

Frequently, home care nurses provide treatments for clients and then assist the client or family to complete the treatment at some future date. Complexity varies. In some instances,

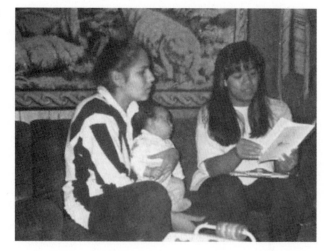

Figure 12-3 Teaching plays a major role in home care. Here a young woman is taught infant care by the community-based nurse involved in home care.

the nurse may teach a simple dressing change by demonstration. In other cases, the family may have to learn to administer treatments with complex equipment. For example, a client with brittle diabetes may develop a large leg ulcer. The nurse changes the dressing, monitors the diabetes, and determines the learning and teaching needs of the client and family. If the client and family are capable, the nurse teaches them to change the dressing and monitor the diabetes. It is not unusual for a client with complex technical equipment to be the recipient of intermittent home visits of 30 to 90 minutes. After instruction from the home care nurse, family members often provide daily intravenous line changes and irrigation, as well as infusions of intravenous fluids, medications, or hyperalimentation through peripheral or central venous lines. They may also insert a Foley catheter or nasogastric tube or carry out tracheotomy care, including suctioning. Each year, more complex treatments and related equipment are available through home care. This trend requires home care nurses to provide teaching for increasingly complex treatments and to rely on the client and family to perform procedures with a high degree of competence, identifying complicating issues and appropriately notifying the home care nurse, nurse practitioner, or physician if problems arise.

Medication

Most of what is known about medication errors is the additional health care costs associated with preventable incidents. Medication errors in the hospital result in an annual cost of $3.5 billion a year, while the cost from errors in ambulatory care is estimated at $887 million a year (Aspden, Wolcott, Bootman, & Cronenwett, 2007). Mager and Madigan (2010) reported that almost half of home care clients contacted had at least one medication error during a 3-week period. A thorough assessment of the client or family's ability to set up medications is the essential first step to this important intervention. The assessment is initiated with a complete review of the medications the client is taking, compared with the most recent orders from the physician(s).

The need for assistance with medications will vary from client to client according to diagnosis, age, and competency in self-care. For example, clients recently diagnosed with diabetes or those with advanced congestive heart failure (CHF) may have complex learning needs for medication administration. Clients may need to learn about using a sliding scale for their insulin dosage based on taking a daily blood sugar level, drawing up the medication correctly, and injecting themselves. Some clients have a large number of medications with complicated doses that they must take several times a day. The more medications prescribed, the more likely the client is to not follow the prescribed regimen. Comprehensive teaching enhances compliance with the home care client.

CASE MANAGEMENT

As a manager of home care services, the nurse must apply leadership knowledge by performing the functions of planning, organizing, coordinating, delegating, and evaluating care for a group of clients. The nurse must coordinate, through case management, an interdisciplinary team of practitioners, the client, family, physician, and various community providers (such as Meals On Wheels and equipment vendors). The nurse's role as case manager depends on the scope of services provided by the agency and the specific providers outside the agency who are involved in the care of the client. Continuity of care is accomplished by effective communication among all members of the interdisciplinary team. To ensure comprehensive quality care, management also includes delegation and evaluation of care provided by paraprofessional caregivers, such as home health aides or homemakers and the family, as well as other professionals.

PHYSICAL CAREGIVING/DELEGATED MEDICAL FUNCTIONS

Although one of the primary functions of the home care nurse is physical caregiving, the nurse is required to be flexible in this role. This means allowing the family to participate in caregiving whenever possible. Before doing a procedure, the nurse must explain to the client and the family what is being done and why, adjusting the instruction to their particular developmental

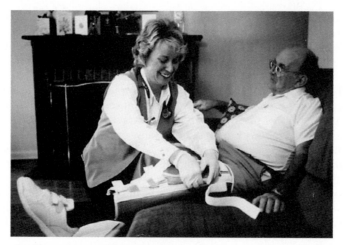

Figure 12-4 Home health nurses combine effective communication skills with their knowledge base of physical caregiving as they provide care for their clients.

stage and cognitive abilities (Fig. 12-4). It is essential for the nurse to know his or her own strengths and weaknesses performing the skill before attempting to demonstrate it. Confidence is not instilled in the client if the nurse is inept and unable to provide skilled care proficiently.

The nurse should always role model keeping the work area neat and clean by carefully disposing of laundry, trash, and equipment. Medical researchers have known for centuries that handwashing decreases transmission of pathogens between clients. People who receive nursing care in the home are at risk of acquiring infections, just as they are in the acute care setting. Thorough handwashing on entering the home, after procedures, and before leaving the home is an essential aspect of good care.

The Centers for Disease Control and Prevention (CDC) Healthcare Infection Control Guidelines recommend either antimicrobial or non-antimicrobial soap and water be used when hands are visibly soiled or contaminated with blood or other body fluids. An alcohol-based hand rub may be used routinely for decontaminating hands that are not visibly soiled in the following clinical situations:

- Before and after direct contact with clients
- Before and after contact with a client's nonintact skin and wound dressings
- Before and after using gloves
- Before inserting an indwelling urinary catheter, peripheral vascular catheters, or other nonsurgical invasive devices (CDC, 2010)

THE HOME VISIT

All nurses working in the community should master the competencies required of home visiting. School nurses and occupational health nurses to name a few sometimes provide nursing care in the home. Where clients will often disclose information not obtained in other ways.

The main components of the home visit follow the nursing process. Assessment in skilled home nursing care is guided and reimbursed by Medicare following the Outcome and Assessment Information Set (OASIS) format, which is explained in the next section. Nursing diagnoses (or problem statements) allow the nurse to work with the client and family to formulate joint plans and establish goals. Following through with these plans helps reinforce therapeutic relationships.

Preparation

In preparation for the initial visit, the referral information is reviewed for basic information about the new client. Referrals come from a variety of sources, including hospitals, clinics, health care providers, physicians, nurses, individuals, and families. The client is contacted

> **BOX 12-2** **Essential Supplies and Equipment for a Home Visit**
>
> 1. Handwashing equipment: disinfectant foam for hands, soap in container, paper towels, old newspapers (to set bag on in the home)
> 2. Assessment equipment: thermometer, sphygmomanometer, stethoscope, tape measure, penlight, urine and blood testing equipment
> 3. Treatment supplies: dressings, sterile and clean gloves, tape, alcohol swabs, scissors, lubricant jelly, forceps, syringes
> 4. Occupational health and safety supplies: eye shields, mask, apron, gloves, plastic bag to double bag, sharps containers, disinfectant spray and clean-up supplies for spills, disposable scrubs, airway/mask
> 5. Printed materials: map, agency forms, business cards
> 6. Laboratory supplies: specimen containers, tubes, and equipment for venipuncture, culture, or urine specimen

by telephone or perhaps in some cases by e-mail to inform him or her of the referral and to make an appointment for the first visit. The nurse identifies himself or herself, gives the name of the agency, and describes the purpose of the visit. A basic overview about the cost of services, eligibility, and alternative sources of financial support should also be discussed at this time. When applicable, the nurse alerts the client that he or she will need an insurance card or other evidence of coverage from a third-party payer, Medicare, or Medicaid on the first visit.

Unlike the acute care setting where a quick trip to the supply cart or utility room satisfies most equipment needs, the nurse must carry supplies in home health care. Before the first visit, the nurse asks about supplies and determines what is needed. All home health care nurses use a bag to carry essential supplies to every home visit. This consists of supplies and equipment the nurse uses daily for all clients, along with additional supplies. Each day, the nurse reviews the needs of the clients to be visited that day and add specific items. Box 12-2 lists essential supplies and equipment often suggested for a home visit.

Beginning the Visit

After introductions, the visit usually begins with a short period of casual, social conversation to put the client and family at ease. The length of this introductory phase varies depending on the cultural background of the family. In some cultures, the family will place a great deal of weight on getting to know the nurse before they will allow the admission assessment to commence. One nurse who specializes in transcultural home visiting states "I know that the family is ready to begin the admission interview when they offer me tea and food." A friendly, warm manner helps as the nurse begins to ask the client questions about specific health care needs. It is important to begin building a trusting relationship from the first greeting.

During the initial interview, the nurse outlines a contract stating the purpose of the visit. The nurse uses a variety of communication tools to assist the client and family to understand the need for nursing care in the home.

Assessment

Assessment on a home visit differs from that of the acute care setting (Fig. 12-5). Assessment is a core function of home care nursing (Fieldsmith, Van Sell, & Kindred, 2009). The nurse incorporates the general elements of community-based care into the process and follows specific guidelines for documenting the status of each client receiving service. The general elements guide the nurse to consider the issue of self-care by determining what the client's perceptions of his or her condition is and what the client identifies as personal problems and strengths. The client's ability to perform self-care and the family's acceptance of responsibility for care are explored. All assessments are made in the context of the family and community resources and support. Culture must also be considered. Continuity of care among various physicians and other professionals caring for the client is evaluated.

Figure 12-5 Home visits enable the nurse to assess whether the client can safely manage important self-care tasks such as cooking.

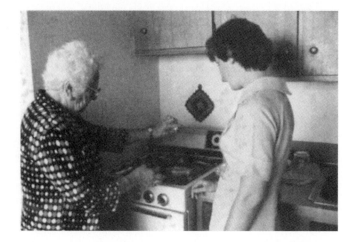

A preventive focus, keeping in mind the principles of continuity of care, is used. The nurse assesses the client and family's knowledge of the client's condition, care, and treatment. Learning needs are assessed.

The specific elements of the first visit are defined by the OASIS, which is an assessment tool developed to measure outcomes of persons receiving home health care. During the first visit, the nurse fills out the (OASIS) form to guide the plan of care and to meet the requirement for reimbursement for Medicare-certified home care. The OASIS data provide a consistent format and standardized points in time for documenting client care status. Payment to home care agencies is based on outcomes determined by comparing admission outcomes to discharge outcomes (Fieldsmith et al., 2009).

In 2010, the OASIS system was revised to include process measures and renamed OASIS-C. This modified assessment added measures related to administration of vaccinations, standardized pain assessment, pressure ulcer risk assessment, fall risk assessment, depression screen, medication management and education, inclusion of specific best practices in the physician-ordered plan of care, timely notification of the physician in certain circumstances, and implementation of best practices as appropriate to all to home care patient (Niewenhous, 2010).

One example of how the new OASIS-C requirements have changed home care nursing practice is seen in depression screening. Historically, the Medicare Home Health Benefit has not focused on depression or any other mental health condition as the basis for eligibility and coverage. Rather, the Medicare Home Health Benefit has focused on short-term, intermittent physical health needs that require skilled nursing or physical therapy and can be treated and discharged. But now, with the new OASIS-C, if the nurse in charge of discharge planning in the hospital identified Risk for Loneliness as a potential nursing diagnosis for a client, this would guide the clinic nurse on need for follow-up. In addition to the possible interventions with this nursing diagnosis under the old OASIS, the revised OASIS-C allows the home care nurse to expand depression care with the requirement of a depression screen when deemed appropriate (Cabin, 2010). Given the high prevalence of depression among the general elderly population as well as among elderly receiving home health care, this is an important change in focus.

Physical Assessment

Specifics of the physical assessment vary according to the client's needs. In most cases, the initial physical assessment will determine if the client is appropriate for home care services, what type of services are indicated, how long these services are likely to be needed, and who will pay for the care.

On the initial visit, and regularly throughout care, the nurse takes vital signs and conducts a full physical assessment of the client, including a review of all systems and a focused assessment of the client's presenting condition. During this assessment, the nurse collects information about the client's physical condition, functional status, ability to leave the home unassisted, ability to do self-care, and ability to perform ADL independently, using the OASIS format as required. Blood or urine specimens are sometimes collected and sent to the laboratory.

Family Assessment

Because community-based care is provided in the context of the client's family and community, assessment of the family is an essential ingredient to the success of home care nursing. Family structure, stage of illness, developmental stage, and family functions may be assessed. The nurse also determines if the client is isolated physically or socially from other members of the family or if the family is a close-knit, nurturing, and supportive family or kinship network.

Financial Assessment

Information about the costs of home care services, insurance payment, and other financial concerns of the client and family are discussed on the first visit. **Financial assessment** and options to reduce the cost of care while continuing the provision of safe, quality care should be explored. Some clients are insured 100% for home care services as long as the services are provided within the parameters of coverage. Others may have little or no insurance coverage. Clients and families may have little knowledge about their home care coverage and may be unaware that the number of visits may be limited or that they have a lifetime maximum as stipulated in the particular health insurance policy. All of these issues are explored in the financial assessment.

Determination of Needs and Planning Care

After assessment, the nurse, client, and family discuss the nursing care needs and develop a plan of care. They also determine who will be responsible for particular aspects of the care until the next nursing visit. The family support person may be responsible, or other professional health care or home care providers may be needed. Expected outcomes are developed and plans are made for a follow-up visit. Home health agencies have to demonstrate the client's progress toward achievement of desired outcomes. Medicare and insurance do not reimburse for a home visit if quality improvement and outcomes are not achieved following the OASIS-C format.

Implementation

Physical care, including delegated medical functions, teaching, counseling, and referrals are completed according to the plan of care. Because home care often replaces hospitalization in meeting acute medical needs, home care focuses on physical care of the client. Short visits of 30 minutes to 2 hours focus on hands-on care of the client; incorporate a large variety of nursing skills. These include giving injections, performing venipunctures for laboratory work, doing dressing changes, giving medications, teaching the client and family how to do the care on an ongoing basis, and being the eyes and ears for the nurse practitioner or physician in observing the client's progress toward recovery. While the nurse is performing skilled nursing care, he or she is also teaching, assessing, counseling, and acting as a consultant for client and family.

Termination of the Visit

The nurse reviews the purpose of the visit, outlines what was learned in the assessment phase, and reviews the mutually agreed on plan of care. The time and purpose of the next visit are discussed. The nurse may end the visit with a very short period of casual conversation. Especially if the client lives alone, conversation will be anticipated and appreciated.

Follow-Up Visits and Evaluation

A thorough initial assessment allows for comprehensive planning for productive follow-up visits. Each visit has specific goals with plans implemented to meet those goals. Subsequent visits allow the nurse to build a trusting relationship with the client, which may lead to identification of additional nursing needs. In community-based nursing, the overall goal of every home visit is to maximize health functioning and self-care.

The nurse, client, and family or caregivers evaluate the visit and the care plan. Physical care, teaching, counseling, and referrals are discussed, and suggestions are made for ways to improve the care provided. The client may be asked to complete an evaluation survey (Assessment Tool 12-1).

DOCUMENTATION

Generally, documentation for home visits follows specific regulations of OASIS and establishing homebound status. To ensure that the agency will qualify for payment for the visit, the client's needs and the nursing care given are documented. This includes the client's homebound status and the need for skilled professional nursing care with Medicare, Medicaid, and most other third-party payers. If documentation is not done correctly, the agency may not be reimbursed for the visit.

At the beginning of this chapter, the Medicare coverage criteria that must be met for home care services to be reimbursed were discussed (Box 12-1). Formerly, all states followed this requirement, but now the definition of homebound status allowing clients to receive skilled nursing care through Medicare varies from state to state. This requires the

Assessment Tools 12-1
Client Satisfaction Survey

To evaluate our services and continue our excellent standards of care, we need to hear from you. Please take a few minutes to complete this form and return it to us in the enclosed stamped envelope. Thank you!

1. Home health care services were provided in a timely manner when I needed them:

    _____ Very good _____ Satisfactory _____ Unsatisfactory

2. Home was the best setting for the care given to me for my comfort and recovery:

    _____ Very good _____ Satisfactory _____ Unsatisfactory

3. The number and frequency of visits provided were adequate to meet my needs:

    _____ Very good _____ Satisfactory _____ Unsatisfactory

4. The care I needed to improve my condition was received from home health care:

    _____ Very good _____ Satisfactory _____ Unsatisfactory

5. The nurse included me and my family (if applicable) in planning, implementing, and evaluating care:

    _____ Very good _____ Satisfactory _____ Unsatisfactory

6. The nurse considered my culture when planning care:

    _____ Very good _____ Satisfactory _____ Unsatisfactory

7. The nurse considered my community when planning care:

    _____ Very good _____ Satisfactory _____ Unsatisfactory

8. I am now able to care for myself with the procedures and instructions provided by the staff:

    _____ Very good _____ Satisfactory _____ Unsatisfactory

9. The home health care staff was courteous and respectful:

    _____ Very good _____ Satisfactory _____ Unsatisfactory

10. The names of community service agencies were given to me as needed and their services explained:

_____ Very good _____ Satisfactory _____ Unsatisfactory

11. I felt my wishes about care were supported by the staff of the home health care agency:

_____ Very good _____ Satisfactory _____ Unsatisfactory

12. I would use home health care services again:

_____ Yes _____ No

13. Home health care provided me with the following services:

_____ Home health care _____ Hospice _____ Private duty

14.   Comments (Please write on a separate sheet if more space is needed):

_____

_____

_____

_____

nurse be familiar with the specific regulations in his or her state. However, in most states, it is absolutely imperative that all of the homebound criteria are met and documented. The nurse is responsible for documenting that the client is homebound. The primary dimensions of homebound status are that absences from the home are infrequent and, for the purpose of receiving medical treatment, that leaving home requires considerable and taxing effort. If the individual is driving at all, they are *not* considered homebound. Homebound status must be documented in objective and measurable terms and include the following information about a client leaving home:

- How often
- For how long
- For what reason
- The effort and assistive devices required

Clients who leave the home to receive medical care not available in the home may still be considered for homebound status for the following reasons:

- Physician office visits
- Outpatient kidney dialysis services
- Attendance at adult day centers to receive medical care
- Outpatient chemotherapy or radiation
- Attending religious services

Documentation should always be focused on the client's illness and safety, centering on the: statement of the problem(s); the skilled care provided to deal with the problem(s); and outcomes expected and achieved from the care provided.

Sometimes the perception is that following OASIS will always protect one from liability. However, in some instances, OASIS requires an ambiguous response, while in other instances, it allows staff to cover an issue without having to state precisely what should be done. To protect oneself from liability, it is necessary that documentation should clearly state what is and what is not expected. Using OASIS competently requires not only precise and consistent language and care plans but also following the documented plan of care (Newfield, 2006). A complete documentation of the care plan is important not only for reimbursement and legal issues, but it is also critical to the evaluation of competent nursing practice used in quality assurance.

COMMUNITY-BASED NURSING CARE GUIDELINES 12-1

Personal Safety Checklist for the Home Care Nurse

- Get to know the community, especially the differences between neighborhoods.
- Dress in sensible shoes and simple clothing, avoid long necklaces, expensive jewelry, or pins of a political or religious nature.
- Get to know your client and family and determine if there is a history of violence.
- Know your agency policies and procedures and follow them.
- Keep your supervisor informed of any potential violent situations with your caseload.
- Have safety accessories in your car: a working cell phone; a flashlight; and have a well-maintained car.
- Lock up equipment and your purse or valuables in the trunk of the car before leaving the agency or your home.
- Attend a course on safety, self-defense, or self-protection.

CONFIDENTIALITY

Confidentiality is essential to quality care and ethical practice in community-based settings. Sometimes nurses may work in their own community and may care for someone they know or a friend or relative of someone they know outside of their professional role. Just as in the hospital setting, nurses must never discuss individual situations or the health status of clients and families with anyone except other professional staff within professional discussions.

SAFETY ISSUES FOR THE NURSE

The nurse should know the destination for the visit and have a route mapped out to get there. Depending on the neighborhood, asking directions can prove dangerous. When entering the client's neighborhood, the nurse begins an environmental assessment by doing a brief windshield survey (see Chapter 5). The purpose of the survey is to collect information about the community where the client lives and to determine if the neighborhood is safe. Occasionally, the nurse may not feel safe entering a client's home. In some areas, the nurse may need to be accompanied by a policeman or security officer. No nurse should ever disregard personal safety in an effort to visit a client. See Community-Based Nursing Care Guidelines 12-1 for a checklist of safety points to be followed by home care nurses.

Support of the Lay Caregiver

Because less time is spent in hospitals and more time at home prior to and following surgery and acute exacerbation of chronic illness compared to the past, the home care environment has become the site of major caretaking activities. Not only is the use of families, relatives, and other support systems such as caregivers on the rise, but client conditions are more serious and less stable. In fact, **lay caregiving** is one of the world's fastest-growing unpaid professions. It is estimated that almost 80% of home care services are provided by family members or other unpaid assistance. Approximately one in every five adults is a lay caregiver, or about 44 million people in the United States. More than 40% of caregivers are men. Family caregivers care for their loved ones an average of 8 years, with many being caregivers for over 10 years (Agency for Healthcare Research and Quality, 2011).

Lay caregivers may have responsibilities for people at both ends of the age spectrum: children and older people with chronic health problems. "Parent caring" is the term used in the literature for sons and daughters caring for older parents. These caregivers are predominantly women. The "typical caregiver" is a middle-aged, married woman who is employed at least part time and is also spending about 18 hours a week caring for her mother who lives nearby (Reinhard, Given, Petlick, & Bemis, 2009).

Caregiving includes providing emotional support, direct health services, and financial support; mediating with health and social service organizations; and sharing a household. It may include tasks such as bathing, toileting, shopping, preparing food, feeding, maintaining a household budget, and housekeeping. Family dynamics can be different from household to household. The nurse must be sensitive to this variety of family dynamics and work with the family and caregivers without being judgmental regarding their decisions.

STRESS ON THE CAREGIVER

Caring for a family member who has acute needs that require complicated technological devices can be difficult. Family caregivers often feel unprepared to provide care and receiver inadequate guidance from formal health care providers, a situation that may weigh heavily on the family caregiver. For several decades, studies have documented the strain of caregiving on the caregiver's physical and psychological health. Adult children who serve as informal caregivers for older family members with long-term-care needs experience negative outcomes such as increased social isolation and decreased preventive care (Robison, Fortinsky, Kleppinger, Shugrue, & Porter, 2009). A woman's hospitalization increases her husband's chances of dying within a month by 35%. A husband's hospitalization boosts his wife's mortality risk by 44% (Christakis & Allison, 2006). Further, family caregivers experiencing extreme stress have been shown to age prematurely. As family responsibility grows, parental distress increases. The nurse provides not only client care and treatment but also support for the family caregiver.

In practice, the transition from visiting a family member in the hospital, where other people are responsible for care, to being a "paraprofessional" caregiver happens almost overnight. All too frequently, hospital discharge is determined and completed within an hour or two. Suddenly the lay caregiver has 24-hour responsibility for tasks for which he or she has little or no knowledge and experience. The lay caregiver may have full- or part-time employment and other family members to care for. The strain on caregivers can be great, and risks for depression and illness are high. Pre-existing psychosocial problems raise the risk. The family may already have other challenges such as mounting bills with a mortgage and utilities,or living in an unsafe neighbourhood. Transportation may be a problem, especially if the person requiring care was the family's means of transportation. Drug abuse on the part of a family member may add to the burdens. The lay caregiver may have no support person or outlets on which to rely.

Twenty-four-hour responsibility for the client's care means more than supplying physical care for the client. It requires that the lay caregiver constantly have the client and his or her care in mind. The role is unrelenting with every day organized around the care activities and needs of the client particularly if the client cannot be left alone and must be under constant observation. Many times, the client's personality, which may have changed with illness, places heavy demands on the caregiver's time and energy. The difficulty of the role of lay caregiver has been associated with low levels of life satisfaction, high levels of depression, and symptoms of stress. In cases where care is to be provided temporarily, the stress may not be as great. If the length of time for care, however, is indefinite, as in chronic care, additional stress may be felt by the lay caregiver. Because the strain on these lay caregivers is tremendous, community-based nurses must consider this fact as they plan care. Although their clients are their main concern, holistic nursing means that nurses also think about the needs and strengths of family and other support persons.

ASSESSMENT

The first home visit is an important time to discuss and clarify the relationship between the client and the caregiver. The OASIS-C provides items to assess caregiver presence, availability, and type of assistance needed. It is also essential to assess the caregiver's knowledge and physical and psychological status. Caregiver needs must also be assessed because

> ### BOX 12-3   Caregiving Tasks and Training Interest of Family Caregivers of Medically Ill Homebound Older Adults
>
> The author stated that the purpose of this study was to assess caregiving activities and training interests of family caregivers of medically ill older adults without dementia who receive home health care. One hundred participants completed a sociodemographic questionnaire as well as a survey that elicited measures of caregiver tasks and training interest. The researchers found that caregiver interest in training had no relationship to the type of caregiver tasks they were to provide for their own family member. Race and age predicted interest in training. Younger caregivers as well as those caregivers who were Black indicated a higher level of interest in training. There was a range of care provision and interest in receiving education to improve caregiving skills. There is a need for additional research to determine specific training needs and the impact that caregiver education may have on client outcomes.
>
> From Wilkins, V., Bruce, M., & Sirey, J. (2009). Caregiving tasks and training interest of family caregivers of medically ill homebound older adults. *Journal of Aging & Health, 21*(3), 528–542. doi: 10.1177/0898264309332838. Retrieved from CINAHL Plus with Full Text database.

of the caregiver's increased risk for health problems. Better understanding of the needs and training interests of caregivers is the first step in developing targeted and effective interventions (Box 12-3).

INTERVENTIONS FOR LAY CAREGIVERS

Nursing interventions may enhance quality of life for both the client and caregiver by ensuring that everyone has adequate preparation for ongoing care needs. Health care professionals need to be sensitive to caregivers, who handle multiple roles such as working outside the home or caring for other dependents in addition to being a caregiver. These individuals are often stressed, burdened, and depressed, as compared to those who have a single caregiver role.

The nurse who initially establishes rapport with both the client and caregivers and builds trust is the most likely to successfully support the family caregiver. Three critical components that contribute to successful family caregiving are communication, decision making, and reciprocity. Promoting communication and decision making takes various forms. The nurse helps caregivers cope by sharing realistic prognostic information, discussing alternative levels of care, and providing information regarding **respite care**. If the caregiver is open to the notion, a community day care program may be available to relieve the lay caregiver of constant responsibility. Some community resources assist with housekeeping provisions or meal programs. Churches may have volunteers who can provide respite care. Additional resources for caregivers are found at the end of this chapter in What's on the Web.

Reciprocity encompasses interactions between the family caregiver and individual receiving care. Mutual satisfaction is seen as both parties receive support from and provide assistance to one another as successful reciprocity incorporates empathy, listening, and partnership. In some cases, working with the client to perform more self-care activities will relieve the caregiver of some responsibilities while providing more teaching may help relieve the caregiver's feelings of inadequacy about ability to perform caregiving tasks or of being overwhelmed.

Other interventions to encourage communication, decision making, and reciprocity skills include educational and support programs, burden-reducing programs, psychotherapeutic interventions, and self-help groups. Even a busy caregiver can find time in the schedule to attend a support group if it is deemed worthwhile. In these groups, people share their experiences and report on strategies that have or have not worked for them. Just knowing that other people are in the same situation or have the same feelings is helpful. Box 12-4 provides suggestions for identifying and intervening with caregiver stress.

> ## BOX 12-4   Family Caregivers: Caring for Older Adults, Working With Their Families
>
> It is not always obvious who the primary caregiver is for a client. Sometimes the person who is at the bedside is not the family member who will be responsible for the actual care once the client goes home. Approaches for accurately identifying, sufficiently communicating with, and supporting the individual family member who will be in charge of the care at home vary by setting. For instance, for the nurse working in the hospital, it may be helpful to delay discharge instruction until the primary caregiver arrives. If someone other than the primary caregiver is transporting the client home from the hospital the nurse may consider getting the name of the primary caregiver and calling them with discharge instructions. In the nursing home, establishing a trusting relationship and expressing appreciation for the caregiver's efforts to visit and do "little extras" for the family member may promote and support family caregiving. In ambulatory care, once permission is granted, it supports the family caregiver if that person is invited (with consent of the client) from the waiting room to the exam room to participate in the review of the client's health status. This is a good time to provide instructions for new treatments. Home care nurses may find that it is helpful to determine the client and caregiver's preferences for time, day, and method (in person, by phone, or e-mail) of communicating. Further, the nurse may want to suggest periodic family meetings to evaluate progress and to keep all members updated on progress and changes.
>
> Long-distance caregiving creates challenges for the caregiver, client, and nurse. Long-distance caregiving is defined as care provided by those living 1 hour or more away from the care recipient. Long-distance caregivers may only be present intermittently but may play an important role in the mutual decision making, and advocacy aspects of caregiving. Strategies to enhance the success of long-distance caregiving may be initiated by conducting a family assessment with the client to identify long-distance caregivers and determine their availability. Developing a plan for communicating with the long-distance caregiver is important as is providing them with contact information for the agencies and team members involved in the client's care.
>
> From Schumacher, K., Beck C. A., Marren, J. M. (2006). Family caregivers: Caring for older adults, working with their families. *American Journal of Nursing, 106*(8), 40–49.

Respite care provides a temporary break for the caregiver. The care may include someone coming into the house for an hour or two so the caregiver can shop, do errands, or keep his or her own doctor's appointments. Respite care is also an important aspect of hospice care. Another form of respite care occurs with the client's temporary visit to a nursing home or other facility. While the client is cared for in other surroundings, the caregiver and family are free to vacation, perform household maintenance duties, or simply relax.

✴ CLIENT SITUATIONS IN PRACTICE

Planning and Implementing a Home Care Visit

The discharge planning nurse calls your home care agency with the following information on a referral. Mrs. Gothie is an 85-year-old woman with severe congestive heart failure (CHF). She cared for her husband, who had dementia, for 7 years. He died 4 years ago. Mrs. Gothie has lived in the same third-floor apartment for 50 years. Although she has no children, she is close to her younger sister and brother, and numerous nieces and nephews, who all live out of state. Her family is devoted to her, visiting her frequently, but most of her lifelong friends are no longer living. She has one friend who is able to help her on a limited basis, but most of her friends are aging.

When she came to the clinic 2 weeks ago, before being admitted to the hospital, her vital signs and laboratory values were as follows:

Temperature: 98.6°F
Blood pressure: 128/88 mm Hg

Respirations: 26 breaths/min
Lung sounds: rales in all lung fields
Lab values: prothrombin 4 times normal
Digoxin level: 0.1 ng/mL

Mrs. Gothie stated the following at the clinic visit:

I have had a terrible time getting my breath, especially at night. My ankles are three times as big as they used to be. I quit taking my water pill because it made me have to go to the bathroom all the time, and I couldn't sleep at night. I don't have any appetite, but I do eat fruit. Most days, I don't even bother to get dressed or take a shower because I'm so tired. What's the use—I never go anywhere—I'm always too tired. I have had a lot of bruises on my arms and legs.

She was admitted to the hospital for acute CHF. After 3 days in the hospital, she was discharged to Goodhue County Home Health Care Nursing Service. You are assigned to be the case manager for Mrs. Gothie's care. After reviewing the referral form plan your first visit with Mrs. Gothie.

◌ *List the points you will cover when you telephone Mrs. Gothie to set up an appointment for the first visit.*

You would call Mrs. Gothie to introduce yourself, give the name of the agency, and mention the purpose of the visit. If the visit is partially reimbursed by insurance, you may want to tell her that you will need to see her insurance card at the visit. You may also want to know if anyone will be home with her after she is discharged and if that person will be present at the visit. You may want to inquire if she has any concerns that she would like you to address during the visit so you can bring the appropriate supplies and educational materials.

◌ *Determine the primary purpose of the first visit and the focus of your physical assessment.*

The primary purpose of the first visit will be determined by the policies and procedures of the agency you are working for and the insurance coverage or Medicare requirements. In the latter case, the OASIS-C initial assessment would be initiated. The same goes for the focus of the physical assessment. You would be particularly concerned with the assessment of her cardiovascular status and any other assessment related to the symptoms of CHF. In her case, you would make sure that you assess her appetite as she said at her last clinic visit that she doesn't have an appetite. She states that she is too tired to go anywhere, so you assess fatigue and what helps with that. Is she depressed? What about the bruises on her legs and arms? Was there a follow-up blood test done when she was in the hospital to explore this issue? Another concern will be what kind of support she needs to be safe at home. Then, you will assess the support she has and fill in the void with referrals. Obviously, you will be very concerned about the home environment and potential safety issues.

◌ *Identify your key areas of concern when you do your psychosocial and family assessment.*

You will do an assessment of the family structure, developmental stage, and functions. Another question you may have is whether Mrs. Gothie is physically or socially isolated from family or whether the family or her support network is close, nurturing, and supportive. Some of her statements at her last clinic visit indicated as much. You explore whether or not a depression screening should be completed.

◌ *List the people who can provide support for Mrs. Gothie.*

According to the referral form, her sister accompanied her home when she was discharged. She also has one friend, but many of her friends are now deceased. You may want to determine the role that her sister may take as a long-distance caregiver. You will want to assess the breadth and depth of any other support network. Does she need or want a home health aide for personal care and meal preparation?

◌ *Identify learning needs you will assess in the first visit.*

You note that she has had CHF for 20 years, with increased symptoms the last year. You learn that her sister will be with her for a month. You will assess the learning need of both Mrs. Gothie and her sister. The first need that you will assess is their understanding of the disease processes of CHF, her medications, and the use of oxygen. According to the notes from Mrs. Gothie's last clinic visit, it sounds like she is not taking the furosemide (Lasix) because she says that it makes her have to go to the bathroom too frequently to get adequate sleep at night. You assess when she takes the Lasix and recommend that she do so in the morning. You will also determine what her knowledge base is regarding the high-protein diet.

> *What referrals would you make?*

Your priority concerns are as follows:

1. Can she manage at home safely and make a reasonable recovery given her support system, her abilities, and other factors related to her living situation?
2. What will she do when her sister goes back to her home in another state?
3. Does she need assistance managing her medications? Does she need someone either in her family or in the community to do this for her?
4. Does she understand the high-protein diet? Does she need to see a nutritionist?
5. How does she do grocery shopping? Are there services in the community to help her with this?
6. Is she open to home-delivered meals, once a day, such as Meals on Wheels?
7. Is congregate dining available in her community and transportation provided to the site?

> *What social opportunities would she consider?*

She states that she has no energy to go anywhere. Once she has more energy, what referrals could you make to address her social isolation (e.g., church, community senior programs, and other senior programs)?

The Future of Home Care

There are several trends in home care. First, there is more focus on practice, including client care, pharmacology, best practices, and cost-saving clinical approaches to client care. Agencies are improving standards of practice through the educational strategies of practice rounds, journal clubs, increased library holdings, expansion of orientation, and teleconferences. Changes that emphasize care to accentuate empowerment with families and clients and individualize the care plan is another trend. With this shift, the view that the home visits should follow what the client and family needs rather than what is typically expected for the diagnosis is gaining more legitimacy.

With the demographic changes in the United States, it is anticipated that home care will assume an increasingly important role in community-based care in the future. Trends in employment in home care are shown in Figure 12-6.

As complexity of health care delivery and concern for cost containment continue, the client advocate role will remain a central element of both. Flexibility and accountability will remain fundamental as the pressure to meet professional practice standards intersects with the pressure to contain costs. Challenges facing home care nurses will require that the nurse keep up with ever-changing regulations regarding coverage, as well as the documentation requirements that will follow. In addition, nurses will be called on to counsel, teach, and act as a consultant for clients and families as they have increasing responsibility for acutely ill family members at home. Of course, as in all nursing specialties, it will be vital for home care nurses to welcome the increased use of technology.

Due to the recession at the end of the decade, states faced severe budget shortfalls. One shortsighted strategy was to cut home care services for the elderly or the disabled, programs that have been shown to save states money in the long run because they keep people out of nursing homes. Nurses must advocate at the city, county, and state levels to advocate for these cost-effective programs to be reinstated.

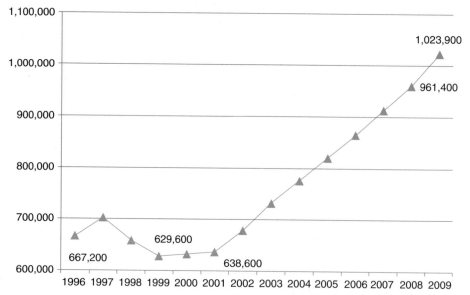

Home Health Care Services: Total Employment, 1996–2009*

Source: U.S. Department of Labor, Bureau of Labor Statistics: Employment, Hours, and Earnings from the Current Employment Statistics Survey (National), www.bls.gov (March 2010).
Notes: *Annual number for 2009 is projected.
Excludes hospital-based and public home care agency employees. Annual data for 1996–2009 is based on the North American Industry Classifications System (NAICS).

Figure 12-6 Home health care services play an increasingly important role in community-based care.

Conclusions

The setting for the provision of health care and nursing care has shifted several times from the late 1800s to the present. Care of the ill in the home was at one point primarily physician care. Then the setting for medical care moved from the home to the hospital or acute care setting in the mid-1900s. In the last 30 years, it has now relocated back to the home and community. The major roles of home care are to educate, reinforce learning, and encourage clients and families to provide ongoing self-care. In home care, the family and client experience a loss of privacy and an interruption in normal decision making, but the advantages for the client and family outweigh the disadvantages when compared with inpatient care. Regardless of the client's diagnosis, the nurse in home care encourages self-care with a preventive focus, which is provided in the context of the client's family and community and follows the principles of continuity of care.

What's on the Web

Administration on Aging (AoA)
INTERNET ADDRESS: http://www.aoa.gov/
   The mission of AoA is to develop a comprehensive, coordinated, and cost-effective system of home and community-based services that helps elderly individuals maintain their health and independence in their homes and communities. This Web site presents information on AoA and its programs. Resources for practitioners, statistics, and consumer information on obtaining services and age-related issues are included.

Canadian Home Care Association
INTERNET ADDRESS: http://www.cdnhomecare.ca/
   The Canadian Home Care Association promotes excellence in home care through leadership, awareness, and knowledge to shape strategic directions. The Canadian Home Care Association is dedicated to the accessibility, quality, and development of home care and community support services that permit people to stay in their homes and communities with safety and dignity. The Web

site contains information on publications, related sites, employment opportunities, and education programs, as well as information related to the organization.

Centers for Disease Control and Prevention, Hand Hygiene in Healthcare Settings
INTERNET ADDRESS: **http://www.cdc.gov/handhygiene**

Hand Hygiene in Healthcare Settings provides health care workers and patients with a variety of resources including guidelines for providers, patient empowerment materials, the latest technological advances in hand hygiene adherence measurement, frequently asked questions, and links to promotional and educational tools published by the WHO, universities, and health departments.

Family Caregiver Alliance
INTERNET ADDRESS: **http://www.caregiver.org/caregiver/jsp/home.jsp**

Family Caregiver Alliance is a public voice for caregivers, illuminating the daily challenges they face, offering them the assistance they so desperately need and deserve, and championing their cause through education, services, research, and advocacy. This site focuses on information and services to families and professionals caring for adults with cognitive disorders, as well as fact sheets and tool kits on topics applicable to a variety of caregivers.

National Association for Home Care & Hospice
INTERNET ADDRESS: **http://www.nahc.org**

NAHCThe National Association for Home Care & Hospice (NAHC) is a professional organization that represents a variety of agencies providing home care services, including home health agencies, hospice programs, and homemaker or home health aide agencies. The Web site contains news and information about home care and hospice, including publications, statistics about home care and hospice, a job search vehicle, and a locator for hospice and home care agencies and their affiliates. It also has information about NAHC membership, meetings and conferences, grassroots activities, and state associations.

National Family Caregivers Association
INTERNET ADDRESS: **http://www.nfcacares.org/**

The National Family Caregivers Association educates supports, empowers and speaks up for the more than 65 million Americans who care for loved ones with a chronic illness or disability or the frailties of old age. NFCA reaches across the boundaries of diagnoses, relationships, and life stages to help transform family caregivers' lives by removing barriers to health and well-being. Free membership is available to any family caregiver. Both the newsletter and Web site provide good resources for "caring for the caregiver" information.

Visiting Nurse Associations of America
INTERNET ADDRESS: **http://www.vnaa.org**

The Visiting Nurse Associations of America (VNAA) is a national association that supports, promotes and advocates for community-based, nonprofit home health and hospice providers that care for all individuals regardless of complexity of condition or ability to pay. The mission of VNAA is to support, promote and advance the nation's network of VNAs, home health care, and hospice providers who provide cost-effective and compassionate home health care to some of the nation's most vulnerable individuals, particularly the elderly and individuals with disabilities. Services include advocacy, education and collaboration.

References and Bibliography

Agency for Healthcare Research and Quality. (2011). *The characteristics of long-term caregivers.* Retrieved from http://www.ahrq.gov/research/ltcusers/ltcuse.htm

Anthony, A., & Milone-Nuzzo, P. (2005). Factors attracting and keeping nurses in home care. *Home Healthcare Nurse, 23*(6), 372–377.

Aspden, P., Wolcott, J., Bootman, J. L., & Cronenwett, L. R. (2007). *Preventing medication errors: Quality chasm series.* Washington, DC: National Academy of Sciences. Retrieved from http://books.nap/catalog/11623.html

Cabin, W. (2010). Lifting the home care veil from depression: OASIS-C and evidence-based practice. *Home Health Care Management & Practice, 22*(3), 171–177. doi:10.1177/1084822309348693.

Centers for Disease Control and Prevention. (2010). Guideline for hand hygiene in health-care settings. *MMWR, 51*(RR16), 1–44. Retrieved from http://www.cdc.gov/handhygiene; http://www.cdc.gov/mmwr/preview/mmwrhtml/rr5116a1.htm

Centers for Medicare & Medicaid Services. (2010). *Medicare and home health care.* Retrieved on from http://www.cms.hhs.gov/center/hha.asp

Christakis, N. A., & Allison, P. D. (2006). Mortality after the hospitalization of a spouse. *New England Journal of Medicine, 354*(7), 719–730.

Ellenbecker, C., Porell, F., Samia, L., Byleckie, J., & Milburn, M. (2008). Predictors of home healthcare nurse retention. *Journal of Nursing Scholarship, 40*(2), 151–160. Retrieved from CINAHL Plus with Full Text database.

Fieldsmith, R., Van Sell, S., & Kindred, C. (2009). Home assessment. *RN, 72*(3), 26–29. Retrieved from CINAHL Plus with Full Text database.

Kenneley, I. (2010). Infection control and the home care environment. *Home Health Care Management & Practice, 22*(3), 195–201. doi:10.1177/1084822309348695.

Leff, B., Burton, L., Mader, S., Naughton, B., Burl, J., Greenough, W., & Steinwachs, D. (2009). Comparison of functional outcomes associated with hospital at home care and traditional acute hospital care. *Journal of the American Geriatrics Society, 57*(2), 273–278. doi:10.1111/j.1532-5415.2008.02103.x

Leff, B., Burton, L., Mader, S., Naughton, B., Burl, J., Koehn, D., et al. (2008). Comparison of stress experienced by family members of patients treated in hospital at home with that of those receiving traditional acute hospital care. *Journal of the American Geriatrics Society, 56*(1), 117–123. Retrieved from CINAHL Plus with Full Text database. doi: 10.1111/j.1532-5415.2007.01459.x.

Mager, D., & Madigan, E. (2010). Medication use among older adults in a home care setting. *Home Healthcare Nurse, 28*(1), 14–23. Retrieved from CINAHL Plus with Full Text database.

McGarry, J. (2009). Defining roles, relationships, boundaries and participation between elderly people and nurses within the home: An ethnographic study. *Health & Social Care in the Community, 17*(1), 83–91. Retrieved from CINAHL Plus with Full Text database.

National Association for Home Care & Hospice. (2010). *Basic statistics about home care.* Washington, DC: Author. Retrieved from http://www.nahc.org/facts/10HC_Stats.pdf

Newfield, J. S. (2006). Documentation: Focusing on better rather than more. *Home Health Care Management & Practice, 18*(3), 247–249.

Niewenhous, S. (2010). OASIS-C: New process measures promote best practices. *Home Health Care Management & Practice, 22*(3), 221–234. doi:10.1177/1084822309355903.

Reinhard, S., Given, B., Petlick, N., & Bemis, A. (2009). Supporting family caregivers in providing care. In: *Patient safety and quality: An evidence-based handbook for nurses* (AHRQ publication no. 08-0043). Rockville, MD: Agency for Healthcare Research and Quality. Retrieved from http://www.ahrq.gov/qual/nurseshdbk/

Robison, J., Fortinsky, R., Kleppinger, A., Shugrue, N., & Porter, M. (2009). A broader view of family caregiving: Effects of caregiving and caregiver conditions on depressive symptoms, health, work, and social isolation. *The Journals of Gerontology Series B: Psychological Sciences and Social Sciences, 64B*(6): 788–98. doi: 10.1093/geronb/gbp015.

Schumacher, K., Beck, C. A., Marren, J. M. (2006). Family caregivers: Caring for older adults, working with their families. *American Journal of Nursing, 106*(8), 40–49.

Wilkins, V., Bruce, M., & Sirey, J. (2009). Caregiving tasks and training interest of family caregivers of medically ill homebound older adults. *Journal of Aging & Health, 21*(3), 528–542. doi: 10.1177/0898264309332838. Retrieved from CINAHL Plus with Full Text database.

LEARNING ACTIVITIES

JOURNALING ACTIVITY 12-1

The Home Visit

1. In your clinical journal, reflect on a home visit you have made. Identify the nursing skills and competencies you used as you provided care or observed if you worked with another nurse.

2. What did you expect the visit to be like and how did the actual visit compare?

3. Describe your experience caring for a client in the home. How was it different from an acute care setting? How was it similar? What did you do differently in the home setting?

4. What did you learn from this experience?

5. How will you use this information in your future practice?

Lay Caregiver

1. In your clinical journal, reflect on an experience you have observed or a client you have cared for in clinical who has been cared for by a lay caregiver for an extended period of time. Ask the person to tell you about their experience as a caregiver. Outline the situation into a case study.

2. Discuss what you observed with this situation and how it applies to the theory in the text or other readings you have done on the topic.

3. How did or would you support the caregiver based on what you learned reading the text or other reading you have done?

4. How will you use what you learned from this experience in your future practice?

5. Remove any identifiable information from the case study you created along with the client names and substitute others. You will be participating in small group discussion and sharing your paper with your classmates.

CLINICAL REASONING ACTIVITY 12-2

Consider the psychosocial needs of home care clients in the following situations. Comment about the likelihood of their condition to produce anxiety or social isolation. Give a reason for your answer. What nursing interventions would you use to address each need for each specific situation?

1. A 50-year-old retired government employee with a 10-year-old son who is caring for his 50-year-old wife who has severe dementia.

2. A 20-year-old woman caring for her 5-month-old baby, who has frequent episodes of apnea. The apnea has required frequent immediate action and, on one occasion, necessitated cardiopulmonary resuscitation to revive the baby.

3. A 70-year-old woman caring for her husband, who has terminal lung cancer.

4. An 80-year-old woman with severe chronic obstructive pulmonary disease who lives alone and is homebound.

5. A 60-year-old single man with congestive heart failure who has frequent episodes of shortness of breath at night.

CLIENT CARE ACTIVITY 12-3

Jose Martinez is an 85-year-old man who lives in a rural area of Texas. He was discharged 2 days ago from a hospital in Austin after breaking his hip while herding his sheep into the corral behind his house. His wife died last year, and he has lived alone since that time. He has eight children; all of whom live in and around the small rural town where Jose has resided since he emigrated from Mexico 20 years ago.

Since fracturing his hip, Mr. Martinez has not been able to care for himself and is upset about his inability to tend to his sheep and be independent. His family has gathered to meet with the home health care nurse about plans for Mr. Martinez.

1. Discuss assessment questions related to culture that the nurse could ask when establishing a relationship with this family.

2. Identify some important questions the home health care nurse could ask during the client conference.

3. Determine what options exist for Mr. Martinez in your community

4. State ways the nurse can address Mr. Martinez's desire to be independent.

5. Determine Mr. Martinez's primary health care needs.

6. Given all the options, summarize the ideal placement for Mr. Martinez at this time.

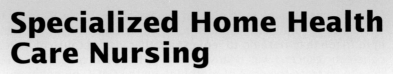

Chapter 13

Specialized Home Health Care Nursing

ROBERTA HUNT

Learning Objectives

1. Identify five specialized roles for home health care nurses.
2. Outline the role responsibilities for each specialized role discussed in the chapter.
3. Utilize a pain assessment tool.
4. Identify trends for specialized roles for home health care nursing.

Key Terms

disease management
home infusion therapy
hospice care
hyperemesis

pregnancy-induced hypertension (PIH)
telehealth
telehomecare
wound care

Chapter Topics

Disease Management in the Home

Telehomecare—Telehealth in Home Care

Infusion Therapy

Wound Care

Maternal–Child Home Care

Pain Management

Hospice Care

Conclusions

The Nurse Speaks

One day when I came in to pick up my assignments, I was asked to visit Mrs. Black, whom I had just seen for the first time the day before. She had called in to triage that morning to request another visit because of increased pain from pancreatic cancer. I was relatively new to **hospice care**, so I reviewed the procedure to increase the dose of morphine on the CADD pump (ambulatory infusion pump). As I drove to her home, I was thinking about the home visit I had made to Mrs. Black the day before for pain management and anxiety issues. I remembered that at that time, she did not want the dosage of morphine or lorazepam increased. During that visit, I noticed the sadness in her eyes and had taken time to sit down next to her and hold her hand to ask her to tell me about her life. She reached under her bed and pulled out her wedding album and talked about the joy she felt on that particular day. I could tell there was sadness and worry behind the words she spoke that she was not willing to share.

When I arrived at her home, I expected that this second visit in as many days would be very short and would be focused on increasing the morphine on the CADD pump. After a pain assessment, I decided to increase the morphine to 2 mg/h more than she had been receiving. As we sat side by side on the sofa, I concentrated fully on the unfamiliar procedure and tuned out the words she was speaking. In fact, I remember wishing that she would be quiet so I could finish the task at hand. But there was something in the sound of her voice that jolted me into hearing her words. I realized that she was sharing deep regrets about choices she had made in her life that could not be easily rectified in the time she had left. A sudden overwhelming feeling washed over me. What could I do about this information? I stopped fumbling with the pump and listened for a long time, acknowledging her pain and her suffering but offering no solutions or answers. She seemed to gain in personal strength as she shared. This experience reminded me to never lose sight of the compassionate and caring role of the nurse in the alleviation of suffering.

Kathleen Dudley, MSN, RN,
Hospice Nurse, Assistant Professor
St. Catherine University

In the last 20 years, home health care has become more specialized and complex as nursing care is increasingly provided in community-based settings. As in basic home health care, nurses must be competent in communication, teaching, management, and physical and emotional caregiving. In addition, they must develop expertise in a specialized area. Specialized home health care nursing, which is discussed in this chapter, includes home telemedicine, disease management, infusion therapy, wound care, maternal–child home care, pain management, and hospice care.

Disease Management in the Home

Interest in disease management has increased dramatically since the mid-1990s. **Disease management** is "a system of coordinated health care interventions and communications for populations with conditions in which patient self-care efforts are significant" (Bott, Kapp, Johnson, & Magno, 2009). Disease management programs encompass providers across the health care continuum, including home care following the basic premise that coordinated, evidence-based interventions can be applied to clients with conditions that are high-cost, high-volume. The goal of disease management in the home is to improve clinical outcomes and lower overall costs. Outcome data are the fundamental element to the success of this approach to client care.

THE ROLE OF THE NURSE IN DISEASE MANAGEMENT

Disease management focuses on chronic conditions that are difficult to manage and costly to treat. These conditions include but are not restricted to congestive heart failure, asthma, coronary disease, diabetes, osteoporosis, stroke, and chronic wounds. Through case findings, the nurse has an important role in identifying individuals who could benefit from disease management. Once the client is identified, all interventions are based on evidence-based practice guidelines for the condition(s). As in all community-based care, collaboration among physicians, care providers, client and family, support service, and providers is key. The nurse's role in promoting the client and families' self-care skills through consultation, counseling, and health education is vital to successful disease management. As with any intervention, disease management necessitates evaluation of outcomes as well as application of the findings to a revised plan of care. Throughout the process of disease management, using routine reporting and feedback loops between and among all involved parties protects the integrity of the process (Disease management programs, 2010).

TRENDS IN DISEASE MANAGEMENT

One trend in disease management entails using technology to develop new connections with clients, particularly those who are elderly. Where home care in the past has been delivered by "high touch" through home visits, disease management uses "high-tech" **telehealth** by telephone, Internet, and various monitors. Intensive use of telephone follow-up has been found to reduce cost and hospitalization for diabetes (Rosenzweig et al., 2010). Telehealth will be more fully discussed in the next section on telehomecare.

Being a relatively new concept in home care, one of the primary trends at this time is to expand utilization of disease management with rigorous evaluation research to establish the efficacy of new programs and models. A severe information deficit exists about disease management in home care, making quality monitoring difficult. To successfully apply evidence-based guidelines to practice, it is necessary to have access to timely information and collaboration among a multidisciplinary team. Home care nurses face many challenges in this area but are well-positioned to influence the issue (Bowles, Pham, O'Connor, & Horowitz, 2010). Through this process, evidence-based practice in the area of disease management will be established.

Telehomecare—Telehealth in Home Care

Telehomecare is an interactive, two-way process that allows home care nurses to have contact with homebound clients to monitor clinical progress. This is accomplished wholly or partly through electronic means, which may include using telephones, televisions, Internet, and videoconferencing to monitor vital signs, heart and lung sounds, blood glucose, and oxygen saturation. Many aspects of case management, chronic disease treatment, hospice care, postsurgical care, and rehabilitation are possible through telehomecare.

From the inception of this form of health care delivery, its main advantage has been cost savings. Telenursing allows nurses to care for many more clients within the same time frame. While nurses average 4 to 8 traditional in-home visits per day, it is possible to complete 20 or more telehomecare visits per day. Agencies receiving reimbursement under Medicare's Prospective Payment System as well as a number of health insurance plans cover telehomecare visits according to the American Telemedicine Association (2010). However, agencies may not substitute telehealth service for physician-ordered Medicare-covered services.

It is more difficult to practice relationship-based care via telecommunication. Without cautious use of thoughtfully developed guidelines, telehealth has the potential to mechanize the delivery of nursing care. Further, telehomecare creates some distinct ethical challenges, the most obvious being confidentiality and informed consent. The American Nurses Association (ANA) has developed core principles on telehealth. The first principle states that the "basic standards of professional conduct governing each health care profession are not altered by the use of telehealth technologies" (ANA, 1999). "High tech" should not replace "high touch" in the provision of nursing care as both are essential to quality care.

ROLE OF THE NURSE

The role of the nurse in telehealth varies depending on the application but often fall into three categories: monitoring, managing, and motivating. The delegated medication function of monitoring health and activities can be accomplished by the nurse 24/7, reducing emergency department visits and allowing for rapid intervention at the first sign of health changes or decline in health status. The nurse utilizing telehealth technology is able to act as a case manager and identify and prioritize clients requiring remote or home-based interventions with information technology. Software that contains embedded risk models can allow the nurse to triage, review, and assess client progress. Case management allows more efficient use of both human and financial home care resources through referral, follow-up, and consultation. The final role for the nurse in telehomecare involves motivating the client and family by engaging, educating, and empowering them in self-care. Motivation encompasses the nursing interventions of counseling and health teaching. As a result, the client and family are able to better manage the existing condition and engage in activities related to tertiary prevention (Research in Community-Based Nursing Care 13-1).

TRENDS IN TELEHEALTH/TELEHOMECARE

Due to future demographic trends and economics, the values of strategies to contain cost are obvious. As the population ages and new technologies are developed, telehealth is one strategy that will be used in the next decade with wide application. The most common use will be for disease management. Rapidly advancing technologies will become more widely available and more affordable. For example, there are small, passive sensors that can seamlessly detect and report vitals; care management systems that can improve adherence to diet and medication guidance; communication systems to improve collaborative decision making between clients, families, and caregivers. These are promising technologies that will soon become more widely available.

There is a scarcity of research focused on client safety in telehealth. This may be due to lack of understanding about possible safety issues associated with telehealth and telenursing. Safety issues associated with telehealth are complex, given potential malfunctioning equipment creating adverse effects on client management from delayed or missing information,

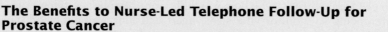

RESEARCH IN COMMUNITY-BASED NURSING CARE 13-1

The Benefits to Nurse-Led Telephone Follow-Up for Prostate Cancer

As the population ages, the continuing increase in prevalence of prostate cancer has significantly intensified the pressure on health care providers to improve service delivery and highlights the importance of effective management with effective follow-up. Follow-up services after surgery after surgery in an outpatients department are time consuming and dependent on client motivation. Nursing services have been found to be efficacious in the management of this chronic disease. In particular, telephone consultations have been shown to provide improvements in service delivery. The purpose of the study was to determine client participation and satisfaction with nurse-led telephone follow-up after surgery for prostate cancer. Telephone follow-up protocol was developed and implemented to increase efficiency in client follow-up an uro-oncology outpatient clinic. Between 2005 and 2009, a total of 67 patients were recruited into the program. Patient satisfaction was elicited using a questionnaire in a telephone interview. Overall, 90% of clients stated that they were very satisfied with the service provided.

Source: Anderson, B. (2010). The benefits to nurse-led telephone follow-up for prostate cancer. *British Journal of Nursing, 19*(17), 1085–1090. Retrieved from CINAHL Plus with Full Text database.

misunderstood advice, or inaccurate findings. There is a need for additional research in the arena of client safety in telehealth practice (Schlachta-Fairchild, Elfrink, & Deickman, 2009).

There are also unique legal and ethical considerations related to telehomecare. There are legal implications because some agencies provide telecare across state borders. How telecare is provided is governed by the law where the client resides, not by where the agency is located. Nurses must keep this in mind when providing care for clients residing in another state. Telephonic communication creates many opportunities for issues related to client autonomy, confidentiality, and privacy to arise. Lack of face-to-face contact may interrupt nurse assessment of the client's ability to make informed decisions. This calls for the nurse to carefully assess whether those receiving telehealth service are mentally competent to make decisions. Protecting client privacy and confidentiality is difficult when information is shared by multiple means but must always be a central consideration (Lorentz, 2008).

Some of these technologies allow for more comprehensive data collection, which can in turn be used to evaluate and analyze the efficacy of these interventions. All of these strategies will contribute to further developing evidence-based nursing practice in home care. This is important because the primary application of telehealth will be disease management where outcome data are the central element to client care. The challenge for the nurse will be to preserve the trusting relationship by maintaining relationship-centered care.

CLIENT SITUATIONS IN PRACTICE

Ruth Loewen is an 85-year-old woman who had a double-bypass surgery 10 years ago. Eventually, she developed congestive heart failure and has received disease management home care services partially provided by telehealth for the last 3 years. Each morning, Ruth weighs herself, takes her blood pressure, pulse and blood oxygen levels with equipment provided by the home care agency. This information is sent by a telemonitoring system to a cardiac specialist in a nearby city. If any of these findings suggest that her condition is changing, a nurse will go to her home to assess her that day. If her vital signs remain stable, a nurse is scheduled to come to her home to perform a more comprehensive assessment every week. At these weekly visits, the nurse sets up Ruth's medication and does a head-to-toe assessment to determine if there have been any changes in her condition. If she experiences some changes in her health indicators, Ruth and the nurse discuss what may have contributed to these changes and what might be done for corrective action in the future.

Infusion Therapy

Home infusion therapy is a broad area, incorporating chemotherapy, pain management, fluid replacement therapy, immunosuppressive drug therapy, inotropic therapy, and blood and platelet transfusion. These medications and blood products are infused by a variety of methods. The actual administration of the therapy is performed by home infusion nurses or self-administered by clients or their caregivers. Because infusion therapy has become widely utilized as a cost-containment strategy, reimbursement criteria are strict. Preauthorization is essential before any home infusion therapy is initiated, or the result could be nonpayment for the services provided. Increasingly, family members are expected to administer medications and fluid via a central line (Craven & Hirnle, 2009).

ROLE OF THE NURSE

It is imperative that nurses who seek employment in infusion therapy have sharp problem-solving and interpersonal skills, detailed knowledge of the therapies and their effects, and technical skill in working with equipment. Although all nursing roles are important in this specialized area, the primary one is that of direct caregiving or delegated medical function. Before the visit, the nurse must be sure that the visit has been preauthorized and that the medication dosage, rate, route, and site-change frequency are all indicated in the physician order. In addition, all necessary equipment and supplies must be in the home or brought to the home by the nurse. Box 13-1 details the numerous safety requirements of this type of therapy.

> **BOX 13-1**
>
> ## Safety Requirements for Infusion Therapy in the Home
>
> - Emergency plan and access to functional phone and list of emergency phone numbers
> - Three-prong grounded outlet to maintain proper grounding of the machine
> - Adequate refrigeration capacity to store medication requiring cool storage and chemical spill kit in the home
> - Notification to the fire and police departments and telephone and electric companies of person on life support equipment or medically necessary oxygen or infusion
> - Systems established to ensure adherence to a complex medication regimen
> - Information on medications, including dosage, adverse effects, interactions, and safe storage
> - Identification and correction of environmental hazards and patient-specific concerns
>
> Adapted from Craven, R., & Hirnle, C. (2010). *Fundamentals of nursing: Human health and function.* Philadelphia, PA: Lippincott Williams & Wilkins.

Another important nursing function involves completing a full assessment, including intake and output, weight, and any signs of a reaction to therapy. This assessment should also include the infusion site, operation of the infusion pump, care for the access site, signs of infection, allergic response, fluid overload, and dehydration or other signs of complications. Response to the therapy must always be assessed and documented. Although this role is highly technical, as in all nursing care, it is imperative to never lose sight of the importance of compassion and caring (Fig. 13-1)

Reimbursement for home care infusion therapy is often limited because it is expected that all clients and their families will assume some or all aspects of the care. It is more common for the infusion therapy nurse rather than the nurse in charge of discharge planning to teach the family caregiver or client how to perform the infusion. It is important that the nurse teach the client and family regarding the safe infusion of the medication. In the rare case when teaching is done before discharge from the hospital, the client and family members are often so overwhelmed and anxious that they may have difficulty learning the

Figure 13-1 It is imperative never to lose sight of the importance of compassion and caring in the alleviation of suffering in our role as nurses.

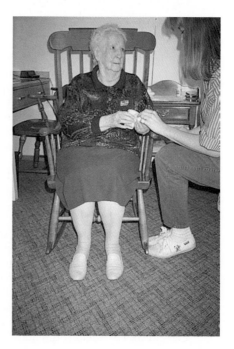

procedure. Often the client or family is unable to complete the skill independently once they are home. The content of this teaching incorporates using proper technique for infusions and solving common problems related to intravenous (IV) therapy, site care, and use of the infusion pump, as well as the purpose, route, and dosage of the medications. The family must also know how to document the rate and time of all infusions, symptoms of IV infiltration and infection, and times to call or contact the nurse or physician (Craven & Hirnle, 2009).

TRENDS IN INFUSION THERAPY

Patient safety is a major issue in infusion therapy. As previously mentioned, nurses who seek employment in this specialized area must possess a sophisticated skill set. Although not required at this time, there is some interest in requiring certification for employment as an infusion therapy nurse. Currently, the Joint Commission on Accreditation of Healthcare Organizations states that nurses must be appropriately qualified and competent in the infusion field to be employed as an infusion nurse. Orientation, training, and validation of the competency of nurses working in infusion therapy are essential for safe patient care. Competencies should include venipuncture and the assessment skills of the nurses related to the therapy and vascular access devices. This educational training is the responsibility of the agency. Some research indicates that certified nurses experience fewer adverse events and errors in care than their noncertified counterparts. There is a trend to require agencies to hire nurses who are certified through the Infusion Nurses Certification Corporation and maintain this certification to be reimbursed for services. The benefit is that certified infusion nurses make fewer errors in administration. One study found an 8% increase in complications or mortality when uncertified registered nurses provided infusion therapy compared to certified infusion nurses (Joint INS/INCC Position Paper, 2009). The downside to requiring home infusion therapy nurses to become certified is that it may create a shortage of such nurses and consequently limit access to home infusion care.

Wound Care

Wounds are responsible for significant suffering and morbidity in home and hospice care (Hindelang, 2006). **Wound care** is a common specialized home care function. Wounds are categorized broadly as acute or chronic, with all wounds being considered acute at the onset of the injury. If the process of healing is prolonged beyond the expected trajectory, the wound is classified as chronic (Greener, 2010).

A variety of problems can occur in wound healing, stemming from a combination of factors and situations. These include the client's general health, nutritional status, skin texture and turgor, body weight, and mobility, all of which impact healing (Craven & Hirnle, 2009). Wound care is not simply a technique of dressing application. There is a discipline of specialized practice for wound care that includes advanced training, education, and certification. There is a lack of wound care specialists, caused by area-specific shortages and the expense of contracting for such services.

ROLE OF THE NURSE

In wound care, the role of the nurse involves an ongoing evaluation of the wound and any particular risk factors for healing. Before the first visit, the nurse must be familiar with the type of wound, wound care orders, cleaning method, and frequency of dressing change, as well as any pressure-relieving or support devices, dietary restrictions and caloric allowance, medications, and activity orders and restrictions. The nurse's main interventions fall within delegated medical functions, consultation, counseling, collaboration, and health education. Mobility enhancement and pain assessment should be initiated at the first visit and done periodically as needed. Scrupulous documentation following the Outcome and Assessment Information Set (OASIS) assessment or the agency policy is an essential aspect of wound care. For additional information on the OASIS documentation, see Chapter 12. Box 13-2 outlines other safety considerations. Every year, numerous new products are developed for

BOX 13-2	Safety Considerations for Wound Care

- Universal precautions for infection control and disposal of sharps and used dressings
- List available to the client and all caregivers of signs and symptoms to report to the nurse or physician
- Documentation of medications and allergies
- Identification and correction of environmental hazards and patient-specific concerns

From Craven, R., & Hirnle, C. (2009). *Fundamentals of nursing: Human health and function.* Philadelphia, PA: Lippincott Williams & Wilkins.

wound care, requiring the nurse to stay abreast of these developments through continuous review of the literature and in-service education.

It is important that the nurse is comfortable educating the client and caregivers in wound care skills. Lay caregivers must become competent in several aspects of wound care, as they often are the main care providers. They need to be able to describe and demonstrate wound care and signs and symptoms of infection. Knowledge of the importance of medicating 30 minutes before a painful dressing change is essential. Nutritional practices profoundly impact wound healing, and one way to monitor this is through a dietary log. The client should be encouraged to participate in an activity as appropriate for the condition. For those with limited mobility, caregivers must understand range-of-motion exercises and initiate them at least three times a day. Techniques for turning and positioning the client every 2 hours to alleviate pressure are also essential caregiver skills.

TRENDS IN WOUND CARE

Interdisciplinary teams and networks of wound care centers are becoming vital to the coordination of wound care. Care conferencing occurs where all team members meet to discuss specific cases and the need for revisions to the plan of care. Most agencies have identified criteria for cases that must be examined by a care conference. It is important that these criteria explore the causes or factors contributing to the wound, and how the plan of care addresses these. The past and current status of the wound and the current orders for the dressing and treatment must also be clearly documented and must be compatible. The client or caregiver's role in the wound plan of care must be examined, as should the frequency of physical therapy visits. The barriers to wound healing should be identified and addressed. Discharge goals and time frame should be realistic.

Through technology, new tools are being developed, along with different, targeted approaches to provide more effective care to those with wounds that require advanced care and supervision. The first trend is the use of telehealth for wound care. Home-based telewound care can involve teleconsulting, conferencing, reporting, and transmitting. For example, telewound care, using an ordinary digital camera to document the status of a wound for tracking and planning, is becoming commonplace. An ongoing photographic history of the wound provides excellent continuity between the home, clinic, and hospital.

Another example of telewound care is specialty wound services delivered directly to the home via a computer screen. The photographs of the wound are transmitted to a specialty wound care service that provides consultation for management of difficult wounds. These virtual specialists work together with the home care nurse to assess and plan care. In some cases, the wound photography is standardized using the wound electronic medical record (Rennert, Golinko, Kaplan, Flattau, & Brem, 2009). Both of these trends are offering hope for healing difficult wounds in a more cost-effective manner. It is anticipated that the need for home care nurses with skills in wound care will continue to grow as the demographics shift, with an increasing percentage of the population becoming older and more obese and developing diabetes.

Maternal–Child Home Care

Recipients of maternal–child home care fall into three main categories: high-risk pregnant women, high-risk infants, and children. The main advantage of home care for high-risk pregnancy is that it reduces costs by preventing hospitalization as well as decreasing the percentage of low birth weight infants. With more than 9% of hospital charges attributable to pregnancy, delivery, and neonatal care, there is considerable opportunity for savings (Cross, 2006). Women who are identified as having high-risk pregnancies may require home care for several pregnancy complications, including preterm labor, **pregnancy-induced hypertension (PIH)**, and **hyperemesis** gravidarum. Increasingly, women experiencing these complications from pregnancy require high-technology care, such as infusion therapy or telemedicine in the form of home monitoring.

High-risk infants may receive specialized home care including infants receiving palliative care, infants who are technology-dependent, and stable premature infants requiring intensive home support. Children with acute or chronic conditions or children requiring palliative or hospice care also may be home care recipients.

Prior to health care reform of 2010, home care service for pregnant women and ill children were only available to individuals with health insurance. Access to perinatal health care services for women living in poverty is complicated by factors such as being underinsured, language and cultural barriers, lack of transportation, and limited health literacy. High rates of premature births, low birth weight infants, and maternal and infant deaths result. Evidence shows that health and social services delivered in the home improve pregnancy outcomes (Temple, Lutenbacher, & Vitale, 2008). Health care reform includes provisions to address these deficiencies by expanding home care and home visiting services.

ROLE OF THE NURSE

Nursing roles depend on the client's condition. In the case of high-risk maternal visits, hyperemesis, or protracted vomiting with weight loss and fluid and electrolyte imbalance, IV replacement therapy at home is sometimes required to maintain hydration. In women at risk for preterm labor, home care may prevent premature birth. Nursing roles include assessment of the mother's weight, fetal heart tones, fundal height, nutrition, psychosocial status, compliance with the plan of care, and knowledge of signs and symptoms of preterm labor.

Hypertensive disorders are the second leading cause of maternal mortality in the United States with 8% of all pregnancies complicated by this condition (Gibson & Carlson, 2010). Hypertensive disorders of pregnancy include (a) chronic hypertension, (b) preeclampsia/eclampsia, (c) preeclampsia with chronic hypertension, and (d) gestational hypertension. Home monitoring of individuals experiencing pregnancy-induced hypertensive disorders has been shown to reduce mortality and health care costs. Skilled nursing care includes assessment of the mother's weight, presence of edema and hyperreflexia, signs and symptoms of a worsening condition, fetal heart tones, compliance with the plan of care, nutrition, psychosocial status, and knowledge of symptoms.

HOME CARE OF HIGH-RISK INFANTS

As discussed in Chapter 8, the number and percentage of low birth weight and premature infants has been on the increase in the United States over the last decades. Low birth weight infants who are discharged from neonatal intensive care units (NICUs) sometimes require home care services. Some low birth weight infants are stable at discharge but progress more successfully with intensive home support. Infants who are technology-dependent when they are discharged from the NICU may have need of home visiting. Infants with congenital conditions for which there is no treatment may be discharged home with palliative or hospice care. Some of the primary roles and considerations for the role of the nurse in these cases are discussed in the section in this chapter on hospice care.

RESEARCH IN COMMUNITY-BASED NURSING CARE 13-2

Enduring Effects of Prenatal and Infancy Home Visiting by Nurses on Maternal Life Course and Government Spending

This randomized controlled trial examined the effects of prenatal and infancy home visiting by nurses on maternal life course over 12 years. A total of 594 urban high-risk mothers enrolled in a public system of obstetric and pediatric care participated in the study. Outcomes measured were mothers' cohabitation with and marriage to the child's biological father, intimate partner violence, duration of partner relationships, role impairment due to alcohol and other drug use, cost of welfare benefits, arrest, child foster care placement, and cumulative subsequent births. The outcomes of the women receiving home visiting and not receiving home visiting was measured at the time the firstborn child was 12 years old. Nurse visited mothers compared to control subjects reported less role impairment owing to alcohol and the use of drugs, longer partner relationships, and greater sense of mastery. Further, there was less government spending per year on food stamps, Medicaid, and Aid to Families with Dependent Children and Temporary Assistance for Needy Families during the 12 year period. Overall, there was a saving of $12,300. The researchers concluded that the program improved maternal life course and reduced government spending.

From Olds, D., Kitzman, H., Cole, R., Hanks, C., Arcoleo, K., Anson, E., et al. (2010). Enduring effects of prenatal and infancy home visiting by nurses on maternal life course and government spending: Follow-up of a randomized trial among children at age 12 years. *Archives of Pediatrics & Adolescent Medicine, 164*(5), 419–424. Retrieved from CINAHL Plus with Full Text database.

PRENATAL/POSTPARTUM/WELL-BABY HOME CARE

Maternal and infant home visiting programs first began in the 19th century. Postpartum well-baby care was a component of these. For several decades, there has been an impressive body of research that documents the long-term value of nurse home visiting for perinatal care. Recent studies document long-term benefits to the mothers and children participating in this type of program (Research in Community-Based Nursing Care 13-2 and 13-3).

RESEARCH IN COMMUNITY-BASED NURSING CARE 13-3

Long-Term Effects of Prenatal and Infancy Nurse Home Visitation on the Life Course of Youths

The purpose of this randomized trail study was to examine the effects of prenatal and infancy nurse home visitation on the life course development of 19-year-old youth whose mothers received home visiting service. Three hundred and ten youths from 400 families were randomly assigned to either a treatment group who received home visiting service or control group who received standard care. Outcomes measured after 19 years included youth self-report of education achievement, reproductive behaviors, welfare use, and criminal involvement. As compared to the control group, girls whose mothers received home visiting were less likely to have been arrested and convicted and had fewer lifetime arrests and convictions. Girls whose mothers received home visiting had fewer children and less Medicaid use compared to the control group. The researchers concluded that prenatal and infancy home visitation reduced the proportion of girls entering the criminal justice system but few program effects for boys were found.

From Eckenrode, J., Campa, M., Luckey, D., Henderson, C., Cole, R., Kitzman, H., et al. (2010). Long-term effects of prenatal and infancy nurse home visitation on the life course of youths: 19-year follow-up of a randomized trial. *Archives of Pediatrics & Adolescent Medicine, 164*(1), 9–15. Retrieved from CINAHL Plus with Full Text database.

In the last decade, postpartum home care has become a growing area of perinatal services. It is common for insurers to reimburse at least one visit for families after early discharge in the presence of high-risk factors. In some communities, this service is provided for any client deemed high risk regardless of whether or not the family has insurance. High risk may include conditions such as hyperbilirubinemia, low birth weight, and failure to feed well or gain weight appropriately. Any woman who manifests signs of postpartum depression merits a referral for follow-up with a home care nurse after discharge. Again, the role of the nurse involves assessing and monitoring postpartum status and referring for follow-up as appropriate.

PEDIATRIC HOME CARE

The need for home care services for the pediatric client has grown substantially in recent years. Most of these services are for postsurgical clients who are released from the hospital early and who require skilled nursing care at home through the rehabilitation phase of care. A second common group—children with chronic conditions such as bronchial pulmonary dysphasia, cystic fibrosis, and cancer—are now being cared for at home rather than in the hospital setting. A third category is vulnerable children who have survived prematurity and are born with congenital anomalies (Cervasio, 2010).

All of these children may require some of the same nursing care that has already been discussed: infusion therapy, wound care, or other high-technology care. All of the general principles and guidelines discussed in Chapter 12 that apply to the home care of adults also apply to children. It is particularly important when caring for children that all nursing functions are formulated, implemented, and evaluated in collaboration with the parents or caregiver. For example, a common pediatric home care service that may be the only alternative to hospitalization is home enteral nutrition (HEN). Children with malnutrition due to a number of different diseases are candidates for HEN. The nutritional team, pediatrician, home care staff, and hospital specialist collaborate with the family to determine the treatment plan to implement in the home (Nanneth & Abbate, 2008).

TRENDS IN MATERNAL–CHILD HOME CARE

Over the last decade, the trends in home care of high-risk pregnancy include use of telemedicine for the management of preterm labor. Home monitoring devices have become increasingly sophisticated and simple to use. One example is a device that allows pregnant women to keep track of the fetal heart rate (FHR) at home. This device allows the pregnant client to check the FHR whenever she has doubts about the welfare of her infant and contact the physician if she has concerns. The FHR can be transmitted to a digital display. Another new device is a smart monitor that can be used in any setting as a wireless system. This offers nondirective supportive therapy from the client's home and may be integrated with other home telehealth services to monitor high-risk clients who otherwise would have to be admitted to the hospital. Another trend is to use a case manager model of care that saves $2 to $5 for every $1 spent on home care and improves pregnancy and neonatal outcomes. Programs that are "high touch" and "high tech" prevent preterm deliveries and C-section births (Cross, 2006).

Standard practice is to follow medically complex patients through the prenatal period. Over time, technology has allowed increasingly complex clients to be monitored at home. Recently, there has been a shift to concentrate effort to ensure that the pregnancy continues to full term of 39 or 40 weeks. Modified bed rest is more commonly seen in home care clients. Another trend is early intervention with home care services for hyperemesis with the goal to prevent hospitalization and to avoid the need for total parenteral nutrition (TPN).

Although pediatric home health care represents a small portion of all the home health care services, increasing technological advances and the continued movement of health care from the acute care to the community setting is expected to lead to higher use. Studies of case load management to determine reasonable staffing ratios to maximize quality care for pediatric home care clients are now reported in the literature (Lewis & Pontin, 2008). There is a continuous stream of new research delineating the cost-effectiveness and efficacy of specialized home care for maternal–child populations.

PAIN MANAGEMENT

For many conditions, pain management is central to effective nursing care. It is common for clients and their caregivers to fear uncontrolled pain. They may need frequent reassurance that pain control can be achieved. At the same time, unfortunately, all too often, pain is underestimated and inadequately treated.

ROLE OF THE NURSE

Many factors contribute to successful assessment and management of pain, but the relationship and trust between the nurse and the client is central to this process. Caring and compassion is essential to this relationship. Effective pain management is based on a comprehensive pain assessment. In the home environment, where the nurse may see the client for very limited periods of time, it is imperative that the nurse develops skills in assessment and management of pain. Because pain is a subjective and an individual experience, the client's report of pain must be considered accurate and valid. When measuring pain, it is essential that a standardized scale that is easy to use and document and has high validity and reliability is used (Ruder, 2010). Assessment Tools 13-1 contains a method for assessing pain. Generally, acute pain is defined as pain that lasts less than 6 months, whereas chronic pain lasts more than 6 months.

Common barriers to effective pain management in home care include beliefs based on misinformation about the use of analgesics, side effects, fatalism, and communication. Issues related to pain management vary across the life span with individuals over the age of 75 reporting beliefs about the use of analgesics and communications with staff as most troublesome. Younger clients identify greater concerns about sleep disturbance due to pain and anxiety as top barriers to pain management (Closs, Chatwin, & Bennett, 2009). As in all community-based nursing care, prevention and early intervention is always the first consideration in the assessment and management of pain.

The pharmacologic interventions for the management of pain are too numerous to address in this chapter. Most medical–surgical textbooks comprehensively discuss the common interventions for pain management, including delegated medication functions,

Assessment Tools 13-1
Pain Assessment

Describe any pain you have now.

What makes it worse?

What makes it better?

When does it occur? How often? How long does it last?

What else do you feel when you have this pain?

Show me on this drawing (or figure) where you have pain.

Rate your pain on a scale of 1 to 10, with 10 being the most severe pain. (Have a child use the Oucher scale, with faces ranging from frowning to crying.)

Has pain impacted your daily activities? How has your pain affected your activities of daily living?

Adapted from Weber, J., & Kelly, J. (2009). *Health assessment in nursing* (4th ed.). Philadelphia, PA: Lippincott Williams & Wilkins.

Table 13-1 Internet Resources for Information About Pain Management
American Academy of Pain Medicine: http://www.painmed.org/
American Pain Society: http://www.ampainsoc.org/
American Pain Foundation: http://www.painfoundation.org/
American Chronic Pain Association: www.theacpa.org
City of Hope Pain Resource Center: http://prc.coh.org/
Medline Plus-Service U.S. National Library of Medicine and National Institute of Health: http://www.nlm.nih.gov/medlineplus/
National Center for Complementary and Alternative Medicine: http://nccam.nih.gov/
National Pain Foundation: http://www.nationalpainfoundation.org/
Pain Resource Center: http://prc.coh.org/
WebMD Pain Management Center: http://www.webmd.com/pain-management/default.htm
World Health Organization's Pain Relief Ladder: http://www.who.int/cancer/palliative/painladder/en/

health education, consultation, case finding, referral, and counseling. Sometimes physical pain-relief techniques can be used with success; positioning and good hygiene often relieve pain for those individuals who spend long hours in bed. Cutaneous stimulation, such as massage, vibration, heat, and cold, is often effective for temporary relief from pain. Anticipatory guidance, distraction, guided imagery, and hypnosis also contribute to pain management. There are also behavioral pain-relief techniques including relaxation and meditation. Resources for information about pain management are found in Table 13-1.

Home care nurses need ongoing pain management education as they are often the client's only advocate and source of information (Fig. 13-2). The home as a setting for practice presents unique challenges (Vallerand, Hasenau, & Templin, 2010). Barriers to pain management occur if home care nurses do not discuss caregiver's perceptions or concerns related to pain management (Oliver et al., 2008). A thorough assessment of caregiver knowledge, skills, and beliefs about pain medication allows the nurse to tailor specific education related to particular pain management issues facing the caregiver. This approach is most easily accomplished through an interprofessional team approach. Additional barrier to pain management are seen in Table 13-2.

Figure 13-2 Intravenous therapy and other technologic treatments contribute to pain management in the home.

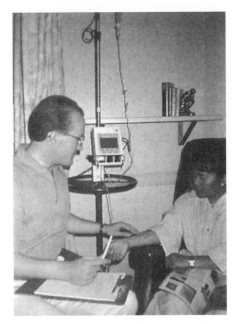

Table 13-2 Barriers to Pain Management	
Barrier	**Description**
Inadequate assessment skills	Not asking about pain Using only subjective assessment Believing what the client says about the level of his or her pain is less likely to be considered by the nurse compared to other data Nurse not aware of or not comfortable using standardized pain scale Lack of knowledge of ethical and legal responsibilities related to pain management
Inadequate intervention skills with pain management	Underuse of opioids due to concern that use of opioids will result in addiction or induce respiratory depression
Inadequate communication	Between nurse, MD, and pharmacist related to role responsibilities for pain management

From Ruder, S. (2010). Seven tools to assist hospice and home care clinicians in pain management at end of life. *Home Healthcare Nurse, 28*(8), 458–470. Retrieved from CINAHL Plus with Full Text database.

TRENDS IN PAIN MANAGEMENT

One trend in pain management is the increasing use of complementary therapies. A great deal of research documents the benefits of alternative therapies for pain management. National Center for Complementary and Alternative Medicine (2010) authorities recommend that practitioners use relaxation and meditation for pain management, given their low cost and demonstrated health benefits, and judge them as among the best complementary therapies for widespread use.

Increasingly, various technologies are used to improve pain management in the home. One pilot study explored the efficacy of teaching parents to use an electronic alarm for around-the-clock symptom management following their child's tonsillectomy. The around-the-clock symptom management group administered significantly more analgesics by the second postoperative day compared to the control group but both groups reported similar pain intensity. The mean hours for nighttime sleep did not differ between groups (Wiggins, 2010). There is also a trend to use personal digital assistant to wirelessly control an internal pump that streams medication directly to its target inside the body for pain control at home (Hachizuka et al., 2010).

There is considerable research at the National Institutes of Health (NIH) assessing the efficacy of various pain management strategies. One area of current research focuses on chronic pain that has lasted at least 6 months. Other studies are comparing different health care approaches to the management of acute low back pain (standard care versus chiropractic, acupuncture, or massage therapy). These studies are measuring symptom relief, restoration of function, and patient satisfaction. Other research is comparing standard surgical treatments to the most commonly used standard nonsurgical treatments to measure changes in health-related quality of life among patients suffering from spinal stenosis (NIH, 2010).

As in other areas of medical research, there is a great deal of work focusing on the role of medication in pain management. Notable among these are researchers working to develop a morphine-like drug that will have the same pain-deadening qualities without the drug's negative side effects. Another group is working to develop pain medications that take advantage of the body's natural ability to block or interrupt pain signals (National Institute of Neurological Disorders and Stroke, 2010).

Hospice Care

Hospice care provides an essential alternative for the terminally ill client. Dr. Cecily Saunders founded the hospice movement in London in the late-1960s. Dr. Sylvia Lack established the first hospice in the United States based on the model developed in

Great Britain. Since 1982, when the Medicare hospice program was established, the number of hospices has grown dramatically. According to the Hospice Association of America (HAA, 2010), there were 31 Medicare-certified hospices in 1984. In 1985, there were 151. In 1991, there were 1,011, and by 2009, the number had increased to 3,407. In addition to all the other benefits to clients and family provided by hospice care, the daily cost is substantially less than the cost of stays in the hospital and in skilled nursing facilities.

Agencies that provide hospice care are committed to maintaining supportive social, emotional, and spiritual services to the terminally ill, as well as support for the client's family. Caring for the terminally ill includes informing clients, family, and caregivers about the benefits of hospice care and the importance of early referral (Research in Community-Based Nursing Care 13-4). Care varies according to the client and family's needs; however, the focus is always on the client and family as the unit of care. Hospice care is often interdisciplinary care that reaffirms the right of every individual and family to participate fully in the final stage of life.

When a client is diagnosed with a terminal illness and has 6 months or less to live, the client qualifies for hospice care through Medicare. Payment for hospice services under Medicare is based on four levels of care:

1. Routine home care

2. Continuous home care (24 hours in a crisis situation)

3. Inpatient respite care not to exceed 5 days at a time

4. General inpatient care at a Medicare-certified hospital, skilled nursing facility, or inpatient unit of a hospice (HAA, 2010)

Hospice care is offered in a variety of settings. These include the freestanding hospice house, where inpatient hospice services are provided at the end of life; hospital- and home-based services provided by freestanding hospice agencies; and home care–affiliated hospice agencies. Most of the programs in the United States are provided through autonomous, community-based, in-home hospice programs. Nurses develop and supervise many hospice agencies.

Intermittent hospice care is provided in the home by nurses; medical social workers; physical, occupational, and speech therapists; home health aides; and homemakers. Hospice programs also provide short periods of continuous care in which a client is provided with shift nursing and aides for an acute episode and respite care for the family by placing

---

RESEARCH IN COMMUNITY-BASED NURSING CARE 13-4

Patients' and Families' Misperceptions About Hospice and Palliative Care: Listen as They Speak

Late referrals to hospice continue to be a common occurrence. This article examines the issue of late referrals to palliative care and hospice for individuals facing life-limiting disease/illness. The study had two purposes: To examine barriers to timely referral to palliative care and to explore the impact of late referral on the quality of life for palliative care patients and their families (p. 107). The author used a phenomenological research design with qualitative interviews of 13 patients and six family members completed. Interviews were tape recorded, transcribed, and analyzed. Patients and family members reported lack of knowledge about palliative care services and its benefits. This researcher concluded that patients and families experience unnecessary burden when referral to palliative care is delayed. This study provides additional incentive for nurses to be persistent in listening to and advocating for what families and patients say about end-of-life care. This information can be used to plan comprehensive teaching about the benefits of palliative and hospice care.

From Melvin, C. (2010). Patients' and families' misperceptions about hospice and palliative care: Listen as they speak. *Journal of Hospice & Palliative Nursing, 12*(2), 107–115. doi:10.1097/NJH.0b013e3181cf7933.

the client in a nursing home for a few days. Hospice-trained volunteers provide emotional and physical support for clients and families by assisting with transportation, household care, child care, errands, and companionship. Volunteers also provide a vital link between the client and health care providers.

THE ROLE OF THE NURSE

Death with dignity is the dictum of hospice as the focus of care shifts to palliative care and strengthening the client and family's quality of life as the client faces death. The goal of hospice in the home is to make the dying process as dignified as possible while providing physical, emotional, and spiritual comfort. Nursing care strives to assist the client and family to define their needs at the end stages of life and to have the resources necessary to carry out their wishes. Home hospice care means individuals can remain in the comfort of their own home, surrounded by family and loved ones, and die peacefully without fear of major medical intervention and resuscitative measures.

The specific role of the nurse varies according to the client's diagnosis and the wishes of the client and family. It is clear that the client is vulnerable at this time, and family members are vulnerable as their loved one is dying. It is very important in this specialization that the nurse is skilled in therapeutic communication and responsive to psychological needs. It is common for the client to experience anxiety, depression, and delirium at the end of life. Each of these conditions can occur as a result of the primary disease, concurrent physical conditions, inadequate pain management, medication side effects, or a combination of all of these.

End-of-life care requires sharp assessment skills to determine necessary delegated medical functions and comfort measures. It is essential that all hospice nurses are knowledgeable about various types of pain management techniques in order to anticipate medication needs. As in any situation providing direct physical and psychological care; the nurse must carefully assess the particular needs of the client, family members, and caregivers. This assessment should be holistic as well as follow the main premises of this book. In other words, the nurse should consider the needs of the client within the context of his or her family, culture, and community. Transcultural nursing principles is an important consideration as the nurse assists families in the decision-making process (Research in Community-Based Nursing Care 13-5).

Even at the end of life, the focus of care should be on maximizing the quality of life for the individual through health promotion and disease prevention. For example, the simple

---

RESEARCH IN COMMUNITY-BASED NURSING CARE 13-5

Factors That Impact End-of-Life Decision Making in African Americans With Advanced Cancer

There is disparity in the use of end of life care between African Americans and Whites with African Americans less likely to use hospice and more likely to die in the hospital. There is a lack of research exploring the factors that lead African Americans to choose options for end-of-life care. A qualitative, descriptive design study interviewed two groups of African Americans with advanced-stage cancer. The researchers discovered that end-of-life decisions were largely guided by clinical factors including: patient-related physical, emotional, and cognitive symptoms stemming from the underlying disease or medical treatments. The health care provider most likely to be involved in the decision making with patients, family members, and caregivers continues to be the physician. Individual factors including personal beliefs influenced this process. Religion and spirituality did not consistently influence decision making while personal beliefs did. The researchers recommended that future studies should explore in depth with family members, caregivers, and health care professionals factors that impact end-of-life decision making.

From Campbell, C., Williams, I., & Orr, T. (2010). Factors that impact end-of-life decision making in African Americans with advanced cancer. *Journal of Hospice & Palliative Nursing, 12*(4), 214–224. doi:10.1097/NJH.0b013e3181de1174.

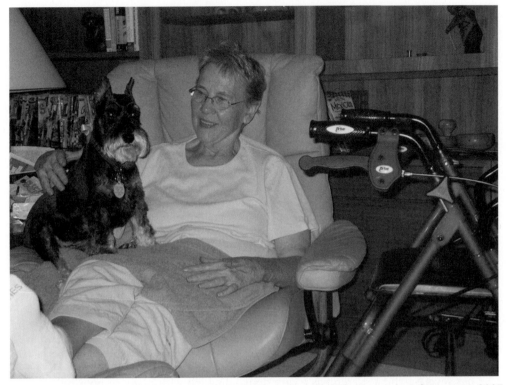

Figure 13-3 Pet therapy provides comfort and support at the end of life. Copyright Roberta Hunt, 2007.

intervention of good hand washing can prevent an infection that could cause pain and suffering during the client's last days. Encouraging activity that the client finds pleasurable promotes health, even when death is near. For instance, if the client enjoys animals, pet therapy may provide benefit (Fig. 13-3). Planning for medication needs to always ensure an adequate supply of meds is another role in comfort care with end-of-life care. These situations should be anticipated before such a need arises by careful advance planning and assessment. Hospice nursing requires excellent pain management skills. Adequate pain relief is assured by the following measures:

- Obtaining and maintaining a standing order for analgesia that incorporates consideration of increasing pain levels
- Assessing for all causes of pain, including anxiety, positioning, and environment
- Documenting every medication dose and any changes in dose, response to medication, and nonpharmacologic interventions that are effective for pain relief for this individual

Following the death of the client, bereavement counseling and support for the family continue for a year. Spiritual counseling is a common aspect of care. Spirituality expressed through the religious beliefs of the client and family can be a useful tool in the care of people who are dying.

TRENDS IN HOSPICE CARE

Public and political consciousness, allocation of research dollars to end-of-life issues, emphasis on personal choice, and increased public awareness of the limits of medical technology have all amplified interest in hospice care. Recognition of the importance of pain management, along with an increase in collaboration between palliative care and hospice, has also contributed to increased availability and quality of pain management in hospice care. It is anticipated that hospice care will assume an even more important role in community-based care in the future (HAA, 2010).

CLIENT SITUATIONS IN PRACTICE

Maria's Story of Transcultural Nursing in Hospice Care

I work for a home care agency that provides various specialized services. Most of my work is in infusion therapy and hospice care. Several years ago, I cared for a woman who was Chinese American. Up to that point, I had never worked with an individual with this cultural background. The experience was so interesting while at the same time challenging and frustrating that I decided I wanted to develop my skills in transcultural nursing.

I met May Lin on December 21. I remember the date because she did not have a Christmas tree in her home and I concluded that May Lin was probably not Christian. I learned from the referral that May Lin was 76 years old and a widow. She had been diagnosed with breast cancer the prior January. She had a mastectomy, three rounds of chemotherapy, and radiation. In the last 3 months, she had visited the clinic multiple times because she was losing weight, was unable to eat, and was also very run down from the chemotherapy treatment. The referral I received was for TPN infusion twice a day via central line. The treatment plan was to teach a family member to do the infusions on the first visit. I would continue to monitor May Lin a few times a week.

She appeared to understand what I was saying to her but she spoke limited English. She was, however, able to communicate most of her needs and answer the questions on the admission form. In the intake interview, I learned that May Lin moved to the United States in 1960. For 30 years, she and her husband owned and ran a restaurant in the Chinese community where they lived in a large metropolitan city. She told me that she is the mother of two adult children. Her son, Alex, is a business lawyer with a busy practice and lived several states away from May Lin. Her daughter, Karen, lives in an apartment about 10 minutes from May Lin. Karen, a physician and neuroscientist has two teenage children, one of whom has severe asthma. Karen has a very demanding job with many responsibilities as the head of an academic department in a large university. Karen's husband had a stroke 1 year prior to her mother becoming ill. He is no longer working and had significant physical limitations.

Karen was unable to be present at the first home visit. Her son had suffered a severe exacerbation of asthma triggered from the respiratory flu the night before and she had to take him to the emergency department. Subsequent to this visit, he was hospitalized for several days. The treatment plan to teach Karen to do the infusions would not be possible for at least another week. The first visit went well, with one exception. May Lin was experiencing pain in her back. She was very stoic about the pain, and I only learned about it when I noticed that when she sat down or changed positions she grimaced. When I asked if she was having pain, she denied it at first. When she continued to show nonverbal evidence of pain, and I asked again if she was uncomfortable, she admitted that she had been having severe pain for several months. I suggested she try a heating pad to relieve the discomfort and make an appointment to see her oncologist later in the week.

The next week, Karen became ill with the flu. Due to May Lin's compromised immune system, Karen and I decided that I would do the treatment for the next week. We scheduled a teaching session with the expectation that Karen would begin to do the infusions before and after work. During the visits in the second week, May Lin continued to move very carefully, as if she was experiencing considerable discomfort with any movement. When she tried to sit during the infusion, she would frequently adjust positions as if it were impossible to be comfortable. I asked if she had seen her oncologist or made an appointment about her back pain. She indicated that she had not. When I asked if she was having any difficulties sleeping, she indicated that she was. I asked her if she would like my assistance to call her physician's office, and she indicated that she did. I dialed the number and assisted her in making the appointment for the beginning of the next week.

The next week, Karen called and said that she was not able to come to the teaching visit to learn about the central line. Her husband had fallen and broken his foot. I told her about her mother's back pain and that we had set up an appointment for her to see her physician. Karen indicated that she would accompany her mother to the visit.

A week later, I received a referral from the oncologist's office that May Lin's plan of care had changed. The pain in her back was bone cancer. A magnetic resonance image scan revealed extensive disease, with a large questionable area in her liver. Liver function tests had been done, but the results were not yet available. I was to continue the infusion therapy. The family had been given information about hospice care. I was to follow-up to determine if the family had any questions about hospice.

I went to May Lin's home that day to teach Karen about the infusions. When I asked May Lin about how the clinic visit went, she said it went fine and that the pain in her back was from arthritis. Puzzled that May Lin had reached a conclusion very different from the one that I had about her conditions, I looked at Karen. She did not make eye contact. I was perplexed and decided I would follow up with a phone call.

The next day, I called Karen and asked what the physician had told them about the results of the tests and what her understanding was about the source of her mother's back pain. She indicated that the physician had told her that May Lin had widespread bone cancer and her liver function tests were abnormal. The physician stated that her disease was very advanced, and there was no chemotherapy available for her condition. I told her that her mother told me that the source of the pain was arthritis. I asked her if she thought that her mother understood what the physician had told them, and she said, "My brother and I did not tell mother that she has a terminal disease." I was shocked and concerned by this news but I knew that I would abide by Karen's desire not to inform her mother for the time being.

I continued to care for May Lin as her primary nurse. Increasingly, I was bothered by the fact that May Lin did not know that she was terminally ill. Why would this family choose not to inform their mother about her condition? Was this situation where a client is not informed about her condition ethical? Was I enabling the family to hide information from their mother, thus also practicing without following ethical practice guidelines? I decided to call Karen and meet with her. I could not continue to support the family's desires without considering my client's rights and interests. It appeared to me that she needed an advocate.

When Karen and I met, I asked her, "Tell me about how you made the decision not to tell your mother about her diagnosis." She replied, "In my family's culture sharing a terminal diagnosis is unnecessarily cruel. My mother holds traditional Chinese values, and telling her that she has a terminal illness would be impolite and disrespectful." I was shocked by her response. While I had concluded that this family was secretive or denying their mother's condition and not advocating for their mother, rather their reaction stemmed from a norm in their culture that was inconsistent from what is considered "best practice" in my own culture. At that moment, I realized how dominant cultural norms are to one's worldview. I had scrutinized this family's reaction through my own definition of the "right way" and made assumptions without clarifying on what basis this family had made this judgment.

I continued in my role as May Lin's primary nurse and cared for her until her death (Fig. 13-4).

There were several decisions related to May Lin's care that were debated in the next 3 months. Asian families are often patriarchal, which was true for May Lin's family. This meant that despite the fact that Karen was the primary family caregiver and a physician, Alex, May Lin's son, was the family decision maker in May Lin's end-of-life decisions. Although this meant a somewhat cumbersome communication process and patience on the part of the hospice nurses, it worked for the family. When it came to decisions related to do-not-resuscitate (DNR), Karen provided Alex with many resources to educate him about the advantages and disadvantages. At first, Alex was opposed to suspending any treatments but, in the end, decided that May Lin should have a DNR order, to suspend any life-prolonging treatments, and shift to palliative care. May Lin died a peaceful death at home, with her son and daughter at her side. Karen said, "Mother's death was dignified and the type of death she wanted."

Trends in Specialized Home Care

In the next 5 years, health care reform requires reimbursement changes are projected to increase demand for home health care ("Reimbursement changes to affect all home

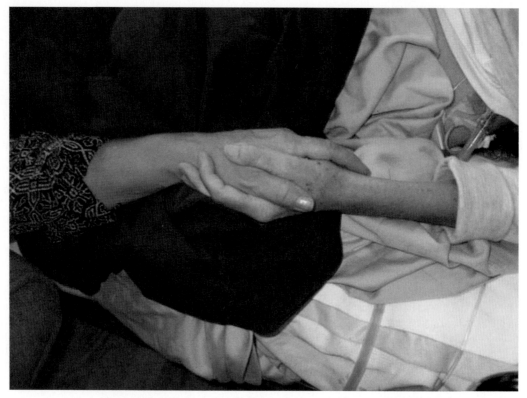

Figure 13-4 Comfort at end of life. Copyright Stephen Hunt, 2011.

health services," 2010). In the future, the way home care is provided may change, but more individuals will have health insurance, increasing access to services such as home care. Health care reform penalizes hospitals for preventable readmissions, creating incentive for collaboration between hospitals and home care agencies and other providers. Given that chronic conditions are frequently the reason for hospital readmissions, there will be more demand for community-based chronic care management programs that keep people at home. These types of services will be well positioned to work in partnerships with hospitals and insurance companies.

Conclusions

Both specialized home care and hospice care will be important settings for practice in the future. The client advocate role will continue to be a central element of community care as complexity of health care delivery and concern for cost-containment continue. Flexibility and accountability will remain fundamental as the pressure to meet professional practice standards intersects with pressure to contain costs. Challenges facing home care will require that the nurse keep up with ever-changing regulations regarding coverage, the documentation requirements that will follow, and the evolving certification requirements for nurses in these specialties. In addition, nurses will be called on to teach and support clients and families because of increasing responsibility for caring for acutely ill family members at home. As in all nursing specialties, it will be vital for specialized home care and hospice nurses to welcome the increased use of technology. Likewise, the need for well-honed skills in chronic care management will continue to accelerate. Balancing "high tech" and "high touch" will continue to be the practice imperative in all areas of specialized home care.

What's on the Web

American Society for Pain Management Nursing (ASPMN)
INTERNET ADDRESS: http://www.aspmn.org/
This organization of nurses is dedicated to promoting and providing optimal care for individuals with pain, including the management of its sequelae. All of this is accomplished through education, standards, advocacy, and research. Online education modules can be found on this site.

Infusion Nurses Society
INTERNET ADDRESS: http:/www.ins1.org/
INS promotes excellence in infusion nursing through standards, education, advocacy, and outcome research. They are committed to supporting access to the highest quality, cost-effective infusion care for all individuals. INS achieves this mission by providing opportunities for advanced knowledge and expertise through professional development and resource networking.

Wound, Ostomy and Continence Nurse Society
INTERNET ADDRESS: http://www.wocn.org/
The WOCN Society is a professional nursing society that supports its members by promoting educational, clinical, and research opportunities to advance the practice and guide the delivery of expert health care to individuals with wounds, ostomies, and incontinence.

Pediatric Home Care Association of America (PedHCAA)
INTERNET ADDRESS: http://www.nahc.org/PedHCAA/home.html
This site provides valuable information about this affiliate of the National Association for Home Care and Hospice (NAHC). One of the goals of this organization is to strengthen communication between pediatric hospices and home care providers. It also represents the interests of pediatric hospice and home care providers before the U.S. Congress and regulatory bodies. Another goal is to develop pediatric resources and educational opportunities at national, regional, and local organization meetings.

End-of-Life Educational Consortium (ELNEC)
INTERNET ADDRESS: http://www.aacn.nche.edu/ELNEC/about.htm
This site provides nursing educators with training in end-of-life care. Content includes a module devoted to cultural consideration.

References and Bibliography

American Nurses Association. (1999). *ANA's core principles on telehealth.* Retrieved from http://www.acnpweb.org/i4a/pages/index.cfm?pageid=3471

American Telemedicine Association. (2010). *Telemedicine defined.* Retrieved from http://www.americantelemed.org/i4a/pages/index.cfm?pageid=3333

Anderson, B. (2010). The benefits to nurse-led telephone follow-up for prostate cancer. *British Journal of Nursing, 19*(17), 1085–1090. Retrieved from CINAHL Plus with Full Text database.

Basso, O., Rasmussen, S., Weinberg, C. R., Wilcox, A. J., Irgens, L. M., & Skjaerven, R. (2006). Trends in fetal and infant survival following preeclampsia. *JAMA, 296*(6), 1357–1362.

Bennett, M., Closs, S., & Chatwin, J. (2009). Cancer pain management at home, I: Do older patients experience less effective management than younger patients? *Supportive Care in Cancer, 17*(7), 787–792. Retrieved from CINAHL Plus with Full Text database.

Berberabe, T. (2010). Home infusion therapy covered well by insurers. *Managed Care, 19*(7), 8–10. Retrieved from CINAHL Plus with Full Text database.

Bott, D., Kapp, M., Johnson, L., & Magno, L. (2009). Disease management for chronically ill beneficiaries in traditional Medicare. *Health Affairs, 28*(1), 86–98. doi:10.1377/hlthaff.28.1.86.

Bowles, K., Pham, J., O'Connor, M., & Horowitz, D. (2010). Information deficits in home care: A barrier to evidence-based disease management. *Home Health Care Management & Practice, 22*(4), 278–285. doi:10.1177/1084822309353145.

Bradley, M., & Rivera, J. (2010). Development and implementation of an advanced wound management class: Preparing for OASIS-C. *Home Healthcare Nurse, 28*(3), 154–166. Retrieved from CINAHL Plus with Full Text database.

Campbell, C., Williams, I., & Orr, T. (2010). Factors that impact end-of-life decision making in African Americans with advanced cancer. *Journal of Hospice & Palliative Nursing, 12*(4), 214–224. doi:10.1097/NJH.0b013e3181de1174.

Cervasio, K. (2010). The role of the pediatric home healthcare nurse: One case study approach in New York City. *Home Healthcare Nurse, 28*(7), 424–431. Retrieved from CINAHL Plus with Full Text database.

Closs, S., Chatwin, J., & Bennett, M. (2009). Cancer pain management at home, II: Does age influence attitudes towards pain and analgesia? *Supportive Care in Cancer, 17*(7), 781–786. Retrieved from CINAHL Plus with Full Text database.

Craven, R., & Hirnle, C. (2009). *Fundamentals of nursing: Human health and function.* Philadelphia, PA: Lippincott Williams & Wilkins.

Cross, M. (2006). Pregnancy + birth = $$$. *Managed Care.* February. Retrieved from http://www.managedcaremag.com/archives/0602/0602.birthcosts.html

Disease management programs. (2010). Retrieved on http://www.andreini.com/PDFs/Disease_Management_Programs.pdf

Eckenrode, J., Campa, M., Luckey, D., Henderson, C., Cole, R., Kitzman, H., et al. (2010). Long-term effects of prenatal and infancy nurse home visitation on the life course of youths: 19-year follow-up of a randomized trial. *Archives of Pediatrics & Adolescent Medicine, 164*(1), 9–15. Retrieved from CINAHL Plus with Full Text database.

Gibson, P., & Carlson, M. (2010). *Hypertension and pregnancy.* Retrieved from http://emedicine.medscape.com/article/261435-overview

Greener, M. (2010). A new approach to wound management. *Nurse Prescribing, 8*(4), 169–172. Retrieved from CINAHL Plus with Full Text database.

Hachizuka, M., Yoshiuchi, K., Yamamoto, Y., Iwase, S., Nakagawa, K., Kawagoe, K., et al. (2010). Development of a personal digital assistant (PDA) system to collect symptom information from home hospice patients. *Journal of Palliative Medicine, 13*(6), 647–651. doi:10.1089/jpm.2009.0350.

Hindelang, M. (2006). Caring for wounds: More than just cuts and scrapes. *Home Healthcare Nurse, 24*(2), 112–114.

Hospice Association of America. (2010). *Hospice facts and statistics.* Retrieved from http://www.nahc.org/facts/HospiceStats10.pdf

Hummel, P., & Cronin, J. (2004). Home care of the high-risk infant. *Advances in Neonatal Care, 4,* 354–364.

Joint INS/INCC Position Paper. (2009). The value of certification in infusion nursing. *Journal of Infusion Nursing, 32*(5), 248–250. Retrieved from CINAHL Plus with Full Text database.

Kitzman, H., Olds, D., Cole, R., Hanks, C., Anson, E., Arcoleo, K., et al. (2010). Enduring effects of prenatal and infancy home visiting by nurses on children: Follow-up of a randomized trial among children at age 12 years. *Archives of Pediatrics & Adolescent Medicine, 164*(5), 412–418. Retrieved from CINAHL Plus with Full Text database.

Lewis, M., & Pontin, D. (2008). Caseload management in community children's nursing. *Paediatric Nursing, 20*(3), 18–22. Retrieved from CINAHL Plus with Full Text database.

Lorentz, M. (2008). Telenursing and home healthcare: The many facets of technology. *Home Healthcare Nurse, 26*(4), 237–243. Retrieved from CINAHL Plus with Full Text database.

Masoorli, S. (2005). Legal issues related to vascular access devices and infusion therapy. *Journal of Infusion Nursing, 28*(3, Suppl), S18–S21.

Melvin, C. (2010). Patients' and families' misperceptions about hospice and palliative care: Listen as they speak. *Journal of Hospice & Palliative Nursing, 12*(2), 107–115. doi:10.1097/NJH.0b013e3181cf7933.

Nanneth, G., & Abbate, B. (2008). Home enteral nutrition and organizing models: Organization and risks of pediatric home enteral nutrition. *Nutritional Therapy & Metabolism, 26*(1), 32–35. Retrieved from CINAHL Plus with Full Text database.

National Center for Complementary and Alternative Medicine. (2010). *Mind-body medicine: An overview.* Retrieved from http://nccam.nih.gov/health/whatiscam/

National Institute of Neurological Disorders and Stroke. (2010). *Pain: Hope through research.* Retrieved from http://www.ninds.nih.gov/disorders/chronic_pain/detail_chronic_pain.htm?css=

National Institutes of Health. *Fact sheet: Pain management.* Retrieved from http://www.nih.gov/about/researchresultsforthepublic/Pain.pdf

Olds, D., Kitzman, H., Cole, R., Hanks, C., Arcoleo, K., Anson, E., et al. (2010). Enduring effects of prenatal and infancy home visiting by nurses on maternal life course and government spending: Follow-up of a randomized trial among children at age 12 years. *Archives of Pediatrics & Adolescent Medicine, 164*(5), 419–424. Retrieved from CINAHL Plus with Full Text database.

Oliver, D., Wittenberg-Lyles, E., Demiris, G., Washington, K., Porock, D., & Day, M. M. (2008). Barriers to pain management: caregiver perceptions and pain talk by hospice interdisciplinary teams. *Journal of Pain & Symptom Management, 36*(4), 374–382. Retrieved from EBSCOhost.

Reimbursement changes to affect all home health services. (2010). *Hospital Home Health, 27*(6), 61–64. Retrieved from CINAHL Plus with Full Text database.

Rennert, R., Golinko, M., Kaplan, D., Flattau, A., & Brem, H. (2009). Clinical concepts: Standardization of wound photography using the Wound Electronic Medical Record. *Advances in Skin & Wound Care, 22*(1), 32–38. Retrieved from CINAHL Plus with Full Text database.

Reichmann, J. (2009). Home uterine activity monitoring: An evidence review of its utility in multiple gestations. *Journal of Reproductive Medicine, 54*(9), 559–562. Retrieved from CINAHL Plus with Full Text database.

Rosenzweig, J., Taitel, M., Norman, G., Moore, T., Turenne, W., & Tang, P. (2010). Diabetes disease management in Medicare Advantage reduces hospitalizations and costs. *American Journal of Managed Care, 16*(7), e157–62. Retrieved from CINAHL Plus with Full Text database.

Ruder, S. (2010). Seven tools to assist hospice and home care clinicians in pain management at end of life. *Home Healthcare Nurse, 28*(8), 458–470. Retrieved from CINAHL Plus with Full Text database.

Schlachta-Fairchild, L., Elfrink, V., & Deickman, A. (2009) Patient safety, telenursing, and telehealth. In: *Patient safety and quality: An evidence-based handbook for nurses* (AHRQ Publication No. 08-0043). Rockville, MD: Agency for Healthcare Research and Quality.. Retrieved from http://www.ahrq.gov/qual/nurseshdbk/

Stephenson, N., Dalton, J., Carlson, J., Youngblood, R., & Bailey, D. (2009). Racial and ethnic disparities in cancer pain management. *Journal of National Black Nurses Association, 20*(1), 11–18. Retrieved from CINAHL Plus with Full Text database.

Temple, P., Lutenbacher, M., & Vitale, J. (2008). Limited access to care and home healthcare. *Clinical Obstetrics & Gynecology, 51*(2), 371–384. Retrieved from CINAHL Plus with Full Text database.

Vallerand, A., Hasenau, S., & Templin, T. (2010). Improving cancer pain management in the home. *Journal of Pain Management, 3*(1), 41–51. Retrieved from CINAHL Plus with Full Text database.

Weber, J., & Kelley, J. (2009). *Health assessment in nursing* (4th ed.). Philadelphia, PA: Lippincott Williams & Wilkins.

Wiggins, S. (2009). Family exemplars during implementation of a home pain management intervention. *Issues in Comprehensive Pediatric Nursing, 32*(4), 160–179. Retrieved from CINAHL Plus with Full Text database.

Wingert, S. (2010). Meeting the unique needs of the pediatric home care patient—Lessons from a full-service provider. *Infusion, 16*(5), 21–25. Retrieved from CINAHL Plus with Full Text database.

LEARNING ACTIVITIES

JOURNALING ACTIVITY 13-1

In your clinical journal, respond to the following questions.

1. Discuss your own attitudes and beliefs regarding pain control. How do you think your own assumptions and beliefs could impact the way that you provide pain control for your clients? What do you think that you can do to prevent your own attitudes about pain from interfering with the needs of your clients?

2. How would you handle pain control for someone who is a self-reported drug addict? What issues do you think could arise? What would you do to address these issues?

3. Discuss what you thought was important content in Chapter 13 and how it fits into what you have learned so far about the role of the nurse in the community.

4. How has your view of the nursing role in the community changed after reading this chapter (and observing a specialized role of the nurse in the community)?

CLIENT CARE ACTIVITY 13-2

Maureen is a 57-year-old widow who was referred to hospice home care. She was diagnosed with liver cancer 3 months ago. After extensive surgery and chemotherapy, she is not improving. Her referral states that she has almost constant pain. Her daughter lives in another state and has three preschool children. Her son is living temporarily in Africa for 6 months. You are the home care nurse doing the admission intake by following the agency forms. However, you have some particular concerns that are not addressed in the intake form given what you read on Maureen's referral form:

1. On what do you concentrate assessment beyond the admission form?

2. What questions do you use to assess these issues?

3. What combination of interventions do you use to help keep Maureen comfortable (both pharmacologic and other methods)?

4. What safety considerations do you have and how do you assess them?

PRACTICAL APPLICATION ACTIVITY 13-3

Contact an agency that employs nurses to work in one of the roles described in this chapter. Arrange to observe a nurse working in the setting. After the observation, arrange for a short interview with the nurse. Develop several questions before the observation and interview. You may decide to use some of the following questions as a part of the interview:

1. What do you enjoy about this type of work?

2. What is difficult?

3. How has the role changed over the last 5 years? 10 years?

4. How do you use the concept of self-care in your practice?

5. What place does health promotion and disease prevention have in your daily work?

6. What do you need to know about families, culture, and community to do this type of work?

7. What type of special training is now required or would you recommend in preparation to perform this specialized role?

8. Do you have any recommendations for a new graduate who may be interested in entering this type of work in the future?

   ▪ Send a thank you note to the nurse and agency after the visit. (Not only is this a great strategy for getting a job in the future, but you are also building goodwill with people you may work with in the future in the community. It is also just plain good manners.)

   ▪ Summarize your observation and interview in a 2-to 3-page paper.

PRACTICAL APPLICATION ACTIVITY 13-4

Find an article or book on the Internet on CINAHL or MEDLINE about one of the specialized settings and roles from the chapter that interests you. Get the article or book (pick a chapter) and respond to the following:

1. What was the main point of the article or chapter from the book?

2. What did you think was the most important aspect of the article or chapter for your learning?

3. How do you think that you can use this new information in the future?

CLINICAL REASONING ACTIVITY 13-5

Identify a topic related to one of the specialized home care settings or roles discussed in this chapter. If you have discovered a specialized home care role not included in the chapter, it can also be used as the topic for this activity. Some examples could be the following:

1. Should certification be required to practice in the specialty home care roles (e.g., pain management, infusion nursing, pediatric home care, high-risk obstetrics home care, hospice home care)?

2. What are the current issues in one of the settings or roles? (e.g., in high-risk home care, one issue is whether home uterine monitoring prevents preterm birth. In pediatric home care, one issue is how to work with the parents to plan and implement care.)

3. How has the nursing shortage impacted these specialized roles?

4. What issues related to reimbursement impact the availability of specialized care?

Chapter 14

Mental Health Nursing in Community-Based Settings

BARBARA CHAMPLIN

Learning Objectives

1. Describe the historical evolution of the care and treatment of people with mental illnesses.

2. Discuss the significance of caring for people with mental illnesses in the community.

3. Describe the characteristics and behaviors associated with the major mental illnesses.

4. Review the components of a mental health assessment.

5. Define the nursing skills and competencies needed in community-based mental health care.

6. Describe community-based mental health care for selected vulnerable populations.

7. Identify agencies that serve people with mental illnesses and their caregivers.

8. Summarize the challenges to providing successful community-based mental health care.

key Terms

deinstitutionalize
institutionalization
mental health assessment
psychotropic medications

suicidal ideation
serious mental illness
stigma
vulnerable populations

Chapter Topics

Historical Perspectives

Significance of Community Mental Health

Nursing Competencies and Skills in Mental Health Nursing

Mental Health Assessment

Community-Based Mental Health Care With Vulnerable Populations

Community Mental Health Agencies and Related Services

Challenges to Successful Community-Based Mental Health Care

Conclusions

The Nurse Speaks

We have a behavioral unit in the county health and human services department in a rural community. In my role as a psychiatric nurse clinician in this community-based service, I follow about 25 to 30 clients on a regular basis and a number of others periodically. One young man had multiple inpatient hospitalizations and a psychotic break that resulted in aggression toward another person. Additionally, he would experience profound depressive episodes and had planned suicide on numerous occasions. When I began seeing this client he was working remotely with a psychiatrist and a social worker. He saw me every 2 weeks for a depot antipsychotic injection and to pick up mediplanners filled with many psychotropic medications. In the beginning he was quiet and guarded, but over time we began to talk. Through care collaboration we narrowed down his huge array of medications eliminating five medications. Over 1½ years we talked about our families and our goals. He wished to have a family one day. He had begun losing weight and had been symptom free for over 1 year. I was supportive of him managing his own medications, and there were plans of discontinuing the injection.

Everything was going in the right direction until I came to work one morning to discover that my client had used a gun to take his life. There was no note. He had been completely compliant and optimistic regarding treatment recommendations. We had rescheduled his injection and made a plan regarding his next psychiatry appointment in 1 month. I was completely blind-sided! What could I have done differently? Why did he do it? How long had he known? How impulsive had his decision been to end his life?

All I know is how much I miss him and our brief encounters. Our therapeutic relationship had grown so much over time. Despite this tragic outcome, his death has only reinforced how much I love my job. I so enjoy working with these clients and the complexity of their symptoms and of their lives. I like to think I made some difference in his life and that the positive progress he appeared to be making was real. Unfortunately, one of the most dangerous times for these clients is when they are truly on the road to recovery. Hopefully, in the future a client such as this will make a phone call first and who knows, perhaps it will be to me.

Sommer Charles, RN
Marin County Health and Human Services

Historical Perspectives

In primitive cultures, the pervasive belief was that mental illnesses were caused by forces acting outside of the body. As a result of these beliefs, treatments included things such as rituals, magic, and exorcisms, all of which were intended to rid the body of evil spirits and cure the victim of their mental illness. When these efforts failed, people with mental illnesses were viewed as outcasts and were to be feared.

Throughout the 17th and 18th centuries, people with mental illnesses continued to be treated in brutal and inhumane ways. Maltreatment included things such as confining people with mental illnesses in cages, chaining them to walls, running them out of town, and beating them into submission. Often people who exhibited unusual behaviors were viewed as witches, demons, or devils. Thus, witchcraft, demonology, and sorcery were employed as treatments. Additionally, at this time there was a sharp contrast in care that was based on whether or not a person had the financial means to seek care for mental illnesses. Those who did not have money were rejected by society.

Early in the 19th century, the interest in providing more humane care to people with mental illnesses grew. During this time, people with mental illnesses were segregated in large state-funded institutions. Initially, the belief was that **institutionalization** would allow for more humane care and treatment, and that in time people would be "cured" and return to live in the community. However, this ideal was never recognized and in time the institutions became overcrowded and inadequately staffed.

The 20th century brought the move to **deinstitutionalize** people with mental illnesses. It was believed that people with mental illnesses had the right to live freely in the community and that care in the community would be less expensive. In addition, there had been pharmacological advances in the treatment of mental illnesses and federal monies had been designated to establish community mental health centers, both of which would help facilitate treatment in the community. Unfortunately, people who were released from the institutions were inadequately prepared for life in the community and the vision of creating multiple community health centers never materialized. Thus, once again, meeting the care needs of people with mental illnesses fell short of the initial vision.

Today, the struggle continues for how to best meet the needs of people with mental illnesses living in the community. Despite severe cuts in state and federal programs, the current trend is to provide care in the community, with hospitalization for acute exacerbation of symptoms and then only if the individual is deemed dangerous to one's self or others. Recent advances in research support an understanding of mental illnesses as diseases of the brain which, along with other treatment modalities, can be successfully treated with **psychotropic medications**.

The impact of early care, institutionalization, and deinstitutionalization all influenced how people with mental illnesses are cared for at the present time. Prior to reform, the aim of treatment was to drive the mental illness out of the person or to drive the person out of the community. As treatment of people with mental illnesses became more humane, reforms first brought institutionalization and then deinstitutionalization. Today, most people with mental illnesses reside in and receive health care in community-based settings. The 21st century brings an opportunity for community health nurses to play a significant role in ensuring that successful care and treatment is provided to all people with mental illnesses.

Significance of Community Mental Health

Historically, in Western medicine, the mind and body have been treated as separate entities. More recently the mind–body connection has been made and mental and physical functions are seen as parts of a whole. The U.S. Congress declared the 1990s the "Decade of the Brain," and mental illnesses were viewed as brain disorders. Current advances in research support a neurobiological view of mental illness. Examples of risk factors that contribute to mental illnesses are shown in Box 14-1.

The Surgeon General's Report (1999) on mental health estimates that approximately 20% of the U.S. adult population is affected by mental disorders during a given year (U.S. Department of Health and Human Services, Office of the Surgeon General, 1999a). The report also estimates the annual prevalence of mental disorders in children and adolescents to be about 20% of that population (U.S. Department of Health and Human Services, Office of the Surgeon General, 1999a). A subpopulation of about 5.4% of mentally ill adults is considered to have a **serious mental illness** (U.S. Department of Health and

---

BOX 14-1   **Examples of Risk Factors That Contribute to Mental Illnesses**

Biologic/genetic factors: having other biological relatives with mental illnesses.
Socioeconomic factors: poverty, economic hardship, overcrowded living conditions.
Environmental factors: head injury, poor nutrition, exposure to toxins (lead and tobacco smoke), exposure to viruses in utero.
Social factors: severe parental discord, history of parental mental illness, abuse, neglect, criminal history of parents, death of family member or close friend, divorce, exposure to violence, chronic medical conditions, lack of friendships/healthy relationships, combat, or exposure to other traumatic events.

Human Services, Office of the Surgeon General, 1999b). This means that one out of every five people in the United States has a mental illness. Although statistics are not readily available, the prevalence is believed to be similar internationally.

The cost of inpatient mental health treatment has come to the forefront with a move away from high-cost, hospital-based treatment to community-based care of people with mental illnesses. Health insurance and the economic challenges of payment for mental health services continue to move toward greater reimbursement of community mental health services. Consequently, today the majority of mental health issues are dealt with in the community and the need for community mental health nurses continues to grow.

Based on the prevalence of mental illnesses and the location of care in community-based settings, well-prepared community health nurses are in demand. Successful provision of community-based mental health nursing care requires a broad knowledge base and understanding of mental illnesses.

Nursing Competencies and Skills in Mental Health Nursing

Nurses are bound by the Code of Ethics for Nurses (ANA Web site) to care for all people, including individuals, families, groups, and communities in a variety of settings. Nurses see clients with mental illnesses in hospitals, but also in clinics, schools, long-term care facilities, and elsewhere in the community. Thus, nurses working in all settings need to be knowledgeable and competent to work with individuals who have mental health issues.

Knowledge of the most prevalent mental illnesses is important in understanding the behaviors that are associated with mental illnesses. A guideline for diagnosing mental illnesses, published by the American Psychiatric Association (2000), is the *Diagnostic and Statistical Manual of Mental Disorders (DSM-IV-TR)*. The manual clarifies mental illnesses and provides diagnostic criteria for approximately 300 mental disorders. Although primarily developed as a tool for physicians, the information provided in the manual can also be useful for nurses as they plan care for their clients.

The Public Health Intervention Wheel as described in Chapter 2 is a practice model that is also useful in planning community-based mental health nursing care. Several of the public health interventions and examples of their application in the community are presented in Box 14-2. In addition to the examples provided, community health nurses can educate the general public about mental illnesses and develop policy that is intended to improve the lives of people with mental illnesses.

The proposed Healthy People 2020 objectives in the topic area of mental health and mental disorders can guide community health nurses as they plan care for their clients in community-based settings. The proposed objectives are listed in Box 14-3. The focus of the proposed objectives on health promotion and disease prevention fits well with the community nursing interventions as described in the Intervention Wheel. Specifically, the proposed objectives emphasize assessment of depression and suicidality, access to care and treatment, and the need to increase services to **vulnerable populations** such as individuals who are experiencing homelessness, children and adolescents, elderly populations, and people with diverse cultural beliefs and practices.

In the next section, several of the most prevalent major mental disorders are discussed. Prevalence, signs and symptoms, assessment, and important community-based nursing interventions are included.

MAJOR DEPRESSIVE DISORDER

Major depressive disorder is one of the most common mood disorders. According to the National Institute of Mental Health Web site, major depressive disorder affects approximately 14.8 million adults, age 18 and older, in the United States in a given year. It is the leading cause of disability in the United States for ages 15 to 44. Major depressive disorder also occurs in children, adolescents, and the elderly. There is growing concern regarding depression in the elderly as high suicide rates are found in white men over age 65. It is

---

BOX 14-2 **Examples of Public Health Interventions in Community-Based Mental Health Nursing**

Screening: a community health nurse completes a depression screening inventory on each of the clients that she sees at a neighborhood health fair.

Referral and Follow-up: a community health nurse refers the spouse of her client to a support group in the community. The nurse follows-up regarding the referral on the next home visit.

Case Management: a community health nurse arranges for a tutor at school, homework help at home, and connects an adolescent client with homework help at the public library.

Delegated Functions: a community health nurse administers a depot injection of the client's prescribed antipsychotic medication on her home visit.

Health Teaching: a community health nurse completes medication teaching with the family members of a client who has recently been prescribed an antidepressant medication.

Counseling: a community health nurse facilitates a discussion of a client's feelings regarding the loss of her son in a motor vehicle accident.

Consultation: a community health nurse contacts a dental clinic to arrange for a free dental check-up for the client he sees at a local homeless shelter.

Collaboration: when a client expresses an interest in losing weight, a community health nurse makes arrangements for her to join an exercise class at the community center. In addition, she sets up a meeting with the dietitian at the clinic.

Advocacy: A community health nurses assists a client in filling out an application to participate in an after-school club.

---

important to note that many people who are experiencing depression do not seek help, although for most the illness can be successfully treated using a combination of treatment modalities.

Nurses need to be aware of the signs and symptoms of major depressive disorder. According to the *DSM-IV-TR*, the signs and symptoms include five of the following for at least 2 weeks: depressed mood or loss of interest or pleasure, weight loss or gain, insomnia or hypersomnia, psychomotor agitation or retardation, fatigue, feelings of worthlessness, and impaired concentration or thoughts of death/suicide. The symptoms may be mild to moderate and in some cases severe. Typically, a person will experience more than one episode of depression over his or her lifetime.

It is important that community health nurses complete a **mental health assessment** (see Box 14-6) with each of their clients. Doing so will reveal important information that may indicate major depressive disorder. In addition, nurses may elect to complete a depression rating scale. There are many depression rating scales that nurses can use to determine the intensity and severity of a client's depressive symptoms. One that is easily administered by a health care professional is the Beck Depression Inventory. It consists of a series of 21 questions and takes 5 to 10 minutes to complete. Each response is assigned a score, from zero to three. The sum of the item scores indicates the intensity of a person's depressive symptoms.

Nursing interventions in depression include assessing psychological and physical symptoms, maintaining a safe environment, and facilitating the expression of feelings. The overall goal is to increase coping and decrease a client's symptoms of depression. It is equally important to assess the client's resources and support systems as these things can be significant in successful recovery. Based on the biological view of major depressive disorder, current outpatient treatments for depression may include antidepressant medications such as selective serotonin reuptake inhibitors (SSRIs) or electroconvulsive therapy. Medication therapy or electroconvulsive therapy would be used in conjunction with other treatment modalities, that is, individual, family, or group therapy.

Proposed Healthy People 2020 Objectives: Mental Health and Mental Disorders

Objectives Retained As Is From Healthy People 2010:

1. Reduce the suicide rate.
2. Reduce the rate of suicide attempts by adolescents.
3. Increase the proportion of homeless adults with mental health problems who receive mental health services.
4. Reduce the proportion of adolescents who engage in disordered eating behaviors in an attempt to control their weight.
5. Increase the proportion of primary care facilities that provide mental health treatment onsite or by paid referral.
6. Increase the proportion of children with mental health problems who receive treatment.
7. Increase the proportion of juvenile residential facilities that screen new admissions for mental health problems.
8. Increase the proportion of counties served by community-based jail diversion programs and/or mental health courts for adults with mental health problems.
9. Increase the number of states and the District of Columbia that track consumers' satisfaction with the mental health services that they receive.
10. Increase the number of states, territories, and the District of Columbia with an operational mental health plan that addresses cultural competence.
11. Increase the number of states, territories, and the District of Columbia with an operational mental health plan that addresses specialized mental health services for elderly persons.
12. Increase the proportion of persons with serious mental illness (SMI) who are employed.

Objectives Retained But Modified From Healthy People 2010:

13. Increase the proportion of adults with mental disorders who receive treatment.
14. Increase the proportion of persons with co-occurring substance abuse and mental disorders who receive treatment for both disorders.

Objectives New to Healthy People 2020:

15. Increase depression screening by primary care providers.
16. Decrease the annual prevalence of major depressive episode (MDE).

From *Proposed Healthy People 2020 objectives: Mental health and mental disorders*. Retrieved July 31, 2010, from http://www.healthypeople.gov/hp2020/

Ongoing assessment of suicide is an important aspect of working with the depressed client. To be comfortable with suicide assessment, the nurse must address any misconceptions or fears he or she has about it. Suicidal thoughts or actions can occur at anytime in the course of depression. One important time in the course of treatment that is a high-risk period of time for suicidal clients is when they start on medications and begin to feel some energy. This energy can make them more vulnerable to the risk of acting on a suicidal plan. Awareness of the risk of suicide allows nurses to set up a safety plan for the client during his or her most vulnerable time. The next section addresses further aspects of suicide.

SUICIDAL BEHAVIORS

Suicide is a major preventable public health issue. In 2006, the National Institute of Mental Health identified suicide as the 11th leading cause of death in the United States. More men than women die by suicide as they typically select more lethal means such as hanging or using a firearm. It is important to note that the majority of people who kill themselves have a diagnosable mental illness, often depression or a substance abuse disorder. Other risk factors for suicide include a prior suicide attempt, family history of mental illnesses or suicide, family violence, and access to firearms.

Community health nurses are in a prime position to screen for **suicidal ideation** (thoughts of suicide) and behaviors. Signs to look for when assessing for suicide risk are recurrent thoughts of or preoccupation with death, ongoing suicidal ideation with or without a plan, a sense of hopelessness or a sudden change from being depressed to being upbeat. Other major factors are possession of the means to commit suicide and a history of or recent suicide attempt.

As a nurse, the first aspect of suicide assessment that must be understood is that asking someone if they are suicidal does not give them the idea, and it does not make a person any more likely to act on suicidal thoughts. Rather, it offers them an opportunity to talk about how they are feeling and to ask for help if needed. It may be reassuring to the person to know that there are resources and support available to them. If a client states that he or she has suicidal thoughts, the next question to ask is, does he or she have a plan? If the client says he or she has a plan, nurses need to ask about the plan, availability of the method, and lethality of the method. For example, a client who plans to shoot himself and owns a gun is at a high immediate risk compared to the client who tells the nurse that he or she wants to overdose but doesn't have ready access to the pills. If the client presents with a lethal method and a means, immediate hospitalization may be necessary. Examples of suicide assessment questions can be found in Box 14-4.

Nurses working in community-based settings can play an important role in the prevention of suicide. They can participate at the primary, secondary, and tertiary levels of prevention. For example, at the primary level of prevention, nurses can educate the general public about risk factors and warning signs, and suggest interventions. At the secondary level of prevention, nurses can work directly with clients who are suicidal to get them the necessary help to prevent suicide. And, at the tertiary level of prevention, they can intervene with friends and family members of people who have killed themselves to ensure that they receive the help and support needed to cope with the situation. Improving outreach to at-risk groups of people is also within the scope of the role of community health nurses. Lastly, nurses can be involved in policy development and enforcement that is aimed at suicide reduction and prevention.

BOX 14-4   Suicide Assessment Questions

General Questions

- Are you feeling like you want to hurt yourself?
- Are you feeling like ending it all?
- Do you have thoughts of wanting to end it all?
- Do you ever feel like it would be easier to not go on?
- Does this feel so overwhelming that you do not feel like living?

Additional Questions

- If there is an answer of yes to any of the above, additional questions are needed.
- How often do you feel this way?
- Have you had any thoughts about how you would end your life?
- What thoughts have you had about ending it all?
- When you feel this way, what do you feel like doing?

Assess Lethality

Assess how lethal the methods are and the availability of those methods.

Lethality has to do with how easy it is to rescue someone as well as what access he or she has to the means.

✳️ CLIENT SITUATIONS IN PRACTICE

Assessing suicidal ideation

The assessment of suicidal ideation can be challenging, especially in situations when clients do not directly state that they are feeling suicidal. I first met Richard, a 78-year-old Caucasian male, on a home visit. He had been diagnosed with lung cancer within the last year and had recently returned home following surgery.

Richard lives alone in a small house in a rural area. His wife died 2 years ago following a progressive debilitating illness. Richard has one daughter who lives out of state. He talks to her on the telephone about once a week, but she seldom visits due to her work schedule. The goals of my visit were to assess Richard's current condition and to follow up regarding his medication regimen.

Upon arrival for the weekly visit, I notice that the drapes on the front window are drawn and there are several newspapers sitting on the front porch. I knock several times before Richard answers the front door. He is still in his pajamas, although it is 2 PM, his hair is uncombed, and it appears that he has not shaved for several days. During the visit, Richard reports that he doesn't have much energy and has been sleeping a lot more. He adds that sometimes it is difficult for him to get out of bed. During the conversation, he states the following: "I miss my wife. We used to do so much together. It just is not the same without her." Later in the conversation he states, "Sometimes I feel like I am backed into a corner and I feel like there is no way out." Richard's vital signs are stable: BP 120/80 mm Hg, P 88, T 98.8, R 20, and his current weight is 155 lb (discharge weight was 167 lb).

During the visit, I place a call to Richard's daughter, Connie. She states that she has been concerned about her father because he has stopped calling her. Connie says that she has had contact with him on the phone two times since he was discharged from the hospital, but she initiated the calls. When she talks to him, she adds that he sounds down and says that he is not getting out of the house nor socializing with her friends from church, which he has done regularly in the past. In addition, she adds that sometimes when she talks to him, she has wondered if he has been drinking.

After completing a mental health assessment, I am concerned that Richard is depressed. **What risk factors support this?**
What data did I gather that support this?
Is Richard at risk for suicide?
I place a call to Richard's primary care physician.
What information should I include in my report to the physician?

POSTPARTUM DEPRESSION

Postpartum depression (PPD), a complication of childbearing, is a significant health concern affecting up to 20% of new mothers in a given year. It may occur within days of delivery or at any time in the next 12 to 18 months. The signs and symptoms include tearful episodes, fatigue, feeling overwhelmed, inability to concentrate, overconcern or lack of concern for the baby, loss of interest in activities, feelings of hopelessness/worthlessness, and feeling sad, anxious, or irritable. There are several things that are risk factors for this disorder, that is, a history of depression or other mood disorders, lack of support, stressful life events, a traumatic birth, hormonal shifts, and substance abuse. In rare instances, when PPD is left untreated it may lead to postpartum psychosis. Signs and symptoms of postpartum psychosis include the following: disordered thinking, loss of reality, paranoia, hallucinations, delusions, and thoughts of suicide or infanticide. Postpartum psychosis is a serious condition and requires immediate medical attention, possibly hospitalization.

It is important for community health nurses to carefully assess all new mothers for the signs of PPD. Along with conducting a thorough mental health assessment, nurses may select to complete a PPD assessment tool. The Edinburgh Postnatal Depression Scale (EPDS) has been used as a successful screening tool for PPD. The EPDS asks mothers to respond to 10 questions regarding how they have felt in the previous 7 days. The tool is easy to administer, available in several languages, and has cross-cultural validity. In addition to assessment, community health nurses who are visiting the client in her home are in a position to observe the mother as she cares for and interacts with her baby. The observations can also provide pertinent data about how the mother is functioning in her day-to-day living.

Treatment of PPD is likely to include medication therapy as well as individual or group therapy. Community health nurses need to be aware of the supportive resources that are available in the client's community. This will ensure that appropriate referrals are made. There also are a number of informative books regarding PPD that nurses can recommend to clients and their family members. Additionally, Postpartum Support International offers many educational and informational materials on its Web site.

BIPOLAR AFFECTIVE DISORDER

Bipolar affective disorder (BPAD) is a mood disorder that affects approximately 5.7 million adults in the United States each year. It is a disorder that includes variation in moods with alternating lows (depression) and highs (mania). The course of the illness varies from person to person, although for most it is a chronic mental illness that involves ongoing treatment and follow-up. Community health nurses need to be able to recognize the mood fluctuations in their clients diagnosed with BPAD, in order to plan for successful care and treatment in the community.

The prevalence, signs and symptoms, assessment, and community-based nursing interventions related to depression have been discussed above. In this section, information on mania is presented. According to the *DSM-IV-TR*, the signs and symptoms of the manic phase of BPAD include three of the following for at least a week: grandiosity, decreased need for sleep, pressured speech, flight of ideas, distractibility, psychomotor agitation, and excessive involvement in pleasurable activities without regard to negative consequences. Grandiosity is a heightened belief in one's identity, and flight of ideas is a pattern of speech in which a person jumps from topic to topic.

Nursing interventions include providing for safety from self-harm and balanced psychologic and physiologic functioning. The first-line treatment for mania is the use of medication, including mood stabilizers such as lithium or anticonvulsants. Community health nurses can help educate their clients and families regarding the importance of medication compliance. It is important to emphasize that medication should not be stopped during periods when the client is feeling better. Lithium has a narrow therapeutic range, so nurses need to be aware of the signs and symptoms of lithium toxicity. Signs of toxicity include the following: tremor, confusion, nausea, vomiting, diarrhea, excessive thirst, edema, frequent urination, and more. Community health nurses can help to educate clients and their families regarding the importance of medication compliance, the importance of routine labs to check for lithium levels, and the signs of lithium toxicity.

During periods of mania, providing a safe environment with minimal stimulation is also critical. In fact, persons who are experiencing severe mania often need to be hospitalized for safety and to prevent exhaustion. Clients in the community who become manic may be resistant to the suggestions offered by the nurse. It is appropriate for nurses working with manic clients to set limits on behaviors that are hostile or demanding. In addition, clients may be sexually inappropriate; they may speak so loudly and rapidly that it is impossible to get a word in, or they may become exhausted. At any of these times, it will take a team approach that involves mental health professionals as well as other community persons who can collaborate to prevent both self-harm and harm to others. If the person is thought to be a danger to self or others, they will need to be hospitalized.

Developing and maintaining a working relationship with professionals in the community becomes essential for positive outcomes. Recovery for persons with BPAD requires acceptance of the illness and understanding that medication must not be stopped when a manic cycle begins and the client feels "on top of the world." This can be a lifelong learning process for individuals. Prevention of relapse is a primary goal as symptoms become worse and recovery more difficult with each successive relapse.

GENERALIZED ANXIETY DISORDER

Generalized anxiety disorder (GAD) affects about 3% to 4% of the U.S. population per year, and it primarily affects women. The symptoms of the disorder may be mild to moderate or even severe. Persons with GAD may present with physical symptoms and other disorders, such as major depression, panic disorder, and substance addictions. In some cases, people with GAD may resort to self-medication with drugs, alcohol, or prescription medications in an attempt to ease their symptoms. The general characteristics of GAD are persistent anxious or worried feelings, restlessness, easily fatigued, difficulty concentrating, irritability, disturbed sleep patterns, muscle tension, and increased blood pressure, pulse, and respirations. The symptoms often begin in childhood and continue into adulthood.

Nursing interventions involve awareness of the behaviors that may indicate an underlying anxiety disorder. This means going beyond the physical symptoms, exploring a client's history, and focusing on the client's anxieties, fears, and concerns. Another aspect of effective nursing intervention when working with anxious clients is awareness of the nurse's own reactions to the client. Anxiety is contagious, and nurses can easily become excited and anxious, particularly when clients are experiencing high levels of anxiety and panic. Awareness involves taking a deep breath and centering awareness on remaining calm. A nurse's ability to be calm and focused can be an effective nursing intervention.

As with other psychiatric disorders, nurses need to maintain the client's safety. Other therapeutic techniques to consider are relaxation techniques, cognitive restructuring, and role playing. Nurses can encourage activity involvement at a level that can be tolerated by the client. This can be increased as the symptoms of anxiety diminish with treatment. Medications are often a part of the treatment regimen for an individual diagnosed with GAD. Benzodiazepines may be prescribed. However, they are used cautiously with clients as there is a potential for addiction and withdrawal if the medication is stopped. There are some antidepressant medications, particularly the SSRIs, that can provide relief from anxiety and depression.

PHOBIAS

A phobia is a severe, persistent, and irrational fear of a specific object or situation. The person is generally aware that the fear is unreasonable and that it interferes with daily functioning, but he or she is unable to control it and will do everything he or she can do to avoid the situation or object that triggers the fear. The objects or situations that cause phobias include almost anything: animals, lightening, public speaking, and crowds, to name a few. In addition to specific phobias, there are other fairly common phobias. Agoraphobia is a fear of being in settings where a person feels there is no place to hide or no easy means of escape. In severe cases, the afflicted person may not feel comfortable leaving his or her home. Social phobias involve situations where a person feels that he or she might be criticized. Phobias generally start in childhood and early adulthood and affect approximately 13% of the population, making them the most common type of anxiety disorder.

Treatment may include a behavioral technique called desensitization. In this case, the person is exposed to the feared object or experience and is taught to alter his or her responses to the object or experience. In addition, people with phobias may participate in individual or group therapy. Along with these treatments, an antianxiety medications may be prescribed. Specific nursing interventions are assessment of the disability caused by the phobia, referrals as needed, and helping the client to manage his or her daily activities.

POSTTRAUMATIC STRESS DISORDER

Posttraumatic stress disorder (PTSD) was first diagnosed in 1980. The incidence of PTSD in the general population is about 7%, with 50% of high-risk populations experiencing PTSD. A real and devastating event or events in one's life cause PTSD. Events that are beyond the individual's control, such as natural disasters, crime, sexual abuse, acts of terror, war, combat or being the witness of trauma, mutilation, or death, may cause PTSD. A primary feature of this disorder is that the person continues to reexperience the event by having recurrent, persistent, and frightening thoughts and memories of the experience. Symptoms of depression, feelings of emotional detachment and emotional numbness, anxiety, anger, sadness, and rage may also occur. The diagnostic criteria for PTSD include the existence of a recognizable stressor, recollections/dreams/flashbacks of the traumatic event, and avoidance of the stimuli.

PTSD is treated with antianxiety and antidepressant medications. Psychotherapy and group therapy are needed for the individual to work through the experience and regain a sense of security. Family involvement in treatment is recommended. Recovery is variable, with some people recovering within 6 months. For others, it may take longer and for some, PTSD can become a chronic disorder.

Nursing interventions with PTSD require assessment to determine the magnitude of symptoms. It is also important to assess for co-occurring conditions such as depression, suicidal ideation, substance abuse, and sleep disorders. Nurses can teach family members about the disorder and suggest ways in which they can support their family member. Often referral to mental health professionals allows the client options such as medication and individual and/or group therapy.

SCHIZOPHRENIA

Schizophrenia is a thought disorder that is characterized by a disturbance in how one thinks, feels, and relates to others and the environment. This disorder affects 2.4 million people in the United States in a given year and remains one of the least understood and least accepted of the mental illnesses. Lifetime risk is about the same for men and women, although there is difference in the age of onset with males being affected at younger ages (ages 16–25) than females (ages 25–30). It is now known that schizophrenia is a neurobiological disorder of the brain. This knowledge has led to major advances in the treatment of schizophrenia. Newer antipsychotic medications offer individuals treatment with fewer side effects, which contributes to better compliance and treatment outcomes.

Signs and symptoms of schizophrenia include positive and negative symptoms. The positive symptoms of this illness are any variety of the following: delusions, hallucinations, disordered thinking, and motor changes, that is, posturing, rituals, and catatonia. Delusions are fixed, false beliefs. The beliefs may be grandiose in nature; for example, the person may think that she is the Queen of England. In other cases, they may believe that their thoughts are being broadcast or inserted into the brain of another person. Hallucinations are incorrect sensory perceptions. Auditory hallucinations are the most common type of hallucinations. In this case, a person is responding to an internal voice that he or she feels is speaking to them and in some cases may be commanding them to do certain things. The negative symptoms of this illness are flat affect, lack of drive to perform, social withdrawal, and lack of interest or ability for follow-through. The behaviors disrupt a person's life in several major areas of functioning, that is, relationships, self-care, and work. Care is taken in the process of assessing and diagnosing schizophrenia as it is considered to be a serious persistent mental illness with long-term repercussions.

Community health nurses should bear in mind that many people with schizophrenia are not receiving treatment. This may be due to a lack of health insurance or it may relate to denial that they are ill and need help. Whatever the cause, nurses are in a position to assess people in the community and to arrange referrals as needed. As is the case, when working with people diagnosed with one mental illness, it is important to assess for other co-occurring conditions such as depression or substance abuse.

Medication management is a priority, as are housing and economic management. Health issues and safety concerns may need to be addressed in relation to issues of paranoid or delusional thinking, hallucinations, lack of self-care, and vulnerability. Community-Based Nursing Care Guidelines 14-1 outlines nursing interventions specific to schizophrenia.

COMMUNITY-BASED NURSING CARE GUIDELINES 14-1

Nursing Interventions Specific to Schizophrenia

Clients with schizophrenia may exhibit unusual or bizarre behaviors; they may have very limited communication; and they may demonstrate altered thinking. These behaviors may make developing a therapeutic relationship particularly challenging.

Interventions for Developing a Relationship

- Approach in a calm, genuine, and accepting manner.
- Spend short periods of time with clients, even if they interact very little.
- Call by name, approach from the front, and use touch cautiously, if at all.
- Demonstrate interest and concern for how clients perceive their illness.
- Speak clearly and distinctly with short sentences and with one thought per sentence.
- Encourage the client to identify and discuss feelings and concerns.
- Reinforce reality. Get a good description of delusions and/or hallucinations. Then focus on reality, that is, current events, activities, and tasks.

Ongoing Assessment Factors to Observe

- Disturbance in the client's thought processes
- Response and adherence with medication regimen
- Behavioral changes in hygiene, isolation or withdrawal, and lack of motivation
- Support network
- Suicide assessment

EATING DISORDERS

There are several types of eating disorders including anorexia nervosa and bulimia nervosa. They are quite common in the United States, and affect significantly more females than males. More recently, obesity has come to the forefront as an additional major public health concern. Nurses working in community-based settings will encounter clients with eating disorders. In most cases, eating disorders will require lifelong vigilance and community health nurses can play a significant role in providing care to these individuals. Anorexia nervosa, bulimia nervosa, and obesity are discussed below.

Anorexia Nervosa

Anorexia nervosa has a prevalence rate of 1% to 2% of the general population in the United States. A person with this disorder has an intense fear of gaining weight, even when underweight. There is a refusal to maintain a body weight that is above a normal minimum for their height and weight. In females, there is also an absence of at least three consecutive menstrual cycles. The ratio of females to males is 20:1.

Community health nurses need to be familiar with the signs and symptoms of anorexia nervosa as it has a high mortality rate. Some of the specific diagnostic criteria are weight loss of at least 25% of original body weight (15% if younger than 18), distortions in attitudes toward eating and weight, denial of illness, fear of weight gain, and refusal to maintain weight. There is no other cause for the symptoms such as a medical illness or another psychiatric disorder. There may be other physical characteristics such as dry skin, constipation, abdominal distress, hair loss, lanugo (fine, soft body hair), peripheral edema, and feeling cold.

Nurses need to first and foremost deal with the malnutrition. In severe cases, clients may need to be hospitalized for stabilization before they can be cared for in the community. Follow-up and aftercare are critical once the person is discharged from the hospital. Individual, group, and family therapy have all been used successfully to treat people with anorexia nervosa. The client may also be on a behavioral contract that aims to facilitate weight gain to an appropriate target weight. Nutritional counseling is important in the care and treatment of this disorder. Cognitive–behavioral strategies are effective in dealing with some of the distorted thinking that is characteristic of anorexia nervosa. Medication therapy may be indicated to treat co-occurring psychiatric disorders such as depression or anxiety. In many cases, anorexia nervosa is a chronic condition that will require long-term care. Some people diagnosed with anorexia nervosa will go on to develop bulimia nervosa.

Bulimia Nervosa

Bulimia nervosa has a prevalence rate of 3% to 8% of the general population in the United States. The ratio of females to males is 9:1. It is a common disorder in secondary schools and on college campuses. Bulimia nervosa includes episodes of rapid ingestion of large quantities of food (binging) in a short period of time. It includes a purging and a nonpurging type. A person with the purging type of disorder engages in self-induced vomiting and use of laxatives in an attempt to lose weight following the binge. People with bulimia tend to be of normal weight. Bulimic clients often feel tense before they binge, and relieved after the binge. However, the relief is short-lived and as anxiety regarding the binge increases, the person participates in self-induced vomiting. The vomiting provides a sense of relief.

Characteristics of bulimia nervosa include normal weight or slightly overweight, perfectionism, fear of obesity, and problems with impulse control. People with bulimia nervosa are more likely to admit that they have a problem than people with anorexia nervosa. There are a number of medical complications that are associated with bulimia nervosa including dehydration, enamel erosion, sore throat, facial puffiness, irregular menses, and hypokalemia (low potassium). Major depressive disorder and substance abuse are common co-occurring disorders.

The primary goal of treatment for bulimia is to reduce or eliminate binge eating and purging behaviors. Outpatient programs are often a successful option for treating bulimia nervosa. Individual, group, and family therapy are all useful in treating the disorder. As with anorexia nervosa, nutrition counseling, behavioral therapy, cognitive therapy, meditation, and relaxation therapy are also helpful. Medications such as the SSRIs have been used in conjunction with other therapies to treat bulimia nervosa.

Obesity

According to the World Health Organization, obesity has reached epidemic proportions internationally. It estimates that more than 1 billion adults and 17.6 million children under age 5 are overweight (World Health Organization, 2010). Many of the people who are overweight meet the criteria for obesity (body mass index greater than 30 kg/m^2). Being overweight or obese contributes to many serious, often chronic, health conditions. Examples include cardiovascular disease, type 2 diabetes, some types of cancer, and gall bladder disease. There are a number of less life-threatening complications that are associated with obesity such as respiratory problems, osteoarthritis, and infertility. All of these health problems contribute to the global burden of disease and disability, increase the risk of premature disease, and impact overall quality of life.

While obesity is not classified as a mental disorder, there are aspects of obesity that are significant from a psychological perspective. Community health nurses can play a significant role in the prevention of weight problems by participating in population-based strategies focused on prevention and health promotion. They can screen at-risk groups for weight problems. There is particular concern related to the increase in the number of overweight children and adolescents. Nurses can screen children and adolescents at school and develop weight management programs that are age-appropriate. Additionally, nurses can provide education to all age groups that includes information on healthy eating, weight loss and maintenance, and the importance of participating in daily moderate physical activity. Lastly, community health nurses have a role in the development and enforcement of public policies that promote the availability of healthy foods, encourage effective weight management, and support healthy lifestyles.

SUBSTANCE ABUSE

The economic costs to society of substance abuse are estimated to be in the billions. This includes alcohol and drug-related loss of productivity as well as alcohol and drug-related crime. The psychological cost to the individual who is addicted and his or her family members, friends, and society as a whole is both devastating and immeasurable. When a person becomes addicted, emotional and maturational growth becomes limited. All actions of the addicted individual are focused on the drug of choice: how to get it, when to use it, and how to get more of it.

Three major unconscious psychological defenses are used by persons who are addicted: denial, rationalization, and projection. Denial is the addicted person's insistence that he or she does not have a problem despite concrete evidence to the contrary. Contrary evidence such as driving under the influence arrests, missed days of work or school, and obvious concerns of others are ignored and denied. Rationalization is a means of justifying one's addictive behavior. An example is the statement: "I am not an alcoholic because I only use on weekends." Projection is the blaming of external forces, such as a nagging spouse, stressful job, or impossible boss, as a reason to use and abuse substances. These defenses affect the addicted individuals, and their family, as well as society as a whole. Community health nurses must not be afraid to recognize and confront the use of these defenses and educate the individual struggling with substance abuse, as well as the family members, about the dynamics of substance abuse.

Nurses need to be aware of the signs and symptoms of drug and alcohol use and abuse. They need to ask screening questions related to drug and alcohol use with each client that they encounter. It is important to ask specific questions in a direct manner. It may be helpful to first ask about the use of nicotine and caffeine, and then to move on to questions regarding the use of other types of drugs. Another question to include is to ask clients, what impact has their drug or alcohol use had on their lives? Addicted persons present in every setting in health care and may present with intoxication or withdrawal at any time. Drug and alcohol withdrawal may lead to a medical emergency in some cases. See Box 14-5 for signs and symptoms of drug and alcohol intoxication and withdrawal.

BOX 14-5 **Symptoms of Drug and Alcohol Intoxication and Withdrawal**

All conditions of drug and alcohol intoxication and withdrawal present a medical emergency and may require hospitalization.

- Alcohol Intoxication: impaired judgment, slurred speech, double vision, dizziness, volatile emotional changes, stupor, and unconsciousness
     Alcohol Withdrawal: anxiety, insomnia, tremors, and delirium tremors, which include confusion and convulsions (a hospital emergency)
- Sedative-Hypnotic and Anxiolytic Intoxication: slurred speech, slow, shallow respirations, cold, clammy skin, weak, rapid pulse, drowsiness, and disorientation
     Sedative-Hypnotic and Anxiolytic Withdrawal: anxiety, insomnia, tremors and convulsions that may occur up to 2 weeks after stopping use
- Opioid Intoxication: sedation, hypertension, respiratory depression, impaired function, constipation, and constricted pupils with watery eyes
     Opioid Withdrawal: restlessness, irritability, panic, chills, sweating, cramps, watery eyes with dilated pupils, nausea, and vomiting
- Cocaine Intoxication: irritability, anxiety, hyperactivity, hypervigilance, slow and weak pulse, shallow breathing, sweating, and dilated pupils
     Cocaine Withdrawal: agitation, depression, and suicidal ideation
- Amphetamine Intoxication: agitation, hyperactivity, and paranoia, dilated pupils, headache, and chills
     Amphetamine Withdrawal: prolonged periods of sleep, disorientation, and major depression
- Hallucinogen Intoxication: bizarre behavior with mood swings and paranoia, nausea and vomiting, tremors, panic with aggression, and possibly flushing, fever, and sweating
     Hallucinogen Withdrawal: depression, irritability, and restlessness

The symptoms of substance disorders include the consistent use of alcohol or other mood-altering drugs until the client is high or intoxicated, or he or she has passed out. There is an inability to stop or cut down use, despite wishes to do so or negative consequences from use. There is denial that substance use is a problem, despite feedback from significant others stating that the abuse is negatively affecting them. The abuse continues despite recurrent and persistent issues with physical, legal, vocational, social, or relationship problems directly related to the chemical use. Addicted individuals also consume a substance in greater amounts and for longer periods than intended.

Since alcohol use is common, nurses in all settings need to carefully assess every client regarding their use. The CAGE questionnaire offers four questions to ask a client when assessing for their alcohol use. The questions are as follows: (a) Have you ever felt you ought to CUT down on your drinking? (b) Have people ANNOYED you by criticizing your drinking? (c) Have you ever felt bad or GUILTY about your drinking? and (d) Have you ever had a drink the first thing in the morning to steady your nerves or to get rid of a hangover? (EYEOPENER). In addition to assessing for alcohol use, nurses need to be very familiar with the signs and symptoms of alcohol intoxication and withdrawal. Signs of intoxication include slurred speech, impaired judgment, emotional changes, dizziness, and double vision. Alcohol withdrawal must be taken seriously as it can be life threatening. The early signs of alcohol withdrawal begin within a few hours of reducing or stopping ingestion of alcohol. The early signs include irritability, anxiety, insomnia, and tremors. Early withdrawal may progress to alcohol withdrawal delirium. The signs and symptoms include anxiety, insomnia, tachycardia, diaphoresis, elevated blood pressure, hallucinations, and delusions. Alcohol withdrawal delirium is considered to be a medical emergency and must be treated accordingly.

Recovery and abstinence from drug or alcohol addiction is a lifelong process that requires changes in one's life. Old routines that activate drug and alcohol use behaviors have to be replaced with new and productive patterns of coping. Without the use of the substance, individuals must confront long-standing anger, resentments, and unresolved grief. Changing social networks and where one lives are aspects of the challenges of recovery. Resources for recovery tend to be highly structured, with an emphasis on self-awareness, limit setting, group therapy, skill development, and family treatment. They may include behavioral and family therapy, and various group therapy options such as involvement in a social skills group, loss and grief group, support group, mental illness/chemical dependency group (for those with a dual diagnosis), and self-help group. Self-help groups such as Alcoholics Anonymous, Cocaine Anonymous, and Narcotics Anonymous use a 12-step program to help the addict develop a different lifestyle and lend support to those in recovery.

It is important for nurses to bear in mind that relapse is common. Suspending personal feelings and judgment regarding relapse is important in maintaining therapeutic relationships with clients. It is best for nurses to view relapse as a situation from which the client has the opportunity to learn and to move forward in their treatment and recovery process. Nurses can view relapse as a time of renewed effort toward changing maladaptive behaviors.

Mental Health Assessment

As a community health nurse, you will assess individuals in a variety of environments. There are a number of useful assessment tools that have been developed for the assessment of specific disorders or for use with specific groups of people. These are readily available online and can be used as appropriate with clients. The main categories of data that are included in a **mental health assessment** are presented in Box 14-6. This can serve as a guide to nurses as they work with clients in community-based settings. The purpose of completing the mental health assessment is to gather a comprehensive history of the presenting complaint as well as to begin to establish a therapeutic alliance with a client. The data that are gathered during the assessment will provide a foundation from which to create an individualized plan of care.

BOX
14-6

Mental Health Assessment

Personal Information: name, sex, age, occupation, allergies, chief complaint, psychiatric history, health history, substance abuse, legal history, and family history of mental illnesses

General Description: height and weight, appearance, grooming, motor activity, speech, and general attitude.

Emotions: mood and affect.

Thought Processes and Content: delusions, suicidal (plan and access to plan) or homicidal ideation, disorganized thinking, or flight of ideas.

Perceptual Disturbances: hallucinations or illusions.

Cognition: orientation (time, place, person, circumstances), memory, concrete/abstract thought, consciousness and attention.

Impulse Control: ability to control impulses.

Judgment and Insight: ability to make decisions and solve problems.

Spirituality: affiliation, spiritual beliefs/activities, and religious activities.

Cultural Practices: beliefs, values, and practices.

CLIENT SITUATIONS IN PRACTICE

Assessing the Mentally Ill Patient

Mary Smith is a 29-year-old woman who has never been married. The history she provides is somewhat vague; however, she says that she comes from the West and that her family is very dysfunctional. She makes several references to rape and her crazy family, but there are no further details offered.

Mary says that she was diagnosed with bipolar affective disorder (BPAD) when she was a teenager. Mary was taking lithium for several years, but how long she took it and how much is unclear. She dropped out of school when she was a junior because she says that the voices she was hearing in her head made it too hard to concentrate on her studies. She was diagnosed with schizophrenia and was prescribed Haldol. She took the Haldol for a while, but because she didn't like the side effects, she was off medications for most of her 20s.

Mary has seen a doctor in the last month and is currently taking 200 mg of quetiapine fumarate (Seroquel). She recently became homeless for a time, but then was able to find an apartment. I first met Mary in a group for the homeless at our clinic.

What further information would you pursue?

The issue of being raped would be an important one to consider in terms of when and what degree of assault. The diagnoses of schizophrenia and BPAD would lead to questions about hallucinations or delusions and mood swings, as well as her level of functioning.

What symptoms is she having and to what degree are they affecting her?

It would also be important to assess her use of her medication Seroquel. Is Mary taking it as prescribed? Is she having any side effects? Does she feel it is helping?

On my first community visit to Mary, I found her living in a relatively safe part of the city, in a secure building. Her room was on the top floor, which meant a four-flight walk up. Her apartment was a room, about 8 × 10 ft, with a small closet with no door. She had a sink, stove, and refrigerator, and two large windows that faced another building about 5 ft away. Mary had many drawings hung on the walls, and she had also painted her windows. She was pleasant and friendly. Mary was dressed in a tee shirt that did not cover her protruding stomach and blue plaid pants. She proceeded to talk about all the things she was planning to tell me and in doing so became disorganized, moving from topic to topic: "I feel great. I'm having a good day. Do you suppose we could get some milk? Could you pray for me? I am joining that rape support group, you know. My refrigerator is working good, and I have bread."

I asked Mary: "Is there any man trying to hurt you now? Are you afraid?" Mary replied, "No, oh, no, I am not dating. There is a nice man down the hall; he helped take out my garbage the other day. How do you like my apartment, isn't it nice? I really want to stay here ...."

What are the major safety issues for Mary?

Mary is proud of having her own apartment, meager as it is. She displays disorganized thinking. The biggest concern is for Mary's vulnerability because she is pleasant and friendly and talks to anyone. She appears to have been the victim of sexual assault in the past. Mary needs to be protected from dangerous situations in the future.

What behavior would you reinforce?

We decided to take a walk to a nearby grocery store. On our walk back to her apartment, I encouraged Mary to be sure to take her medicine as prescribed and to see me again in 3 days.

What steps would you take?

Because my visit was on a Friday, I left the crisis line phone number with Mary, in case she needed someone over the weekend. On Monday morning, I phoned a service called Early Intervention to get Mary a mental health case manager. I will also make referrals for Mary for day treatment and social programs where she can interact with others safely. After letting her psychiatrist know of my concerns, we arranged for an appointment with Mary and her psychiatrist to reevaluate her medication. My biggest concern for Mary is her vulnerability and her safety.

Providing Care to Vulnerable Populations in the Community

There are some groups of people with mental illnesses who have been underserved for various reasons. These groups are referred to as at-risk or **vulnerable populations**. They present with unique needs that are often not adequately met in current health care systems. These populations include, but are not limited to, populations without permanent housing, caregivers, the elderly, adolescents, and racially and ethnically diverse populations.

POPULATIONS WITHOUT PERMANENT HOUSING

The number of homeless people in the United States is difficult to accurately measure. However, the National Coalition for the Homeless estimates that approximately 3.5 million people experience homelessness in a given year. It goes on to say that 20% to 25% of the homeless population have serious mental illnesses. Serious mental illnesses impact social relationships, the ability to complete activities of daily living, employment opportunities, physical health, and household management. Nurses in the community are in a position to provide care for mentally ill homeless people.

Ploeg, Hayward, Woodward, and Johnston (2008) described an intervention program for elderly people who were homeless or at risk for becoming homeless. In addition to being homeless or at risk, the participants had chronic illness, mental illness, and substance abuse. Several factors were significant to the success of the Homeless Intervention Programme (HIP) including the establishment of an ongoing therapeutic alliance with participants and provision of holistic health care services over time. Community health nurses have the expertise to provide outreach and case management for vulnerable populations such as those in the HIP. Another study explored the impact of homelessness on individuals in the HOMES (Housing and Outreach, Mobile and Engagement Services) Program (Kirkpatrick & Byrne, 2009). Participants in the program had a history of homelessness and mental illness. The HOMES Program provided safe, affordable housing and many supportive services available 7 days a week/24 hours a day. Stable housing and treatment for illnesses allowed the participants to reintegrate into the community. The authors identified nurses as crucial in the success of the HOMES Program. Specifically, nurses provided services, collaborated with other providers, referred participants to services, and conducted education.

Clearly, community health nurses have a role in advocating for people who are homeless and mentally ill. The holistic nursing process and focus on individualized care provides a sound foundation for this work.

CAREGIVERS OF PEOPLE WITH SERIOUS MENTAL ILLNESSES

A great deal has been written about the impact of providing care for people with serious mental illnesses on an ongoing basis. Most often care is provided in the community by caregivers who are relatives or close friends. Champlin (2009) found the experience of *being there* day after day for a family member or close friend with a serious mental illness to be challenging and isolative (Research in Community-Based Nursing Care 14-1).

Additionally, evidence supports that female caregivers experience greater levels of perceived burden when compared with males. Moller, Gudde, Folden, and Linaker (2009) conducted a study that examined gender differences among caregivers for people with serious mental illnesses and the association of self-reports of their experience of burden. The authors indicate a strong association between poor mental well-being and caregiver burden. They also found that females experienced higher levels of burden and negative feelings than male relatives in the caregiving experience.

In another study, Zauszniewski, Bekhet, and Suresky (2008) report a more specific finding saying that female family members who are mothers of a mentally ill person experience even greater feelings of burden than other female family members, that is, sisters, daughters, or wives, when providing care. They also found that female caregivers who lived with

RESEARCH IN COMMUNITY-BASED NURSING CARE 14-1

Mental illnesses are prevalent in the United States and internationally. Most often care is provided in the community, and usually by family members and close friends who are not health care professionals. It is important for nurses to explore the experience of providing care to a loved one with mental illness on a long-term basis from the perspective of family members and close friends. Once the experience is better understood, nurses will be better able to provide support to family members and others who are in the experience.

Champlin (2009) sought to gain a deeper understanding of the experience of *being there* for another with a serious mental illness. Twelve people, each with a mentally ill family member or close friend, participated in audiotaped and transcribed interviews. A descriptive phenomenological approach was used in data analysis. The findings reveal the general structure of the experience to be one that includes periods of tensely waiting and sometimes taking action to keep the loved one and others safe, times of confidence and also of self-doubt. There is ambiguity and unpredictability in the experience and often no clear end is in sight. All these aspects are woven together with knowing, accepting, and caring for the other in an intimate and enduring bond. Specifically, the following constituents emerged as central to this experience: accepting the changed other and grieving the loss of who the other once was; taking action in challenging circumstances; recognizing the ongoing, never-ending, and sometimes unpredictable nature of the experience; feeling isolated; having ambiguity of the heart; experiencing the tension of waiting; knowing the other well; and caring for the other.

This study suggests that community health nurses are in a prime position to support the family members and close friends who provide care to their family members or close friends with mental illnesses. They can act as advocates, provide the general public with accurate information related to mental illnesses, and work toward the development of policies that are intended to improve the care and treatment of people with mental illnesses.

RESEARCH IN COMMUNITY-BASED NURSING CARE 14-2

Fujino and Okamura (2009) conducted a study in Japan that explored the sense of burden felt by family members caring for people with mental illnesses at home. They found that the patients' satisfaction with life and their ability to perform activities of daily living decreased the feeling of burden for their caregivers. The results of the study suggest that care and support need to be provided to both the person with mental illness and their families. Nurses can promote independent functioning and increase the quality of life for the person with mental illness. At the same time they can work with the family caregivers to ensure that they have the resources and support that they need to care for their family members.

Many families serve as the primary caregivers for their mentally ill family members. Research suggests that often these caregivers have unmet needs and do not receive adequate support. Community health nurses are in a key position to provide care and support to caregivers in the community. They can even direct their primary efforts toward high-risk groups, such as women, specifically mothers who are living with their mentally ill family member and caring for them over long periods of time. Nurses can plan interventions directed at easing the burden of the care giving experience. Public health interventions such as counseling, case management, screening, advocacy, health teaching, and referral and follow-up will be useful. By supporting the client who is mentally ill, nurses can indirectly support the caregivers, and improve the lives of both groups of people.

the mentally ill person experienced higher burden than those who did not. Interestingly, Fujino and Okamura (2009) discovered that efforts directed at improving the quality of life of patients with mental illnesses had the added benefit of decreasing the sense of burden felt by the family members who were caring for them (Research in Community-Based Nursing Care 14-2).

CARING FOR OLDER ADULTS: DEPRESSION AND SUICIDE

The life expectancy for people residing in the United States is 77.7 years. As people live longer, they are likely to have increased health care needs, including mental health needs. Therefore, nurses working in community-based settings need to be aware of and qualified to intervene as needed regarding mental health concerns for older adults. Depression is prevalent across the life span and is often not diagnosed or treated. Untreated depression plays a significant role in suicide. In fact, according to the National Institute of Mental Health, in 2006, 14.2 out of 100,000 people in the United States, age 65 and older, died by suicide. Currently, non-Hispanic White men have the highest suicide rate (48 deaths per 100,000 each year). Interestingly, they add that many of the older adults who die by suicide had visited their medical doctor in the month prior to their death.

Persistent feelings of depression that interfere with activities of daily living are not a normal part of aging. Signs and symptoms of major depressive disorder include depressed mood or loss of interest or pleasure, weight loss or gain, insomnia or hypersomnia, psychomotor agitation or retardation, fatigue, feelings of worthlessness, impaired concentration, and thoughts of death/suicide. Some health care providers mistake these things for other medical illnesses or as a response to a physical illness. This may prevent or delay treatment. The most effective treatment for older adults who are experiencing depression is a combination of individual therapy and medication. Antidepressant medications called SSRIs are commonly prescribed as they have fewer side effects than some of the older antidepressant medications. It is important for nurses to remind the clients that they are working with that antidepressant medications take time to reach a therapeutic level in the blood. It may take 4 to 6 weeks until the client feels better. Clients may need encouragement to stay on the medication long enough to determine whether or not it is efficacious.

Suicide is a preventable illness and there are many things that community health nurses can do to prevent it. Nurses need to assess all of the clients that they come into contact with for the signs and symptoms of depression and suicide. Important questions to ask relate to mood, affect, eating and sleeping patterns, energy and activity level, and suicidal ideation. There are depression inventories that have been specifically developed for use with elderly clients. Public education is needed to emphasize the preventable nature and to encourage people to seek help if they are feeling depressed or suicidal. Educational efforts should be directed at several groups including older adults, their family members, and primary health care providers. Oyama et al. (2008) reviewed five studies and concluded that prevention programs using community-based depression screening and health education reduced the risk of completed suicide among older adults. They state that follow-up with a psychiatrist rather than a general practitioner yields better results with at-risk individuals. An example of a successful education strategy is a project called "Prevention is the Only Cure: Raising Awareness to Prevent Suicide in Older Men" developed by Bartlett, Travers, and Cartwright (2008). The project utilizes presentations about suicide and depression, and an information kit that includes tools for use with at-risk individuals. Nurses can also be involved in public policy development and enforcement that is aimed at suicide prevention. One example of a social marketing strategy is the use of billboards and television advertisements that focus on suicide prevention.

CARING FOR ADOLESCENTS: SUICIDE PREVENTION

The prevalence rate for adolescent suicide in the United States is high. In 2006, it was the third leading cause of death for adolescents ages 15 to 24. More males than females die each year by suicide, in part because they select more lethal methods. There is an urgent need to target suicide prevention efforts with adolescent populations.

Mental health assessment with adolescents is similar to that in adults; however, with adolescents, it is also important to ask about developmental milestones, social relationships, school performance, and participation in extracurricular activities. It is ideal if parents or guardians can be interviewed regarding their view of the adolescent's behaviors as well as interviewing the adolescent client.

The signs and symptoms of depression and suicide have been presented in previous sections of the chapter. However, it is important to note that sometimes adolescents and children may present with signs and symptoms that are not the same as those adults present with. Nurses need to be aware of these differences and watch for things such as the following: extreme sensitivity, increased irritability, persistent boredom, frequent complaints of physical illness, school absences, alcohol or drug use, reckless risk taking, and threats to run away from home. Adolescents who are getting in trouble at school may actually be depressed and may need to be evaluated by a health care professional.

As is the case with most mental illnesses, there are multiple etiologies when depression and suicidal behaviors are diagnosed in adolescents. Thus, treatment should include a combination of treatment modalities. For example, an adolescent may take a prescribed medication and also attend individual and family therapy. Similar to adults, the primary goal of treatment is to decrease symptoms and increase adaptive functioning.

There are community-based programs aimed at suicide prevention. One innovative community-based suicide prevention program led by nurses included three strategies: developing a wallet-size card, creating a resource brochure, and providing suicide prevention (Pirruccello, 2010). The project aimed to eliminate suicide, to raise community awareness about youth suicide, and to provide youth with easy access to crisis intervention resources. One year later, the adolescent suicide rate in the community was recorded as zero. The author suggests that this is a model that can be individualized and implemented in other communities.

Once again, nurses are in a position to be in the forefront when it comes to the prevention of suicide. As demonstrated above, nurses can take a leadership role within their communities in developing successful programs.

CARING FOR RACIALLY AND ETHNICALLY DIVERSE POPULATIONS

According to the Surgeon General's Report (U.S. Department of Health and Human Services, Office of the Surgeon General, 2001), there are disparities in mental health care for racial and ethnic minorities when compared with whites. Specifically, the report identifies that minorities have less access to mental health services, are less likely to receive mental health services, receive poorer quality of care, and are less represented in the research. Alexandre, Younis, Martins, and Richard (2010) examined the disparities between whites and nonwhite adolescents in receiving adequate mental health care for major depressive episodes over a 1-year period. They found that 36% of whites received adequate mental health care as compared to 28% for nonwhites.

While evidence confirms that disparities exist, other studies search for reasons why it exists. A community-based participatory research project conducted by Shattell, Hamilton, Starr, Jenkins, and Hinderliter (2008) identified factors that affect access and use of mental health services by a Latino population. Factors included the following: lack of health insurance coverage, differences in beliefs regarding the cause of mental disorders, suspiciousness of health care providers, language barriers, and the high cost of health care. The authors suggested that health care providers work toward improving services by setting up sliding-scale programs for services, increasing the number of bilingual providers, learning more about the Latino culture, and participating in efforts to reform the current health care system.

Community health nurses need to take an active role in eliminating disparities in mental health services. There are a number of things that nurses can do to work toward this end. First, they can lead efforts to improve access to mental health treatment. This will include efforts to combat **stigma** as well as efforts to decrease the cost of services. Second, nurses can work to improve the quality of mental health services. Lastly, they can participate in all efforts to promote mental health.

Community Mental Health Agencies and Related Services

Community support services are public and privately funded resources to assist persons who are mentally ill. The resources promote mental health, prevent mental illness, and serve the needs of the mentally ill and their family members. Some of the services provided include crisis intervention, mental health treatment, case management, advocacy, and supportive services for living and working. Three areas of support, community mental health agencies, housing, and human needs support, are discussed here.

COMMUNITY MENTAL HEALTH AGENCIES

Community mental health agencies are funded primarily through public dollars and offer a variety of services. As a community mental health nurse, you may be employed by one of these agencies and refer a variety of services to your clients. If you are not connected to an agency through employment, it is important that you learn what community mental health agencies exist, what services they offer, and how they can best serve your clients. Some of the following services are offered through community mental health agencies:

- Individual psychotherapy
- Group therapy
- Mental health assessment, diagnosis, and treatment
- Chemical health assessment, diagnosis, and treatment
- Medication management
- Vulnerable adult protection

HOUSING

Housing options include battered women's shelters, homeless shelters, halfway houses, transitional housing, and other supportive housing options. Shelters for battered women offer safety to women and their children who are in abusive living situations. These shelters offer services to both mothers and their children, including school transportation and case management for women seeking safe housing. Homeless shelters are of two kinds: overnight shelters with check-in from 5:00 to 8:00 PM and checkout by 7:00 AM, and 24-hour shelters where people can stay in during the day. Halfway houses and transitional housing are both temporary housing but are generally longer-term living situations than shelters for persons who are not ready to live independently. Supportive housing is long-term housing that offers intensive case management to clients who are unable to live independently. This type of housing is ideal for persons with chronic mental illnesses who are unable to live independently. The greatest difficulty with housing services is the acute shortage of supportive housing options available for people with mental illnesses.

HUMAN NEEDS SUPPORT

Human support services for the mentally ill include self-help groups, community drop-in centers, clothes closets, food shelves, services to immigrants and victims of abuse and crime, legal assistance, job training and placement, education programs, and advocacy programs. It is the nurse's responsibility when working with mentally ill clients in the community to know the resources offered in the community. Familiarity with the available resources will facilitate appropriate referrals. In cases where there is a lack of support for people with mental illnesses living in the community, nurses have an opportunity to work to effect political awareness and change.

Challenges to Providing Community-Based Mental Health Care

After a year of study, the President's New Freedom Commission on Mental Health (2003) published a report that confirmed that there are unmet needs and barriers to receiving mental health services in the United States. Specifically, it identified stigma, fragmentation of services, high unemployment for people with serious mental illnesses, lack of care for older adults, and lack of a national suicide prevention program as obstacles. The Commission emphasized that mental illnesses are treatable and that more individuals could recover if they had improved access to treatment and care in the community. Health care professionals, including community health nurses, can be instrumental in efforts to meet the needs of people with mental illnesses and to remove barriers to receiving treatment.

Despite advances in the care and treatment of people with mental illnesses, stigma persists. Oftentimes people with mental illnesses and their family and friends are secretive about mental illnesses due to the injustices that may occur if people knew. Those affected feel they may face negative repercussions in their social and work relationships if they are open about their illnesses. Additionally, they feel that they may face discrimination in employment, housing, and health insurance coverage. The direct consequence of this is that many people with mental illnesses do not seek treatment for their mental illnesses. If mental illnesses were viewed in a less negative light and not as something to be ashamed of, more people would receive appropriate care.

Community-based education is one strategy to consider in the effort to decrease the stigma of mental illness. Educational programs could present accurate information about the causes of mental illnesses and the treatment options. The fact that mental illnesses can be successfully treated could be the overall focus. Information regarding access to resources and support could be available. Community health nurses have the knowledge and expertise to actively participate in educational efforts aimed at decreasing the stigma that is associated with mental illnesses. Pinto-Foltz and Logsdon (2009) state that nurses can take part in stigma reduction activities by participating in letter writing campaigns to address the concern and by watching for inaccurate portrayal by the media of people with mental illnesses and presenting correct information. A study conducted by Chambers et al., (2010) compared mental health nurses' attitudes toward mental illnesses in five European countries. They found that overall the nurses' attitudes were primarily positive (sympathetic and compassionate). The authors regarded this finding as encouraging as it suggests that nurses will then be likely to promote independent living for people with mental illnesses living in community settings.

Improving collaboration between the providers of care and treatment of people with mental illnesses has the potential to decrease the fragmentation of services. Efforts to consolidate services in one place or to assist with transportation if needed would also be important. Community health nurses can also direct clients to resources that can assist with employment and housing. Lastly, as discussed previously, improving mental health services for older adults and increasing suicide prevention strategies are within the role of community health nurses.

Conclusions

The evolution of mental health care has exploded in the last two decades. Understanding the origins of mental illnesses has contributed to major breakthroughs in medication management and treatment. These advances have also helped to eliminate some of the myths about mental illnesses. Community health nurses are in a position to play a significant role in improving mental health care.

Concern for the care and treatment of people with mental illnesses needs to be an ongoing priority worldwide. Nurses need to look beyond the physical issues and consider clients' stories and how they are coping. The gift of relationship is what community mental health nursing is all about. Being in relationships with clients, their families, and other mental health professionals enables community health nurses to achieve the best possible outcomes for clients.

What's on the Web

The American Psychological Association (APA)
INTERNET ADDRESS: http://www.apa.org
This professional and scientific organization for the practice of psychology has several brochures and fact sheets for consumers and health professionals. Write or call APA Public Affairs, 750 First Street, NE, Washington, DC 20002-4242; (800) 374-2721.

Centers for Disease Control and Prevention (CDC)
INTERNET ADDRESS: http://www.cdc.gov/mentalhealth/
This site is managed by the CDC Mental Health Workgroup. The group is committed to advancing the field of mental health by providing information on statistics, resources, and publications.

The National Alliance for the Mentally Ill (NAMI)
INTERNET ADDRESS: http://www.nami.org
This site has a medical information series that provides clients and families with information on several mental illnesses and their treatments. NAMI state affiliates provide emotional support and can help find local services. Find your local NAMI on the Web site under State and local NAMIs.

The National Institute of Mental Health (NIMH)
INTERNET ADDRESS: http://www.nimh.nih.gov
This site offers information and publications on all the mental health disorders. Contact the Information and Resources and Inquiries Branch, NIMH, Room 7C-02, MSC 8030, Bethesda, MD 20892-8030.

The National Mental Health Association (NMHA)
INTERNET ADDRESS: http://www.nmha.org
The NMHA publishes information on a variety of mental health issues. It also provides referrals and support. Write or call the NMHA Information Center, 1021 Prince Street, Alexandria, VA 22314-2971; (800) 969-6642.

Postpartum Support International
INTERNET ADDRESS: **http://www.postpartum.net/**
 Postpartum Support International helps women suffering from perinatal mood and anxiety disorders including postpartum depression. It also provides education to families, friends, and health care providers regarding perinatal disorders.

Suicide Awareness Voices of Education
INTERNET ADDRESS: **http://www.save.org/**
 SAVE is a nonprofit volunteer organization with staff who are dedicated to the prevention of suicide. The site provides resources and products intended to promote awareness that suicide is preventable.

References and Bibliography

Alexandre, P. K., Younis, M. Z., Martins, S. S., & Richard, P. (2010). Disparities in adequate mental health care for past-year major depressive episodes among white and non-white youth. *Journal of Health Care Finance, 36*(3), 57–72. Retrieved from CINAHL Plus with Full Text database.

American Psychiatric Association. (2000). *Diagnostic and statistical manual of mental disorders* (4th ed., text rev.). Washington, DC: Author

Bartlett, H., Travers, C., & Cartwright, C. (2008). Evaluation of a project to raise community awareness of suicide risk among older men. *Journal of Mental Health, 17*(4), 388–397. doi:10.1080/09638230701506010.

Chambers, M., Guise, V., Valimaki, M., Rebelo Botelho, M. A., Scott, A., Staniuliene, V., et al. (2010). Nurses' attitudes to mental illness: A comparison of a sample of nurses from five European countries. *International Journal of Nursing Studies, 47*, 350–362. doi:10.1016/j.ijnurstu.2009.08.008.

Champlin, B. E. (2009). Being there for another with a serious mental illness. *Qualitative Health Research, 19*, 1525–1535. doi:10.1177/1049732309349934.

Fujino, N., & Okamura, H. (2009). Factors affecting the sense of burden felt by family members caring for patients with mental illness. *Archives of Psychiatric Nursing, 23*(2), 128–137. Retrieved from CINAHL Plus with Full Text database.

Kirkpatrick, H., & Byrne, C. (2009). A narrative inquiry: Moving on from homelessness for individuals with a major mental illness. *Journal of Psychiatric and Mental Health Nursing, 16*, 68–75. Retrieved from CINAHL Plus with Full Text database.

Minnesota Department of Health, Division of Community Health Services, Public Health Nursing Section. (2001). *Public health nursing interventions: Application for public health nursing practice.* Minneapolis, MN: Author.

Moller, T., Gudde, C. B., Folden, G. E., & Linaker, O. M. (2009). The experience of caring in relatives to patients with serious mental illness: Gender differences, health and functioning. *Scandanavian Journal of Caring Sciences, 23*, 153–160. doi:10.1111/j.1471-6712.2008.00605.x.

National Coalition for the Homeless. (2009a). *How many people experience homelessness.* Retrieved August 4, 2010, from http://mentalhealth.samhsa.gov/

National Coalition for the Homeless. (2009b). *Mental illness and homelessness.* Retrieved August 4, 2010, from http://mentalhealth.samhsa.gov/

National Institute of Mental Health. (2010a). *The numbers count: Mental disorders in America.* Retrieved July 30, 2010, from http://www.nimh.nih.gov/health/publications/the-numbers-count-mental-disorders-in-america/index.shtml

National Institute of Mental Health. (2010b). *Suicide in the U.S.: Statistics and prevention.* Retrieved July 31, 2010, from http://www.nimh.nih.gov/health/publications/suicide-in-the-us-statistics-and-prevention/index.shtml

National Institute of Mental Health. (2010c). *Older adults: Depression and suicide facts.* Retrieved July 31, 2010, from http://www.nimh.nih.gov/health/publications/older-adults-depression-and-suicide-facts-fact-sheet/index.shtml

Oyama, H., Sakashita, T., Ono, Y., Goto, M., Fujita, M., & Koida, J. (2008). Effect of community-based intervention using depression screening on elderly suicide risk: A meta-analysis of the evidence from Japan. *Community Mental Health Journal, 44*, 311–320. doi:10.1007/s10597-008-9132-0.

Pinto-Foltz, M. D., & Logsdon, M. C. (2009). Reducing stigma related to mental disorders: Initiatives, interventions, and recommendations for nursing. *Archives of Psychiatric Nursing, 23*, 32–40. doi:10.1016/j.apnu.2008.02.010.

Pirruccello, L. M. (2010). Preventing adolescent suicide: A community takes action. *Journal of Psychosocial Nursing, 48*(5), 34–41. Retrieved from CINAHL Plus with Full Text database.

Ploeg, J., Hayward, L., Woodward, C., & Johnston, R. (2008). A case study of a Canadian homelessness intervention programme for elderly people. *Health and Social Care in the Community, 16,* 593–605. doi:10.1111/j.1365-2524.2008.00783.x.

Proposed Healthy People 2020 objectives. Mental health and mental disorders. Retrieved July 31, 2010, from http://www.healthypeople.gov/hp2020/

Shattell, M. M., Hamilton, D., Starr, S. S., Jenkins, C. J., & Hinderliter, N. A. (2008). Mental health service needs of a Latino population: A community-based participatory research project. *Issues in Mental Health Nursing, 29,* 351–370. doi:10.1080/01612840801904316.

The President's New Freedom Commission on Mental Health. (2003). *Executive summary.* Rockville, MD: Author. Retrieved August 1, 2010, from http://www.mentalhealthcommission.gov/reports/reports

U.S. Department of Health and Human Services, Office of the Surgeon General. (1999a). *Mental health: A report of the Surgeon General.* Washington, DC: Author. Retrieved July 1, 2010, from http://www.surgeongeneral.gov/library/mentalhealth/home.html

U.S. Department of Health and Human Services, Office of the Surgeon General. (1999b). *Epidemiology of mental illness.* Washington, DC: Author. Retrieved July 1, 2010, from http://www.surgeongeneral.gov/library/mentalhealth/chapter2/sec2_1.html

U.S. Department of Health and Human Services, Office of the Surgeon General. (2001). *Mental health: Culture, race, and ethnicity.* Washington, DC: Author. Retrieved July 1, 2010, from http://mentalhealth.samhsa.gov/cre/toc.asp

World Health Organization. (2010). *Obesity and overweight.* Retrieved July 31, 2010, from http://www.who.int/dietphysicalactivity/publications/facts/obesity/en/

Zauszniewski, J. A., Bekhet, A. K., & Suresky, M. J. (2008). Factors associated with perceived burden, resourcefulness, and quality of life in female family members of adults with serious mental illness. *Journal of the American Psychiatric Nurses Association, 14,* 125–135. doi:10.1177/1078390308315612.

LEARNING ACTIVITIES

JOURNALING ACTIVITY 14-1

Before your first clinical caring for individuals with mental illness, respond to the following questions in your journal:

- Describe an encounter you have had with an individual who was mentally ill.
- What do you think the client you care for will be like?
- Describe what you think it will be like to care for an individual with mental illness.
- What do you feel when you think about your first encounter as a nurse caring for someone who has a mental illness?
- What questions do you have for your instructor before you begin clinical?
- In your clinical journal, discuss a situation you have encountered in one of your clinical experiences with a client who is having difficulties with a mental illness.
- Describe your feelings and reactions to what you saw and heard.
- Reflect on your preconceptions and compare them to what you experienced when working with individuals with mental illness.
- What was the most important thing you learned about mental illness?

JOURNALING ACTIVITY 14-2

Contact a community mental health center in your community and find out about the volunteer opportunities available for nursing students. Once you find something that appeals to you, volunteer for a month, several months, or longer. Keep a journal about your experiences as a volunteer.

PRACTICAL APPLICATION ACTIVITY 14-3

Volunteer at a homeless shelter in your community. Take time to visit with at least one person who is staying at the shelter. Before the visit, find information about homelessness in your community including the scope of the issue, trends, programs, and policy that has been developed to address the need. After volunteering write about what you learned about homelessness in your community.

PRACTICAL APPLICATION ACTIVITY 14-4

With a group of students, assist with the serving of a meal in a homeless shelter. Before you go, identify an article in a nursing journal about homelessness, poverty, or mental illness and homelessness. While at the shelter, have at least one interaction with one of the people you are serving. For example, ask someone if you can sit down and have a cup of coffee and visit with him or her. After the interaction, discuss the following:

- What are your feelings and reactions to what you saw and heard?
- What did you expect that this experience would be like? What did you actually experience?
- What did you learn from speaking to the person with whom you interacted?
- Discuss the article you read and how it relates to what you saw.
- Identify the most important thing you learned during this experience.
- What did you learn that may be helpful to you once you begin working as a nurse?

PRACTICAL APPLICATION ACTIVITY 14-5

Contact a mental health nurse working in a community setting. Interview him or her and ask the following questions:

- Describe your primary responsibilities as a nurse in this setting.
- Discuss the challenges and benefits of this type of work.
- Outline the goals and missions of your agency.
- Would you recommend this type of work to a new graduate?
- Identify additional coursework or continuing education that would be beneficial in preparation for doing this type of work.

Chapter 15

Global Health and Community-Based Care

JOAN BRANDT AND ROBERTA HUNT

Learning Objectives

1. Discuss the relationship between community-based nursing and global health.
2. Identify roles that the community-based nurse has in global health.
3. Discuss the relationship between global health and environmental health.
4. Develop a global perspective on disparity.
5. Consider the global nature and global consequences of natural disasters, epidemics, and terrorism.
6. Consider the needs of immigrants, refugees, and victims of societal violence.
7. Understand the impact of the global shortage of RNs on global health.
8. Appreciate the need for nursing advocacy in global health.

Key Terms

advocacy
disasters
emergency preparedness
environmental health
environmental quality
global health disparity
globalization

immigrants
natural disaster
pandemic
physical environment
refugees
social environment
undocumented workers

Chapter Topics

Developing a Global View of Nursing

Millennium Development Goals

Environmental Health

Global Health Disparity

Emergency Preparedness

Immigrants and Refugees

Nursing Advocacy in Global Health

Global Nursing Shortage

Conclusions

The Nurse Speaks

Katrina Response—One Nurse's Story

Be ready for anything. Drop your job description and egos at the door. Plan to bring closure to the Operation Minnesota Lifeline service to the Gulf Coast area following the "cosmic slap" delivered by the Katrina and Rita hurricanes. Such were the instructions given to us during orientation as 28 of us—health care providers, clerical, and logistical workers—prepared to bus down to Louisiana to do whatever was necessary for the 16 days we were scheduled for service with evacuees of the hurricanes.

I have been a nurse for 40 years. I worked in the hospital for 5 years, in community/public health practice for 15 years, and as a nurse educator for 20 years. This experience was an odyssey where collaboration and teamwork came to life for me as never before.

The environment in which we served was every bit as tumultuous as the media portrayed. Homes, churches, and schools were totally destroyed. At the same time—6 weeks posthurricanes—I was amazed at the resilience of people as they worked to put lives back together in the midst of turmoil. To alleviate total school disruption, districts worked together. Schools that remained intact would have classes for their respective students in the morning; schools that were destroyed would bus their students in for afternoon classes in the same intact building. The plan was to have school year round.

Amidst this backdrop, our team set out each day to provide health services to the region. Working out of vans, we set up wherever there were people—trailer parks, motels, road crossings, at the local market, domes, emergency medical technician headquarters, and campgrounds.

As one might predict, many of our "stops" included immunization "clinic." I was touched by the gratitude of all of the people who received services. After immunizing one mom and her family of four, I was hugged and the mom expressed her appreciation in these words—"Honey, I loves you, I loves you like a pig loves corn!;" Ah-the colloquial expressions of the Louisiana people!;

As I reflect back, two areas of nursing practice stand out—that of assessment and presence. Assessment of all ages was carried out—for respiratory, skin, eye, and mental health concerns among many. We can only hope that our team of primary providers made a dent in the health needs and that referrals made were indeed available and followed.

A particularly poignant experience was illustrative of the human-to-human presence that characterized much of our work among the crowds.

During one of the campground stops, 7-year-old "Jimmy" came bounding up to us, followed by his dog. He grabbed our hands and asked if he could get "a shot." As we skipped along with him to find his mother, we talked about his family "camping out." He was so eager to stay with us as he told us it was kind of fun, but nobody could find his grandma. Then without missing a beat he held our hands tighter, pulled up his sleeve ready for his shot, and said "can you stay with us all day?" That encounter was one of many transforming experiences of healing presence for all of us.

Romana Klaubauf, MSN, RN, Public Health Nurse,
Assistant Professor, College of St. Catherine

Globalization is defined as the development of an increasingly integrated global economy marked especially by free trade, free flow of capital, and the tapping of cheaper foreign labor markets (Merriam-Webster, 2010).

Globalization has become a major challenge for the nursing profession. An illness is no longer contained by geographic boundaries nor is anyone protected from events occurring in distance places. For example, an epidemic in New York may quickly spread to Thailand. One person with influenza who travels by plane to an international conference may be responsible for exposing numerous individuals attending the conference to the virus. If several conference attendees become ill and return home, each may serve as a vector and spread the illness to colleagues and family in their respective countries. With increasing air travel, epidemics are easily transmitted throughout the world. Or, toys that are made in China are the source of lead poisoning for young children in the United States. Multiple factors influence the spread of infectious diseases on an international level (Box 15-1). Another example is seen in the ways that nursing knowledge is becoming global. The World Wide Web has made information from around the word instantly available at our fingertips. Additionally, there has been an increase in participation in international nursing confer- ences as well as publications of studies conducted by nurses worldwide over the last two decades. As a result, nurses in Sioux Falls, South Dakota, may be using a model of practice developed in Sweden. Nurses in Budapest, Hungary, may use a model of community-based care conceived by a nurse in St. Paul, Minnesota.

In this chapter, community-based nursing is considered from the perspective of global health. Increasingly, nurses must be competent to consider health as a comprehensive con- cept that requires an understanding of **environmental health, global health disparity**, and **emergency preparedness**. Once health is understood as a global concept, our professional responsibility to consider and address issues of global health follows. Our scope of **advocacy** broadens as we develop a sense of social responsibility for the health of new Americans and citizens of other countries.

Developing a Global View of Nursing

In order to develop a global view of nursing, it is helpful to look to professional standards as a guide. The *Nursing Code of Ethics* delineates professional responsibility to global health and the international community. Nursing commitment to health promotion, welfare, and safety extends to all persons. This requires consideration of not only individual clients but also broader health concerns for community, national, and international issues. These issues may include world hunger, environmental pollution, lack of access to health care, and inequitable distribution of nursing and health care resources. To address these professional responsibilities, nurses may participate in interdisciplinary planning and collaborative partnerships among health professionals and others at the community, national, and inter- national levels (American Nurses Association, Code of Ethics, 2001).

There are numerous avenues for developing a global view of nursing. First, it is impor- tant to become informed about local, national, and international health issues. Once

 BOX 15-1   **Factors Impacting the Emergence of Infectious Diseases**

- International trade and commerce
- Human demographics and behavior
- Human susceptibility to infection
- Poverty and social inequality
- War and famine
- Breakdown of public health measures
- Technology and industry
- Changing ecosystems
- Climate and weather
- Microbial adaptation and change

Adapted from Institute of Medicine. (2010). *Infectious disease movement in a borderless world.* Washington, DC: National Academies Press.

acquainted with the issues, speaking out and informing others is the next step. Attending international conferences develops a global view of nursing, with a modest commitment of time and resources. International conferences provide ample opportunities to meet other attendees and, in some cases, begin a connection that evolves into a collaborative relationship. Volunteering internationally is a powerful way to learn about both oneself and health care from another cultural perspective. For additional resources, there are some Web sites of volunteer opportunities listed at the end of the chapter. Working abroad in developing countries provides opportunities to share clinical expertise while learning new approaches to health and illness. There are numerous student exchange programs that offer study abroad. Immersion experience exposes one to the language, religion, art, customs, and traditions along with health care systems. Most universities and colleges offer study abroad programs.

Millennium Development Goals

Just as *Healthy People 2020* is a guide for community health in the United States, the Millennium Development Goals (MDG) provide a framework for global health. Developed by the United Nations (UN), in cooperation with several international organizations, such as the World Health Organization (WHO), the World Bank, and the World Food Organization, the eight goals offer concrete benchmarks for tackling poverty, hunger, maternal and child mortality, disease, inadequate shelter, environmental health, and gender inequality (United Nations Development Programme [UNDP], 2006a). Box 15-2 outlines the eight goals.

Environmental Health

Environmental health is defined by the WHO as the study of "the effects of various chemical, physical, and biological agents, as well as the effects on the health of the broad physical and **social environment**, which includes housing, urban development, land use and transportation, industry, and agriculture" (World Health Organization [WHO], 2010b). The **environmental quality** of both the physical and social environments plays major roles in the health of individuals and communities. The **physical environment** includes the air, water, and soil through which exposure to chemical, biological, and physical agents may occur. The **social environment** reflects where individual live and work and has a profound influence on one's health. It includes housing, transportation, urban development, land use, industry, and agriculture, along with issues related to work-related stress, injury, and violence. The inequity in access to health care and education, their living and working conditions, their neighborhoods, and cities all impact an individual and family's ability to thrive in life. These conditions of daily life reflect the majority of health inequities between and within countries (WHO, 2010a).

BOX 15-2 **Millennium Development Goals**

Goal 1: Eradicate extreme poverty and hunger
Goal 2: Achieve universal primary education
Goal 3: Promote gender equality and empower women
Goal 4: Reduce child mortality
Goal 5: Improve maternal health
Goal 6: Combat HIV/AIDS, malaria, and other diseases
Goal 7: Ensure environmental sustainability
Goal 8: Develop a global partnership for development

Source: United Nations Development Programme. (2006b). *What are the millennium development goals?* Retrieved July 20, 2010, from http://www.undp.org/mdg/learnmore.shtml

It is not possible for individual nations to completely regulate and ensure environmental quality because climate change or some of the elements of air and water pollution are not contained by geographical borders. Climate change affects access to safe water, clean air, and adequate food and shelter (WHO, 2010b). Air pollution is thought to cause close to 2 million deaths per year (WHO, 2008a). With international trade, food and goods cross borders, and with them, the potential for transmission of chemical, biological, and physical agents exists. Thus, environmental quality and environment health is a global issue that depends on interstate and international cooperation and agreements. It is important to remember that the quality of both the immediate and the broader environment impacts the health status of individuals, families, and communities. This chapter discusses the concept of environmental health as it relates to the health of populations in the United States as well as globally.

ENVIRONMENTAL HEALTH IN THE UNITED STATES

The goals of Healthy People 2020 address health equity for all groups, with the elimination of health disparities; achieve higher quality lives across the life span through health promotion and disease prevention; and "create social and physical environments that promote good health for all" (U.S. Department of Health and Human Services, 2010). It is clear that there is a relationship between the environmental quality and health.

Assessing the contribution that quality of the immediate physical environment has on health is an important role for the nurse in community settings. An example is seen when a nurse does a home assessment for the presence of lead in a home where there are infants or children living. If the nurse discovers that there is evidence of lead, an abatement process commences to improve the environmental quality of the home. Because of this type of public health programs, childhood lead exposure has been significantly reduced in the United States. Asthma is an example of a chronic condition common among children and adults in the United States that is impacted by environmental quality. Nurses play an important role in the assessment and intervention of factors that contribute to asthma in individuals, families, and populations. This includes advocating for policies that improve the environmental quality of the communities they serve (Research in Community-Based Nursing Care 15-1).

A commonly discussed issue related to the environmental health of communities and populations is the relationship between air pollution and health. Air pollution is an environmental quality that characterizes the broader physical environment. In the United States, air pollution is associated with health problems such as asthma and pulmonary or heart disease leading to increased rates of hospitalization (National Resources Defense Council, 2008). Air pollution is related to increased risk for cardiovascular disease (American Heart Association, 2010) and an increased incidence of asthma, bronchitis, and emphysema as well. The financial burden of asthma due to repeated emergency department (ED) visits and hospitalizations, the cost of medications, and lost work and schools days is significant (Bahadori et al., 2009). As with other health indicators, there is disparity in the ways that environmental quality impacts health. Children of color and poor children face greater health risks due to pollution (Environmental Protection Agency, 2008). Black children are two times more likely to have asthma than White children; additionally, they are two times more likely to be hospitalized due to asthma and four times more likely to die from it (Environmental Protection Agency, 2008).

The Surgeon General recently called for a renewed public health effort focusing on the importance of healthy homes for U.S. residents (U.S. Department of Health and Human Services, 2009). Just as air pollution has a significant impact on health, poor quality indoor air contributes to some types of cancer, heart disease, and asthma. Poor water quality can lead to gastrointestinal illness, and certain chemicals that are in and around the home can have a toxic effect on physical health. Through specific multilevel community actions, such as ensuring accessible and affordable homes that are healthy, safe, and environmentally friendly and promoting health literacy, which increases the public's understanding of the relationship between health and housing, individual, family, and community health will ultimately be improved (U.S. Department of Health and Human Services, 2009).

RESEARCH IN COMMUNITY-BASED NURSING CARE 15-1

Asthma and ED Visits

More than 20 million adults and 9 million children are diagnosed with asthma in the United States. There is strong evidence that secondhand tobacco smoke is an environmental trigger for asthma symptoms in both children and adults. The number of ED visits for asthma increased from 1.6 million in 2001 to 1.7 million in 2005. A growing number of states and local communities have passed laws prohibiting smoking in workplaces, restaurants, and bars. This study examined the impact of the implementation of a smoke-free law on ED visits for asthma in Lexington, Kentucky. During the study period, there was a 22% decline in ED visits after implementation of the smoke-free public places law in Lexington. Researchers suggest that policy and legislative efforts banning smoking in public places and in workplaces in all communities is the only way to reduce the likelihood of exposure to secondhand smoke, thus reducing ED visits related to asthma.

Rayen, M. K., Burkhart, P. V., Zhang, M., Lee, S., Moser, D. K., Mannino, D., et al. (2008). Reduction in asthma-related emergency department visits after implementation of a smoke-free law. *Journal of Allergy and Clinical Immunology, 122*(3), 537–541.

ENVIRONMENTAL HEALTH AS A GLOBAL ISSUE

The MDG 7 addresses the assurance of environmental sustainability through ensuring sustainable access to safe drinking water and basic sanitation, as well as attending to the needs of at least 100 million of the world's slum dwellers (UNDP, 2010). While progress has been made in improving access to safe drinking water, this is an area of disparity, as 8 out of 10 individuals worldwide who do not have access to clean water live in rural communities (UNDP, 2010). An estimated 25% of preventable illnesses and over one third of childhood illnesses worldwide can be attributed to poor environmental quality. Almost 2.6 billion people globally continue to lack access to safe sanitation facilities (see Fig. 15-1).

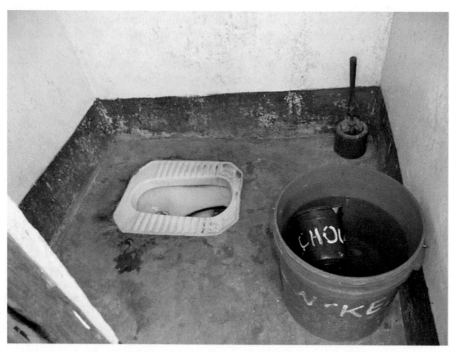

Figure 15-1 Enclosed bathroom in rural Tanzania (2009).

Nearly 48% of the population is without basic sanitation, and over 828 million people live in slums, without access to waste management (UNDP, 2010). Air pollution is estimated to cause over 2 million deaths globally every year. As mentioned earlier, the fact that air and water pollution are not contained by national boundaries contributes to the global nature of environmental issues. Further, as increasing numbers of people and products cross national borders, health risks such as infectious diseases and chemical hazards often follow. An example is seen in pesticides that are not registered or are restricted for use in the United States but that may be imported in the fruits, vegetables, and seafood produced abroad.

Over 1.2 million people die and between 20 and 50 million people are injured every year in traffic accidents worldwide. The majority of deaths occur in low- and middle-income countries, where less than half of the world's vehicles are located. Almost half who die in traffic accidents are pedestrians, cyclists, or people driving motorized two-wheelers. Road traffic deaths are projected to be the fifth leading cause of death by the year 2030, surpassing human immunodeficiency virus/acquired immunodeficiency syndrome (HIV/AIDS), tuberculosis (TB), and diarrheal diseases (WHO, 2008b) (Box 15-3). The direct and indirect impact on health care costs, including rehabilitation services, is significant. Family burden is high; the emotional toll is great, in addition to the responsibility for the medical and/or funeral costs and the costs resulting from the loss of the victim's income.

BOX 15-3 **Leading Causes of Death Worldwide, 2004 and 2030 Compared**

2004 Disease/Injury Rank	2030 Rank Disease/Injury
1 Ischemic heart disease	1 Ischemic heart disease
2 Cerebrovascular disease	2 Cerebrovascular disease
3 Lower respiratory tract infections	3 COPD
4 Chronic obstructive pulmonary disease (COPD)	4 Lower respiratory tract infections
5 Diarrheal diseases	5 Road traffic accidents
6 HIV/AIDS	6 Trachea, bronchial, and lung cancers
7 TB	7 Diabetes mellitus
8 Trachea, bronchial, and lung cancers	8 Hypertensive heart disease
9 Road traffic accidents	9 Stomach cancer
10 Prematurity and low birth weight	10 HIV/AIDS
11 Neonatal infections and other*	11 Nephritis and nephrosis
12 Diabetes mellitus	12 Self-inflicted injuries
13 Malaria	13 Liver cancer
14 Hypertensive heart disease	14 Colon and rectum cancers
15 Birth asphyxia and birth trauma	15 Esophageal cancer
16 Self-inflicted injuries	16 Violence
17 Stomach cancer	17 Alzheimer and other dementias
18 Cirrhosis of the liver	18 Cirrhosis of the liver
19 Nephritis and nephrosis	19 Breast cancer
20 Colon and rectum cancers	20 TB
21 Violence	21 Neonatal infections and other*
22 Breast cancer	22 Prematurity and low birth weight
23 Esophageal cancer	23 Diarrheal diseases
24 Alzheimer and other dementias	24 Birth asphyxia and birth trauma
	25 Malaria

*Includes other noninfectious causes which occur during the perinatal period.
Adapted from World Health Organization. (2008c). *Ten highlights in health statistics.* Geneva: World Health Organization. Retrieved August 12, 2010, from http://www.who.int/whosis/whostat/EN_WHS08_Part1.pdf

Less than half of the countries worldwide have legislation related to preventive factors such as speed, drinking and driving, use of helmets, seat belts, and infant or child car seats. For those countries that do have legislation addressing these risk factors, enforcement is inconsistent at best (WHO, 2009). Community health nurses can be on the frontline of assuring that this issue is on the agenda of federal, state, and local policy makers.

Nurses are increasingly the primary contact for clients, families, and communities concerned about health problems related to the environment both locally and globally. Nursing is well positioned to assess, prevent, and mitigate the impact of environmental hazards on the health of populations.

Global Health Disparity

There are increasing **global health disparities** between the developed and developing world. Although there is no standard designation of "developed" and "developing" countries, North America, Europe, Australia, New Zealand, and Japan are considered "developed" countries. More recently, Singapore, Hong Kong, Taiwan, and South Korea, along with Israel, Cyprus, and Slovenia, have emerged as newly industrialized economies (International Monetary Fund, 2009). Countries emerging from the former Yugoslavia, except Slovenia, are treated as developing nations (United Nations Statistics Division, 2010). Least developed countries are considered the poorest and weakest countries, where extreme poverty, weak economies, and infrastructure weaknesses impede efforts to improve the quality of life for their people (United Nations Office of the High Representative for the Least Developed Countries, Landlocked Developing Countries and the Small Island Developing States [UN-OHRLLS], 2010). At the present time, 49 countries are classified as least developed, and the majority (33) of these countries are located in Africa (UN-OHRLLS, 2010).

Global disparities include differences in health and access to health care services by gender, age, race or ethnicity, education or income, disability, geographic location, or sexual orientation. An example is seen in life expectancy. Life expectancy ranges from 38 years of age in Angola to almost 90 years of age in Morocco (Central Intelligence Agency, 2010). Over the past 50 years, average life expectancy at birth has increased globally by almost 20 years. Life expectancy reflects the quality of health care in a country, including the rates of infant mortality and HIV/AIDS infection. Many countries have made significant improvement in achieving the health related goals of the MDG, while many countries are falling behind due to high rates of HIV/AIDS, economic hardship, or conflict (WHO, 2010c). While progress has been made toward achieving the MDG of reducing infant and child mortality, as annual childhood deaths have dropped by 30% since 1990, there is still more work to do. Maternal mortality remains a concern as progress is not being made at the projected rate due to the shortage of skilled birth attendants worldwide, as well as fewer women having access to the recommended number of prenatal visits (WHO, 2010c).

Currently, high blood pressure, tobacco use, uncontrolled or untreated diabetes, physical inactivity, and overweight/obesity are the leading global risks for mortality. Globally, most deaths now are from cardiovascular disease (Mathers, Boerma, & MaFat, 2009). However, drug-resistant strains of disease, particularly TB, malaria, and pneumonia, are of growing concern. Approximately 440,000 new cases of drug-resistant TB are diagnosed annually. For individuals between 10 and 24 years of age, the majority of the causes of death are preventable and treatable. Road traffic accidents, complications during pregnancy and child birth, suicide, violence, HIV/AIDS, and TB are the major causes of death for young people worldwide (WHO, 2009).

Although mortality from cardiovascular disease has declined steadily to 250 per 100,000 in the European Union (EU) since 1970, the rate in the former Soviet Union is almost three times this level, over 750 per 100,000. The use of cigarettes and other tobacco products is responsible for 5 million deaths in the EU each year, mostly in poor countries and poor populations. In the next 20 years, without effective intervention, this toll is expected to double. Across the world, poorer children are at higher risk of dying. The leading cause of maternal mortality is hemorrhage and hypertension. While maternal mortality is improving in many countries, access to skilled birth attendants remains an issue in sub-Saharan Africa and southern Asia. Significant disparities exist between the wealthiest and poorest women in developing countries, where the wealthiest women are three times more likely to receive professional health care during birth (United Nations, 2010a). Child mortality rates in countries in the developed world are improving at a faster rate, while a child born in a developing country is over 13 times more likely to die in the first 5 years of life (UNDP, 2010). Pneumonia, malaria, diarrhea, and AIDS accounted for 43% of all deaths in children under age 5 during 2008 (United Nations, 2010b). The availability of low-cost prevention and methods of treatment such as mosquito nets, antibiotics, and drugs to treat malaria could reduce the number of deaths among children in these countries.

During 2008, approximately 17.5 million children under the age of 18 years lost one or both parents to AIDS (United Nations, 2010). Children whose parents have died of AIDS are at a greater risk for poor health, abuse and neglect, or sexual exploitation than children who are orphaned from other causes (United Nations, 2010).

Just as nurses have a role in the issue of health disparity in their own community and country, there are contributions to be made toward addressing the issue of global disparity. Most obvious is to become informed about the issues, speak out, and inform others. Box 15-4 provides an interesting illustration of the magnitude of the issue of worldwide disparity.

Emergency Preparedness

What does an outbreak of H1N1, a public water supply contaminated with potentially deadly levels of *Cryptosporidium* protozoa, an earthquake in Haiti, a war in Iraq, an outbreak of a highly contagious spinal meningitis on a college campus, and a bioterrorist attack have in common? All require a major population-based response. The difference in these issues is the level from which the response occurs. H1N1 is likely to be addressed through individual city or state efforts, while public water supply may be within the auspice of

---

 BOX 15-4   **A View of World Citizenship**

If we could shrink the earth's population to a village of 100 people, with all existing human ratios remaining the same, it would look like this:

- There would be 57 Asians, 21 Europeans, 14 from the Western Hemisphere (North and South), and 8 Africans
- 52 would be female; 48 would be male
- 70 would be persons of color; 30 would be White
- 10 would be gay, lesbian, or bisexual
- 6 would be over the age of 65
- 33 would be children, with special needs
- 30 would be Christian
- 6 people would own half of the village's wealth and all 6 would be citizens of the United States
- 9 would speak English
- 50 would suffer from malnutrition
- 80 would be living in substandard housing
- 70 would be unable to read
- 66 would not have access to clean, safe drinking water
- 1 would have a college education
- 1 would be near death; 1 would be near birth

When one considers our world from such a compressed perspective, the need for tolerance and understanding becomes glaringly apparent.

Diversity Journal. (1997). Brookline, MA: Office of Diversity, Harvard Pilgrim Health Care.

municipalities or cities. The chaos, violence, and death created by any war or an earthquake may require an international response through organizations such as the UN, Red Cross, United Nations Educational, Scientific and Cultural Organization, or Doctors Without Borders. The college or state or county health department would be the intervening body for an outbreak of spinal meningitis. Bioterrorism has become the focus of national governments as well as multinational efforts such as the North Atlantic Treaty Organization and the UN.

The equivalent of prevention, as it relates to natural **disasters**, epidemics, and terrorism, is emergency preparedness. **Emergency preparedness is** defined as the development of plans and capabilities for effective disaster response, which includes coordinating, planning, and communicating with the public in order to promote understanding of and response to public health emergencies. Potential public health threats include bioterrorism, chemical hazards, radiation emergencies, mass casualties, **natural disasters** and weather, and epidemics (Centers for Disease Control and Prevention [CDC], 2010). In the following section, epidemics, natural disasters, and terrorism are discussed. Further, the role of the nurse in addressing the related health concerns and the role of emergency preparedness are outlined.

DISASTERS

Disasters are unpredictable but occur with regularity. **Natural disasters** include such events as earthquakes, fires, hurricanes, tornados, tsunamis, and wildfires. They take tens of thousands of lives and cause billions of dollars in damage. Man-made disasters such as airline crashes, wars, chemical explosions, and other mishaps with other hazardous material also take thousands of lives each year. Both natural and man-made disasters impact the health of individuals, families, and communities by devastating the environment and significantly disrupting daily life. To mitigate these consequences, the need for preparedness is imperative.

In January 2010, an earthquake in Haiti killed over 220, 000 people and injured 300,000 more. Some 2.3 million people were displaced. Recovery efforts were delayed for days, as first responders were hindered by a lack of passable roads, the loss of bridges, and the loss of any means of communication. More than one half of the government, economic, administrative infrastructure was destroyed. Nearly one fourth of all homes in the capital city were damaged beyond recovery and had to be demolished, nearly half of all hospitals were damaged or destroyed, and nearly one fourth of all schools were destroyed or damaged (United Nations Office for the Coordination of Humanitarian Affairs, 2010). Haiti's endemic poverty contributed to the government's inability to plan or prepare for such a devastating natural disaster.

Here in the United States, this same demonstration of the vulnerability of low-income, and racial and ethnic minorities during a disaster was seen as a result of Hurricane Katrina in 2005. The resulting displacement of over half a million of the most vulnerable people taught the importance of local community planning before a disaster strikes. Early response and rescue work is the job of local health care and emergency workers, as well as ordinary citizens. Nurses can and should be at the forefront of these initiatives. Community preparedness must include consideration for and outreach to the most at-risk populations, including the development of culturally sensitive information related to vaccine safety, in the event of a **pandemic** (Trust for America's Health, 2010). As nurses and advocates for the vulnerable, it is our professional and social responsibility to educate and guide policy makers to develop emergency preparedness to minimize harm to people and property.

EPIDEMICS AND PANDEMICS

One of the great epidemics of modern times occurred during the last 6 months of World War I in 1918. In pockets across the globe, a new enemy erupted—influenza—that at first seemed as benign as the common cold but eventually became the major pandemic of modern history. A **pandemic** is an epidemic or outbreak of an infectious disease that occurs over a wide geographic area and affects an exceptionally high proportion of the population (Dictionary.com, 2010). In the 2 years that followed, the virus infected one fifth of the world's population. Unlike the typical pattern for influenza, which is most deadly for young children and the elderly, this strain was most fatal to people between 20 and 40 years of age. It infected 28% of all Americans. An estimated 675,000 Americans died of influenza during the pandemic, 10 times as many as in the World War.

An influenza pandemic has the potential to cause more death and illness compared to any other major disaster. The experience of the H1N1 pandemic during 2009 demonstrated the importance of multiple levels of advance planning and preparation for such an event. Early reports of the incidence of H1N1 occurred in California in April 2009, with outbreaks quickly being reported throughout North America. The CDC worked closely with international organizations such as the WHO and the Pan American Health Organization, Canada and Mexico. The virus quickly spread around the world and by June 2009, WHO declared H1N1 a pandemic, with 74 countries and territories reporting confirmed cases of the influenza virus (WHO, 2009). By the time the pandemic was declared over in August 2010, most countries in the world and all 50 states in the United States had documented cases of H1N1.

Within the United States, the CDC worked closely with state and local health departments to conduct epidemiological investigations to trace the source of the infection as it occurred. Of significant concern to investigators was the fact that the virus was leading to patterns of illness and death not normally identified with influenza. Most of the deaths from H1N1 occurred in young people, most of whom were otherwise healthy. As the influenza spread worldwide, CDC worked to develop a vaccine, and in October 2009, the U.S. government launched the national influenza 2009 H1N1 vaccination campaign. Globally, between 20% and 40% of populations in some areas were infected by the virus (WHO, 2010d); in the United States, it is estimated that between 43 and 89 million people were infected, resulting in somewhere between 8,870 and 18,300 deaths (CDC, 2010). When the WHO Director General declared that the H1N1 pandemic was over, he cautioned that no two pandemics are alike and are, therefore, unpredictable (WHO, 2010d). Because of this, it is essential to maintain local, state, national, and international vigilance. The international preparation and coordination assisted in early detection and reporting, thus averting an even more disastrous outcome (WHO, 2010d).

There are contributions that nurses can make to minimize the mortality, morbidity, and other losses in the event of a pandemic. An immunized health care staff is one defense strategy to minimize the spread of infectious agents. It is estimated that seasonal influenza accounts for 250,000 to 500,000 deaths worldwide annually and impacts between 5% and 20% of the U.S. population annually, resulting in more than 225,000 hospitalizations and 36,000 deaths. Health care workers are known to be a reservoir and vector of the influenza virus, yet less than 50% of health care workers are vaccinated annually (Rice, 2010). A yearly vaccine not only helps protect the nurse but also his or her family, patients, and the community from getting the flu. Further, a yearly vaccine reduces absenteeism and allows the nurse to continue to provide patient care in the event of an epidemic or a pandemic. Maintaining a low nurse/patient ratio is known to reduce mortality and improve patient outcomes.

Once again, assessment skills are essential in early identification and intervention with emerging epidemics. Nurses are in a position to notice patterns and trends in the conditions clients present with in clinics and hospitals. An upsurge in the number of clients with respiratory illness or symptoms that follow a pattern not seen in past years always requires additional exploration. Keen clinical skills along with an open, curious attitude toward clinical care can lead nurses to question what they observe. This may lead to the early identification of a new virus as well as early vigilance with an emerging epidemic, as was seen with H1N1. One nurse contacting the local or state department of health with a question or concern may be enough to identify an early case of a communicable disease. Further, the nurse may intervene by investigating the disease, gathering and analyzing the information regarding the threat to the health of populations, ascertaining the source of the threat, and determining control measures. These actions may serve to protect a community from a pandemic.

Community health nurses are uniquely situated to assist with disaster planning, response, and support. Participating in local emergency preparedness task forces for pandemics or volunteering on the National Disaster Medical System or on a local Medical Reserve Corps are just a few ways that nurses are involved in community health preparedness. In addition, nurses are often the professionals who develop educational materials and facilitate the training to ensure that communities are ready to respond should a community-wide emergency occur. All of these actions contribute to containing an influenza epidemic. Nurses may also participate in training in behavioral techniques to cope with grief, exhaustion, stress, and fear. This expertise allows nurses to assist patients, other employees, families, and communities with the psychological aspects of care during and after an emergency.

TERRORISM

The events of September 11, 2001, as well as other acts of terrorism worldwide have heightened awareness of the need for bioterrorism preparedness. The most important role played by community health nurses is that of disease surveillance. In terms of being a real threat to the health and welfare of large numbers of individuals, bioterrorism has, up to this point, caused limited mortality as compared to natural disasters and epidemics. However, preparedness for any emergency protects the citizenry. The elements of bioterrorism preparedness and management are essentially the same as those already mentioned.

Clinical Situation: Hurricane Katrina—Failure to Rescue

Prevention is a central component to community-based care. The inadequacy of the current system seen in the lack of emergency preparedness that would have minimized or avoided damage to New Orleans from Hurricane Katrina was not taken. Despite warnings from the Army Corps of Engineer, federal funding to shore up the sinking levee that protected New Orleans from Lake Pontchartrain was slashed. Despite enormous allocation of resources into biopreparedness, public officials were days too slow in responding. The inadequate command of the situation by the local, state, and federal officials was obvious. Likewise, the emergency response was poorly coordinated. Multiple inadequate systems and leadership compounded the devastation. The most heart-wrenching aspect of the entire disaster was seen in the photos and films of the aftermath of the event. These exemplified the disparity of services in the United States and illustrated the racial and class divide. Katrina profoundly brought to light that disparity is real in the United States. Nurses were some of the heroes of this disaster, providing leadership through organization, coordination, advocacy, teamwork, and support for patients, families, staff, and peers (Danna & Matthews, 2010).

Immigrants and Refugees

The plight of **refugees** and **immigrants** has been a phenomena throughout human history. Famines, floods, and other natural disasters, as well as human-created disasters of war and domination, are documented in the holy books of the Old Testament and Torah. All of these events have forced, and do force, human relocation at great loss of life and severe disruption of quality of life.

In the United States, there are three categories of newcomers: legal immigrants, refugees, and **undocumented workers**. Although there are some similarities between these categories, there are important distinctions. Most newcomers to the United States are legal **immigrants** who come here by choice, while **refugees** are typically fleeing from their country of origin. In most cases, despite the harsh circumstances surrounding the immigrant or refugees' life in their country of origin, their experience is colored by loss and uncertainly following relocation.

There are an unspecified number of **undocumented workers** in the United States who enter the country illegally mainly for employment opportunities. Most of these individuals leave their country of origin to escape abject poverty. Despite their contribution to the U.S. economy through taxes, they are barred from many rights that most citizens take for granted: the legal right to work, hold a driver's license, and collect Social Security payments. Understandably, reluctant to have any contact with government or state officials, they often avoid health or legal services.

The varied needs of this diverse population present a challenge to health care providers. One is access to systems of care. They often encounter numerous barriers to care, stemming from their own cultural norms toward certain types of care from their country of origin. For many refugees, preventive care is a new concept, which they were not afforded in their country of origin. Lack of knowledge and understanding of the U.S. health care system results in a reluctance to seek care, particularly for mental health services or prenatal care. Along with many other Americans, newcomers often lack any or adequate health insurance. Unfortunately, health care services are not always culturally sensitive, resulting in their not being appealing or appearing relevant to the newcomer. Cultural norms both of the newcomer and of the nurse create powerful barriers to care. The language barriers are often obvious but create ongoing barriers to care. Specific suggestions to deal with these obstacles are discussed in Chapters 3 and 6.

Nurses can learn a great deal about international health by seeking out experiences with new Americans in their own communities. One way to do this is by requesting to care for these clients when they come to the unit, clinic, or agency where the nurse works. Developing expertise in caring for new Americans in one's own community is another approach to understanding global health. Listening to the life stories of new Americans is another, as our clients are often our most important teachers.

Nursing Advocacy in Global Health

Advocacy is to "plead someone's cause or act on someone's behalf, with a focus on developing the individual, family's, or community capacity to plead their own cause or act on their own behalf" (Public Health Nursing Interventions, 2001, p. 262). The principles of advocacy in global health are the same, whether in one's own neighborhood or in a distant land. Obviously, because issues related to global health often occur some distance away, some of the strategies for advocacy are different, as compared to those in our own community. To act as an advocate for someone suffering from a famine in Africa, we may think that the only way to impact their condition is to go to central Africa or to donate to a charity. Too far, we may say, to make a difference. However, awareness campaigns and membership in groups supporting international efforts are ways to participate in international advocacy. As mentioned, one way to broaden practice skills and knowledge is to become familiar with, and eventually act as an advocate for, new Americans in our own community. Another strategy is to become involved in international health organizations.

There is wide variation in the size, organization, and funding of international health organizations. Sometimes getting involved in an organization creates opportunities to learn about the organizations' goals and missions. It is prudent to use care before giving time or money to any cause. The agenda of some of these organizations may be self-serving and work against improving the health status of a population the organization seeks to serve. An example would be an organization offering free samples or selling formula to women who are breast-feeding. Unless contraindicated because of certain infectious diseases, it is generally in the infant and mother's best interest to continue breast-feeding. Another example would be if in a country where most citizens are Muslim, a Christian organization requires that recipients of humanitarian aid participate in Christian religious services.

The trend in international health organizations is to focus more on preventative services and sustainability. Agencies are concentrating on the development of rapid response teams that use short-term assignments to target specific health issues. Once you have clarified that the agency you are interested in becoming active in represents an approach consistent with your own values, you may decide to become more involved. Some international health organizations are listed in What's on the Web at the end of the chapter.

Global Nursing Shortage

The nursing shortage is a global problem. It is occurring in health systems around the world, creating a serious crisis in terms of adverse impact on health and well-being of populations. Achievement of the MDG will be impacted by the shortage of health care providers globally. One recent report states there is a shortfall of more than 4.3 million health care workers worldwide, including the need for over 600,000 nurses to meet the need in sub-Saharan Africa alone. Although there have been a shortage of nurses in the past, currently the health systems are suffering from pressure exerted on both supply and demand. Further, the future need for nurses will continue to escalate as the worldwide population ages, the health care provider workforce ages, and the growth for alternative careers for woman continues. Multiple critical issues contribute to the current shortage, including poor deployment practices, international migration, high attrition, HIV/AIDS, a shortage of nursing faculty worldwide, and an underinvestment in human resources. For many people globally, the necessary higher education for entry into health care is unachievable due to poverty and family demands. And, while the shortage of health care providers increases, health care demands also increase, contributing to an international workforce crisis.

Nurses make up the largest group of health care providers in every country in the world. Because nursing services are essential to the provision of safe and effective care, addressing these issues is imperative to thwart a major crisis in health care. Nursing is often on the frontline in the provision of health care in areas of greatest need. In sub-Saharan Africa, the shortage is so critical that even basic health care services for infants, children, and woman are not readily available. In a world where global issues become local issues, a global nursing shortage has implications for citizens in every country.

The nursing shortage brings up interesting questions related to advocacy at the global level. This plays out in a variety of ways with numerous implications. Rather than further marginalize fledgling health systems, wealthy nations could act as advocates by not actively recruiting nurses from developing countries. Nurses in developed countries have a professional responsibility to advocate, not to actively recruit nurses from developing countries into developed countries. The intent would be to avoid exacerbating disparity between developed and developing countries and prevent further marginalizing of health systems that are struggling.

Conclusions

Globalization requires that the profession of nursing expand the scope and emphasis of community-based care to include the global community. It is imperative that nurses be informed and competent in the areas of environmental health, global health disparity, and emergency preparedness. The need for international advocacy intensifies as the nursing shortage worldwide simultaneously transpires while the health needs of the world intensify. These challenges call for all nurses regardless of their nationality or ethnicity to reflect on the world as the client.

What's on the Web

World Health Organization
INTERNET ADDRESS: **http://www.who.int/en/**
   The WHO is the United Nations agency for health. It was established to focus on the attainment by all peoples of the highest possible level of health. Health is defined in WHO's Constitution as a state of complete physical, mental, and social well-being and not merely the absence of disease or infirmity.

United Nations Millennium Development Goals
INTERNET ADDRESS: **http://www.undp.org/mdg**
   The Millennium Development Goals are eight concrete goals established by world leaders and adopted by multiple international organizations to address local and global development needs, including reducing world poverty and hunger, improving women and children's health, reducing infant mortality, and ensuring environmental sustainability.

Global Health
INTERNET ADDRESS: **http://www.globalhealth.gov/**
   The U.S. Department of Health and Human Services Web site is dedicated to global health issues, including current topics in refugee health, global health, specific health information by country, and information relevant for international travel.

International Health Volunteers
INTERNET ADDRESS: http://www.globalvolunteers.org/

As a nongovernmental organization (NGO) in special consultative status with the United Nations, Global Volunteers mobilizes some 150 service-learning teams year-round to work in 20 countries on six continents and is the internationally recognized leader in this field of work. Global Volunteers continues to work to help lay a foundation for world peace through mutual understanding.

Cross-Cultural Solutions
INTERNET ADDRESS: http://www.crossculturalsolutions.org/

Cross-Cultural Solutions offers international volunteers an opportunity to make a meaningful contribution working side-by-side with local people and sharing in the goals of a community. This experience allows one to gain new perspective and insight into the culture and themselves.

Peace Corps
INTERNET ADDRESS: http://www.peacecorp.gov

The Peace Corps traces its roots and mission to 1960, when then-Senator John F. Kennedy challenged college students to serve their country in the cause of peace by living and working in developing countries. From that inspiration grew an agency of the federal government devoted to world peace and friendship. Since that time, more than 182,000 Peace Corps Volunteers have been invited by 138 host countries to work on issues ranging from AIDS education, information technology, and environmental preservation.

Centers for Disease Control and Prevention/Emergency Preparedness & Response
INTERNET ADDRESS: http://www.bt.cdc.gov/

This site provides information and links for bioterrorism, mass causalities, chemical emergencies, natural disasters, radiation emergencies, and recent outbreaks and incidents (epidemics). There are numerous other topics found on this site along with the most recent research and resources such as videos and slides.

Emergency Preparedness
INTERNET ADDRESS: http://www.ready.gov/

This Web site provides linkages to information for individuals and businesses in order to prepare for disasters. It includes a linkage to state-specific information, as well as local resources to volunteer for and/or assist with community emergency preparedness.

New York Consortium for Emergency Preparedness Continuing Education (NYCEPCE)
INTERNET ADDRESS: http://www.nycepce.org/default.htm

The mission of the NYCEPCE is to strengthen the competency of health professionals to respond effectively to emergency events of all kinds through competency-based continuing education. There are numerous resources on the Web site that can be used for training purposes including an emergency preparedness course for hospital clinicians.

The National Center for Disaster Preparedness
INTERNET ADDRESS: http://www.ncdp.mailman.columbia.edu/training.htm

This is a resource for free, online courses related to public health and disaster preparedness. There are webinars, slides, videos, and printed resources.

National Nurse Emergency Preparedness Initiative
INTERNET ADDRESS: http://www.nnepi.org

Sponsored by George Washington University, George Mason University, and the Department of Homeland Security, this is a centralized resource of online learning resources for nurses, organized by type of employment.

References and Bibliography

American Heart Association. (2010). *Air pollution, heart disease and stroke.* Retrieved August 10, 2010, from http://www.americanheart.org/presenter.jhtml?identifier=4419

American Nurses Association. (2001). *Nursing code of ethics.* The Center for Ethics and Human Rights. Retrieved July 30, 2010, from http://nursingworld.org/ethics/code/protected_nwcoe629.htm

Bahadori, K., Doyle-Waters, M., Marra, C., Lynd, L., Alasaly, K., Swiston, J., et al. (2009). Economic burden of asthma: A systematic review. *Pulmonary Medicine, 9*(24), 1–16.

Centers for Disease Control and Prevention. (n.d.). *National environmental public health tracking network*. Retrieved August 10, 2010, from http://ephtracking.cdc.gov/showHome.action

Centers for Disease Control and Prevention. (2010). *Emergency preparedness and response*. Retrieved August 8, 2010, from http://emergency.cdc.gov/planning/

Central Intelligence Agency. (2010). *Country comparison: Life expectancy at birth. The World Factbook*. Retrieved August 2, 2010, from https://www.cia.gov/library/publications/the-world-factbook/rankorder/2102rank.html

Danna, D., & Matthews, P. (2010). Experiences of nurse leaders surviving Hurrican Katrina, New Orleans, Louisianna, USA. *Nursing and Health Science, 12*, 9–13.

Dictionary.com. (2010). Retrieved August 12, 2010, from http://www.dictionary.reference.com/browse/pandemic

Diversity Journal. (1997). Brookline, MA: Office of Diversity, Harvard Pilgrim Health Care.

Environmental Protection Agency. (2008). *Children's environmental health disparities: Black and African American children and asthma*. Retrieved August 10, 2010, from http://yosemite.epa.gov/ochp/ochpweb.nsf/content/HD_AA_Asthma.htm/$File/HD_AA_Asthma.pdf

Merriam-Webster online dictionary. (2010). Retrieved August 10, 2010, from http://www.merriam-webster.com/dictionary/globalization

Institute of Medicine. (2010). *Infectious disease movement in a borderless world*. Washington, DC: The National Academies Press.

International Monetary Fund. (2009). *World economic outlook: Database—WEO groups and aggregates information*. Retrieved August 2, 2010, from http://www.imf.org/external/pubs/ft/weo/2009/02/weodata/groups.htm#ae

Mathers, C. D., Boerma, T., & MaFat, D. (2009). Global and regional causes of death. *British Medical Bulletin, 92*(1), 7–32.

Minnesota Department of Health, Division of Community Health Services, Public Health Nursing Section. (2001). *Public health nursing interventions: Application for public health nursing practice*. Minneapolis, MN: Author.

National Resources Defense Council. (2008). *Global warming and our health: Addressing the most serious impacts of climate change*. Retrieved August 10, 2010, from http://www.nrdc.org/health/effects/globalwarming-map/gwhealth.pdf

Rayen, M. K., Burkhart, P. V., Zhang, M., Lee, S., Moser, D. K., Mannino, D., et al. (2008). Reduction in asthma-related emergency department visits after implementation of a smoke-free law. *Journal of Allergy and Clinical Immunology, 122*(3), 537–541.

Rice, R. (2010). Is it ethnically permissible to mandate influenza vaccination for health care workers? *Journal of the American Academy of Physician Assistants,33*(8), 27–30. Retrieved August 12, 2010, from http://www.jaapa.com/is-it-ethically-permissible-to-mandate-influenza-vaccination-for-health-care-workers/article/171485/

Trust for America's Health. (2010). *Ready or not? 2009*. Retrieved August 10, 2010, from http://healthyamericans.org/reports/bioterror09/

United Nations. (2009). *The United Nations and road safety*. Retrieved August 2, 2010, from http://www.un.org/en/roadsafety/

United Nations Development Programme. (2006a). *Millenium development goals*. Retrieved July 20, 2010, from http://www.undp.org/mdg/basics.shtml

United Nations Development Programme. (2006b). *What are the millenium development goals?* Retrieved July 20, 2010, from http://www.undp.org/mdg/learnmore.shtml

United Nations Development Programme. (2010a). *The Millenium development goals report*. Retrieved July 20, 2010, from http://mdgs.un.org/unsd/mdg/Resources/Static/Products/Progress2010/MDG_Report_2010_En.pdf

United Nations Development Programme. (2010b). *The Millenium development goals report*. Retrieved July 20, 2010, from http://mdgs.un.org/unsd/mdg/Resources/Static/Products/Progress2010/MDG_Report_2010_En.pdf

United Nations Office for the Coordination of Humanitarian Affairs. (2010). *Haiti earthquake: Six months later*. Retrieved August 22, 2010, from http://ochaonline.un.org/tabid/6412/language/en-US/Default.aspx

United Nations Office of the High Representative for the Least Developed Countries, Landlocked Developing Countries and the Small Island Developing States [UN-OHRLLS]. (2010). *Least developed countries*. Retrieved August 2, 2010, from http://www.unohrlls.org/en/ldc

United Nations Statistics Division. (2010). *Composition of macro geographical (continental) regions, geographical sub-regions, and selected economic and other groupings*. Retrieved August 2, 2010, from http://unstats.un.org/unsd/methods/m49/m49regin.htm#ftnc

U. S. Department of Health and Human Services. (2009). *The Surgeon General's call to action to promote healthy homes*. Rockville, MD: U. S. Department of Health and Human Services, Office of the Surgeon General.

U. S. Department of Health and Human Services. (2010). *Healthy People 2020 framework*. Retrieved August 1, 2010, from http://www.healthypeople.gov/hp2020/Objectives/framework.aspx

World Health Organization. (2008a). *Air quality and health*. Retrieved August 3, 2010, from http://www.who.int/mediacentre/factsheets/fs313/en/index.html

World Health Organization. (2008b). *Closing the gap in a generation: Health equity through action on the social determinants of health*. Retrieved July 17, 2010, from http://whqlibdoc.who.int/hq/2008/WHO_IER_CSDH_08.1_eng.pdf

World Health Organization. (2008c). *Ten highlights in health statistics*. Geneva, Switzerland: World Health Organization. Retrieved August 12, 2010, from http://www.who.int/whosis/whostat/EN_WHS08_Part1.pdf

World Health Organization. (2009). *Road accidents, suicide and maternal conditions are leading causes of death in young people*. Retrieved August 2, 2010, from http://www.who.int/mediacentre/news/releases/2009/adolescent_mortality_20090911/en/index.html

World Health Organization. (2010a). *Climate change*. Retrieved August 3, 2010, from http://www.who.int/mediacentre/factsheets/fs266/en/index.html

World Health Organization. (2010b). *Environmental health*. Retrieved August 3, 2010, from http://www.who.int/topics/environmental_health/en/

World Health Organization. (2010c). *Millennium Development Goals: Progress towards the health-related Millennium Development Goals*. Retrieved July 27, 2010, from http://www.who.int/mediacentre/factsheets/fs290/en/index.html

World Health Organization. (2010d). *H1N1 in post-pandemic period*. Retrieved August 12, 2010, from http://www.who.int/mediacentre/news/statements/2010/h1n1_vpc_20100810/en/index.html

LEARNING ACTIVITIES

JOURNALING ACTIVITY 15-1

In your clinical journal, respond to the following:

- What has surprised you about the information presented in this chapter?
- As you consider the MDGs, what do you believe are the barriers to achieving these goals by 2015?
- Discuss your own attitudes and beliefs regarding global health.
- How have your views about global health been influenced by the media?
- What are the roles that nurses play in international health? How do these roles reflect your understanding of nursing?
- How has your view of the nursing role in the community changed after reading this chapter (and observing the role of the nurse in the community)?

PRACTICAL APPLICATION ACTIVITY 15-2

Find the WHO Web site (http://www.who.int/en). Click on the Countries site. Choose at least two countries and compare the statistics, health expenditures, and provisions/coverage. Choose at least one developing country and compare it to a developed country.

- What did you learn? What surprised you?
- What were the leading causes of mortality? Or morbidity? How does this compare to the United States?
- How does this information help you in your practice?
- What do you think that nurses should or can do about the issues you have identified?

PRACTICAL APPLICATION ACTIVITY 15-3

Choose one of the countries from Practical Application Activity 15-2. Select one health priority for that country and develop a health plan, using population-level interventions from the Minnesota Department of Health Public Health Nursing Intervention Wheel to address the priority. As a part of your plan, identify an international organization that you could collaborate with to implement your intervention.

CLINICAL REASONING ACTIVITY 15-4

Review the MDGs at http://www.un.org/millenniumgoals/ and http://www.undp.org/mdg/.
Respond to the following questions.

1. What is the intent of this initiative?
2. Why is this initiative important for global health?
3. What is the connection between improving access to education and health? Between eradicating poverty and health?
4. Why is it important for the health of citizens in the United States?

CLIENT CARE ACTIVITY 15-5

Marie is a Central American woman in her mid-30s. She comes to your clinic with a wound on the top of her hand that is red, draining copious green and yellow pus. As you remove the dirty bandage that is covering the wound you ask her what happened to her hand. She looks down and does not answer your question. You ask her again. When she does not reply, what do you do?

YOU WONDER IF SHE HEARS YOU OR IF SHE DOES NOT SPEAK ENGLISH.

You ask her in Spanish if she speaks or understands English. She indicates that she does not speak English but understands. You contact an interpreter.

The interpreter arrives 1 hour later. In the meantime you have cleaned and débrided the wound and applied ointment. How do you proceed with the interpreter? (Hint: see Community-Based Nursing Care Guidelines 6-1 Working With Interpreters.)

JOURNALING ACTIVITY 15-6

Reread Client Care Activity 15-5. In your clinical journal, respond to the following:

- How would you feel if you discovered Marie is an undocumented immigrant?
- Would it matter if Marie has been in the United States for less than 1 year? Would it matter if she has been employed in the United States for the past 10 years?
- How would you feel if Marie has children who were born in the United States, and, therefore, are U.S. citizens?
- How might these feelings influence your nursing practice?

JOURNALING ACTIVITY 15-7

In your clinical journal, respond to the following:

- How do you feel about nurses being mandated to report during a disaster?
- What might prevent you from being willing to report to a disaster?
- How do you feel about mandatory vaccinations for health care workers during a pandemic? How might this influence your practice?

SIMULATION ACTIVITY 15-8: OUTBREAK AT WATERSEDGE

http://www.mclph.umn.edu/watersedge/
Follow the link and complete this interactive game. It provides an opportunity to learn about how a disease outbreak is handled by a public health agency. It is an entertaining way to learn what nurses and other public health professionals do in the event of a disease outbreak. Learn how nurses play an important role in determining the source of disease outbreaks in most communities.

Source: Centers for Public Health Education and Outreach (CPHEO) at the University of Minnesota School of Public Health.

SIMULATION ACTIVITY 15-9: DISASTER IN FRANKLIN COUNTY

http://cpheo.sph.umn.edu/umncphp/franklincounty.html
Complete this simulation, where you will assume the perspective of various public health professionals responding to a natural disaster. You will make decisions as would a county public health director, a public health nurse, an environmental health specialist, and other public health professionals. By approaching the emerging public health issues from these perspectives, you will gain a deeper understanding of the issues at hand, the decisions that colleagues in other disciplines face, and how those decisions impact nursing.

Source: Centers for Public Health Education and Outreach (CPHEO) at the University of Minnesota School of Public Health.

LEARNING MODULE ACTIVITY 15-10: ENVIRONMENTAL HEALTH ONLINE

http://cpheo.sph.umn.edu/mclph/courses/ehn.html
Complete the first section, *Introduction to Environmental Health and Nursing.* This will assist you to develop a framework for integrating environmental health concepts into nursing practice.

Source: Centers for Public Health Education and Outreach (CPHEO) at the University of Minnesota School of Public Health.

UNIT V

Implications for Future Practice

Nursing is a profession that is constantly evolving. Any nurse, whether he or she has practiced for years or is just entering the profession, needs to think ahead. What will the trends and patterns in society hold for the future of community-based nursing care? How can you best prepare yourself to give quality care in your future practice?

Chapter 16 reviews anticipated future trends in health care and implications for community-based nursing care. The role of the nurse, including educational preparation, is discussed at length. Cost containment will remain a prominent deciding factor in health care delivery, but it must also be weighed in relation to maintaining quality care. The implications of technological developments and the information age, and their profound impact on everyday nursing care, are discussed. All of these issues are considered in light of the shift in demographics in the United States.

Chapter 16 ◈ **Trends in Community-Based Nursing**

Chapter 16

Trends in Community-Based Nursing

ROBERTA HUNT

Learning Objectives

1. Discuss how current trends in community-based nursing will affect the role of the nurse in the future.

2. Determine how market-driven economic policy affects the delivery of nursing care.

3. Discuss the implications of technological developments on health care in general and on the nursing profession specifically.

4. Identify trends in knowledge explosion related to alternative and complementary therapies.

5. Outline how the shift in demographics affects the role of the nurse.

6. Develop a plan for your personal goals as a nurse in community-based settings.

Key Terms

Chapter Topics

The Nursing Student Speaks

Completing a rotation in the community has definitely made me realize that I am no longer going to be Elizabeth Wright. I am going to be Elizabeth Wright, RN, and along with that title comes a piece of responsibility. I am no longer just a name; I am a person with a title. In other words, when you think of Dr. Smith, you automatically think that there is an air of power with that title, and I fully intend to use my new power. This is something that became more apparent to me this last semester when I was doing my community rotation. Yes, people look up to someone with a title. I am a role model for people. And I have to be very careful and deliberate in my actions. But it is also very exciting. I always wanted to be a nurse, and I have always wanted to do good and make a positive difference. I have always known that that was possible through nursing. But I think being at a shelter and working as a student in the community has made it much more real for me.

Elizabeth Wright, Nursing Student
St. Catherine University

Trends in Health Care

Forces affecting health care in the future will also affect the role of the nurse. One can only speculate about what that future will be. Some broad changes can almost certainly be predicted. These include emphasis on cost containment resulting from market-driven economic policy, advancements in technology, **knowledge explosion**, expanded use of alternative and **complementary therapies**, and demographic shifts.

Anticipating these trends is imperative to maintaining quality and appropriate nursing service. Curricula in schools of nursing and staff education in the service arena are faced with preparing nurses to meet these changing requirements. Content related to cost containment will be essential. It will be a given that nurses are technologically competent and able to keep up with new ways of accessing and using information. The knowledge explosion requires that nurses develop skills in evaluating the legitimacy, efficacy, and importance of information and new treatments. All of these changes will occur within the context of shifting demographics for a population that is older, more diverse, and living with more chronic conditions. A shortage of nurses and nurse educators creates additional challenges. In this chapter, all of these are addressed within the context of community-based care.

The Future of Nursing Care

Nurses in practice in the 21st century face new responsibilities and new challenges as clients, and family members have a larger role in administering complex treatment regimes, usually under distant medical supervision. As the complexity of these interventions increases, so does the need for a skilled nurse able to use surveillance to identify early changes in the client's physical and mental condition. In the future, the evolving role of the nurse in all settings calls for well-developed clinical reasoning skills and clinical judgment and effective communication and collaborating skills. While the role of the nurse will continue to demand a service orientation of cost-containment, these must be accompanied by accountability for clinical outcomes accomplished through continuous improvement of care. Increasingly, nurses must combine population-based approaches with an ethic of social responsibility. In order to meet these robust expectations, all nurses must make a commitment to continual learning in professional development (Benner, Sutphen, Leonard, & Day, 2010).

In the future, nurses must be prepared to use clinical reasoning skills to solve problems and make independent clinical judgments regarding care based on the most recent evidence.

They must be knowledgeable about making appropriate referrals to other disciplines and community agencies. Because more acute care will be provided in the home and clinics, nurses must be able to autonomously perform complex, precise, and diverse technological interventions and must be adept at detailed documentation to ensure payment for services. As a larger number and percentage of the population are older, living with chronic conditions and managing symptoms at home, there will be a need for competent, skilled nursing practitioners who are comfortable practicing independently in the area of disease management.

Flexibility will be important because cost-containment measures require decreased specialization. Administrators are introducing multiskilled health care providers who are cross-trained to practice in a **"seamless care"** environment, in which practitioners provide care in different facilities or settings. With the trend away from specialization of health care personnel, nurses will be called on to perform more tasks and to cross discipline lines. In home care nursing, this is evidenced by nurses doing venipuncture (a laboratory technician's role) and teaching and monitoring administration of oxygen (a respiratory therapist's role). To prepare for the home care role, nurses must be competent case managers and health educators.

Nurses have a responsibility for advocating for clients as well as taking the lead in shaping health care in the future. Nurses are fortunate to belong to a profession that commands a high level of credibility and respect seen in the fact that they have consistently been the highest rated profession in Gallup's "honesty and ethics" survey since 1999. When polled, an overwhelming majority of leaders from insurance, corporate, health services, government, and industry as well as university faculty say that nurses should have more influence on health systems and services (Robert Wood Johnson, 2010). This extends from reducing medical errors, to increasing the quality of care, to promoting wellness, to improving efficiency, and to reducing costs. While these leaders also viewed nurses as having less influence on health care reform compared to government, insurance, and pharmaceutical executives, a majority said that nurses should have more influence than they do now on health policy, planning, and management.

This high degree of public support begs the following question: "How can nurses use this asset to advocate on behalf of our profession and the clients, families, and communities we serve?" Every day elected officials make decisions that impact our profession and the clients for whom we care. Registered nurses (RNs) have the largest number of professionals of all health care professions. There is power in numbers. If nurses were to become involved in the political, legislative, and regulatory processes of government, they could have a significant impact on policy. Nurses should not only know who their elected Representatives and Senators are but also educate these officials about health and the status of health care. Nurses observe on a daily basis clients and families without insurance and the impact that poor health has on individual and family life. Nurses may be forced, because of policy or

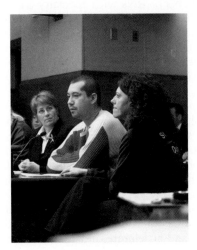

Figure 16-1 Erin Murphy, RN, a state legislator in Minnesota, brings the perspective of nursing to the political process. Source: Erin Murphy, 2011, used by permission.

lack of insurance, to discharge clients with inadequate resources at home. Nurses often hear anecdotes from clients and families of rehospitalizations resulting from the lack of sufficient health teaching, case management, or continuity. Both anecdotal accounts of what is seen in practice and research findings can be shared with officials to affect future legislation on health care reform (Fig. 16-1).

In the last decade, our profession has made major progress in several areas of public policy. The issue of delegating duties to nonlicensed personnel has been addressed and continues to need clarification. In some states, hospitals are mandated to maintain a safe level of staffing RNs based on the research on staffing ratio and hospital mortality. Today, advanced practice nurses (APNs) can bill directly through Medicare and, in most states, can prescribe medication. The Affordability Act further expands opportunities for APNs in community-based settings. Increasingly, concern about the number and the percentage of Americans without health insurance has led more states to devise plans to provide primary care to the **underinsured** or **uninsured**. The Affordability Act improves access to care by increasing funding for community health centers and establishing new programs to support school-based health centers and nurse-managed health clinics (Kaiser Family Foundation, 2010). All of these policies were shaped by the lobbying efforts of various nursing organizations, groups concerned about equity in access to health care, along with the efforts of numerous individual citizens.

There are several ways that nurses can be involved in the political process. The first is to be informed about issues that impact health care and the nursing profession. Obviously, once informed, everyone must remember to vote. It would require only a fraction of our nation's almost three million RNs to create a collective voice and an unstoppable force for change for our profession, our patients, and our nation's crumbling health care system.

EDUCATIONAL PREPARATION AND ADVANCED PRACTICE NURSING

As discussed, if current trends continue, the outlook is that nurses will perform a wider range of responsibilities. This will require both increased knowledge and skill because community-based care demands a more proficient and autonomous practitioner. The current number of nurses educated at each level of preparation does not support this growing demand. Forty-five percent of all new nurses graduate from an associate degree program, 34% receive baccalaureate degrees, and 20% from hospital-based programs (U.S. Department of Health and Human Services [DHHS], 2010). The need for nurses with a baccalaureate degree will exceed the supply in this second decade of the 21st century. The fastest growing nursing programs for undergraduate preparation are those offering a BA/BS in nursing for RNs with an ADN degree and those offering a major in nursing for individuals who have already completed a BS or BA in another discipline.

Currently, there is a great deal of support for APNs or RNs with specialty training at the master's degree level to provide primary care. As early as the 1980s, studies showed that when comparing the same type of clients, nurse practitioners have as good or better outcomes as physicians. During the early 1990s, state laws broadened the authority of nurse practitioners by allowing prescriptive authority and third-party billing. As a result, nurse practitioners can establish independent practices paralleling those of primary care physicians. This trend is expected to continue.

Specialty areas of nurse practitioners have expanded to numerous subspecialties in the last three decades. These include adult, gerontology, neonatal, occupational, pediatric, psychiatric, school or college student, and women's health. Nurse practitioners work in both rural and urban areas, from rural North Dakota to New York City. They practice in diverse settings such as community health centers, hospitals, college student health clinics, physician offices, nurse practitioner offices, nursing homes and hospices, home health care agencies, and nursing schools.

The most severe shortage of graduate prepared nurses is in nursing education, particularly those with a PhD. With a large percentage of nurse educators anticipated to retire in the next decade, this trend is expected to continue and accelerate and remain a primary contributor to the nursing shortage. Further, there is an established need for faculty who are nurse practitioners with an interest in research and advanced practice at the master's and doctoral levels. Nursing administrators must be educated and trained in management, finance, and the economic and social implications of our changing population as it affects the health care system.

Trends call for all nurses to be well prepared for the current and future practice roles, which again highlight the need for nurses to view education as a lifelong process. Continuing education is essential as the care delivery system demands more nurses with baccalaureate, graduate, and postgraduate degrees.

Cost Containment

The U.S. health care system is the most expensive in the world, using over 15% of the gross national product, yet ranks behind most other industrialized countries in virtually every measure of health (World Health Organization, 2011). Further, only half of U.S. adults receive preventive and screening tests. Every industrialized nation, except the United States, has a national health plan in place that covers all citizens. However, in the United States, health care is not a right but a commodity available to those who can purchase it, sold as a part of a **market-driven economy**. In a market-driven economy, consumer demand drives production regarding which services will be created and consumed and in what quantity. Keeping costs down and profits up is always the key aspect of a market-driven economy. Managed care has increasingly become an important provider of care because its central element is cost containment. Thus, cost containment as an important element of health care is here to stay. Consequently, nurses must continue to be aware of the financial aspects of the work they do, whatever the setting or position, now and in the future.

Technology and Information

TECHNOLOGIC DEVELOPMENT

The health care system of the future will continue to be driven by technology and information. Technology is the tool to extend human abilities, manage information, and make decisions about care. These tools may include using cell phones, televisions, Internet, and other means of electronic transmission and video-conferencing to monitor vital signs and an array of other measurements such as heart and lung sounds, blood glucose, and oxygen saturation. Many aspects of case management, chronic disease treatment, hospice care, postsurgical care, and rehabilitation are possible through telehealth. Technology assists functions such as delivery of medications, assessment processes, completing procedures, monitoring medical devices, and other electronically based systems that support care delivery. At this time, the most promising advances are associated with high-speed telecommunications and portable computers and devices. Nurses will program, operate, and troubleshoot a variety of technological devices. Because models evolve constantly, the potential for improving continuity is an important aspect of nurse-managed technology.

Several trends are shaping technology in health care. One trend is that of globalization. This started at the beginning of the 20th century with the invention of the telephone and was expanded at the end of the 20th century with the development of the wireless telephone and other devices, expansion of personal computers, and the creation of the Internet. Gradually, national borders have dissolved as the world has become one. Thanks to cell phones, telecommunications, and telemedicine, nurses are now able to practice across geographic and national borders. Physicians and **health care organizations** are using globalization to export expertise, a practice that has accelerated because of concerns for cost and profit. Through the construction of systems, health care providers, intermediaries, and consumers are able to collaborate and share information. Further, through technology, we now have the capability to maintain comprehensive health care databases for creating disease-management programs and clinical protocols. In addition, through telemedicine and remote-monitoring technologies, health care providers are able to access health information 24 hours a day, 7 days a week.

Electronic health records are one important application of multiple technologies. The value of personal health records was evident after Hurricane Katrina in 2005 when hundreds of thousands of health records were destroyed. The electronic health record is an evolving concept that is commonly defined as a systematic collection of electronic health information about individual clients or groups of clients. Although, in almost every other sector besides health, electronic information exchange is the accepted business model, only 2 in 10 doctors and 1 in 10 hospitals use even a basic electronic record system. Health care reform through the Recovery Act has reduced many of the obstacles that limited the spread of electronic health records in the past (Sebelius, 2010). The expected trend is that electronic health records become the norm throughout the health care system.

KNOWLEDGE EXPLOSION

The **knowledge explosion** has produced what is often referred to as the information age. Genetics is one area in which the information explosion is particularly evident. Because of the completion in 2000 of part of the Human Genome Project, which has mapped the human genetic code, it was expected that treatments would be possible that were not even considered within the realm of possibility in the previous decade. For example, **pharmacogenomics** is the technology of developing and producing medications tailored to specific genetic profiles. In the mid-2000s, it was postulated that the physician or nurse practitioner would be able to draw a genetic blood test that would indicate which medication was right for each person. This theory led to an increased integration of diagnostics and pharmaceuticals in scientific research. Understanding the role for epigenetic modifications in the human genome progressed rapidly over the decade, but by 2010 the science of this theory was being questioned. It had become evident that the science of the theory that medication could be tailored to specific genetic profiles was more complex than first believed. More clinical trials were deemed necessary (Rivera & Bennett, 2010). The speculation surrounding pharmacogenomics exemplified how the development of new technology has an uneven path of progression. Press releases in the media may sound promising for any given treatment, but the development of medical science is a dynamic, ongoing process. This makes it very difficult to advise clients on new treatments.

Technological advances such as the Human Genome Project stimulate emergence of codeveloped products and create a need for new regulations. For example, biotech companies are developing blood tests that reveal disease–gene mutations that forecast an individual's chances of developing a certain condition or disease such as dementia. The rapid development of technology in health care creates numerous ethical questions. Often, the technology is ready for use before these ethical issues are fully explored. Further, the exponential availability of medical technology drives consumer expectations and demands.

Major scientific developments have been occurring so quickly that knowledge overload is common. In the past, clients and families consulted their nurses, nurse practitioners, or physicians for information regarding health and illness. The health care provider carried that information in his or her head or knew where to go to explore the question. Now, an almost infinite amount of information is available to anyone who is computer-literate. This causes difficulty for the consumer as well as the health care provider. Not only is the amount of information overwhelming, but it is also difficult to discern what is outdated, incorrect, or unproven information, and what is not. Therefore, it is important for the health care provider and the consumer to realize that being information-literate is an ongoing process.

NURSING IMPLICATIONS

Computer technology has freed the nurse from some paperwork, allowing more time for client care and teaching about self-care. The expanding implementation of electronic health records allows the preservation of a client's history from birth to death.

Automation and electronic transmission of information in home care and in other community settings is viewed as a way to improve efficiency. A growing number of manufacturers produce this developing technology that integrates data with a central system, facilitates the tracking of specific costs, and allows the client to interact with the system and retrieve information regarding care.

Imagine working as a home health care nurse or in a clinic, transmitting pertinent diagnostic data directly to the attending physician, and having a three-way interaction with the client, physician, and nurse instantly. It has become common for nurses to electronically connect with client databases to obtain information from the client's complete nursing, medical, diagnostic, medication, and treatment history. Nurses are also able to order online prescriptions or home care equipment.

As a result of the explosion in information, people have access to near-infinite amounts of information. Many diagnostic kits will become available in the consumer market requiring the nurse to interpret or explain the results. Misinformation and misunderstanding by the consumer may be possible, resulting in additional consultation. As self-care becomes a social norm, many individuals are finding information related to health promotion, disease prevention, and management on the Web. While there are numerous benefits to this type of resource for health education, issues including the quality and validity of the information are possible. These are outlined in Box 6-7 in Chapter 6.

There are some important questions to ponder regarding the use of technology. Are educational programs preparing nurses adequately for the use of technology? Are nurses comfortable moving into a present and future dominated by information systems? What are the ethical implications of learning technology? Educational institutions must have exit criteria that at a minimum ensure computer skills including ability to use the Internet for accessing health information. Faculty members benefit from continually updating their skills in computers and other technology.

Alternative and Complementary Therapies

Thirty years ago, **alternative** and **complementary therapies** were considered fringe treatments by most Western health care practitioners. However, consumers wanted more choices for treatment and more control over their care. As a result of unpleasant side effects from conventional therapies and a growing skepticism about Western medicine, consumers have turned in larger numbers to other treatment modalities. Large numbers of individuals have used **alternative therapies** for at least the last three decades. In 2009, a report was published estimating the costs of complementary and alternative medicine (CAM) use among U.S. adults (Nahin, Barnes, Stussman, & Bloom, 2009). About 40% of adults and 12% of children under 18 years of age use complementary or alternative therapies. Total out-of-pocket expenditure was estimated at $33.9 billion to CAM practitioners and products. Nearly two thirds of this expenditure was for self-care products, classes, and materials. About three quarters of both visits to CAM practitioners and total out-of-pocket expenses were associated with manipulative and body-based therapies such as chiropractic, massage, or movement therapies. A total of 44% of all out-of-pocket costs for CAM, or about $14.8 billion, was spent on the purchase of nonvitamin, nonmineral, natural products.

NURSING IMPLICATIONS

To follow the holistic perspective, nurses must be knowledgeable about alternative therapies so they can monitor care and treatment and provide information about benefits and potential harm for clients. The National Institutes of Health has categorized alternative modalities and therapies into major types of modalities, as shown in Box 16-1. Nurses benefit from education and training in multiple alternative/complementary therapies.

It is imperative that the client discuss with his or her primary caregiver any over-the-counter medication and alternative or complementary therapies he or she may be taking concurrently with Western medicines or treatments. Many alternative or complementary therapies may either potentiate or diminish the impact of medications or other treatments. To ensure maximum efficacy of all treatment modalities, the use of alternative or complementary therapies and Western medicine should always be coordinated with the primary health care provider.

Major Types of Complementary and Alternative Therapies

Alternative systems are built on theory and practice that have evolved apart from, or even, earlier than, the conventional medical approach used in the United States. Examples include homeopathic, naturopathic, and traditional Chinese medicine.

Mind–body practices focus on the interactions among the brain, mind, body, and behavior, with the intent to use the mind to affect physical functioning and promote health. Many CAM practices embody this concept in different ways. Commonly used mind–body practices include mediation, yoga, and acupuncture. Other examples of mind–body practices include deep-breathing exercises, guided imagery, hypnotherapy, progressive relaxation, and qi gong.

Natural products include the use of a variety of herbal medicines (also known as botanicals), vitamins, minerals, and other "natural products." Many are sold over the counter as **dietary supplements**. (Some uses of dietary supplements—e.g., taking a multivitamin to meet minimum daily nutritional requirements or taking calcium to promote bone health—are not thought of as CAM.)

Manipulative and body-based practices focus primarily on the structures and systems of the body, including the bones and joints, soft tissues, and circulatory and lymphatic systems. They are therapies that are based on manipulation and/or movement of one or more parts of the body. Examples include chiropractic or osteopathic manipulation and massage.

Movement therapies are a broad range of Eastern and Western movement-based approaches used to promote physical, mental, emotional, and spiritual well-being. Examples include Feldenkrais method, Alexander technique, Pilates, and Rolfing. The goal is to encourage health and relieve stress by bringing the body into proper alignment with gravity. According to the 2007 NHIS (National Health Interview Survey), 1.5% of adults and 0.4% of children used movement therapies.

Energy therapies consist of two types. One is biofield therapies that are intended to affect energy fields that purportedly surround and penetrate the human body. Examples are qi gong, reiki, and therapeutic touch. Bioelectromagnetic-based therapies involve the unconventional use of electromagnetic fields, alternating current, or direct current fields.

Source: National Center for Complementary and Alternative Medicine, National Institute of Health (2011). *What is complementary and alternative medicine?* Retrieved from http://nccam.nih.gov/health/whatiscam/

Alternative and complementary therapies have gained respect and recognition from the general public and medical professionals as more is known about efficacy. Medical and nursing educators are beginning to integrate alternative and complementary therapies into medical and nursing curricula. In the future, nurses will increasingly be expected to provide knowledge about and use of alternative therapies. It is crucial that nurses continue to build their knowledge and skill base about alternative therapies. As the population becomes more diverse ethnically, it is anticipated that more knowledge of methods of promoting health and treating illness will be necessary.

For the person who feels intimidated and dehumanized by the sterility and businesslike environment of most Western medical facilities, the warm, personal caring and concern of alternative practitioners may be therapeutic (Fig. 16-2). Because stress and anxiety are major factors in many illnesses, the soothing environment and supportive attitude of alternative practice and practitioners have contributed to their appeal.

Research provides evidence that some alternative therapies enhance health and promote recovery from illness for both the client and family caregivers. While some caregivers still support only Western methods of health care and continue to ignore or repudiate the value of more traditional or alternative methods, the use of these practices has persisted and grown because people find them useful. Acknowledging the full breadth of services that individuals use, and working with them, is more productive than ignoring what the client chooses to do in the quest for wholeness and health.

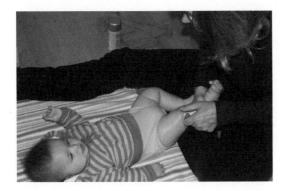

Figure 16-2 One complementary therapy is infant massage. Source: Roberta Hunt, 2011, used by permission.

However, because alternative and complementary therapies are an unregulated industry, care should be taken before recommending or utilizing them. For example, up to half of individuals diagnosed with inflammatory bowel disease use CAM, but the number of high-quality trials of CAM on the topic is extremely limited. Generally, individuals with chronic conditions such as inflammatory bowel disease that are difficult to control through conventional drugs will seek out CAM. Health professionals should be well informed about available CAM and the evidence (if any) of benefit or harm (Hawthorne, 2010).

Empirical research of the benefit and harm of many CAMs is in its infancy. The potential for harm should always be a part of the risk–benefit analysis, with some interventions such as massage and acupuncture presenting less risk as compared with those ingested, such as herbal medications (see Fig. 16-3). Nurses can begin to broaden their perspectives about different health care therapies by addressing their own bodies, minds, and spirit issues. It is possible to work successfully with clients who use alternative approaches.

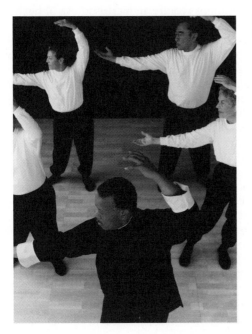

Figure 16-3 Some complementary therapies have low risk for harm. Tai chi photo from CDC.

CLIENT SITUATIONS IN PRACTICE

When the Nurse Has Not Been Exposed to Alternative Therapies

Lisa is a 29-year-old woman who delivered a healthy, 9-lb, 10-oz baby boy 2 weeks ago. The home health care nurse makes a home visit. Lisa complains about continued perineal discomfort with no unusual discharge or odor. The nurse suggests hydrocortisone cream and suppositories. Lisa says that she wants to avoid steroid creams and asks if there is an alternative. The nurse is concerned but states that she cannot provide her with any other suggestions. The only things that work, she says, are hydrocortisone and time, and Lisa should adhere to the medications that are known to be effective. Lisa is left feeling insecure and unsatisfied, without a remedy for her discomfort.

Aromatherapy, the use of essential oils with diverse medicinal qualities, was shown over two decades ago to help in the treatment of a range of conditions, including perineal discomfort. More recently lavender oil has been found to reduce perineal pain (Vakilian, Atarha, Bekhradi, & Chaman, 2011). If the home health care nurse had interest and training in alternative therapies, she may have been better equipped to care for her client. When the nurse is willing to acknowledge the client's philosophy and values, the client may be willing to consider what the nurse has to offer for the client's care.

Shifting Demographics

The number and proportion of older people continues to increase with particularly life expectancies at ages 65 and 85 over the past 50 years. People who live to age 65 can expect to live, on average, nearly 18 more years. Since 1900, the percentage of the population older than 65 years has tripled, and this growth is expected to continue.

In North America, cultural diversity continues to increase. In 1900, about one out of eight Americans was of a race other than white but by 2000, about one out of four Americans was of a race other than white. While minorities currently comprise one third of the population, it is anticipated that whites will become the minority population by 2042 (U.S. Census Bureau, 2008). At the same time, between 1960 and 2010, the health disparity between whites and blacks in the United States, as seen in the mortality rates, has changed very little and worsened for black infants and black men age 35 and over (Agency for Healthcare Research and Quality, 2010). If the black–white health disparity gap were closed, it would eliminate 83,000 excess deaths per year among African Americans (Satcher et al., 2005).

People living longer with more chronic conditions require an increased use of health care resources. This growing segment of the population has health care needs that are different from those of other segments of the population. Of people older than 70 years, 80% have one or more chronic conditions (Administration on Aging, 2010; Centers for Disease Control and Prevention, 2010; Interagency Forum on Aging Related Statistics, 2011). Because the percentages with disabilities increase sharply with age, disability takes a heavier toll on the very old.

This is one of the rationales for more emphasis on health promotion and disease prevention, because without intervention, it is likely that as this group ages, the percentage of the elderly population with chronic conditions will increase exponentially (Administration on Aging, 2010). This growing segment of the population has health care needs that are different from those of other segments of the population.

The nursing shortage is the latest demographic trend that will impact community-based care in the future. The Bureau of Labor Statistics estimates that job opportunities for RNs in all specialties are expected to be excellent with employment of RNs predicted to grow much faster than average for all occupations through 2018. The U.S. Bureau of Labor Statistics anticipate that the need for nurses will increase by 22% by 2018, while at the same time the number of U.S educated nursing school graduates decreased by 10% from 1995 to 2004 (Bureau of Labor Statistics, 2010).

Nurses have reported the negative impact of the shortage on work conditions, believing that some tasks currently assigned to nurses will shift to other staff including unlicensed assistive personnel. Some anticipate the shortage will result in nurses leaving nursing for nonnursing jobs, thus intensifying the shortage. These changes could result in lower quality of care provided.

NURSING IMPLICATIONS

Because community-based nursing practice will be central to the care of a population of aging and chronically ill people, nurses will be confronted with many challenges. Providing nursing care to diverse populations has been discussed throughout this text and will continue to be a challenge for nurses.

In the future, regardless of the nurse's own ethnic background, the nurse must be proficient at transcultural nursing to be an effective caregiver. Nurses will play a major role in promoting self-care and addressing health promotion and disease prevention issues for elderly clients. A larger proportion of the nurse's caseload will include individuals with chronic, disabling conditions. Promoting self-care and health promotion and disease prevention with this population entails skills and knowledge that are different from those needed for clients having an acute episode of a resolvable condition.

Continuity is more complex in cross-cultural nursing. Every decision hinges on the cultural context of the issue. Also, it is often more difficult to enhance continuity with older clients who may have a weak support system or multiple chronic conditions that impair mobility or sensory perception than it is for a middle-aged client with a spouse.

Collaboration is even more important when working with diverse populations. Collaboration across disciplines is always challenging, but it may be more likely to be demanding if the interdisciplinary team members are from several cultural backgrounds.

Social Justice

The Code of Ethics for Nurses charges all nurses with an ethical responsibility to promote community, national, and international efforts to meet health needs (American Nurses Association [ANA], 2001). Nurses are expected to influence social and public policy to promote **social justice** (ANA, 2010). In the United States, health care is a commodity to which a growing number of individuals and families have limited or no access. This growing **underserved population** would benefit from additional opportunities for nursing service. Nurses have a professional responsibility to improve access to care for individuals who are uninsured or underinsured.

One way to meet this professional duty is through volunteerism. Nurses, students, and nursing faculty can make a sustained commitment to community well-being through volunteering. By carefully exploring options, students may find that by volunteering in a community-based setting, they expand their skills and knowledge base in ways not possible in a traditional clinical setting.

A second way to address social justice is through **service learning** experiences that are structured to combine learning and volunteering. Service learning experiences can be valuable to develop empathy, social awareness, and social and cultural competence. Students can take the initiative to learn while volunteering by taking an internship or independent study in an area of community health that interests them.

Another way to become more socially responsible is by understanding the impact that public policy has on the individuals included or excluded from that policy. Many nurses discover that being active in the community creates awareness of issues related to access to care that are not seen when only working with fully insured clients. In turn, this may act as an impetus to speak up about public policy. For example, a nurse volunteers in his community with homeless youth. He sees firsthand the positive impact that having emergency housing in his community has on some of the homeless youth with whom he works. He notes that youth who are referred to certain services in the community are less likely to become permanently homeless, more likely to complete high school, and more likely to adopt a more stable lifestyle. When the funding in his state for emergency housing for homeless youth is proposed to be cut, the nurse sends a letter to his State Legislator and Governor. In this letter, the nurse describes the lives that he has seen changed through participation in the programs at the emergency shelter. He includes some numerical data that support his observations (i.e., number of teens that graduate from high school or technical training as a result of participating in the programs). The nurse relates the impact that the program cuts will have on the youth who do not receive assistance. If the funding for homeless youth in this example was affected by federal policy, the nurse may contact his Senator or Congressman with similar information.

There is a large number and percentage of the population, including individuals of all ages, in many cities, states, and the United States at large who do not receive the basic services and opportunities necessary to sustain health. Basic services include sufficient food, a livable-wage job, safe housing, adequate education, and access to health care. Volunteering provides the opportunity to consider the context in which some of the social issues facing citizens in our society develop and what our responsibility as a RN is to right these wrongs. Ask yourself: What system issues contribute to poor health outcomes in my community?

The Future of Community-Based Nursing Care

Cost containment will continue to be a driving force for health care services, challenging nurses to be flexible, autonomous, and creative in their thinking. The current decrease in specialization calls for flexibility in the performance of roles across disciplines and the articulation of nursing as a profession. This requires the nurse to encourage clients and families to maximize their independence and follow through with self-care in all aspects of their lives. The educational preparation of the nurse will determine the scope of practice; however, this may involve a broad range of activities from the simple to the complex. More education will be necessary for some who are required to perform, teach, and oversee complicated care. Further, as in most professions, nurses benefit from a commitment to lifelong learning and continually updating their skills and knowledge related to all aspects of health care.

SELF-CARE

In the future, the number of clients requiring assistance with self-care will grow as the percentage of the population with chronic disease increases. Self-care requires the nurse to recognize that assessment, planning, intervention, and evaluation revolve around the question, "How much care can the client and caregivers safely provide on their own?" Another issue maybe, "How can I motivate and facilitate self-care through disease prevention and health promotion with this client, family, or community?"

Self-care is especially challenging when the client is older or is from a culture different from that of the nurse. The nurse of the future must be equipped to enhance the self-care skills of the client who is likely to be aging, from a different culture, and coping with several chronic conditions.

Self-care will continue to require mastery of an increasingly complex technology. To manage at home with a chronic health problem, the client and family caregiver will have to use complicated monitors and life-sustaining medical equipment, while the nurse uses sophisticated telecommunications devices to access information and transmit client data to the agency, attending physician, or nurse practitioner to manage care.

PREVENTIVE CARE

The future focus of health care will be on treatment efficacy rather than technologic imperative. This promotes nursing care at all levels of prevention. Focusing on prevention will be particularly challenging as the percentage of the population ages and is living with chronic conditions. Growing trends in alternative health therapies allow more culturally sensitive options in preventive care.

Health care's focus on cost containment challenges the nurse to use prevention strategies to reduce expenses. This is as true in the hospital as in other community-based settings. Rather than being seen as expensive baggage that can be eliminated, nurses need to present themselves as the key to holding down health care costs. This concept has been discussed throughout this book but will require numerous creative applications in the future.

There are different ways that nurses can operationalize the concepts of health promotion and disease prevention in community-based nursing. Nurses can position themselves as the first link between clients and the hospital, through developing long-term relationships. This involves developing systems and models of care that require periodic contact with clients with chronic problems. For example, nurses can develop telephone triage services or create computer-based services, referring clients to more cost-effective services, and reducing the number of unnecessary visits to emergency departments. In addition, nurses can be proactive in developing policies and systems that address primary, secondary, and teriary prevention needs of a community.

CARE WITHIN THE CONTEXT OF COMMUNITY

Earlier chapters explained the value of the community in providing health care, and Chapter 3 discussed the cultural aspects of community-based nursing. Nursing care must be provided within the cultural context of a community, taking into consideration the strengths and resources of the client, family, and community. As the population ages, this challenge will be further complicated by the demands of technology and the health and technology literacy of the community. Acceptance of alternative methods of care delivery respects the context of the client's family and community, including, in many cases, popular and folk healers. Because the racial and ethnic make-up of the nation is changing, nurses will be required to speak languages other than English or to be competent using interpreters. Nurses should also encourage representatives of minority groups to enter the nursing profession.

CONTINUITY OF CARE AND COLLABORATIVE CARE

The hospital of the future may be known as a **health care organization** or an **integrated health care system**. These systems already exist in many parts of the country. More community-based care programs will come from these integrated systems. Another term used is **seamless care**, in which all levels of care are available in an integrated form. Continuity allows quality care to be preserved in a changing health care delivery system. It is an essential component of cost containment and prevents duplication of services, rehospitalization, and inappropriate use of services. An older, more diverse population will provide challenges to the nurse as continuous care becomes the expected norm.

As a result of increased use of alternative therapies, the importance of continuity is evident. It will be essential for traditional and nontraditional providers to respect one another's contributions to the client's care and to communicate and coordinate care effectively.

Conclusions

Cost-effective and quality health care accessible to everyone remains at the forefront of health care goals for the 21st century. In addition, flexibility will be an important aspect of community-based care. Ongoing professional development will be imperative to keep pace with the professional demands of community-based nursing. The nurse of the future must be equipped to care for the client who is likely to be aging, from a different culture, and coping with several chronic conditions. It will be essential for traditional and nontraditional providers to respect one another's contributions to the client's care and to communicate effectively. Trends in alternative methods of healing allow more culturally sensitive options.

The nature and scope of nursing service are broader than any one setting in which care is offered. Nursing care has remained constant in its philosophy over the decades. However, nurses must now adapt their care delivery models to include clients in acute care settings, long-term care, ambulatory settings, and the home. Nurses follow the standards of nursing care in all settings. In the future, this will require a more educated, autonomous, and competent nurse.

What's on the Web

American Botanical Council
INTERNET ADDRESS: http://www.herbalgram.org

This site is dedicated to providing current and accurate information on herbal medicine. There is an educational link that consumers may find helpful. On this site are a variety of accredited continuing education modules for professionals interested in learning more about the safety and efficacy of herbal products.

American Medical Informatics Association
Nursing Informatics Work Group
INTERNET ADDRESS: https://www.amia.org/wiki/biomedical-imaging-informatics/additional-nursing-informatics-resources-and-organizations

This organization's goal is to promote the advancement of nursing informatics within an interdisciplinary context. This goal is pursued in professional practice, education, research, and governmental and other service.

American Nurses Association Political Action Committee
INTERNET ADDRESS: http://nursingworld.org/MainMenuCategories/ANAPoliticalPower/ANAPAC.asp

The American Nurses Association Political Action Committee, ANA-PAC, was established to promote the improvement of the health care system in the United States by raising funds from Constituent Member Associations (CMAs) members and contributing to support worthy candidates for federal office who have demonstrated their belief in the legislative and regulatory agenda of the American Nurses Association.

Online Journal of Issues in Nursing
INTERNET ADDRESS: http://www.nursingworld.org/ojin

This online publication provides a forum for discussion of current issues in nursing.

National Center for Complementary and Alternative Medicine (NCCAM)
INTERNET ADDRESS: http://www.nccam.nih.gov

The NCCAM at the National Institutes of Health (NIH) conducts and supports basic and applied research on complementary and alternative therapies. This site disseminates information on complementary and alternative interventions to practitioners and the public. This is an excellent site for current, reliable information based on research.

General Web Resources

Aetna InteliHealth
INTERNET ADDRESS: http://www.intelihealth.com

This site provides physician-reviewed, consumer-friendly articles, online communities, and a medical dictionary. The "Ask the Expert" feature is popular.

American Heart Association
INTERNET ADDRESS: http://www.americanheart.org

This Web page contains information related to heart health, support group links, licensed products and services, and science and research. There is an excellent client and caregiver education area, "Heart Failure," at http://www.americanheart.org/presenter.jhtml?identifier=1486

American Lung Association
INTERNET ADDRESS: http://www.lungusa.org

This site contains information on lung disease in all forms, with special emphasis on asthma, tobacco control, and environmental health.

National Cancer Institute
INTERNET ADDRESS: http://www.cancernet.nci.nih.gov

Maintained by the National Cancer Institute, this site has extensive credible information on cancer, reviewed by oncology experts and based on research.

Health on the Net Foundation
INTERNET ADDRESS: http://www.hon.ch

This international initiative has a multilingual search engine for information on health and health care.

Health Promotion Online
INTERNET ADDRESS: http://www.hc-sc.gc.ca/hppb/hpo/index.html

This Canadian site addresses a wide range of health promotion and disease prevention programs. It also offers content in French.

Healthfinder
INTERNET ADDRESS: **http://www.healthfinder.gov**
   This site from the U. S. Department of Health and Human Services (DHHS) leads to publications, clearinghouses, databases, Web sites, and support and self-help groups, as well as providing reliable information.

Healthy People 2020
INTERNET ADDRESS: **http://www.healthypeople.gov/2020/default.aspx**
   This site provides access to all of the Healthy People 2020 documents and initiatives.

Lippincott Williams & Wilkins
INTERNET ADDRESS: **http://www.lww.com**
   Lippincott Williams & Wilkins leads in the world of information resources for nursing, medical, and allied health professionals and students.

March of Dimes
INTERNET ADDRESS: **http://www.modimes.org**
   This organization focuses on issues related to prenatal care and prevention of birth defects, infant mortality, and low-birth-weight infants. The Web site includes information on research, programs, and public affairs.

MayoClinic.com
INTERNET ADDRESS: **http://www.mayohealth.org**
   Sponsored by the Mayo Clinic, this site features reliable information on a variety of health issues with resources for each.

Medscape
INTERNET ADDRESS: **http://www.medscape.com**
   This commercial site is a professional site built around practice-oriented information.

National Institutes of Health (NIH)
INTERNET ADDRESS: **http://www.nih.gov**
   The NIH Web site is an excellent all-around resource for nurses from all specialties. It contains news and events, health information, grants, scientific resources, and links to other sites, including the National Institute of Nursing Research and the W.G. Magnuson Clinical Center Nursing Department.

National Institutes of Health, Warren Grant Magnuson Clinical Center Nursing Department
INTERNET ADDRESS: **http://www.cc.nih.gov/nursing**
   This site provides links to federal resources, Internet search engines, and other useful resources. This nursing-specific site provides information from universities, the Centers for Disease Control and Prevention, and the National Institute of Nursing Research.

National League for Nursing
INTERNET ADDRESS: **http://www.nln.org**
   A resource for nursing education, practice, and research, this site has the latest information about the organization and nursing in general.

National Women's Health Information Center (NWHIC)
INTERNET ADDRESS: **http://www.womenshealth.gov**
   The NWHIC is a free information and resource service on women's health issues for consumers, health care professionals, researchers, educators, and students. This bilingual site (English and Spanish) contains a wealth of information on health issues that is free of copyright restrictions and may be copied.

OncoLink
INTERNET ADDRESS: **http://www.oncolink.upenn.edu**
   This site is maintained by the University of Pennsylvania's Abramson Cancer Center. It contains news, education on treatment options, reporting on clinical trials, psychosocial support through an active online community, and resources such as associations, support groups, online journals, and book reviews.

Planned Parenthood
INTERNET ADDRESS: **http://www.plannedparenthood.org**
   In both Spanish and English, this Web site includes legislative updates, statistics, newsletters, and a library with information on family planning.

PubMed
INTERNET ADDRESS: **http://www.ncbi.nlm.nih.gov/entrez/query.fcgi**
This search service of the National Library of Medicine provides access to more than 10 million citations.

Transcultural Nursing
INTERNET ADDRESS: **http://www.culturediversity.org**
This site's goal is to provide information about transcultural nursing to help other nurses understand behavior and its cultural basis.

U.S. Department of Health and Human Services
INTERNET ADDRESS: **http://www.dhhs.gov**
This site provides links to numerous health resources from the federal government.

U.S. National Library of Medicine
INTERNET ADDRESS: **http://www.nlm.nih.gov**
The U.S. National Library of Medicine is the world's largest medical library.

World Health Organization
INTERNET ADDRESS: **http://www.who.int/en**
This is the Web site of the international World Health Organization, which is committed to the attainment of the highest possible level of health for everyone worldwide.

References and Bibliography

Administration on Aging. (2010). *Aging statistics.* Retrieved from http://www.aoa.gov/AoARoot/Aging_Statistics/index.aspx

Agency for Healthcare Research and Quality. (2010). *National health care disparity report.* Retrieved from http://www.ahrq.gov/qual/nhdr09/nhdr09.pdf

American Nurses Association. (2001). *Code of ethics for nurses with interpretive statements.* Washington, DC: American Nurses Association.

American Nurses Association. (2010). *Nursing's social policy statement: The essence of the profession.* Washington, DC: American Nurses Association.

Benner, P., Sutphen, M., Leonard, V., & Day, L. (2010). *Educating nurses: A call for radical transformation.* San Francisco: Jossey-Bass.

Bureau of Labor Statistics, U.S. Department of Labor. (2010). *Occupational outlook handbook, 2010–2011 edition,* Registered Nurses. Retrieved from http://www.bls.gov/oco/ocos083.htm#projections_data

Centers for Disease Control and Prevention. (2010). *The state of aging and health in America.* Retrieved from http://www.cdc.gov/aging/data/stateofaging.htm

Hawthorne, A. (2010). Complementary and alternative therapies in Crohn's disease and ulcerative colitis. *Gastrointestinal Nursing, 8*(3), 32–37. Retrieved from EBSCO*host*.

Interagency Forum on Aging Related Statistics. (2011). *Older Americans update 2010: Key indicators of well-being* (p. 54). Retrieved from http://www.agingstats.gov/agingstatsdotnet/Main_Site/Data/2010_Documents/Docs/OA_2010.pdf

Kaiser Family Foundation. (2007). *Key facts: Race, ethnicity and medical care.* Retrieved June 15, 2010, from http://www.kff.org/minorityhealth/upload/6069–02.pdf

Kaiser Family Foundation. (2010). *Summary of new health reform law. Focus on Health Reform Law.* Retrieved from http://www.kff.org/healthreform/upload/8061.pdf

Nahin, R. L., Barnes, P. M., Stussman, B. J., & Bloom, B. (2009). *Costs of complementary and alternative medicine (CAM) and frequency of visits to CAM practitioners: United States, 2007. National Health Statistic Report, 18.* Retrieved from http://www.cdc.gov/NCHS/data/nhsr/nhsr018.pdf

National Center for Complementary and Alternative Medicine, National Institutes of Health. (2011). *What is CAM?* Retrieved from http://www.nccam.nih.gov/health/whatiscam/

Phillips, K. A. (2006). The intersection of biotechnology and pharmacogenomics: Health policy implications. *Health Affairs (Millwood), 25*(5), 1271–1280.

Rivera, R. M., & Bennett, L. B. (2010). Epigenetics in humans: An overview. *Current Opinions Endocrinol Diabetes Obesity, 17*(6), 93–99.

Robert Wood Johnson. (2010). *Nursing leadership from bedside to boardroom: Opinion leaders' perceptions.* Retrieved from http://www.rwjf.org/pr/product.jsp?id=54350

Satcher, D., Fryer, G. E., Jr., et al. (2005). What if we were equal? A comparison of the black-white mortality gap in 1960 and 2000. *Health Affairs (Millwood)*, 24(2), 459–464.

Sebelius, K. (2010). *The new momentum behind electronic health records*. Kaiser Health News. Retrieved from http://www.kaiserhealthnews.org/Columns/2010/August/082610Sebelius.aspx

U.S. Census Bureau. (2008). *Press release*. Retrieved April 6, 2010, from http://www.census.gov/Press-Release/www/releases/archives/population/012496.html

U.S. Department of Health and Human Services. (2010). *The registered nurse population: 2008 National sample survey of Registered Nurses*. Retrieved from http://bhpr.hrsa.gov/healthworkforce/rnsurvey/2008/

U.S. Department of Health and Human Services. (2011). *Healthy people 2020. Retrieved from* http://www.healthypeople.gov/2020/default.aspx

Vakilian, K., Atarha, M., Bekhradi, R., & Chaman, R. (2011). Healing advantages of lavender essential oil during episiotomy recovery: A clinical trial. *Complementary Therapies in Clinical Practice*, 17(1), 50–53. Retrieved from EBSCOhost.

World Health Organization. (2011). *United States of America: Statistics*. Retrieved from http://www.who.int/countries/usa/en/

LEARNING ACTIVITIES

JOURNALING ACTIVITY 16-1

1. In your clinical journal, discuss a future trend in health care that is of interest to you. Find at least two articles about this trend and summarize each.

2. Follow the summary with two paragraphs in which you discuss the implications for health care, the nursing profession, and nurses' daily practice. What would be possible education needs for the nurse that might come from these implications?

CLIENT CARE ACTIVITY 16-2

The year is 2025—the future is here. You are a case manager in a busy, urban nursing clinic. You have a caseload of clients who live in the community where your center is located. Most of the clients have multiple chronic conditions. You see your clients in the ambulatory clinic, in the client's home, or you communicate with them via computer. Today, one of your clients, Alfred Martinez, who is 64 years old, is having a sigmoid bowel resection with a temporary colostomy by laparoscopic laser surgery at the day surgery center. Home care will be provided by his wife, who will be assisted by their three adult sons on a rotating basis. It is your responsibility to coordinate the disciplines involved in his health care and manage his nursing care.

1. Identify factors that must be addressed when you plan for Mr. Martinez's postoperative recovery at home.

2. List five questions you will ask Mr. Martinez when you assess his care needs. Review the questions.
   - Do these questions view the client holistically?
   - Are they indicative of a contextual approach to identifying the client's needs?

3. Organize topics you will include when you teach Mrs. Martinez and her sons about Mr. Martinez's postoperative care. Compare and contrast current care from the care that would have likely been provided in 1997.

4. State alternative treatments or nursing interventions you included in the plan of care. How would you determine if they are paid for by a third-party payer?

5. Analyze how technology will assist you in Mr. Martinez's care (e.g., in making the assessment, communicating, maintaining a therapeutic relationship, and implementing the plan of care).

PRACTICAL APPLICATION ACTIVITY 16-3

Interview a nurse who has been employed for at least 10 years. The longer the nurse has been working, the more interesting the discussion will be. Use the following questions as a basis for the interview:

- When did you first start working as a registered nurse?
- What was nursing like when you first started working?
- How has health care changed in the last 10 (or 15, 20) years?
- How is nursing different now?
- How many clients did you care for when you first started working as a nurse?
- How are the clients different now than when you first started working as an RN?
- What were your responsibilities for client care when you first started working and how have those responsibilities changed?
- What concerns do you have about how nursing has changed over the last 10 years (or however many decades the nurse has been working)?
- What is better about how nursing care is provided now?
- Summarize the interview in a two page paper. What were the two most important things you learned?

PRACTICAL APPLICATION ACTIVITY 16-4

Interview a middle aged or older adult who has had a chronic condition over a long period of time (best candidate would have this condition for at least 10 years). Ask that person the following questions:

- How have health care services changed over the last 10 years (or however long you have had your health condition)?
- Which of these differences are of particular concern to you and why?
- In the last 10 years has your family taken over more of your care that was previously provided by a health care provider?
- Talk about for a typical day for you and how having a chronic condition impacts (or does not impact) your activities?
- How have your family members been impacted by the fact that you have a chronic illness?

Appendix A

Nutrition Questionnaires for Infants, Children, and Adolescents

Nutrition Questionnaire for Infants

1. How would you describe feeding time with your baby? (*Check all that apply.*)
   - ☐ Always pleasant
   - ☐ Usually pleasant
   - ☐ Sometimes pleasant
   - ☐ Never pleasant

2. How do you know when your baby is hungry or has had enough to eat?

3. What type of milk do you feed your baby? (*Check all that apply.*)
   - ☐ Breastmilk
   - ☐ Iron-fortified infant formula
   - ☐ Low-iron infant formula
   - ☐ Goat milk
   - ☐ Evaporated milk
   - ☐ Whole milk
   - ☐ Reduced-fat (2%) milk
   - ☐ Low-fat (1%) milk
   - ☐ Fat-free (skim) milk

4. What types of things can your baby do? (*Check all that apply.*)
   - ☐ Open mouth for breast or bottle
   - ☐ Drink liquids
   - ☐ Follow objects and sounds with eyes
   - ☐ Put hand in mouth
   - ☐ Sit with support
   - ☐ Bring objects to mouth and bite them
   - ☐ Hold bottle without support
   - ☐ Drink from a cup that is held

5. Does your baby eat solid foods? If so, which ones?

6. Does your baby drink juice? If so, how much?

7. Does your baby take a bottle to bed at night or carry a bottle around during the day?

8. Do you add honey to your baby's bottle or dip your baby's pacifier in honey?

9. What is the source of the water your baby drinks? Sources include public, well, commercially bottled, and home system–processed water.

10. Do you have a working stove, oven, and refrigerator where you live?

11. Were there any days last month when your family didn't have enough food to eat or enough money to buy food?

12. What concerns or questions do you have about feeding your baby?

Source for all questionnaires: Bright Futures at Georgetown University. (2006). Retrieved on July 10, 2006, from http://www.brightfutures.org/nutrition

Nutrition Questionnaire for Children

1. How would you describe your child's appetite?
   - ☐ Good
   - ☐ Fair
   - ☐ Poor

2. How many days does your family eat meals together per week?

3. How would you describe mealtimes with your child?
   - ☐ Always pleasant
   - ☐ Usually pleasant
   - ☐ Sometimes pleasant
   - ☐ Never pleasant

4. How many meals does your child eat per day? How many snacks?

5. Which of these foods did your child eat or drink last week? (*Check all that apply.*)

   Grains
   - ☐ Bread
   - ☐ Rolls
   - ☐ Bagels
   - ☐ Muffins
   - ☐ Other grains: _____
   - ☐ Noodles/pasta/rice
   - ☐ Tortillas
   - ☐ Crackers
   - ☐ Cereal/grits

   _____

   Vegetables
   - ☐ Corn
   - ☐ Peas
   - ☐ Potatoes
   - ☐ French fries
   - ☐ Tomatoes
   - ☐ Greens (collard, spinach)
   - ☐ Other vegetables: _____
   - ☐ Green salad
   - ☐ Broccoli
   - ☐ Green beans
   - ☐ Carrots

   _____

Fruits

☐ Apples/juice
☐ Oranges/juice
☐ Grapefruit/juice
☐ Grapes/juice
☐ Other fruits/juice:

☐ Bananas
☐ Pears
☐ Melon
☐ Peaches

_____
_____

Milk and Other Dairy Products

☐ Whole milk
☐ Reduced-fat (2%) milk
☐ Low-fat (1%) milk
☐ Fat-free (skim) milk
☐ Other milk and dairy products:

☐ Yogurt
☐ Cheese
☐ Ice cream
☐ Flavored milk

_____
_____

Meat and Meat Alternatives

☐ Beef/hamburger
☐ Pork
☐ Chicken
☐ Turkey
☐ Fish
☐ Cold cuts
☐ Other meat and meat alternatives:

☐ Sausage/bacon
☐ Peanut butter/nuts
☐ Eggs

☐ Dried beans
☐ Tofu

_____
_____

Fats and Sweets

☐ Cake/cupcakes
☐ Pie
☐ Cookies
☐ Chips
☐ Doughnuts
☐ Other fats and sweets:

☐ Candy
☐ Fruit-flavored drinks

☐ Soft drinks

_____
_____

6. **If your child is 5 years old or younger, does he or she eat any of these foods?** (*Check all that apply.*)

☐ Hot dogs
☐ Pretzels and chips
☐ Raw celery or carrots
☐ Nuts and seeds
☐ Raisins

☐ Whole grapes
☐ Popcorn
☐ Marshmallows
☐ Round or hard candy
☐ Peanut butter

7. **How much juice does your child drink per day? How much sweetened beverage (e.g., fruit punch and soft drinks) does your child drink per day?**

8. **Does your child take a bottle to bed at night or carry a bottle around during the day?**
☐ Yes   ☐ No

9. What is the source of the water your child drinks? Sources include public, well, commercially bottled, and home system–processed water.

10. Do you have a working stove, oven, and refrigerator where you live?
☐ Yes   ☐ No

11. Were there any days last month when your family didn't have enough food to eat or enough money to buy food?
☐ Yes   ☐ No

12. Did you participate in physical activity (e.g., walking or riding a bike) in the past week? If yes, on how many days and for how long?
☐ Yes   ☐ No

13. Does your child spend more than 2 hours per day watching television and videotapes or playing computer games? If yes, how many hours per day?
☐ Yes   ☐ No

14. What concerns or questions do you have about feeding your child?

Nutrition Questionnaire for Adolescents

1. Which of these meals or snacks did you eat yesterday? (*Check all that apply.*)
☐ Breakfast   ☐ Afternoon snack
☐ Morning snack   ☐ Dinner/supper
☐ Lunch   ☐ Evening snack

2. a. Do you skip breakfast three or more times a week?
☐ Yes   ☐ No

 b. Do you skip lunch three or more times a week?
☐ Yes   ☐ No

 c. Do you skip dinner/supper three or more times a week?
☐ Yes   ☐ No

3. Do you eat dinner/supper with your family four or more times a week?
☐ Yes   ☐ No

4. Do you fix or buy the food for any of your family's meals?
☐ Yes   ☐ No

5. Do you eat or take out a meal from a fast-food restaurant two or more times a week?
☐ Yes   ☐ No

6. Are you on a special diet for medical reasons?
☐ Yes   ☐ No

7. Are you a vegetarian?
☐ Yes   ☐ No

8. Do you have any problems with your appetite, such as not feeling hungry or feeling hungry all the time?
☐ Yes   ☐ No

9. **Which of the following did you drink last week?** *(Check all that apply.)*

☐ Regular soft drinks ☐ Fat-free (skim) milk
☐ Diet soft drinks ☐ Coffee/tea
☐ Fruit-flavored drinks ☐ Tap/bottled water
☐ Whole milk ☐ Juice
☐ Reduced-fat (2%) milk ☐ Sports drinks
☐ Low-fat (1%) milk ☐ Beer/wine/alcohol
☐ Flavored milk (e.g., chocolate, strawberry)

10. **Which of these foods did you eat last week?** (*Check all that apply.*)

Grains

☐ Bread ☐ Cereal/grits
☐ Rolls ☐ Popcorn
☐ Bagels ☐ Noodles/pasta/rice
☐ Crackers ☐ Tortillas
☐ Other grains: _____
_____

Vegetables

☐ Corn ☐ Green salad
☐ Peas ☐ Broccoli
☐ Potatoes ☐ Green beans
☐ French fries ☐ Carrots
☐ Tomatoes
☐ Greens (collard, spinach)
☐ Other vegetables: _____
_____

Fruits

☐ Apples/juice ☐ Peaches
☐ Oranges/juice ☐ Pears
☐ Grapefruit/juice ☐ Berries
☐ Grapes/juice ☐ Melon
☐ Bananas
☐ Other fruits/juice: _____
_____

Milk and Other Dairy Products

☐ Whole milk ☐ Yogurt
☐ Reduced-fat (2%) milk ☐ Cheese
☐ Low-fat (1%) milk ☐ Ice cream
☐ Fat-free (skim) milk ☐ Flavored milk
☐ Other milk and dairy products:

Meat and Meat Alternatives

☐ Beef/hamburger   ☐ Sausage/bacon

☐ Pork   ☐ Peanut butter/nuts

☐ Chicken   ☐ Eggs

☐ Turkey   ☐ Dried beans

☐ Fish   ☐ Tofu

☐ Cold cuts

☐ Other meat and meat alternatives: _____

_____

Fats and Sweets

☐ Cake/cupcakes   ☐ Chips

☐ Pie   ☐ Doughnuts

☐ Cookies   ☐ Candy

☐ Other fats and sweets: _____

_____

11. **Do you have a working stove, oven, and refrigerator where you live?**

☐ Yes   ☐ No

12. **Were there any days last month when your family didn't have enough food to eat or enough money to buy food?**

☐ Yes   ☐ No

13. **Are you concerned about your weight?**

☐ Yes   ☐ No

14. **Are you on a diet now to lose weight or to maintain your weight?**

☐ Yes   ☐ No

15. **In the past year, have you tried to lose weight or control your weight by vomiting, taking diet pills or laxatives, or not eating?**

☐ Yes   ☐ No

16. **Did you participate in physical activity (e.g., walking or riding a bike) in the past week? If yes, on how many days and for how long?**

☐ Yes   ☐ No

17. **Do you spend more than 2 hours per day watching television and videotapes or playing computer games? If yes, how many hours per day?**

☐ Yes   ☐ No

18. **Do you take vitamin, mineral, herbal, or other dietary supplements (e.g., protein powders)?**

☐ Yes   ☐ No

19. **Do you smoke cigarettes or chew tobacco?**

☐ Yes   ☐ No

20. **Do you ever use any of the following?** (*Check all that apply.*)

☐ Alcohol/beer/wine

☐ Steroids (without a doctor's permission)

☐ Street drugs (marijuana/speed/crack/heroin)

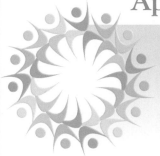

Appendix B

Implications for Teaching at Various Developmental Stages

Age	Physical Development	Language (Cognitive) Development (Based on Piaget)	Psychosocial Development (Based on Erikson)	Nurse's Approach to Teaching
Overview of birth to 1 y		Sensorimotor stage of development	Developmental task: trust vs. mistrust. Learns to trust and to anticipate satisfaction. Sends cues to mother/caretaker. Begins understanding self as separate from others (body image)	Involve caretaker in all aspects of care
1–3 y	Begins to walk and run well. Drinks from cup, feeds self. Develops fine motor control. Climbs. Kneels self-toileting. Kneels without support Steady growth in height/weight. Adult height will be approximately double the height at age 2. Dresses self by age 3	Preoperational stage of development. Has poor time sense. Increasing verbal ability. Formulates sentences of four to five words by age 3. Talks to self and others. Has misconceptions about cause and effect. Interested in pictures Fears: ▪ Loss/separation from parents—peak ▪ Dark ▪ Machines/equipment ▪ Intrusive procedures ▪ Bedtime Speaks to dolls and animals. Increasing attention span. Knows own sex by age 3	Developmental task: autonomy vs. shame and doubt. Establishes self-control, decision making, independence (autonomy). Extremely curious and prefers to do things himself Demonstrates independence through negativism. Very egocentric; believes he or she controls the world. Attempts to please parents. Participates in parallel play; able to share some toys by age 3	Be flexible. Begin any intervention with play period to establish rapport. Be honest. Praise for cooperation. Begin slowly; speak to child. Involve caretaker/parent. Let child hold security object. Allow child to play with stethoscope, tongue blade, flashlight before using on child if possible
4–6 y	Growth slows. Locomotion skills increase and coordination improves. Tricycle/bicycle riding. Throws ball but difficulty catching. Constantly active, increasing dexterity. Eruption of permanent teeth. Skips, hops, jumps rope	Preoperational/thought stage of development continues. Language skills flourish. Generates many questions, such as how, why, what. Simple problem solving. Uses fantasy to understand and problem solve. Fears ▪ Mutilation ▪ Castration ▪ Dark ▪ Unknown ▪ Inanimate ▪ Unfamiliar objects Causality related to proximity of events. Enjoys mimicking and imitating adults	Developmental tasks: initiative vs. guilt. Attempts to establish self like his or her parents, but independent. Explores environment on own initiative. Boasts, brags, has feelings of indestructibility. Family is primary social group. Peers increasingly important. Assumes sex roles. Aggressive, very curious. Enjoys activities such as sports, cooking, shopping. Cooperative play. Likes rules. May stretch the truth and tell large stories	Establish rapport through talking and play. Introduce self to child. Have parent present but direct conversation to child. Games such as "follow the leader" and "Simon says" can be used to elicit necessary behaviors. Explain each intervention in simple language. Ask for child's help and use flattery. Use pictures, models, or items he or she can see or touch. Reserve genital examination for last; drape accordingly

Age	Physical	Cognitive	Psychosocial	Implications
6–11 y	Moves constantly. Physical play prevalent; sports, swimming, skating, etc. Increased smoothness of movement. Grows at rate of 2 inches/7 lb a year. Eyes/hands well coordinated	*Concrete operations stage of development.* Organized thought; memory concepts more complicated. Reads, reasons better, focuses on concrete understanding. *Fears* • Mutilation • Death • Immobility • Rejection • Failure	*Developmental task: industry vs. inferiority.* Learns to include values and skills of school, neighborhood, and peers. Peer relationships important. Focuses more on reality, less on fantasy. Family is main base of security and identity. Sensitive to reactions of others. Seeks approval and recognition. Enthusiastic, noisy, imaginative, desires to explore. Likes to complete a task. Enjoys helping others	Explain all procedures and impact on body. Encourage questioning and active participation in care. Be direct about explanation of procedures, based on what child will hear, see, smell, and feel. (In addition, explain body part involved, and use anatomical names and pictures to explain step by step.) Be honest. Reassure the child that he or she is liked. Provide privacy. Involve parents, but give child choice as to whether parent will stay during exam. Reason and explain. Allow child some choice as to direction of assessment. May be able to proceed as if assessing adult. Praise cooperation
12–18 y	Well developed. Rapid physical growth (early adolescence): maximum growth). Secondary sex characteristics	*Formal operations stage of development.* Abstract reasoning, problem solving. Understanding of multiple cause-and-effect relationships. May plan for future career. *Fears* • Mutilation • Disruption of body image • Rejection by peers	Developmental task: identity vs. role confusion. Predominant values are those of peer group. Early adolescence: outgoing and enthusiastic. Emotions are extreme, with mood swings. Seeking self-identity; sexual identity. Wants privacy and independence. Develops interests not shared with family. Concern with physical self. Explores adult roles	Respect privacy. Accept expression of feelings. Direct discussions of care and condition to child. Ask for child's opinions and encourage questions. Allow input into decisions. Be flexible with routines. Explain all procedures/treatments. Encourage continuance of peer relationships. Listen actively. Identify impact of illness on body image, future, and level of functioning. Correct misconceptions. Involve parent in assessment only if child requests presence

Continued on following page

Age	Physical Development	Language (Cognitive) Development (Based on Piaget)	Psychosocial Development (Based on Erikson)	Nurse's Approach to Teaching
19–30 y		*Formal operations*	*Developmental task: intimacy vs. isolation.* Intimate relationships are ultimate	Involve significant other in care and consider how the client's condition affects the relationship
30–60 y		*Formal operations*	*Developmental task: generativity vs. stagnation.* Concerned with parenthood, mentoring, and guiding the next generation.	Work, family, and children are priorities. Teach with this concern in mind
60 y to death		*Formal operations*	*Developmental task: integrity vs. despair.* Reviews life to bring life events into an integrated life theme	Use life review to help client reduce anxiety and blocks to learning

Adapted from Weber, J. (2008). *Nurses' handbook of health assessment* (6th ed.). Philadelphia, PA: Lippincott Williams & Wilkins.

Appendix C

Cognitive Stages and Approaches to Patient Education With Children

Cognitive Stage	Approach to Teaching
Ages Birth to 2 y—Sensorimotor Development	
Begins as completely undifferentiated from environment	Orient all teaching to parents
Eventually learns to repeat actions that have effect on objects	Make infants feel as secure as possible with familiar objects in home environment
Has rudimentary ability to make associations	Give older infants an opportunity to manipulate objects in their environments, especially if long hospitalization is expected
Ages 2–7 y—Preoperational Developments	
Has cognitive processes that are literal and concrete	Be aware of explanations that the child may interpret literally (e.g., "The doctor is going to make your heart like new" may be interpreted as, "He is going to give me a new heart"); allow child to manipulate safe equipment, such as stethoscopes, tongue blades, reflex hammers; use simple drawings of the external anatomy because children have limited knowledge of organs' functions
Lacks ability to generalize	Do not compare child to other children; this is not helpful, nor is it meaningful to compare one diagnostic test or procedure to another
Has egocentrism predominating	Reassure child that no one is to blame for his pain or other problems; belief that he causes events to happen may result in guilty thoughts that he caused his own pain, hospitalization, and so forth
Has animistic thinking (thinks that all objects possess life or human characteristics of their own)	Anthropomorphize and name equipment that is especially frightening
Ages 7–12 y—Concrete Operational Thought Developments	
Has concrete, but more realistic and objective, cognitive processes	Use drawings and models; children at this age have vague understandings of internal body processes; use needle play with dolls to explain surgical techniques and facilitate learning
Is able to compare objects and experiences because of increased ability to classify along many different dimensions	Relate his or her care to other children's experiences so he or she can learn from them; compare procedures to one another to diminish anxiety
Views world more objectively and is able to understand another's position	Use films and group activities to add to repertoire of useful behaviors and establish role models

Has knowledge of cause and effect that has progressed to deductive logical reasoning	Use child's interest in science to explain logically what has happened and what will happen; explain medications simply and straightforwardly (e.g., "This medicine [insulin] unlocks the door to your body's cells just as a key unlocks the door to your house. By unlocking the door to the cell, the insulin can deliver the food and energy in your blood to the cell.")

Adapted from Kolb, L. C. (1977). *Modern clinical psychiatry* (9th ed., pp. 90–91). Philadelphia, PA: Saunders; London, F. (1999). *No time to teach: A nurse's guide to patient and family education.* Philadelphia, PA: Lippincott Williams & Wilkins; Petrillo, M., & Sanger, S. (1998). *Emotional care of hospitalized children* (pp. 38–50). Philadelphia, PA: Lippincott-Raven.

Index

Note: A "t" following a page number indicates a table; an "f" indicates a figure; and a "b" indicates a box.